# Improve International Manual of Clinical Small Animal Internal Medicine

Volume 2

Improve
International

# Improve International Manual of Clinical Small Animal Internal Medicine

Volume 2

**Verónica Salazar Nussio, Pachi Clemente Vicario, Dolores Pérez Alenza, Sandra Díaz, Chiara Noli, Alejandro Luján Feliu-Pascual, Maria Dolores Tabar Rodríguez, Albert Lloret Roca, Alejandro Bayón del Río, Nick Marsh**

**Translated by Gemma Gaitskell-Phillips**

**Edited by Pippa Elliott**

Improve International

First published 2020



Published by
Improve International Limited
Alexandra House
Whittingham Drive
Wroughton
Swindon
Wiltshire SN4 0QJ, UK
01793 759159
www.improveinternational.com

Complementary to Improve International's 2 year modular programme in small animal medicine, this reference manual covers small animal medicine at practitioner level.

***Important note***
Medicine is an ever-changing science, so the contents of this publication, especially recommendations concerning diagnostic and therapeutic procedures, can only give an account of the knowledge at the time of publication. While utmost care has been taken to ensure that all specifications regarding drug selection and dosage and treatment options are accurate, readers are urged to review the product information sheet and any relevant material supplied by the manufacturer, and, in case of doubt, to consult a specialist. From both an editorial and public interest perspective, the publisher welcomes notification of possible inconsistencies. The ultimate responsibility for any diagnostic or therapeutic application lies with the reader.

A Catalogue record for this book is available from the British Library

ISBN 9781913352103

Book layout by Servis Filmsetting Ltd, Stockport, Cheshire
Printed by Monterreina Comunicación, S.A., Madrid
Photos by the authors unless otherwise indicated; photos in chapter 9 by SYNLAB VPG Exeter
Illustrations by Elaine Leggett

# Contents

# Contributors

**Dolores Pérez Alenza DVM PhD**

Dolores obtained her DVM in 1989 from the Complutense University of Madrid and subsequently her PhD in veterinary medicine from the same university in 1994. She completed her training with various visits to the Universities of Utrecht (Holland), Davis in California and Florida (USA). She is currently Professor in the Department of Animal Medicine and Surgery in the Veterinary Faculty at the Complutense University of Madrid and is Head of the Department of Small Animal Internal Medicine at the University Veterinary Hospital and is responsible for the endocrinology and mammary oncology consult service. She has more than 90 publications in scientific journals and has contributed to various book chapters covering her area of expertise.

**Alejandro Bayón del Río DVM, PhD, Dipl. CLOVE**

Dr. Bayón obtained his PhD in Veterinary Medicine from the University of Murcia, where he is currently Senior Lecturer in the Department of Animal Medicine and Surgery. He undertakes his clinical activities at the Veterinary Hospital of the University of Murcia and is Head of the Ophthalmology Department, in addition to being Head of the Animal Medicine and Surgery Department and has been responsible for coordination of the official Masters degree in "Small Animal Medicine". He is a diplomate of the Latin American College of Veterinary Ophthalmology (CLOVE), and undertook his residency in ophthalmology at the Autonomous University of Barcelona, as well as being AVEPA accredited as an ophthalmology specialist. Dr. Bayón is President of the Ophthalmology working group for AVEPA and member of the examination committee for accreditation. He has spoken and presented and run courses and seminars at both national and international congresses and conferences. His work and research is focused on ophthalmology, particularly pathologies and surgery of the cornea, glaucoma, ocular lesions caused by systemic disease and the treatment of abnormalities of the posterior pole of the eye. He is a collaborative researcher with the Ophthalmobiology Research Group at the University of the Basque Country and has co-directed several Doctoral Theses as part of this role. He is the author of multiple articles in both national and international journals.

**Sandra Díaz DVM, MS, Diplomate ACVD**

Assistant Professor in Dermatology in the Department of Clinical Sciences at the College of Veterinary Medicine at The Ohio State University, Columbus OH, USA. Sandra obtained her DVM in Veterinary Science in 1994 and graduated in Veterinary Medicine in 1996 from the Santo Tomás University in Santiago, Chile. She received her PhD in veterinary sciences in 2006 from the University of Minnesota, USA, where she also completed her residency in dermatology. Before joining the School of Veterinary Medicine at Ohio State University she also worked in Virginia-Maryland Regional College of Veterinary Medicine, Virginia Tech and prior to this at the NYC Veterinary Specialists and Cancer Center in New York, USA. Her research interests include hair growth disorders, canine and feline otitis and allergic dermatitis. She is a member of the American Academy of Veterinary Dermatology and is a Diplomate of the American College of Veterinary Dermatology.

**Alejandro Luján Feliu-Pascual LV MRCVS DipECVN**

Alejandro obtained his DVM from the University of Murcia in 1994. He undertook a general internship at Davis Veterinary Specialists in the United Kingdom (2000–01) and then subsequently completed a residency in neurology and neurosurgery at the Faculty of Veterinary Medicine in Glasgow (2001–04). He has been a Diplomate of the European College of Veterinary Neurology ECVN since 2006 and a European specialist and specialist veterinary neurologist with the Royal College of Veterinary Surgeons (RCVS) in the UK. He was Head of the Education Committee for the ECVN from 2009–2012 and has worked in referral hospitals in the UK (Davis, AHT and the University of Glasgow) and Spain (Ars Veterinary 2008–2015). He is a scientific reviewer for the JSAP, Veterinary Surgery, JFMS, and JVIM journals and co-author of the "Canine and Feline Neurology" book, Multimédica Editions 2012 as well as author of numerous oral communications at both European and national congresses. He is a partner and Head of the Neurology / Neurosurgery department at the AÚNA Veterinary Specialists in Valencia. His main areas of interest include medical and surgical treatment of brain tumours, congenital malformations and neuromuscular diseases.

**Nick Marsh**

Nick Marsh graduated from Bristol University in 1999, and consequently saw in the milliennium whilst on call. He spent four years in mixed practice, and a further twelve years in small animal practice. In 2016, he started a residency in clinical pathology at VPG Exeter, and hopes to pass his final exams in 2020. He is married and is also the co-creator of two small humans. He spends his limited free time playing games, drinking coffee and being cruel to pot plants, as well as occasionally writing biographies for textbooks.

**Chiara Noli DMV, Dip ECVD**

Chiara graduated from the University of Milan in 1990 and has been a specialist in small animal diseases since 1995. Between 1992 and 1995 she attended a course to become a specialist in veterinary dermatology at the University of Utrecht, Holland and in dermatological pathologies at the University of Bern, Switzerland. In 1996 she was the first Italian to become a Diplomate of the European College of Veterinary Dermatology. She was the first female president of the Italian Society of Veterinary Dermatology (SIDEV) and is also a member of the executive council of the International Society of Veterinary Dermatology (ISVD), President of the European Society of Veterinary Dermatology (ESVD), member of the executive council of the World Association of Veterinary Dermatology (WAVD) and member of the executive council of the European College of Veterinary Dermatology (ECVD). She is a regular speaker at both Italian and international congresses and author of more than 100 articles in international scientific journals and various books. She currently works in Piamonte and Liguria as a dermatology consultant in different practices, including the Anubis Moncalieri (TO) and Borgo San Dalmas Cuneo (CN) veterinary hospitals.

**Verónica Salazar Nussio LV, MS, PhD, Dipl. DACVAA**

Verónica received her DVM from the Complutense University of Madrid in 2001 and subsequently obtaining her PhD in Veterinary Medicine from the same university in 2005. She undertook a residency in Anaesthesia at Cornell University (USA) from 2005 to 2008. She has been a Diplomate of the American College of Veterinary Anaesthesiology and Anaesthesia (ACVAA) since 2010 and also achieved a diploma in "University Medical Education" from the University of Dundee (UK) in 2014. She has worked as a clinical anaesthetist at the Animal Health Trust (UK) between 2008 and 2010. Since 2010 she has been the Head of the Anaesthesia Department at the Veterinary Clinical Hospital of the Alfonso X El Sabio University and also coordinates the Anaesthesiology teaching for veterinary undergraduates at the same university. She currently is the coordinator for the master's degree in Anaesthesiology and Resuscitation and is responsible for two residents who are enrolled in this course as well as having supervised several doctoral theses. Among her clinical interests are anaesthesia in critical care and emergency patients and analgesic treatments.

**Maria Dolores Tabar Rodríguez Dip ECVIM-CA, AVEPA Internal Medicine Accredited**

Maria Dolores obtained her DVM from the University of Zaragoza in 2001 and subsequently completed a small animal internship at the University Clinic Hospital at the Autonomous University of Barcelona from 2001 to 2003. She then undertook a residency in internal medicine at the same university and became a Diplomate of the European College of Veterinary Internal Medicine (small animal speciality, Dip ECVIM-CA) in 2010. From 2007 she has been Head of the Internal Medicine Department at the San Vicente Veterinary Hospital (San Vicente del Raspeig, Alicante) and is accredited in Internal Medicine by AVEPA. She is a member of the scientific committee of the internal medicine working group at AVEPA and has been President of the group from 2014 onwards. She has published numerous articles both as main and co-author in both national and international journals and actively participates in talks, oral communications and posters at international and national congresses (ACVIM forum, ECVIM Congress, SEVC-AVEPA, GTA, FECAVA...). Her particular area of interest in internal medicine is infectious diseases.

**Albert Lloret Roca DVM residencia ECVIM, MANZCVS**

Albert obtained his DVM from the Faculty of Veterinary Medicine at the Autonomous University of Barcelona (UAB) in 1990. He worked in veterinary practice from 1990 to 1997 and since 1997 has been a member of the Internal Medicine team at the University Clinic Hospital at the UAB where he is a clinical lecturer. He completed short-stays as a visiting veterinarian at Colorado State University (internal medicine and oncology services) in 1999 and 2002. He was President of the Feline Medicine working group at AVEPA (GEMFE) from 2005 to 2009 and is currently a member of the scientific committee. He is a member of the veterinary committee of the ISFM (International Society of Feline Medicine) and a member of the European Advisory Board on Cat Diseases (ABCD). He is associate Editor of the Small Animal Veterinary Clinical Practice publication (AVEPA) and is accredited in feline medicine by AVEPA. He is a Diplomate in Internal Medicine, ECVIM-CA (European College Veterinary Internal Medicine Companion Animal), after undertaking a residency and has recently been recognized as the only individual in Europe who is actively accredited in feline medicine MANZCVS (Medicine of Cats). He has authored numerous publications in national and international publications and participated as a speaker at internal and feline medicine congresses. His particular areas of interest in internal medicine are feline medicine, infectious diseases and oncology.

**Pachi Clemente Vicario DVM, MS, Dip-ACVIM (Oncology)**
Pachi obtained his DVM from the University of Extremadura in 1993. Since this time, he has worked in small animal medicine, with a particular interest in oncology. From 2003 to 2012 he combined working in clinical practice with teaching as an Associate Professor at the Cardenal Herrera CEU University in Valencia where he was the Head of the Oncology service at the University Hospital. Between 2012 and 2015 he undertook an American College of Veterinary Internal Medicine residency in Medical Oncology at the Ohio State University where he also completed a master's degree in Veterinary Comparative Medicine. From August 2015 he has worked at La Merced Veterinary Oncology in Calpe, Alicante.

# 1 Clinical management of the critical and emergency patient

Verónica Salazar Nussio

## Chapter summary



If there is one certainty about veterinary practice, it is that the veterinarian will regularly have to deal with critical patients and emergencies. This responsibility should weigh heavily on the clinician, because their actions may well play a crucial role on the eventual outcome for that patient.

Indeed, the emergency patient represents a row of dominoes waiting to be knocked over. The aim of treating a critical patient is to bring about stabilisation and prevent dominoes further down the line from being knocked over. To do this, successful therapy depends on anticipating and recognising the various stages of deterioration and counteracting them.

For example, the patient with septic peritonitis undergoes activation of pathways that lead to reduced circulation and hypovolaemia, which in turn reduces the blood flow to the gut and increases gut permeability, which allows pro-inflammatory factors to leak into the lymphatic system and venous circulation. The ultimate result is that the patient enters disseminated intravascular coagulopathy (DIC) and, when the last domino in this cascade topples over, this may prove fatal to the patient.

This chapter aims to help the clinician recognise and understand the cause of complications in the critical patient and feel confident about how best to attempt correction. This includes an overview of the latest thinking in coping with such patients using a multimodal approach to their support that goes beyond aggressive fluid therapy.

### Key learning points

- Understand the pathophysiological changes in an emergency patient and the implications for stabilisation and treatment.
- Understand the types of fluid and rate of administration appropriate for each clinical case.
- Understand efficient and effective triage of the emergency patient.
- Understand the importance of analgesia, and appropriate pain relief strategies for shocked patients.
- Understand effective cardiopulmonary resuscitation (CPR) techniques for patients in cardiopulmonary arrest (CPA).

## Pathophysiological changes in the critical and emergency patient

Critical and emergency patients present with a number of diverse and varied characteristics. However, whatever the cause of the emergency, these patients potentially share a series of pathophysiological changes that often require rapid and potentially complex actions in order to stabilize them.

### *Sepsis*

#### *Definition*

Sepsis is characterized by a severe inflammatory response to an infection (viral, bacterial or fungal). This type of response is called systemic inflammatory response syndrome (SIRS)

#### *Aetiopathogenesis*

Patients with sepsis have at least **one septic focus** that is the source of infection, and this can be varied (including conditions such as pneumonia, pyometra, parvoviral enteritis, pyelonephritis or deep pyoderma), with the most common cause of sepsis in dogs and cats being **septic peritonitis**.

The incidence of septic peritonitis in septic patients ranges from 36 to 71%. The most frequent trigger is the **release of gastrointestinal content into the peritoneum**, normally associated with:

- **ulcers** caused by non-steroidal anti-inflammatory agents (NSAIDs)
- **perforation** due to a foreign body
- gastrointestinal **neoplasia**
- **dehiscence** of enterotomies
- **enterectomy** breakdown.

The most common causative organisms are **Gram-negative bacteria** (of enteric or urogenital origin), although there may also be mixed infections and **Gram-positive bacteria** (especially of dermal or iatrogenic origin from infected intravenous catheters).

#### *Progression*

The initial stage is a systemic inflammatory response as a **defence measure** by the body. Over time, however, the production of **inflammatory mediators** becomes excessive and the **inflammation regulation systems are blocked**, which results in generalised systemic inflammation (SIRS) characterised by the presence of specific clinical signs including:

- tachycardia
- tachypnoea
- leukocytosis or leucopoenia
- hyper- or hypothermia.

In many cases, this situation causes **acute circulatory failure** and persistent arterial **hypotension** (refractory hypotension), which generates a condition known as **septic shock** (mediated by generalised changes in the microvascular endothelium and the activation of the coagulation cascade and complement system). If this is not corrected in time, **multiple organ dysfunction syndrome (MODS)** may develop, with the consequent worsening of the prognosis for the patient and, ultimately, **death**.

**Sepsis and septic shock are the most frequent causes of morbidity and mortality** in both human and veterinary medicine. In the United States septic shock in humans has an incidence of 0.3% with a mortality of 30% (due to progression to multi-organ failure). In veterinary medicine there are no precise data on its incidence, but it is thought that mortality is higher, reaching values of 20–68%.

#### *Clinical signs*

Patients presenting with this type of condition suffer significant changes in different systems.

##### Cardiovascular

Characterised by:

- inability to maintain vascular tone
- greater **permeability of the vascular endothelium** and, therefore, **hypovolaemia**
- decreased myocardial contractility, which causes **decreased cardiac output**.

### Coagulation

Due to alterations in coagulation and fibrinolysis, cases present from initial stages of hypercoagulation to terminal states of consumption coagulopathy characterised by the development of **disseminated intravascular coagulation (DIC)**.

### Respiratory

In patients with septic shock, two types of respiratory syndrome can be observed:

- acute lung injury (ALI)
- acute respiratory distress syndrome (ARDS).

These two syndromes are similar, with a common pathophysiology in epithelial and endothelial lesions derived from the action of inflammatory mediators, **changes in the synthesis and functionality of surfactant** as well as **accumulation in the alveoli** and the interstitial alveolar space of fluid and inflammatory cells.

Such alterations are particularly important in **feline patients**, since the **lung is the main target organ** in this species when symptoms of sepsis occur.

### Gastrointestinal

The gastrointestinal system plays a fundamental role in the evolution of symptoms, even when the focus of origin is elsewhere and the intestinal serosa is intact. In fact, **epithelial permeability increases due to hypoperfusion** and the direct effects of inflammatory mediators on gastrointestinal tissue, so that **absorption occurs of pro-inflammatory factors** into the lymphatic system that end up draining into the venous system. This perpetuates the SIRS and results in the development of **multi-organ failure**.

### Renal

Lesions caused by **ischaemia-reperfusion** can sometimes lead to secondary **acute tubular necrosis**, which may result in acute renal failure.

### Hepatic

The liver is the target organ in canine patients in shock, and therefore the following can occur:

- hypoalbuminaemia
- hypoglycaemia
- coagulopathies
- hepatic encephalopathy.

## SIRS

### *Aetiopathogenesis*

SIRS consists of the generalised release of inflammatory mediators in response to an insult, for example:

- infectious:
  - sepsis
- non-infectious:
  - multiple trauma
- pancreatitis
- heat stroke
- severe burns
- very invasive surgery.

### *Physiopathology*

SIRS describes a **clinical state** rather than a pathology in its own right.

The pathophysiological consequences of SIRS are the result of **disruption of homeostasis** by pro-inflammatory mediators in three areas:

1. **Loss of vascular tone**. Possibly due to excessive production of inducible nitric oxide synthase (i-NOS) and vasopressin deficiency.
2. Alterations to **endothelial barrier permeability**. As a direct consequence of cytokine production.
3. **Coagulation stimulation**. Induced by the expression of tissue factor on the surface of leucocytes, which leads to the **deposition of fibrin in microvasculature** (a phenomenon directly related to organ failure in inflammatory conditions), all of which can deplete endogenous anticoagulant systems, further exacerbating hypercoagulability.

Ultimately, in an attempt to compensate for exaggerated levels of systemic inflammatory mediators, a compensatory anti-inflammatory response is launched which can end up generating an immunosuppressive condition called the **compensatory anti-inflammatory response syndrome (CARS)**. When this syndrome occurs, a direct consequence is increased patient susceptibility to secondary infections, with the complications entailed in weakened animals.

If the natural evolution of this condition is not controlled or treated in time, the result is shock, multi-organ failure and, finally, death of the patient.

### *Diagnosis*

The diagnostic criteria consist of the coexistence of several (**two in dogs and three in cats**) of the following clinical signs (Table 1.1):

Table 1.1. SIRS: diagnostic criteria in dogs and cats.

| | Dog | Cat |
|---|---|---|
| Temperature (°C) | <38 and >40 | <37.7 and >40 |
| Heart rate (bpm) | >120 | <140 and >225 |
| Respiratory rate (bpm) | >40 or $PaCO_2$ <30 mmHg | >40 |
| Leukocytes (GB/µl) | >18,000 and <5,000 | >19,000 and <5,000 |

- hypo- or hyperthermia
- leukocytosis or leucopenia
- tachycardia
- tachypnoea.

It is interesting to note the recent relevance of **certain biomarkers** when determining if the origin of SIRS is septic or not. Since both the course and clinical manifestations are identical, biomarkers can provide results fast than samples submitted for culture. The following are of particular interest:

- **C-reactive protein (CRP)**
- **Procalcitonin (PCT)**. Results are promising, since the utility of this biomarker has been demonstrated when differentiating between septic and non-septic SIRS, and they show a correlation with the severity of the condition, which is of prognostic value.

### Treatment

The treatment of SIRS is based on two fundamental concepts:

- **Correction of the triggering cause** (hence the importance of biomarkers that provide information on the aetiology of the condition).
- **Symptomatic support** therapies in the three areas mentioned above.

Alterations to the endothelial barrier complicate the conservation of water provided by crystalloids within the intravascular space, so that water can accumulate in the interstitial space resulting in clinical signs of **peripheral oedema**. Caution is therefore recommended with the aggressive administration of crystalloids in these cases.

## Shock

### Definition

Shock is defined as a state in which there is **an oxygen deficit in tissues**.

### Aetiopathogenesis

Shock may be due to:

A **decrease in tissue perfusion** that generates **insufficient oxygen delivery** to the tissues and organs. It is what happens in the vast majority of cases. If this **hypoperfusion** is not corrected in time, a cascade of events begins that can eventually end in:

1. changes in cellular metabolism
2. cell death
3. organ failure
4. patient death.

Deficits in the oxygen content of blood (hypoxaemic complications) create problems with **cellular metabolic functioning**, which make it impossible for the cell to take advantage of the oxygen that reaches it.

Pathophysiologically it is understood that the organism needs oxygen delivery to tissues that matches its oxygen demand. At the point when this balance is lost, due either to an increase in demand or a decrease in delivery, an **oxygen deficit occurs at the tissue level** and therefore, shock (Figure 1.1).

In critical or emergency patients, the **demand for oxygen in tissues may be increased** in some very specific and disparate circumstances, including:

- status epilepticus
- heat stroke
- emergence of malignant hyperthermia in patients under general anaesthesia.

However, the most frequent circumstance is when the imbalance is due to a **decrease in delivery**. Oxygen delivery is directly related to perfusion, determined by the following elements:

- cardiac output:
  - heart rate.
- cardiac stroke volume:
  - preload
  - afterload
  - contractility
  - oxygen content in arterial blood ($CaO_2$).

Consequently, changes in any of these factors in the cardiovascular system may be responsible for a deficit in oxygen delivery to tissues:

- vasculature and vascular tone
- cardiac pumping
- blood volume
- oxygen content in arterial blood.

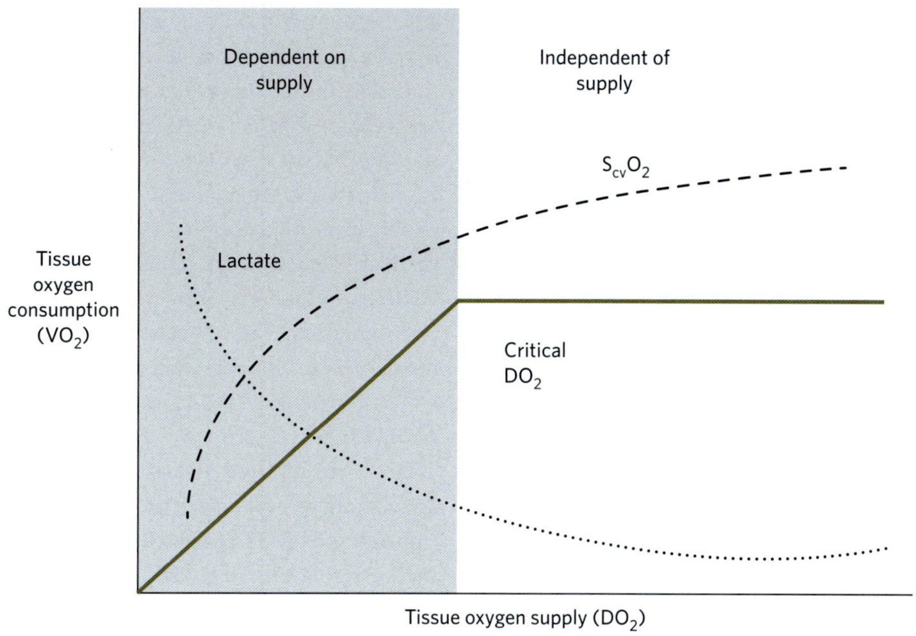


**Figure 1.1.** Equilibrium between the supply (S) and demand (D) of oxygen in tissues.

In fact, one of the classification systems used for the different types of shock is based precisely on its aetiology:

1. **Hypovolaemic shock**: due to an intravascular volume deficit (for example, in the case of haemorrhage).
2. **Distributive shock**: due to the existence of an inadequate vascular tone caused by microcirculation dysfunction, which results in generalised vasodilation (for example, in the case of septicaemia).
3. **Obstructive shock**: due to the obstruction of blood flow both in and out of the heart (for example, in the case of pericardial effusion).
4. **Cardiogenic shock**: due to a failure in heart pumping (for example, in congestive heart failure).
5. **Hypoxaemic shock**: due to insufficient oxygen content in arterial blood.
6. **Metabolic shock**: due to alterations in cellular metabolic machinery.

## Physiopathology

Regardless of the cause that triggers the initial decrease in perfusion, all states of shock go through the same phases:

1. *Compensation phase*. Self-regulatory mechanisms are underway thanks to the release of endogenous catecholamines due to stimulation of baroreceptors which detect decreases in systemic blood pressure. In this phase, catecholamines trigger a series of mechanisms that are aimed at **increasing cardiac output** (increase in heart rate and myocardial contractility) and increasing venous return (promoting water retention). All these compensatory mechanisms need large amounts of energy, so a **hypermetabolic state** is established in cells. Compensation can maintain adequate cardiac output for a limited period of time, after which the body automatically enters the decompensation phase.
   Clinical signs of compensation include:
   - increase in HR
   - increase in RR
   - congested mucous membranes
   - CRT <1 s
   - unaltered consciousness
   - normal or even high arterial blood pressure.
2. *Early decompensation phase*. Begins once all **self-regulatory mechanisms are exhausted** and the body **diverts blood flow to priority organs** (the heart and the central nervous system). This means that the rest of the tissues have to cope with the oxygen deficit entering **anaerobic metabolism**, resulting in **lactic acidosis**. The consequences of this phenomenon on certain organs give rise to the characteristic effects of this condition:

   In the pancreas, myocardial depressant factors are released that cause the appearance of arrhythmias and a decrease in contractility.

   In the kidney, the decrease in blood flow causes tubular necrosis and oliguria.

   During this phase the clinical signs include:
   - hypotension
   - compensatory tachycardia
   - pale mucous membranes
   - CRT >2 s

- hypothermia
- altered consciousness.

3. *Terminal decompensation phase*. Prolonged tissue hypoxia results in a self-regulatory escape situation, which translates clinically into **complete circulatory failure** due to massive vasodilation and loss of chronotropic and inotropic responses in the heart. Clinical signs in this phase include:
   - bradycardia
   - severe hypotension
   - pale or cyanotic mucous membranes
   - absence of capillary refill
   - anuria
   - coma
   - imminent cardiopulmonary failure.

## Acute traumatic coagulopathy

### Definition

Acute traumatic coagulopathy (ATC) consists of a state of endogenous hypocoagulability that occurs in 10–25% of human patients with severe poly-trauma. It is characterised by the early development of hypocoagulability and hyperfibrinolysis in the immediate post-traumatic period (approximately 30 minutes after trauma). It is one of the main causes of mortality in the first 24 hours after trauma in human patients with poly-trauma.

### Aetiopathogenesis

Even today there is a great **controversy** surrounding the aetiology and pathophysiology of ATC, although everything points to three possible development mechanisms:

1. ATC could be a phenotypic **variation of DIC**. This means that in the first 24-48 hours of the post-traumatic period a DIC with a fibrinolytic phenotype occurs, while after 48 hours DIC evolves with a conventional thrombotic phenotype.
2. ATC could develop from a **decrease in thrombin degradation** and an increase in thrombomodulin activity, which leads to activation of the C-protein anticoagulant pathway activated by thrombin–thrombomodulin complex action.
3. Activation of the sympathetic adrenal response and **consequent endothelial injury** that produces the release of anticoagulant and fibrinolytic substances, which could play a fundamental role.

With regard to the underlying pathophysiology, it is known that the trigger factors for ATC are **severe tissue injury together with shock** (and consequent hypoperfusion). However, there are also a number of **contributing factors** that are directly related to the development of ATC, including metabolic acidosis, hypothermia, haemodilution and systemic inflammation. The last of those is considered a key factor, since the relationship between inflammation and coagulation has been clearly demonstrated in the last decade. In fact, it is known that severe trauma and bleeding evoke an immediate, massive release of inflammatory mediators (such as cytokines and tissue necrosis factor, TNF) as well as activation of the complement cascade, phenomena that have been related to the activation of the C-protein anticoagulant pathway.

### Diagnosis

There is **no method** available to identify ATC reliably and definitively. Today, it seems that **visco-elastic tests** (for example, ROTEM and TEG) are the most sensitive methods for early detection of ATC, their main limitation being the lack of availability of such technology in a clinical setting. Therefore, at the present time, identification of ATC is based solely on the presence of indices that suggest its presence, including:

- History of **severe poltrauma** along with a state of **significant hypoperfusion** (low arterial pressures, MAP <60 mmHg, high lactate levels > 5 mmol/l or a defect with very low bases, <–6).
- Presence of **severe bleeding** and haemorrhagic shock.
- Results from visco-elastic tests indicating a clot resistance <40% of the reference value or **coagulation times 1.5 times greater than average**.

### Treatment

Today the **clinical approach remains totally empirical**, with strategies such as hypotensive resuscitation and damage containment surgery. Pharmacologically, the administration of antifibrinolytic drugs (such as aminocaproic acid or tranexamic acid) and concentrated haemostatic factors can be considered, although there are not yet sufficient studies available on their efficacy.

## Critical illness-related corticosteroid insufficiency

### Definition

Since the late 1970s in human medicine, the relationship between a **disrupted hypothalamic–pituitary–adrenal (HHA) axis** and the **increased mortality** of patients with severe sepsis and septic shock has been recognised. In fact, this relationship was what brought to light the existence of a form of **relative adrenal insufficiency in septic patients**.

At the beginning of the 21st century, the term '**relative adrenal insufficiency**' was coined to describe the condition in septic patients who had very **low levels**

**of plasma cortisol** or whose response to exogenous administration of ACTH was considered insufficient despite baseline levels of cortisol (this parameter is called 'cortisol delta concentration', and refers to the difference in plasma cortisol levels one hour after ACTH administration compared to previous baseline cortisol levels). Years later, the American College of Critical Care Medicine replaced this term with '**Critical illness-related corticosteroid insufficiency** (**CIRCI**).

### *Aetiopathogenesis*

The aetiology of CIRCI is tremendously **complex**, given that it seems to involve more than one mechanism and individual variations play an important role. In general, it is believed both the hypothalamus and the pituitary and adrenal glands may be **damaged by high levels of cytokines**, reactive oxygen species and other **inflammatory mediators** from pro-inflammatory states such as sepsis, SIRS or septic shock, giving rise to an **inadequate production of cortisol**.

On the other hand, pro-inflammatory systemic states inhibit the binding of cortisol to its cytoplasmic receptor so that **the action of the cortisol-receptor complex in the cell nucleus is affected**. In short, the mechanisms by which systemic inflammation can affect the production and action of cortisol are numerous and complex, which further complicates its diagnosis.

### *Diagnosis*

A wide variety of diagnostic methods have been proposed (baseline plasma cortisol levels, delta cortisol levels after ACTH stimulation, free fraction levels versus total cortisol and treatment response), although in human medicine a unanimous consensus has not yet been reached on the most reliable method. For practical purposes, diagnosis is still made today by **evaluating the response to treatment with low doses of hydrocortisone**. Nevertheless, very possibly most of the **controversies related to CIRCI are in regard to its treatment**.

### *Treatment*

The latest recommendations of the Surviving Sepsis Campaign team in human medicine suggest avoiding the administration of hydrocortisone provided that fluid therapy resuscitation and vasopressor therapy are effective, **reserving the use of hydrocortisone for patients in septic shock resistant to vasopressor therapy in spite of fluid therapy** resuscitation.

In veterinary medicine the situation is even more unclear, given that reliable clinical trials are lacking and a heterogeneous population with significant differences between species with regard to cortisol metabolism and response to the administration of exogenous steroids. Until now, the corticosteroid that has shown the best results is **intravenously administered hydrocortisone**, although the doses used vary among studies (*0.5 mg/kg/6 h* or *0.08 mg/kg/h*), with no information existing regarding the optimal duration of treatment or the interruption strategy for its administration.

In summary, there are still many uncertainties and controversies regarding CIRCI, especially in the field of veterinary medicine. Fortunately, in 2017 the conclusion from an ambitious large-scale, multi-centre clinical trial on the use of hydrocortisone in septic shock will shed considerable light on different aspects of its diagnosis and treatment.

## Pharmacological agents

### *Sympathomimetics*

Sympathomimetic agents are the most frequently used tool for the clinical management of critical patients that are cardiovascularly unstable.

#### *Mechanism of action*

The mechanism of action of this group of drugs depends on activation of the receptors to which they bind, i.e. **adrenergic receptors** (located in the membranes of the effector cells), with their clinical effect depending on the action exerted by them.

For practical purposes, the **clinically relevant receptors** for the management of haemodynamic stabilisation of the critical patient are:

- $\alpha 1$. Its activation, in general, results in **vasoconstriction**.
- Activation is responsible for increase in heart rate (chronotropism) and cardiac contractility (inotropism).
- $\alpha 2$. Its activation produces **sedation** in addition to **vasoconstriction**.
    - Activation results in **bronchodilation** and glycogenolysis, among other effects.

#### *Classification*

Sympathomimetics are classified based on their nature:

##### Catecholamines

- **endogenous**: dopamine, epinephrine and norepinephrine
- **synthetic**: dobutamine and isoproterenol.

##### Non-catecholamines

- **indirect action**: ephedrine
- **direct action**: phenylephrine.

From a clinical perspective, it is easier to group them **based on their therapeutic uses**:

- **inotropes,** agents capable of increasing myocardial contractility by stimulation of **β1 receptors**
- **vasopressors,** agents capable of increasing vascular tone by stimulation of **α1 receptors**.

## Inotropes

### *Dobutamine*

Synthetic β-adrenergic catecholamine, which has a **higher affinity for β1 receptors** than for β2. Its main clinical effect is an **increase in myocardial contractility**, with little effect on heart rate. It is indicated in patients with **low cardiac output in euvolaemic states**. Its main side effects may include tachycardia, arrhythmias and vasodilation.

### *Dopamine*

Endogenous catecholamine capable of activating different adrenergic receptors depending on the dose at which it is administered:

- At **low** doses *(1–4 μg/kg/min)* it exerts its action on dopamine receptors, leading to diuresis and increased blood flow to the kidneys and gastrointestinal tract.
- At **medium** doses *(5–10 μg/kg/min)* it exerts its action on β1 receptors, causing an increase in myocardial contractility and heart rate.
- At **high** doses *(10–20 μg/kg/min)* it exerts its action on α1 receptors, which causes peripheral vasoconstriction.

The main controversy regarding the clinical action of this drug is based on the **high variability of its plasma concentration** in critically ill patients. This means that, clinically, it is difficult to determine into which dose group the chosen dose falls and, therefore, what pharmacological effect is achieved.

Its main side effects may include the appearance of tachycardia or bradyarrhythmias and excessive peripheral vasoconstriction.

## Vasopressors

### *Epinephrine*

Endogenous α- and β-adrenergic catecholamine, whose pharmacological effects include:

- increased systemic vascular resistance
- increased myocardial contractility
- increased heart rate
- bronchodilation.

Its main side effects include **severe vasoconstriction** and an increase in the oxygen demand of certain tissues, from which both phenomena can give rise to situations of severe tissue hypoxia.

Clinical use is limited to very critical situations of **refractory hypotension** and cardiopulmonary resuscitation.

### *Norepinephrine*

Endogenous α-adrenergic catecholamine with minimal β-adrenergic activity, whose main pharmacological effect is the **increase in systemic vascular resistance**, with a variable increase in myocardial contractility and heart rate. The key advantage of this medication is its ability to **increase blood flow to the heart and kidneys** without causing ischaemia in the rest of the tissues. This characteristic means that it is widely used for the treatment of refractory hypotension in critical patients.

### *Phenylephrine*

Pure direct-acting α-adrenergic agonist, whose only pharmacological effect is **vasoconstriction** (with the appearance of the consequent reflex bradycardia). Adverse effects include excessive vasoconstriction, which can lead to potential ischaemia in the gastrointestinal, hepatic and renal systems, which is particularly significant. Therefore, its **clinical use is limited to situations of refractory hypotension** in which no other α-adrenergic agent has been effective.

### *Ephedrine*

Indirect acting synthetic α- and β-adrenergic agonist, whose pharmacological effects are:

- significant increase in systemic vascular resistance (with consequent reflex bradycardia)
- increased myocardial contractility
- some degree of bronchodilation.

As an indirect action agent, its effectiveness can be limited by the appearance of tachyphylaxis phenomena in the case of depletion of the norepinephrine reserves in the sympathetic terminals. Amongst its side effects are the following:

- risk of marked reflex bradycardia
- severe vasoconstriction that can lead to ischaemia in certain organs
- potential tachyphylaxis phenomena.

### *Vasopressin*

Excellent non-adrenergic vasopressor, whose mechanism of action is based on the stimulation of V1 receptors (completely independent of the adrenergic system), leading to an increase in intracellular calcium as well as the production of nitric oxide, allowing **vascular smooth muscle constriction**.

In addition, it has been shown that vasopressin is capable of **lowering plasma inflammatory cytokine levels** in patients in septic shock, a phenomenon associated with a significant increase in the survival of these patients.

Its clinical use is particularly interesting in **septic patients suffering from cases of refractory hypotension**, given that the vasoconstriction it causes has been shown not to decrease cardiac output and improves the renal function of these patients; and in **critically ill patients whose refractory hypotension may be related to the existence of acidaemia** (catecholamines that act on the adrenergic system are not effective) and whose adrenergic system may suffer depletion of endogenous catecholamines. Therefore, the possibility of increasing vascular tone through a mechanism that is independent of the adrenergic system is of great therapeutic utility. Despite this, its vasoconstrictive capacity should be considered, so among its adverse effects **potential tissue ischaemia** in different viscera should be included, especially if high doses are administered.

Table 1.2 lists the recommended dosages of the above vasopressors.

### *Administration guidelines*

The treatment of hypotension in critically ill patients is complex, and the administration of vasopressors and inotropes is **not without risks** due to their adverse effects (in some cases, of significant clinical importance), which has meant that in recent years a large number of comparative studies have been carried out to evaluate the efficacy and safety of different pharmacological protocols to address this pathology.

Table 1.2. Dosages of the vasopressor and inotrope drugs most frequently administered for the stabilisation of the critical or emergency patient.

| Drug | Dose |
|---|---|
| Dopamine | 5–10 mcg/kg/min (average dose, effect) |
| Dobutamine | 2–20 mcg/kg/min (dog); 1–5 mcg/kg/min (cat) |
| Epinephrine | 0.005–1.0 mcg/kg/min |
| Norepinephrine | 0.05–2.0 mcg/kg/min |
| Phenylephrine | 1–3 mcg/kg/min |
| Ephedrine | 30 mcg/kg/min |
| Vasopressin | 0.5–2.0 mU/kg/min |

In general, the first thing which should be done is to **confirm the presence of adequate intravascular volaemia**. Given a hypotensive condition, even in the presence of normovolaemia, the administration of β-adrenergic agents is usually the first therapeutic option, especially in patients in whom an increase in afterload due to α-adrenergic stimulation causing vasoconstriction (dilated cardiomyopathy) is contraindicated (mitral regurgitation, etc.). When hypotension continues even after administration of inotropes and there are signs of vasodilation, the administration of α-adrenergic agents that allow direct increase in vascular tone and combatting of vasodilation should be considered.

The choice of a vasopressor agent is often accompanied by great difference of opinion, especially in veterinary medicine. In human medicine, a series of clinical recommendations for the treatment of refractory hypotension were issued in 2012 whereby **norepinephrine remains the agent of choice** and **vasopressin can be considered as an adjuvant** to increase systemic blood pressure values or decrease the need for norepinephrine. The administration of high doses of dopamine for vasoconstriction is not recommended.

In veterinary medicine, because similar large-scale studies are not yet available, all the clinical criteria used are directly extrapolated from human studies, with the limitations that this entails.

## The principles of fluid therapy

Fluid therapy is indicated in every patient that needs correction or prevention of the appearance of deficits in circulating **blood volume**, **electrolyte balance** and **blood pH**, or **oxygen delivery** to tissues.

### *Classification of fluids used*

#### *According to their nature*

*Crystalloids*

**Crystalloids are aqueous solutions** containing ions, buffer substances and glucose with varying concentrations, pH and osmolarity. In general, despite generating net movements of water depending on their osmolarity, approximately one hour after administration **85% of their volume is redistributed outside the intravascular space**. That is, water passes into the **interstitial or intracellular space**, which is why it does not remain in the intravascular space for a long period of time. Therefore, crystalloids are usually administered when **deficits in the interstitial space need to be corrected**. Crystalloids include 0.9% or 7.5% NaCl, lactated Ringer's or Isofundin®.

### Colloids

Colloids are solutions containing high-molecular weight particles capable of remaining in the intravascular space. These molecules attract sodium and water, causing a net movement of water from the interstitium into the vessel, and retain water within the vessel owing to the positive charges on their surface. That is, colloids expand plasma volume and maintain it. Therefore, they are usually administered when correction of deficits in the intravascular space is necessary. The main colloids include Hetastarch, albumin and plasma.

### According to pH

All of the above crystalloid and colloid solutions are, in general, **acidic in nature** – that is, their pH is lower than plasma pH (7.35–7.45). Therefore, many of them are formulated including a series of **buffer substances**. These substances are usually anions (such as lactate, acetate, malate or gluconate) capable of donating bicarbonate to the solution.

The mechanism of action of these anions is based on their **oxidative metabolism** in different organs (acetate and malate in muscle, lactate in the liver, etc.), because one of the products of the metabolic reaction that they undergo is the release of bicarbonate into plasma. Thus, based on the presence or absence of buffer substances, the various solutions can be classified into:

- buffered
- non-buffered.

### Buffered

Typically these are solutions containing some type of **bicarbonate anion precursor**. In the case of colloids, they include all colloids that are formulated in buffered crystalloids. Among these are lactated Ringer's, Isofundin® and Isohes®.

### Non-buffered

These solutions **do not include bicarbonate precursors** in their formulation. In the case of colloids, this includes all colloids that are formulated in 0.9% NaCl and Hemohes®.

### Crystalloids

Depending on their osmolarity, compared to that of plasma, crystalloids are classified as (Table 1.3):

- **Isotonic**. With an osmolarity similar to that of plasma.
- **Hypertonic**. With an osmolarity greater than that of plasma, and therefore they are capable of generating a very intense net water movement into the intravascular space.
- **Hypotonic**. With a lower osmolarity than plasma, so they are capable of generating a net movement of water out of the vessels into the interstitial or intracellular space.

### Isotonic crystalloids

*Lactated Ringer's and Isofundin®*

Isotonic crystalloids are indicated in situations where there is **metabolic acidosis**.

*0.9% NaCl*

This has a high chlorine content and acidifying capacity. Indicated in situations where there is **alkalosis associated with hypochloraemia**. It is the fluid of choice in **Addison's disease**, since it allows correction of hyponatraemia and hyperkalaemia. In addition, its high sodium levels favour calciuresis when there is hypercalcaemia.

### Hypertonic crystalloids

*7.5% NaCl*

Its administration is indicated in situations where there is **acute hypovolaemia** (although the increased volaemia is of limited duration), in which a rapid increase in volume is necessary. Hydration and sodium levels should always be monitored, and rapid administration should be avoided (associated with bronchospasm and bradycardia).

### Hypotonic crystalloids

*5% glucose in water*

As it is only water, it is limited to correction of hypernatraemia, **free water deficit or drug reconstitution/dilution**.

## *Colloids*

Colloidal solutions can be classified into the following according to their nature:

- **Natural**. Blood derivatives uses differ depending on composition.
- **Synthetic**. Mixtures of different molecular-weight polysaccharides formulated in different types of isotonic crystalloids, whose administration is indicated in situations where there is **hypovolaemia or decreased colloidal osmotic pressure (COP)** (in both patients with changes in endothelial permeability and those that are hypoproteinaemic).

### Natural colloids

In general, **blood products** are not usually the first option for the correction of volume deficits or haemodynamic alterations. However, they may be indicated for the correction of changes in blood composition,

Table 1.3. Characteristics of different crystalloids.

| | 0.9% NaCl | LR | Isofundin® | 5% Glu H2O | 7.5% NaCl |
|---|---|---|---|---|---|
| pH | 6.0 | 5.0–7.0 | 5.1–5.9 | N/A | N/A |
| Osm (mOsm/l) | 308 | 275 | 309 | 250 | 2400 |
| Na (mmol/l) | 154 | 131 | 145 | X | 1200 |
| Cl (mmol/l) | 154 | 112 | 127 | X | 1200 |
| K (mmol/l) | X | 5 | 4 | X | X |
| iCa (mmol/l) | X | 3 | 2.5 | X | X |
| Glu (g/l) | X | X | X | 50 | X |
| Buffer | X | Lactate | Acetate | X | X |
| Malate | | | | | |
| Uses | Hypochloraemia | Hypokalaemia | Hypokalaemia | Hypernatraemia (gradual correction) | Rapid recovery of IV volume |
| | Hyperkalaemia Hypercalcaemia | Metabolic acidosis (diarrhoea, RI) | Metabolic acidosis (diarrhoea, RI) | Free water deficit | Haemorrhages |
| | Addison's disease | | | Dilution/ reconstitution of certain drugs | ICP increase due to cerebral oedema |
| | Metabolic alkalosis (chronic vomiting) | | | | Hyponatraemia (gradual correction) |
| Contraindications | Metabolic acidosis Hypernatraemia | Co-administration of blood products (Ca citrate) | Co-administration of blood products (Ca citrate) | Any clinical situation that is neither of the two mentioned above | Hypernatraemia Dehydration |
| | Hypokalaemia | Co-administration Na bicarb. (Ca carbonate) | Co-administration Na bicarb. (Ca carbonate) | Never for the treatment of hypoglycaemia | Rapid administration (bronchoconstriction, bradycardia and hypotension) |
| | | Metabolic alkalosis | Metabolic alkalosis | | |
| | | Compromised BBB (cerebral oedema) | | | |

LR, lactated Ringer's; Osm, osmolarity; Glu, glucose; ICP, intra-cranial pressure; BBB, blood–brain barrier.

with respect to **red blood cells and platelets and coagulation factors**. These types of fluids, with the exception of albumin, are described in the section covering transfusions of blood products.

### *Albumin*

Albumin is of human origin and its most frequent commercial format is at a concentration of 20–25%, thus making it a **hypertonic solution**. Its main use is for the correction of **hypoalbuminaemia and low COP levels**.

Formula for the calculation of albumin volume that should be administered:

albumin deficit (in grams)
10 × (desired albumin level – patient albumin) × weight (in kg) × 0.3.

## Synthetic colloids

### *Gelatines*

Substances of synthetic origin **derived from degradation of bovine collagen**. Because they contain small molecular-sized particles, their **half-life and clinical effect are short (approximately 8–12 h)**. The volume expansion they generate is equal only to the volume administered.

There are two commercially available gelatines:

- Haemacell® (urea-linked gelatin, which contains calcium)
- Gelofusin® (calcium free, succinated gelatin).

### *Dextranes*

Linear polysaccharide solutions **synthesised from sucrose** by *Leuconostoc mesenteroides* formulated in 0.9% NaCl. They achieve a plasma volume expansion of approximately 80–100%. Their **half-life and clinical effect last for approximately 24 h**; 40–50% is eliminated by renal excretion while the remainder is metabolised by the plasma enzyme dextranase. Therefore, its **elimination depends largely on correct renal function**. On the other hand, the **incidence of allergic reactions is very high**. In short, today these are **practically obsolete** as there are equally effective but much safer options.

Commercial format: Dextranorm Salino®.

### *Hydroxyethyl starch (HES)*

A fluid that contains a **synthetic polymer derived from amylopectin** using chemical modification. It produces a plasma volume expansion of 70–200%. Its particles are large but heterogeneous – the largest are slowly eliminated by the action of plasma amylase while the smallest are eliminated in the kidneys. **Its half-life is about 25 h and its clinical effect is about 12-48 h.** Most hydroxyethyl starches are formulated in 0.9% NaCl, and they lack buffer substances. The exception is Isohes® fluid, which is formulated in Isofundin® (a balanced solution that also contains bicarbonate precursors such as acetate and malate).

Its main role is in the **correction of hypovolaemia** although its use in critical patients is controversial, mainly due to recent results of various meta-analyses in which the safety of these substances in septic and critical human patients is questioned. In fact, its administration seems to be associated with an **increase in renal dysfunction and mortality** in these types of patient. However, in veterinary medicine these types of studies are not available to date, so all conclusions around its use are directly extrapolated from human studies without sufficient evidence to generate specific recommendations in this regard.

Two commercial formats:

- 10% Hetastarch
- 6% Isohes®.

# Transfusion

## *Introduction*

Critical and emergency patients may have severe systemic pathologies associated with a wide range of physiological changes:

- primary and secondary **haemostasis**
- **plasma protein, red blood cell and platelet concentrations**
- **COP**
- blood volume.

The administration of **blood products is a fundamental therapeutic tool** for correction of many of these problems.

## *Blood-derived products*

### *Red blood cell derivatives*

Red blood cell derivatives increase the oxygen-carrying capacity and thus **improve oxygen delivery** to tissues.

Red blood cell derivatives include:

- fresh whole blood
- preserved whole blood
- red blood cell concentrate.

### *Plasma derivatives*

These provide **plasma proteins, coagulation factors** and, in some cases, **platelets**. They are part of the therapeutic arsenal in patients with coagulation disorders and, to a lesser extent, with hypoproteinaemia.

Plasma derivatives:

- fresh plasma
- fresh frozen plasma
- frozen plasma
- platelet concentrate
- cryoprecipitate.

### *Derived haemoglobin-based oxygen carrier (Oxyglobin©)*

Bovine polymerised haemoglobin formulated in a buffered isotonic crystalloid solution, characterised by its powerful colloidal action that also provides oxygen transport capacity.

## Guidelines

The instructions for the use of blood products vary depending on the product, and its use to correct specific deficiencies. The important thing is to determine exactly what the deficit is and use a product appropriate to this.

In critical and emergency patients the following are common:

- severe haemorrhage
- anaemia
- hypoproteinaemia
- coagulation abnormalities.

### Severe haemorrhage

With regard to the acute loss of large volumes of blood due to severe bleeding, it is important to be aware of the concept of massive transfusion. **Massive transfusion** is defined as **transfusion of whole blood or blood products that involve the replacement of**:

- **large volumes** of the patient's blood volume in a **24-hour period**
- **half of the patient's blood volume** over a **3-hour period**
- **150% of the patient's blood volume** in an indeterminate period of time.

In human medicine, massive transfusion protocols are available to guide the administration of blood products (red blood cell, plasma or platelet concentrates) in predetermined proportions.

The main complications of massive transfusion are due to the rapid supply of a proportionately large volume of blood that has been refrigerated over a period of time. These complications include:

- hypocalcaemia
- anaphylaxis
- hyperkalaemia
- acidaemia
- hypothermia
- acute lung damage.

### Anaemia

With respect to anaemia, there is no haematocrit (Hct) limit that constitutes a cut-off point at which it is necessary to start a transfusion. However, a **Hct of 20%** is usually considered as a reference value around which transfusions potentially may be necessary. Even so, it should be remembered that patients with Hct >20% but with very severe, acute blood loss may need a transfusion, while in patients with chronic anaemia it may not be necessary until Hct levels are <20%. In fact, the decision to transfuse a patient must be based on more than one of the following factors:

- haematocrit
- type of anaemia (chronic or acute)
- haemorrhages which are still active
- existence of clinical signs (main factor), among others:
  - tachycardia
  - tachypnoea
  - pale mucous membranes
  - dazed
  - generalised weakness.

In general, it can be said that:

- Whole blood should be used in haemorrhages where volume and red blood cells need supplementation.
- Red blood cell concentrates should be used to correct anaemia in euvolaemic patients.

### Hypoproteinaemia

The benefit of administrating plasma products is limited to **correction of hypoproteinaemia**, and in particular **hypoalbuminaemia**. There are several ways to calculate an albumin deficit and the plasma units required to correct it. However, provided there are no concomitant active losses, to **increase albumin levels by approximately 1 g/dl around 45 ml of plasma/kg of weight is needed**.

That is, for a patient of about 30 kg with albumin levels of 1 g/dl and that needs a minimum increase of 1 g/dl, approximately 1.3 l of plasma (approximately 6–7 units of plasma) will be necessary. Consequently, since plasma correction requires the administration of large volumes capable of causing volume overload and excessive cost, **the best treatment option to correct hypoalbuminaemia is albumin**.

### Coagulation abnormalities

Finally, conditions such as DIC or traumatic coagulopathies are frequent abnormalities in critical patients. The **element that is deficient should be identified** (in short, the details of the pathogenesis of the coagulopathy) in order to supply the appropriate product:

- Cryoprecipitate in the case of patients with von Willebrand disease or haemophilia A.
- Fresh or fresh frozen plasma in the case of patients with von Willebrand disease or DIC.

## Types of product

### Fresh whole blood

The volume of blood obtained from the donor that is administered directly after collection (<8 **hours**) without refrigeration.

Therefore, the blood obtained contains all the components that are still fully functional:

- red blood cells
- platelets
- labile and stable coagulation factors
- plasma proteins.

Their use is indicated in:

- patients with **severe active bleeding** where an increase in coagulation is needed
- anaemic patients
- hypovolaemic patients.

### Preserved whole blood

This is whole blood stored under **refrigeration for up to 35 days** after collection.

This blood contains:

- red blood cells
- stable coagulation factors
- plasma proteins.

Their use is indicated in:

- anaemic patients
- hypovolaemic patients.

### Red blood cell concentrate

A product that is obtained by centrifugation of fresh whole blood after its separation from plasma. It must be kept **refrigerated for a maximum of 35 days**.

It **contains only red blood cells** and lacks the remaining blood components (platelets, coagulation factors and plasma proteins), which remain in the plasma fraction from which it is separated. It should be taken into consideration that the concentration of red blood cells is significantly higher than in the blood of origin, since the same number of red blood cells is concentrated into a much smaller volume. Therefore, the Hct of red blood cell concentrates ranges **70–80%**. In short, it can be said that the main utility of red blood cell concentrate is its ability to provide the same oxygen transport as whole blood, but with a much smaller volume.

Its use is mainly indicated in:

- euvolaemic anaemic patients
- patients in whom volume overload is contraindicated.

### Plasma

All types of plasma are obtained by **separating whole blood by centrifugation** and, according to the type of processing and storage they receive after obtaining them, they can be classified as:

- fresh plasma
- fresh frozen plasma
- frozen plasma.

### Fresh plasma

Fresh plasma is plasma that, after it is obtained, is stored refrigerated for a **maximum of 24 hours** before administration. Because certain coagulation factors are extremely labile, storage time determines their composition and the presence/absence of platelets.

This plasma contains:

- platelets
- all coagulation factors
- plasma proteins.

Its administration is indicated for:

- thrombocytopenia
- coagulopathy
- conditions causing hypoalbinaemia (with reduced effectiveness).

### Fresh frozen plasma

Plasma that is **frozen before 6 hours have elapsed from its collection**, and stored frozen for a maximum of 12 months before its administration.

This plasma lacks platelets but contains all coagulation factors as well as plasma proteins.

Its administration is indicated for:

- conditions where there is coagulopathy
- conditions causing hypoalbuminaemia (with reduced effectiveness).

### Frozen plasma

Plasma that is **stored frozen for more than 12 months** before administration.

This plasma lacks platelets and more labile coagulation factors (such as factors V, VIII and von Willebrand); however, it contains plasma proteins and coagulation factors dependent on vitamin K.

Its use is therefore only indicated for:

- partial support in certain coagulopathies
- contribution to COP in situations where there is hypoproteinaemia.

### *Platelet concentrate*

Due to the extremely **delicate nature of platelets**, these are obtained from fresh whole blood by special processing. To increase the survival and functionality of platelets, a series of special measures are necessary at all stages of collection and processing: whole fresh blood must be centrifuged at a very low speed and for a very short time; once centrifuged and separated from the red cell concentrate fraction, it should be stored at 20–24°C whilst being gently but continuously agitated. Depending on the concentrate collection system, it can be stored up to 4 h before administration (if collected in an open system) or up to 5 days (if collected in a closed system), since its storage at relatively high temperatures potentially favours bacterial growth. In some countries a form of concentrated and frozen freeze-dried platelets is marketed, which to date has produced very good results in all studies.

The use of platelet concentrates is indicated in situations where there is severe haemorrhage in patients with:

- thrombocytopenia
- thrombocytopathies.

### *Cryoprecipitate*

Obtained from the concentrated plasma fraction.

It contains very high levels of:

- Von Willebrand factor
- factor VIII
- factor XI
- factor XII.

Therefore, moderate volumes are capable of providing **high concentrations of coagulation factors** (concentrations between 5 and 10 times higher than those in plasma).

Their use is indicated in:

- coagulopathies
- cases of bleeding in patients with von Willebrand disease.

### *Oxiglobin®*

A solution of stromal-free polymerised bovine haemoglobin prepared in a modified lactated Ringer's solution. Its **half-life is approximately 24 h**, although its clinical effect depends largely on the patient's pathology (active bleeding, etc.). In the UK, where its use is authorised in dogs and cats, it has been administered anecdotally with very good results. In the last 10 years its commercialisation has suffered, and continues to suffer, numerous interruptions in different countries. Currently it is not available in Spain.

Table 1.4 summarises the uses and limitations of the products described above.

## *Complications associated with transfusions*

Any **unwanted side effects** that occur **during or after** the administration of **transfusion of a blood-derived product** should always be **considered as a transfusion reaction**. The **severity** of these reactions, as well as the implications they entail, are variable depending on the type of reaction that occurs. In general, depending on **whether or not the immune system is involved** in triggering the reaction, they can be classified into two main groups:

1. immune-mediated
2. non-immune-mediated.

### *Immune-mediated*

#### Acute immune-mediated

These are acute haemolytic reactions, are very dangerous and, in some cases, they can cause death. They are characterised as being **type II hypersensitivity reactions** in which **intravascular haemolysis of the donor's red blood cells occurs**. Clinical signs include:

- fever
- tachycardia
- dyspnoea
- vomiting
- haemoglobinaemia and haemoglobinuria
- shock
- DIC
- acute renal failure.

The treatment for this type of reaction is based on:

- immediately stopping the transfusion
- symptomatic treatment
- aggressive fluid therapy
- diuresis monitoring
- systemic pressure monitoring.

It may require the administration of:

- antihistamines
- corticosteroids.

Table 1.4. Main abnormalities that can be found in emergency patients, and the use of different products for correction.

| Condition/ Product | Haemorrhage with hypovolaemia | Anaemia | Thrombo-cytopenia | Thrombo-cytopathy | Von Willebrand | Coagulopathy | Hypo-proteinaemia |
|---|---|---|---|---|---|---|---|
| Fresh whole blood | **Optimal** | **Optimal** (with hypovolaemia) | Acceptable | Acceptable | Acceptable | Acceptable | Minimal benefit |
| Preserved whole blood | Acceptable | **Optimal** (with hypovolaemia) | No benefit | No benefit | No benefit | No benefit | Minimal benefit |
| Red blood cell concentrates | Acceptable (in combination with other products, in certain proportions) | **Optimal** (with euvolaemia) | No benefit | No benefit | No benefit | No benefit | No benefit |
| Fresh plasma | Acceptable (in proportion with other products) | No benefit | Acceptable | **Optimal** | Acceptable | **Optimal** | Acceptable |
| Fresh frozen plasma | Acceptable (in proportion with other products) | No benefit | No benefit | No benefit | No benefit | **Optimal** | Acceptable |
| Frozen plasma | Acceptable (in proportion with other products) | No benefit | No benefit | No benefit | No benefit | No benefit | Acceptable |
| Platelet concentrate | No benefit | No benefit | **Optimal** | **Optimal** | Acceptable | No benefit | No benefit |
| Cryoprecipitate | No benefit | No benefit | No benefit | No benefit | **Optimal** | **Optimal** | No benefit |
| Oxiglobin® | No benefit | **Optimal** | No benefit | No benefit | No benefit | No benefit | No benefit |

### *Acute non-haemolytic reactions*

Type I hypersensitivity reactions – that is, **anaphylactic or anaphylactoid reactions**.

The characteristic clinical signs of this type of reaction include:

- pruritus
- urticaria
- erythema
- vomiting
- oedema of the glottis
- increase in temperature
- vasodilation
- tachycardia
- bronchoconstriction.

The treatment for this type of reaction is based on:

- immediately stopping the transfusion.

Evaluation of the presence of shock, in which case the following should be administered immediately:

- epinephrine
- intravenous fluid therapy
- antihistamines.

If the reaction is mild and has been corrected, a decision can be made **whether to continue the transfusion at 25–50% of the previous rate**.

### *Delayed immune-mediated*

These are haemolytic reactions characterised by the presence of **extravascular haemolysis** that occurs between **2 and 21 days after transfusion**.

The clinical signs are **similar to those of acute haemolytic reactions**, and the only difference is the presence of **bilirubinaemia and bilirubinuria**.

In many cases treatment is not necessary, although it is important that from that point a **mandatory cross-match is performed** whenever the patient is going to receive a transfusion.

## Non-immune-mediated

These occur as a result of the administration of large volumes of products that have been **processed and**

**preserved in different ways** during storage. These abnormalities include:

- **Hypocalcaemia**, due to citrate poisoning.
- **Hyperkalaemia**, because of the release of potassium from the inside of the cells during the conservation time.
- **Acidosis**, due to acidification during storage time.
- **Hypothermia**, due to not properly warming the unit before administration.
- **Dilution coagulopathy**, due to a decrease in concentrations of factors V, VIII and IX and platelets.
- Existence of **microaggregates** that can lead to acute respiratory distress syndrome, if not properly administered through filters that can retain them.

## *Blood groups*

Different blood groups in dogs and cats are determined by the presence of **species-specific antigens on the surface of the red blood cells**. Because these antigens are transmitted genetically, the prevalence of different blood groups varies according to geographic location and breed.

### *Dogs*

Canine blood groups are classified by their **DEA (dog erythrocyte antigen)**, and there are **12 different ones** including three subtypes of the DEA 1 group: DEA 1.1, DEA 1.2 and DEA 1.3. In addition, each group can be **positive or negative**. The group with the **highest antigenic potential is DEA 1.1**. Fortunately there are **no alloantibodies** in the canine species, so a first exposure to a DEA 1.1-positive blood transfusion should not trigger a severe reaction in DEA 1.1-negative patients. However, antibodies capable of causing **a severe acute haemolytic reaction are produced if a second transfusion of DEA 1.1-positive blood** is received, as soon as 4 days after the first exposure to it. In general, and as a rule, the aim should be to ensure that DEA 1.1-negative patients receive only DEA 1.1-negative blood. However, DEA 1.1-positive patients may receive DEA 1.1-positive or -negative blood.

#### Typing

The **typing of donors and recipients** should always be carried out so that the DEA 1.1 status of both is known. The majority of typing tests are based on agglutination techniques, in some of which haemagglutination is observed and in others it is not.

#### Cross-matching

Cross-matching between the blood of the donor and that of the recipient **means that the compatibility of the blood of both individuals can be assessed**. It should be done under the following circumstances:

- Recipients who received a transfusion more than 4 days ago.
- When there is a history of a transfusion reaction.
- When the previous transfusion history of a patient is unknown.

### *Cats*

In cats, blood groups follow the **AB nomenclature** and there are **three groups** (A, B and AB – which is uncommon) of extremely variable prevalence, depending on the breed and even within the same breed, and on the geographic location. For example, studies have shown that:

- Almost 100% of Siamese cats are type A.
- Races such as Persian, Abyssinian, Himalayan and Burmese have a higher prevalence of type B.
- Type AB is usually common in the Ragdoll breed.

In general, the group with the highest prevalence in the common European cat is type A, although an increase in the prevalence of type B has been observed in recent years.

Cats have **alloantibodies against the opposite blood group** from two months of age (i.e. a cat with blood group A has anti-B alloantibodies and vice versa), except for cats with blood group AB (which do not have any type of alloantibody). Therefore, patients with blood group A should receive blood from only a type A donor, while animals with blood group B should receive blood from only a type B donor.

#### Typing

**Typing is always mandatory**, both in the case of the donor and of the recipient.

The most frequently used technique is haemagglutination.

#### Cross-matching

In cats, cross-matching should **always be performed**.

## *Administration*

Blood products are usually **administered intravenously**, although occasionally intra-osseous administration may be necessary; **no other route of administration** should be considered. A specific filter, which usually comes as part of a transfusion set (170–260 μm) (Figure 1.2) should be used. In the case of small patients, there are smaller filters that can be adapted to syringes (18–40 μm) (Figure 1.3).

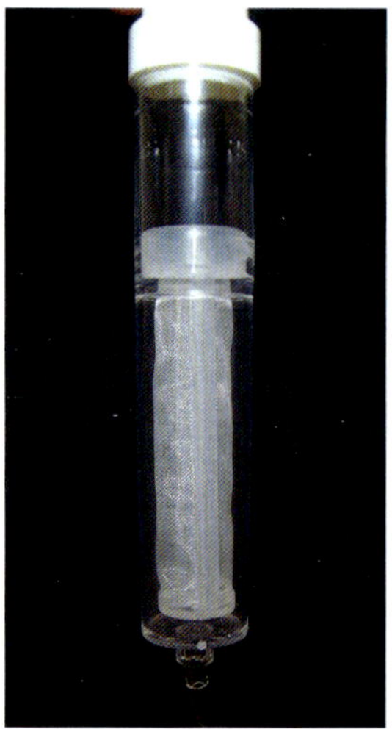

**Figure 1.2.** Filter built into the transfusion system.

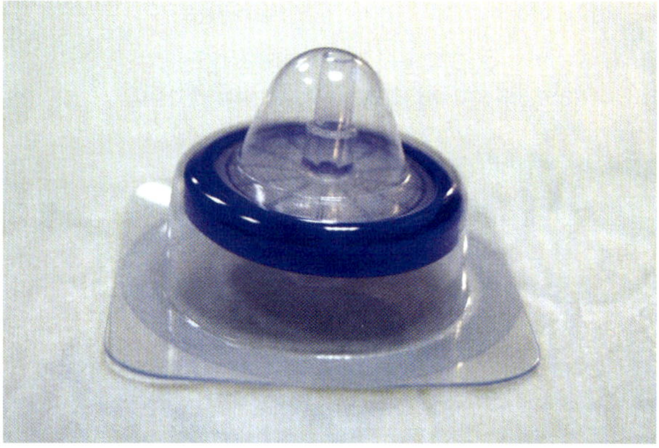

**Figure 1.3.** Filter for transfusion adapted for syringe use.

It is important to remember that the **intravenous route through which the transfusion is administered should be used only for 0.9% NaCl**, since any calcium-containing crystalloid can form microcrystals because citrate reacts with calcium, forming calcium citrate. In general, the administration of food, drugs or **fluid therapy (except for 0.9% NaCl)** during transfusion should be avoided.

Recommended volumes depend on:

- the specific product being administered
- the effect sought with its administration
- the patient's pathology.

Table 1.5 summarises the volumes of transfusion products most frequently used.

Although the final speed of transfusion administration depends on the cardiovascular status of the patient, following these guidelines is generally recommended:

- Initial speed (first 20 minutes): 0.25–1.0 ml/kg/h.
- Final speed: If the patient is cardiovascularly stable, remaining volume over a maximum of 4 h.
- If there is a risk of volume overload: maximum 3–4 ml/kg/h.

**Table 1.5.** Most commonly used transfusion product volumes.

| | Dose | Uses |
|---|---|---|
| Whole blood (fresh or preserved) | 5–20 ml/kg | Haemorrhage, anaemia |
| Red blood cell concentrate | 10 ml/kg | Anaemia |
| Plasma (fresh, fresh frozen or frozen) | 10 ml/kg | Coagulopathies, thrombocytopenia, thrombocytopathies |
| Platelet concentrate | 10 ml/kg | Thrombocytopenia, thrombocytopathies |
| Cryoprecipitate | 1 unit/10 kg | Von Willebrand coagulopathy |
| Oxiglobin® | 15 ml/kg | Anaemia |

## Monitoring

Due to the potential occurrence of transfusion reactions, continuous and thorough patient monitoring is absolutely essential during the procedure. Among the parameters that should be evaluated are:

- temperature
- heart rate
- respiratory rate
- colour of mucous membranes
- capillary refill time (CRT).

All of the above must be monitored with the following frequency:

1. before starting the transfusion
2. every 5 minutes for the first 30 minutes
3. every 15 minutes until the end of the transfusion
4. 1, 12 and 24 hours after the transfusion has finished is also advisable.

Hct and total protein should also be assessed before and a few hours after transfusion.

All the above information should be carefully recorded in a graph (Figure 1.4) that provides a record of what happened during the transfusion and the existence of trends to be assessed, as well as being able to act as soon as possible against potential complications.

| **PRODUCT:** | | | FWB | PWB | RBCC | FP | FFP | PRP | |
|---|---|---|---|---|---|---|---|---|---|
| Administration date: | | | | Donation date: | | | | | |
| **PATIENT:** | | | | **DONOR:** | | | | | |
| Name | | | | Name | | | | | |
| Species | | | | Species | | | | | |
| Case number | | | | Donor no. | | | | | |
| Blood group | | | | Blood group | | | | | |
| Weight | | | | Hct/PT | | | | | |
| Volume needed | | | | Volume | | | | | |
| **CHART MONITORING:** | | | | | | | | | |
| | Time | Infusion speed (ml/h) | Temperature | HR | RR | Mucous membrane colour | S/M/D | Hct | PT |
| Pre-transf. | | | | | | | | | |
| **Start time:** | | | | | | | | | |
| | Time | Infusion speed (ml/h) | Temperature | HR | RR | Mucous membrane colour | S/M/D | Hct | PT |
| 5 min | | | | | | | | | |
| 10 min | | | | | | | | | |
| 15 min | | | | | | | | | |
| 20 min | | | | | | | | | |
| 25 min | | | | | | | | | |
| 30 min | | | | | | | | | |
| 35 min | | | | | | | | | |
| 40 min | | | | | | | | | |
| 45 min | | | | | | | | | |
| 60 min | | | | | | | | | |
| 75 min | | | | | | | | | |
| 90 min | | | | | | | | | |
| 105 min | | | | | | | | | |
| 120 min | | | | | | | | | |
| 135 min | | | | | | | | | |
| 150 min | | | | | | | | | |
| 165 min | | | | | | | | | |
| 180 min | | | | | | | | | |
| 195 min | | | | | | | | | |
| 210 min | | | | | | | | | |
| 225 min | | | | | | | | | |
| 240 min | | | | | | | | | |
| **End time:** | | | | **Comments:** | | | | | |
| **CALCUL ATIONS:** | | Speed (ml/kg/h) | Speed (ml/h) | | | | | | |
| Speed (first 15') '): | | | | | | | | | |
| Speed (Normovol): | | | | | | | | | |
| Speed (Hypovol): | | | | | | | | | |
| Speed (risk of overload): | | | | | | | | | |

**Figure 1.4.** Example of transfusion graph.

## Triage and evaluation of the critical and emergency patient

### Triage

The care of critical patients **requires immediate availability of facilities, equipment and personnel**. The first step is to identify quickly and accurately what care is needed. To do so, it is essential to establish an **automatic protocol** that allows identification, classification and **prioritisation of the urgency**, along with the **intensity of clinical care** a patient requires. This is achieved through triage.

**Triage is a method of selecting and classifying patients** that uses the **type and urgency of their therapeutic needs** as criteria. Its ultimate goal is to **quickly identify those patients whose clinical condition is critical** and whose therapeutic needs require the most urgent medical attention. This prioritisation system has decreased the mortality rate considerably since it was first introduced in human medicine in the 1970s.

In recent decades, different triage protocols have been created in both human and veterinary medicine. For example, indexes such as the Manchester Triage System, the Emergency Severity Index and the Canadian Triage & Acuity Scale have been created and validated for use in the emergency services of many human hospitals.

The first veterinary triage system was the **Animal Trauma Triage** system created by the University of Pennsylvania in 1994, where the aim was to have a survival prediction instrument as well as stratification of poly-trauma patients, based on the urgency of their medical care. More recently, the so-called **Veterinary Triage List** (**VTL**) has been created, based on the adaptation of the Manchester Triage Scale from human medicine, which uses a colour code and allows emergency patients to be categorised into four groups with four different waiting times according to their clinical condition:

- Red. Immediate attention. Examples: severe active bleeding or the presence of seizures.
- Orange. Maximum wait: 15 minutes.
- Yellow. Maximum wait: 30–60 minutes. Example: episode of loss of consciousness already resolved.
- Green. Maximum wait: 120 minutes.

Whichever system is adopted, the final objective is to **optimise the use of the available resources** by **establishing an appropriate waiting time** for each patient. This is especially useful in emergency veterinary medicine, where unfortunately resources are limited and must be optimised to the maximum.

Before starting a physical examination for triage, it is important to **obtain a minimum medical history** for the patient and their pathology which should include:

- signalment
- current problem and development
- treatments received so far
- concomitant pathologies and their treatments.

Right at the start it is also important to obtain an **informed consent signed by the owner**. This allows all necessary procedures for the stabilisation of the patient to be commenced without interrupting clinical care.

### Initial assessment

As a first approach to an emergency patient, a **swift systematic and methodical physical examination** should always be carried out (<2 minutes is recommended), with specific clinical interventions that allow for stabilisation of immediately life-threatening complications. The management of this type of patient is usually carried out using **horizontal resuscitation**, which implies that both the evaluation/monitoring/diagnosis tasks and the instrumentation/stabilisation/treatment tasks are **carried out simultaneously** thanks to the teamwork of several professionals that act at the same time to treat the same patient. For this initial evaluation, following the ABC rule is recommended:

- **a**irway
- **b**reathing
- **c**irculation
- **d**isability
- **e**xternal assessment
- **u**rogenital

#### Airway

The patient's airway should be examined by **ocular inspection and palpation of the oral cavity**, in order to confirm that the airway is not obstructed by the presence of a foreign body. If necessary, immediate clearance of the airway should be performed.

#### Breathing

**Observing the patient's respiratory movements** is essential, as well as auscultating the chest and trachea to confirm the presence of respiratory sounds and that these are normal. If respiratory movements or sounds cannot be appreciated, immediate endotracheal intubation should be performed along with assisted ventilation.

Similarly, a first assessment of respiratory function should be performed by assessing the **colour of the mucous membranes** and **respiratory rate**. If there is cyanosis, tachypnoea or the presence of stridor and wheezing are observed on auscultation, **supplementation with 100% oxygen** should begin immediately using a mask, direct flow or oxygen cage, since these are signs that suggest the presence of hypoxaemia. On the other hand, a **respiratory rate >40 breaths per minute** should be considered as tachypnoeic and all its **differential diagnoses (hypovolaemia, pain, fear, etc.) should be considered**.

Monitoring of blood oxygenation by **pulse oximetry ($SpO_2$)** should be established as soon as possible to provide additional information. $SpO_2$ values <95% indicate the immediate need for supplementation with 100% $O_2$.

### Circulation

Firstly, the **presence of a pulse** should be assessed.

If cardiopulmonary arrest (CPA) cannot be ruled out, **commencing cardiopulmonary resuscitation (CPR)** manoeuvres as soon as possible is recommended. It has been shown that the consequences of delaying its initiation are much more severe than those derived from beginning CPR manoeuvres on patients who are not in CPA.

Next, the **presence of active haemorrhage** should be ruled out. If there is external haemorrhage, direct manual compression is usually sufficient to control minor haemorrhages, but sometimes internal haemorrhages or lacerations of large vessels must be stopped by surgical exposure of the affected arteries and structures. In these cases, **fluid therapy-based resuscitation procedures** should be part of hypotensive resuscitation procedures. At this point it is essential to obtain a first **estimate of the degree of tissue perfusion** through a rapid assessment of:

- mucous membrane colour
- capillary refill time (CRT)
- pulse quality
- heart rate
- cardiac auscultation
- level of consciousness
- temperature of the extremities.

**Electrocardiographic (ECG)** and **blood pressure monitoring** using Doppler should be set up as soon as possible to detect arrhythmias or low systemic pressures (<90 mmHg) that may cause low cardiac output. **Plasma lactate** values are also useful, since values <2.5 mml/l are indicative of hypoperfusion.

### Disability

The **functionality of the nervous system** must be assessed both centrally and in the spine, through a rapid neurological examination and action taken accordingly:

If there are **seizures, anticonvulsant treatment** should be started immediately to avoid cerebral oedema, hyperthermia and irreversible brain damage.

If **cerebral hypertension** is suspected, treatment should be given as soon as possible to avoid irreversible secondary problems such as cerebral ischaemia or herniation through the foramen magnum.

If **traumatic spinal injury** is suspected, the **patient should be immobilised** to prevent further spinal damage.

### External assessment

This examination is particularly important for polytrauma patients, since it allows the assessment of haemorrhage, lacerations, bruises, points which are painful on palpation or open fractures.

### Urogenital

An **evaluation of the bladder by palpation** is essential when assessing the existence of possible urethral obstructions or ruptured bladder. This is vital since, as these conditions can cause **serious arrhythmias**.

Table 1.6 summarises the key findings on initial examination.

It is important to remember certain things that should be taken into account related to this initial examination phase of the critical patient:

In many cases patients are examined in the initial stages of shock in which compensatory mechanisms are still under way, so cardiovascular disorders are either not present or are very mild and an incorrect diagnosis is likely. Therefore, the initial examination must be, as well as rapid, both methodical and careful so that the slightest hint of shock is appreciated.

Table 1.6. Main indicators of compromise that can be found on initial examination.

| Parameter | Value |
|---|---|
| Mucous membrane colour | Pale Cyanotic Congested |
| Capillary refill time | >2 s |
| Heart rate | **Cats** (>220 or <140 bpm)<br>**Large-breed dogs** (>100 bpm)<br>**Small-breed dogs** (>160 bpm) |
| Pulse quality | Dorso-pedal pulse absent and weak at femoral level |
| Systolic arterial pressure | <90 mmHg |
| Respiratory rate | >40 rpm |
| Lactate levels | >2.5 mmol/l |
| Level of consciousness | Depressed |

Patients in whom **potential poisoning** is suspected should receive **priority attention**, even if their condition at the time of presentation is not critical, since **toxin-elimination procedures** (gastric lavage, induction of vomiting, etc.) should be initiated soon as possible.

Every patient who is in **pain should receive analgesia as soon as possible**. A critically ill patient with pain should never be denied analgesia, not only for obvious ethical reasons but also to minimise the negative effects of untreated pain on homeostasis. There are pharmacological (and non-pharmacological) alternatives that can be considered even in the unstable patient. Of course, a neurological examination should be performed before administration since results may be affected after administration of analgesia.

**Blood sampling should always be performed before starting fluid therapy**, so as not to affect results.

## *Diagnostic imaging tests* in situ

(FAST, AFAST, TFAST and VetBLUE)

### FAST: focused assessment with sonography for trauma

**Internal injuries are frequent** in critically ill patients, but their detection on physical examination, with conventional radiology or using sampling by centesis, can be complicated. To overcome this, a new diagnostic tool has been developed in emergency medicine and intensive care, both human and veterinary, in recent years. It is a technique using ultrasound evaluation of the abdominal and thoracic cavity in critical patients called **focused assessment with sonography for trauma, or FAST**.

In fact, since the 1990s, the FAST technique (that is, **ultrasound-focused evaluation for trauma**) has become the initial diagnostic test of choice for the **evaluation of free fluid in the peritoneal, pleural and pericardial spaces** of critical poly-trauma patients with non-penetrating injuries. It has also been used to assess the status of patients with penetrating lesions, aiming to detect those in the retroperitoneal space and in solid organs. Its use can also be combined with evaluation systems for the presence or absence of abdominal fluid, such as the AFS (abdominal fluid scoring system).

This diagnostic instrument is now included in the evaluation protocol of every critical veterinary patient and, since both thorax and abdomen can be evaluated, two different terms have been coined:

- AFAST: FAST for evaluation of the abdominal cavity
- TFAST: FAST for evaluation of the thoracic cavity.

### AFAST

The AFAST method aims for the **early detection of fluid in the intraperitoneal cavity** in critical patients who need a rapid, non-invasive, portable diagnosis that allows **serial evaluation in the event of changes in the general state**. The majority of poly-trauma patients present with **abdominal free fluid**, which is easily detectable using this test. Diagnosis is completed with **fine-needle aspiration and subsequent analysis**. Some studies have demonstrated the usefulness of serial AFAST evaluations along with records from an abdominal fluid evaluation scale (AFS) to detect changes in the evolution of the condition over time.

The AFAST method uses the evaluation of **four windows on the abdomen** following a clockwise direction (Figure 1.5), both in right and left lateral recumbency over an average time of 3–6 minutes:

1. diaphragmatic-hepatic window (DH)
2. spleno-renal window (SR)
3. cysto-colic window (CC)
4. hepato-renal window (HR).

Using this system, the following organs are visualised systematically and in an orderly way:

- diaphragm
- liver
- gall bladder
- spleen
- kidneys
- intestinal loops
- bladder.

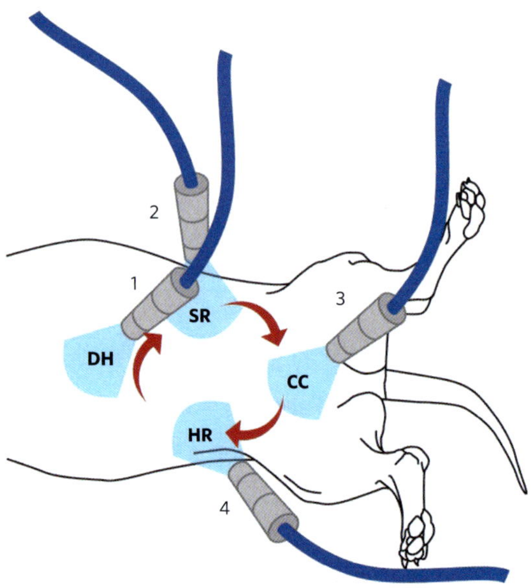


**Figure 1.5.** AFAST: examination windows – diaphragmatic-hepatic window (DH), spleno-renal window (SR), cysto-colic window (CC) and hepato-renal window (HR).

The presence of free fluid is usually seen in the form of **black triangles surrounded by the different organs** (since free fluid is an anechoic substance and therefore appears black).

The AFS is obtained very simply: recording the locations in which the presence of free liquid is detected is sufficient (that is, an AFS of 2 is obtained when it is detected in two locations, while an AFS of 0 is obtained when none is detected in any).

Serial AFAST evaluations can be **performed every 4 hours** to assess the evolution of the condition, as well as the effectiveness of the therapeutic measures used.

## TFAST

The use of TFAST has two objectives:

- detection of a pneumothorax *in situ*
- detection of injuries to the chest wall, pleura or pericardium.

The study is based on the evaluation of five points in each hemithorax (Figure 1.6):

1. **Chest tube site (CTS)**. This is usually the one chosen to assess the existence of pneumothorax and pulmonary pathologies.
2. **Pericardial site (PCS)** (with two perpendicular views). This is usually used to detect pleural or pericardial fluid, evaluate volaemia and detect cardiac abnormalities.
3. **Diaphragmatic-hepatic window (DH).**

The patient should be positioned in **right lateral recumbency** (and sternal recumbency when the opposite hemithorax needs to be examined), since this is the position recommended for AFAST evaluation and can be used to perform both studies simultaneously. **Dorsal recumbency should be avoided**, because it significantly hinders breathing.

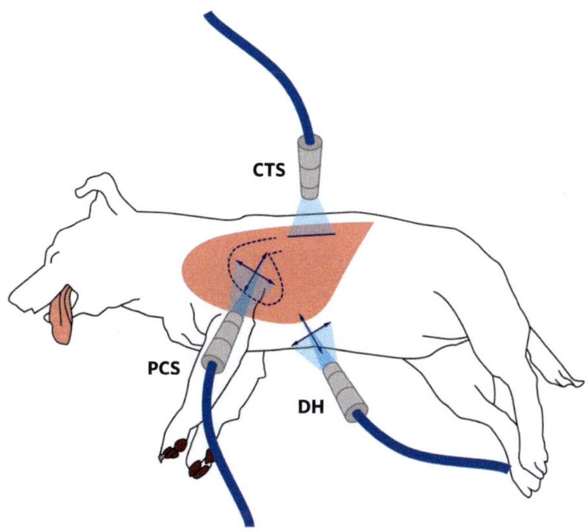


**Figure 1.6.** TFAST: examination windows – chest tube site (CTS), pericardial site (PCS, with two perpendicular views) and diaphragmatic-hepatic window (DH).

**For the diagnosis of pneumothorax**, the following structures should be studied on ultrasound images of the chest tube site (CTS):

- **A-lines** (artefacts of air reverberation).
- **Crocodile sign** (the ribs resemble the eyes of a crocodile looking out of the water).
- **Interface between pleura and lung** (the line that draws the crocodile's nose between the eyes).
- **Sliding sign** (the white arrows that would indicate the movement described by the ribs during the different phases of breathing).

Images of patients with healthy lungs (Figure 1.7a) show all the features mentioned here (clear presence of the pleura–lung interface line and sliding sign); those of animals with pneumothorax have no sign of sliding (Figure 1.7b), and those that have abnormalities in the costal wall or pleura have the step sign at the pleura–lung interface (Figure 1.7c).

## VetBLUE

The technique called **VetBLUE** (**Bedside Lung Ultrasound Examination**; Figure 1.8) is an ultrasonographic study performed *in situ* that is used as the first line of examination for patients that are either compromised or non-compromised from a respiratory point of view. It allows early **diagnosis of areas of pulmonary consolidation** (contusion, oedema and foci of pneumonia) using ultrasound examination at four points on each hemithorax:

1. caudodorsal lung lobe region (CdLL)
2. perihilar lung lobe region (PhLL)
3. middle lung lobe region (MdLL)
4. cranial lung lobe region (CrLL).

This study is based on the recognition of two characteristic patterns:

- The presence of **ULR** (**Ultrasound Lung Rockets**) (pulmonary consolidation; Figure 1.9): intense **hyperechoic lines** that extend from the pleura–lung interface. These **oscillate in a pendular manner** with the different phases of breathing. They indicate the presence of areas of **pulmonary consolidation** (oedema, contusion or pneumonia).
- The presence of sliding signs and A-lines (healthy lung parenchyma).

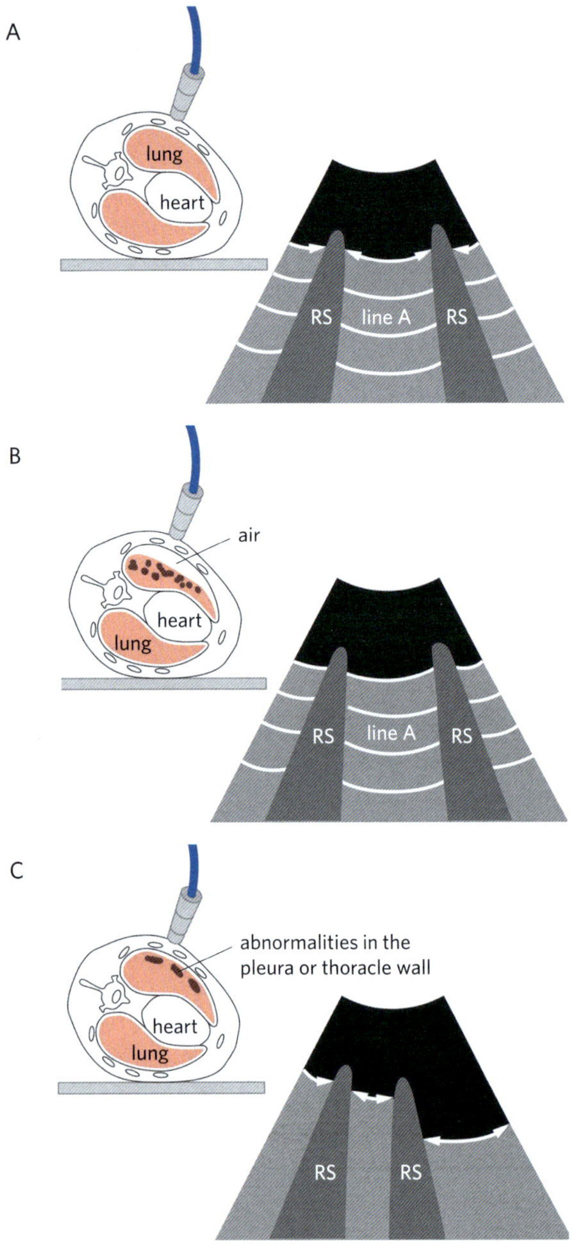


**Figure 1.7.** TFAST, images obtained from the CTS window. a, healthy lung; b, pneumothorax; c, abnormalities in the thoracle wall or the pleura.

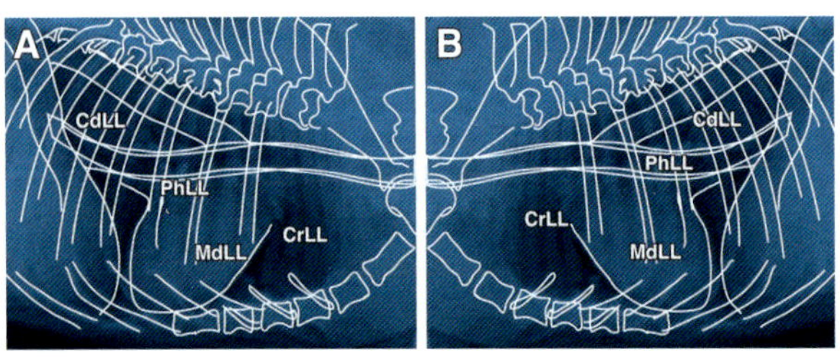


**Figure 1.8.** VetBLUE: areas examined.

Patients in whom no ULRs (or very few) are detected do not usually present with pulmonary abnormalities associated with parenchymal consolidation (oedema, contusion or pneumonia).

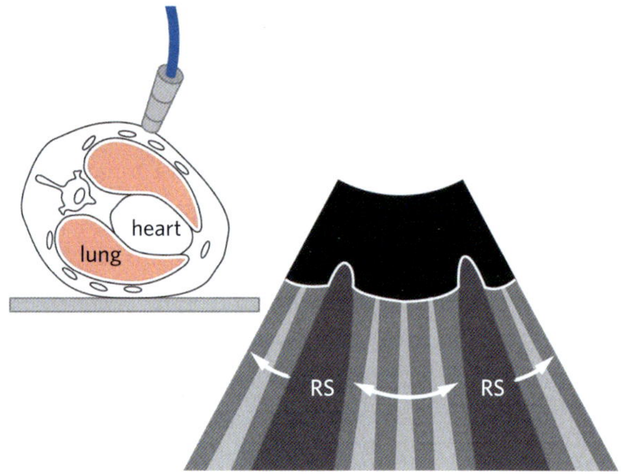


**Figure 1.9.** Characteristics of ULR.

### GFAST

The combination of AFAST, TFAST and VetBLUE is called **Global FAST, or GFAST** and is a fundamental tool used to obtain clinical information in critical patients. By means of a simple, rapid and reliable ultrasound evaluation, potentially fatal abnormalities can be diagnosed in a few minutes without moving the animal, and the efficacy of the clinical management of these patients can be assessed.

## *Initial monitoring*

The initial monitoring should be able to provide information about the haemodynamic functionality of the patient, in order to guide fluid therapy and drug administration quickly and non-invasively. Evaluation of the haemodynamic state is usually based on parameters measured during the physical examination (such as pulse, mucous membrane colour and CRT) as well as the electrocardiogram (ECG) and direct or indirect blood pressure.

With regards to the **respiratory system**, arterial blood oxygen saturation is usually monitored by continuous and non-invasive methods such as **pulse oximetry**.

Likewise, **perfusion** can be evaluated by measuring **lactate levels** and **pH in venous blood**.

### Electrocardiography

**Uninterrupted ECG monitoring** is very useful in critical patients, since it provides continuous and **non-invasive information on heart rate and rhythm**. In this way, arrhythmias that may be infrequent and intermittent can be detected, as well as determining the need for their treatment and its efficacy.

Two methods can be used for electrocardiography:

1. standard
2. telemetric (advantage: less need for wiring, which facilitates patient mobility).

In the case of critical or emergency patients, unlike cardiology patients, what is clinically useful is continuous monitoring rather than specific studies of multiple electrical leads. Its use allows the detection of:

- trends of the abnormality, even if values remain within physiological limits
- abnormalities that occur with characteristic ECG changes, such as certain electrolyte abnormalities (hyper- and hypokalaemia, hyper- and hypocalcaemia, hyper- and hypomagnesaemia)
- hypoxaemia
- pleural effusions.

## Direct and indirect arterial pressure

In these patients, **monitoring of systemic blood pressure** is of vital importance since findings can be used to guide treatment decisions related to fluid therapy and the administration of inotropic or vasopressor agents. So much so, that the administration of these types of agent is completely contraindicated if no system is available that allows continuous or frequent measurement of arterial pressure.

### *Physiological arterial blood pressure values*

In the dog:

- systolic pressure: 150 mmHg
- mean pressure: 105 mmHg
- diastolic pressure: 85 mmHg.

In the cat:

- systolic pressure: 150 mmHg
- mean pressure: 105 mmHg
- diastolic pressure: 90 mmHg.

## Methods for monitoring blood pressure

- indirect (non-invasive methods):
  - Doppler
  - oscillometric instruments
  - directly (invasive methods) through an arterial catheter associated with a pressure transducer.

### *Indirect arterial blood pressure*

Non-invasive measurement systems are based **on inflation of a cuff capable of occluding arterial blood flow**, followed by measuring the pressure at which the flow returns. These are easy to use and require only equipment that is relatively affordable from an economic point of view, but they can provide unreliable values usually due to errors in handling or the selection of an incorrectly sized cuff. It should be emphasised that **cuff selection is absolutely essential**, since one that is larger or smaller than the appropriate one can over- or undervalue arterial blood pressure values:

In the **dog, the width of the cuff should be approximately 40% of the circumference of the limb**; in the cat, 30%.

Other important factors are that the patient is **absolutely still** during measurements and the correct **positioning of the cuff with respect to the heart** (at the height of the right atrium).

### *Doppler*

The Doppler method uses a **10 MHz ultrasound probe** capable of detecting arterial blood flow in a patient's limb. Probe and cuff are placed over the same artery, although the cuff is proximal to the probe. As the pressure of the cuff decreases, blood flow returns to the artery so that the sound it generates is again audible. The pressure at the exact moment of return is considered to be systolic arterial blood pressure.

The Doppler method is used very frequently in:

- small patients
- patients suffering from arrhythmias (in which the oscillometric method does not work).

### *Oscillometry*

The oscillometric method is also based on the use of a **cuff that obstructs the flow of arterial blood**. In this case, it is the oscillations that occur when the blood flow returns under the cuff that determine the different pressures:

- Oscillations of maximum amplitude are associated with mean blood pressure.
- The moment when oscillations are first detected constitutes systolic pressure.
- The moment when oscillations disappear constitutes diastolic pressure.

These types of devices determine the mean blood pressure by oscillometric measurement and then calculate the systolic and diastolic pressures through algorithms included in their software. Despite being used frequently in the veterinary world, the validation of its use still leaves much to be desired and the absolute reliability of results is questioned. However, there is a new system, called **high-definition oscillometry**, capable of calculating the amplitude of the oscillations of the arterial wall in real time so that the values provided of systolic and diastolic pressure are measured, not calculated. In addition, the analysis system of this device is high-speed, so pressures in the presence of arrhythmias and heart rates of up to 500 bpm can be assessed.

*Indirect arterial blood pressure*

Invasive blood pressure measurement is the reference method in both human and veterinary medicine. Its use is particularly indicated in critical patients, since it allows:

- A guide to the replacement of intravascular volume and use of vasopressors and inotropes for the maintenance of systemic pressures through analysis of the curve.
- Assessment of the effect of possible arrhythmias on the generation of a pulse, and guiding the decision on the use of antiarrhythmics.
- A patent arterial route that can be used to obtain serial samples of arterial blood, both to perform arterial blood gas tests and for any other laboratory test that is necessary, without the need to puncture the patient.

However, the morbidity associated with its placement and use must be considered, the main danger being its **accidental disconnection and the potential associated bleeding**.

*Pulse oximetry*

**Pulse oximetry** offers fundamental clinical information on respiratory function in the management of the critical patient, since it is indicative of the **degree of oxygenation of arterial blood**. However, since it is an indirect oxygenation assessment system, it provides only the percentage of saturated haemoglobin in arterial blood ($SpO_2$).

Its principle of action is based on the **non-linear (yet directional) relationship** between the partial pressure of oxygen in arterial blood ($PaO_2$) and the oxygen saturation of haemoglobin in arterial blood ($SpO_2$) through the haemoglobin **dissociation curve**. This is why pulse oximetry can indirectly obtain continuous information about $PaO_2$ non-invasively (rather than arterial blood gas).

Ultimately, pulse oximetry provides only the **percentage of saturated haemoglobin in arterial blood with respect to the total haemoglobin present** in arterial blood, and this information must be subsequently interpreted based on the relationship with $PaO_2$ in order to determine arterial blood oxygenation.

## Immediate stabilisation

In a horizontal resuscitation strategy, an initial examination must be carried out simultaneously alongside a basic immediate stabilisation.

The first step of this primary stabilisation is to establish a **patent intravenous route**. A **peripheral vein** is usually catheterised (such as the cephalic or lateral saphenous vein although, depending on the breed, the atrial vein or, in the case of cats, the medial saphenous vein, can also be considered).

Due to the nature of the cases presented by these patients, sometimes catheterising a peripheral vein is a real challenge; despite this, an attempt should always be made with the **shortest, largest-diameter catheter** appropriate. In this manner, the speed of administration of fluids will be adequate for the state of shock and hypovolaemia (since catheters with these characteristics allow a maximum flow to be achieved and, therefore, a maximum administration rate). If the **large volume of fluids** has to be administered, **catheterisation of multiple peripheral veins** can be contemplated.

On the other hand, when it is **impossible to catheterise a peripheral vein** (very hypovolaemic patients, puppies or very small animals), an **intra-osseous catheter** should be placed, which has the advantage over intravenous routes in significantly hypovolaemic animals of allowing direct access to sinusoids and medullary venous channels (structures not affected by lack of volume and capable of communicating directly with the systemic venous system). These types of catheter require some basic knowledge related to their placement.

Taking advantage of the placement of the catheter, **obtain a blood sample** which allows at least minimum and basic tests to be carried out, including:

- haematocrit
- total protein
- glucose
- blood urea nitrogen.

If possible, the following are also recommended:

- venous blood-gas analysis
- measurement of lactate levels
- measurement of electrolyte levels.

It is important to **take these samples before initiating any stabilisation** or treatment procedures, which may then mask or modify alterations present in the blood.

With reference to the initial **lactate and base excess (BE) levels**, it is important to remember their meaning and clinical utility.

### Lactate

**Lactate is an indicator of tissue perfusion**. Its levels increase above the **normal physiological limit**

**(2.5 mmol/l)** when situations causing tissue hypoxia occur which force cells to enter **anaerobic metabolism** (and generate lactic acid as a by-product of that metabolism). But perhaps its greatest clinical utility lies in its condition as a **guide for resuscitation therapy** (see objective-guided resuscitation section), as well as in its **predictive survival properties** for certain pathologies. For this purpose, recent studies have shown that these predictive values are found in the evolution of the initial value throughout stabilisation and not in the starting value. That is, **lactate values that decrease by >50% in the first 12 hours of presentation and stabilisation constitute a positive predictive** factor for survival. For example, the prognosis of a patient with a lactate of 8 mmol/l which, after aggressive stabilisation procedures, shows a reduction to only 7.5 mmol/l, is much worse than that of a patient with an initial lactate of 10 mmol/l which, after resuscitation and stabilisation procedures, was lowered to 3.5 mmol/l.

A BE has predictive value for mortality and transfusion needs in poly-trauma patients.

## Glucose

The measurement of glucose levels is essential in this type of patient:

**Hypoglycaemia is often associated with sepsis.** The latest recommendations for clinical management of the septic patient in human medicine suggest avoiding hypoglycaemia (**supplementing glucose until maximum values of 180 mg/dl** are reached) as well as very sharp oscillations that reach values >180 mg/dl.

**Hyperglycaemia is accompanied by a higher morbidity-mortality** than hypoglycaemia.

## Total proteins

Levels of total protein are another vitally important factor for management of the critical patient. Hypoproteinaemia is very frequent, mainly due to hypoalbuminaemia phenomena.

**Albumin levels <4 mg/dl** are associated with **increases in morbidity and mortality**, since albumin is responsible for carrying out fundamental biological functions such as determining the free fraction of many drugs and colloidal osmotic pressure. The latter is of great importance, since it is responsible for attracting and retaining water molecules within the intravascular space (a determining factor in the maintenance of volaemia and the prevention of peripheral oedema).

**Hypoalbuminaemic patients may benefit from the administration of natural or synthetic colloids**, although in animals with levels <2 mg/dl it is reasonable to consider albumin transfusions.

## Oxygen

In this first phase of stabilisation, **supplemental oxygen administration** is usually included. Depending on factors such as the $FiO_2$ that needs to be achieved, the condition of the patient and their temperament, the most suitable method will be chosen:

The simplest system is **direct flow administration**, with the oxygen source 1–3 cm from the animal's snout. **Oxygen flow should be 6–8 l/min and the maximum $FiO_2$ 0.25–0.45**. Its main advantage is that it involves minimal stress for the animal, and among its drawbacks are the need to allocate a member of the team solely to hold the source of $O_2$ in front of the patient, the high oxygen expenditure that is generated and the enormous variability (and not very high) $FiO_2$ that is obtained in the best-case scenario.

The use of an **oxygen mask** fitted around the animal's snout, with an oxygen flow of **6–10 l/min, should provide a $FiO_2$ of 0.35–0.55**. Its advantages include the possibility of reaching a potentially greater $FiO_2$ than with the previous method, though in a slightly more invasive way, and its disadvantages, the high oxygen expenditure and the stress that it can generate in the patient.

The use of a **bilateral nasal catheter** allows a **maximum $FiO_2$ of 0.7 with a flow of 1–2 l/min** to be achieved. Its main advantage is the $FiO_2$ that can be reached, while inconveniences include the poor tolerance that some patients present, the damage caused to the nasal mucosa due to the high and continuous flow of oxygen and the potential risk of passage of gas to the stomach, which can lead to gastric dilation.

**Oxygen cages** provide a sealed environment in which both $FiO_2$ and temperature and humidity can be programmed: most of those available today allow up to a maximum **$FiO_2$ of 0.4–0.5, a temperature of 22 °C** and a relative humidity of 40–50% to be reached. Their main advantage is that it is a non-invasive system that provides oxygen to the animal without causing stress, and the main disadvantage is inability to manipulate the patient while it remains inside the cage, which makes it impossible to continue with stabilisation and examination.

## Fluid therapy

Administration of fluid therapy in the initial stabilisation may also be essential for certain patients, and its sole objective is to **return systemic arterial pressures to physiological values** as quickly as possible. For this, both **isotonic crystalloids and colloids** can be used, assessing the possible advantages/disadvantages with respect to the underlying pathology. This is not always possible at the time of initial evaluation and stabilisation, so it is advisable to base the choice of fluid on the analysis of factors such as signs of cardiac abnormalities that may indicate danger of volume overload and potential electrolyte abnormalities, pH and volume associated with the possible differential diagnoses. Regarding the **speed of administration**, the underlying pathology and the risk of volume overload should be taken into account. However, the parameters that constitute the therapeutic references for administration are the same in all patients and include the normalisation (at physiological levels) of:

- heart rate
- pulse quality
- mucous membrane colour
- capillary refill time
- systemic arterial pressure
- temperature
- consciousness.

## Secondary examination

If the primary examination indicates the presence of **respiratory function abnormalities**, a more thorough investigation of **blood oxygenation** levels as well as **arterial carbon dioxide levels ($PaCO_2$)** should be initiated. For this, more invasive and expensive diagnostic tests are used, such as arterial blood gas, which allows measurement of the partial pressure of arterial blood oxygen ($PaO_2$) and carbon dioxide ($PaCO_2$):

- **$PaO_2$ <80 mmHg** indicates the presence of **hypoxaemia** and, therefore, the need for additional therapeutic measures in addition to 100% $O_2$ supplementation (for example, thoracentesis if pleural effusion is suspected).
- **$PaCO_2$ >70 mmHg** is indicative of **hypoventilation**, so the **immediate intubation** of the patient and provision of assisted ventilation is recommended.

In the intensive care of veterinary patients, once the initial examination and stabilisation have been completed, **checklists are widely used**, possibly due to the latest trends in human medicine. One of the most frequently used lists is that proposed by Kirby in 1995. This list includes parameters that are obtained systematically and integrated into the physical examination, clinical observations, laboratory findings and the performance of auxiliary diagnostic tests:

- hydration state
- colloidal osmotic pressure
- glucose
- electrolytic and acid–base status
- oxygenation and ventilation
- consciousness
- perfusion and systemic pressures
- heart rate, rhythm and contractility
- albumin levels
- coagulation
- red blood cells and haemoglobin concentration
- renal function and diuresis
- immune system, selection and dosage of antibiotic treatment
- gastrointestinal motility and mucosal integrity
- metabolism and antibiotic dosage
- nutrition
- analgesia
- nursing care and moving the recumbent patient
- wound care and bandage changes.

## Clinical management of the critical patient

### *Shock*

The clinical management of critically ill patients (especially those with symptoms of septic shock) is based on the strategy called **'Early objective-guided therapy'**, which consists of a series of procedures for monitoring and intervention focused on haemodynamic optimisation of high-risk patients. This clinical focus was introduced in 2001 by the Rivers study published in the *New England Journal of Medicine*.

The concept of clinical monitoring was used for the first time as a guide to therapeutic management. The ultimate goal of this strategy is to **ensure that oxygen delivery matches demand**, in such a way that establishing an oxygen supply dependency that is pathological is avoided – that is, to ensure adequate tissue oxygenation and, therefore, survival. Its main virtue is probably that clinical actions are based on the observations obtained after monitoring both macrovascular and microvascular parameters. **Macrovascular parameters** are all those that provide information about the **circulation responsible for driving blood flow to the small vascular beds** responsible for distributing oxygen adequately to tissues (microvascular circulation). Therefore, macrovascular parameters are indicative of cardiovascular status and include:

- arterial blood pressure (AP)
- central venous pressure (CVP)
- diuresis.

**Microvascular parameters** include those **related to tissue oxygenation**, such as:

- lactate
- central venous saturation ($ScvO_2$)
- BE.

### *Macrovascular parameters*

#### Arterial pressure

This is the **pressure exerted on the vessel walls** resulting from the outflow of blood from the left ventricle. The **elastic distention capacity** of the arterial walls is responsible for maintaining the flow, even during diastole. The **mean arterial pressure (MAP) should always be >65 mmHg**, since that is the pressure below which organs such as the kidney and brain lose the ability to self-regulate their blood flow.

#### Central venous pressure

This is frequently used as an indicator of the patient's volume status. It is a measure of the hydrostatic pressure of the intrathoracic cranial vena cava and should be equivalent to the pressure of the right atrium, and therefore the pressure of the right ventricle at the end of the diastole, which is indicative of the heart preload, that is, **if CVP is adequate, cardiac output and oxygen delivery are also adequate**. Reference values in the dog are 2.2 ± 3.0 mmHg, although in **critically ill patients values of 8–12 mmHg are more likely**.

#### Diuresis

Measurement of diuresis is important when looking for signs of severe systemic pathologies. In fact, **acute renal failure** is one of the first complications in critical patients. In these situations, symptoms of azotaemia – of the loss of ability to concentrate and decrease urine production – are common.

- Diuresis should always be maintained between 1–2 ml/kg/h as:
  - <0.5–1.0 ml/kg/h is compatible with oliguria.
  - <0.5 ml/kg/h is compatible with anuria.

### *Microvascular parameters*

#### Lactate

**Lactate** is a by-product of pyruvate metabolism that is **generated in situations of insufficient oxygen delivery** with respect to tissue oxygen demand – that is, its plasma concentration increases in cases of **tissue anaerobiosis**. It is important to remember that the **prognostic value** of lactate is not based on initial levels but on the ability to decrease levels once adequate resuscitation therapy has been implemented. **Normal reference values range from 1.25–2.5 mmol/l in both dogs and cats**.

#### $ScvO_2$

Indicative of the **oxygenation of venous blood in the vena cava** and is a reflection of the level of oxygen use by tissue: it reflects the balance between the amount of oxygen delivered and extracted from tissues. Therefore, in situations where there is oxygen deficiency, this balance is reduced since oxygen delivery decreases while the extraction is maintained. $ScvO_2$ is monitored by venous blood-gas analysis from blood obtained from the vena cava. **In healthy patients, it is around 65–75%**.

#### BE

This is defined as the **amount of base needed to buffer the pH up to 7.4**, and it is used as an indicator of metabolic acidosis.

## *Stabilisation of macroscopic and microscopic parameters*

When stabilising these types of patient through the objective-guided early-therapy strategy, following a series of precise steps that allow the **stabilisation of abnormal macroscopic and microscopic parameters** is recommended:

#### (1) Achieve a CVP of 8–12 mmHg

The objective of this step is to guarantee optimisation of intravascular volume. For this purpose, the administration of isotonic and hypertonic crystalloids, synthetic colloids or blood products can be used, depending on the characteristics of the clinical symptoms of each patient. However, it is important to take into account some general considerations.

Regarding crystalloids, it should be noted that administration of 0.9% saline solution can be associated with the development of hyperchloraemic metabolic acidosis, so that the administration of **balanced isotonic crystalloids** (such as lactated Ringer's, Plasmalyte or Isofundin®) should be the **first choice for treatment**.

With respect to **synthetic colloids**, recent studies in human medicine should be taken into account that relate the administration of Hetastarch in septic patients to a higher mortality rate due to the occurrence of acute renal failure. There are no veterinary studies that prove the same relationship, although the coagulation abnormalities that occur when Hetastarch doses are high must be taken into account. Therefore, conservative administration is recommended to **avoid doses higher than**:

- 20 ml/kg/d in dogs.
- 10 ml/kg/d in cats.

In cases of **severe albuminaemia** (<2 g/dl), the **administration of human albumin (HSA, human serum albumin), can be considered**, but the **risk of developing hypersensitivity** reactions during administration should be considered. On the other hand, it should also be noted that **HSA is a hypertonic solution**, so its use should be limited in patients with clinical symptoms characterised by lower tolerance to large volumes of fluids.

In general, the choice of the fluid used to replenish the patient's vascular volume is a topic with many differences of opinion. In fact, even the most recent human studies do not recommend a particular fluid, since the important focus should be on the optimisation of the intravascular volume that can be achieved.

### (2) Achieve a MAP of 65–90 mmHg

In many cases, fluid therapy may be sufficient to correct hypotension. However, if after the resuscitation volume the blood pressure remains below the aforementioned limits, the administration of **vasopressor agents and positive inotropes** is recommended. The decision to administer one or another category of drugs depends solely on the underlying pathophysiology:

- In patients with **loss of myocardial contractility**, **positive inotropic drugs** (dopamine or dobutamine) are indicated.
- If hypotension is caused by **loss of vascular tone, vasopressor administration** is recommended, the most common being:
  - phenylephrine
  - norepinephrine
  - vasopressin.

These are very **potent vasopressor medications**, so they should always be administered at the **lowest possible dose** to avoid producing severe vasoconstriction and consequent tissue ischaemia. In any case, there are still many different opinions regarding which vasopressor to select. In veterinary medicine there is not enough evidence to be able to issue definitive conclusions but, in human medicine, norepinephrine is used as the first treatment option. If the administration of additional agents is necessary, the use of epinephrine or vasopressin is recommended. Dopamine is not recommended except in very specific circumstances.

### (3) Achieve $ScvO_2$ >70%

Once the CVP and MAP have been stabilised, performing a **central venous blood gas** on blood obtained from a jugular catheter is recommended. If the $ScvO_2$ is not within the physiological range, **measurement of haematocrit** is recommended, as well as correction of its levels. For this, transfusion of whole blood or red blood cell concentrate can be used until the haematocrit rises to >30%.

### (4) Achieve lactate values <2.5 mmol/l

For this, improved tissue perfusion should be encouraged by volume and cardiac output optimisation – that is, by means of fluid therapy and the administration of vasopressors and/or positive inotropes. **Serial measurement of lactate levels** during resuscitation is essential to guide the effectiveness of the treatment used, as well as to enable consideration of the prognostic value of its evolution over time. In fact, the absence of the normalisation of levels within 24–48 hours after resuscitation is associated with high mortality.

### (5) Achieve diuresis >0.5 ml/kg/h

**Correcting diuresis** can be complicated, since there are many different opinions regarding different aspects of fluid therapy aimed at correcting it (how aggressive treatment should be, choice of fluid type, treatment objectives, etc.); the main **risk is volume overload**. If after the introduction of fluid therapy, overhydration or a lack of improvement in diuresis is observed, the administration of **furosemide, low-dose dopamine** (***2.5–5 mcg/kg/min***) or mannitol should be considered. There is also debate about the efficacy of these treatments, since they increase urine output but not renal recovery.

### *Haemorrhage due to poly-trauma*

**Massive haemorrhage is the loss of more than 40% of blood volume**, and is a leading cause of death in polytrauma patients. The resuscitation and stabilisation of these patients should be focused on achieving a double objective:

- Stop the bleeding.
- Restore effective circulating volume and tissue perfusion.

The following are secondary objectives:

- Avoid the recurrence of bleeding.
- Correct systemic abnormalities caused by trauma, hypoperfusion and resuscitation procedures (metabolic acidosis, hypothermia and acute traumatic coagulopathy).

In recent decades, the approach to the clinical management of this type of patient has changed dramatically. **Formerly, resuscitation was based on volume normalisation by administering large volumes**

**of crystalloids**, causing systemic blood pressure to increase. However, this resulted in coagulation factors being diluted and potential displacement of newly formed, unstable clots, and a decrease in blood viscosity (with consequent increase in bleeding).

However, today a much more complex strategy is followed called **'damage control resuscitation'** (**DCR**). This strategy is based on the simultaneous establishment of:

- hypotensive resuscitation
- haemostatic resuscitation
- damage-control surgery.

The goal is to systematically and quickly reverse:

- acidosis
- hypothermia
- coagulopathy.

### *Hypotensive resuscitation*

In recent decades it has been shown that the previous resuscitation strategy based on the administration of **high volumes of crystalloids is not without complications**. In fact, a link has been shown to abnormalities such as **exacerbation of the inflammatory response** to haemorrhagic shock, induction of **vasoconstrictive dysfunction**, increased red blood cell deformation, **impaired immune system regulation**, increased intestinal permeability and induction of neutrophil sequestration in the lungs. All this gives rise to a phenomenon called **'resuscitation injury'** and is responsible for the increase in mortality in these patients.

Since 1994, from the Bickell study, clinical recommendations tend towards a much more **conservative resuscitation strategy** regarding the volume of fluids administered in poly-trauma patients with active bleeding. This strategy is called '**hypotensive resuscitation**' and is based on obtaining and maintaining **adequate systemic arterial pressures** (capable of guaranteeing perfusion of vital organs and tissue oxygenation) but that are not too high (to **avoid disruption of potential thrombi** in formation or dilution of coagulation factors). That is, the maintenance of relatively hypotensive arterial pressures (SAP of 80–90 mmHg or MAP of 50–60 mmHg) is sought and tolerated until bleeding ceases.

### *Haemostatic resuscitation*

Once the **haemorrhage has been stopped** and the haemodynamic parameters restored, one of the priorities of the DCR should be the **restoration of oxygen delivery** to tissues and cells. For this, the **administration of whole fresh blood** or a combination of different blood products in appropriate proportions is recommended. Preferably, the administration of whole blood is recommended over preserved blood products since the ability of stored red blood cells to transport and deliver oxygen is greatly impaired. It has also been shown that stored products can produce pro-inflammatory and immunosuppressive effects. When administration of whole fresh blood is not possible, then the administration of blood products in specific proportions is recommended:

- haemoconcentrate / fresh frozen plasma / platelets (1 / 1 / 1)
- fresh frozen plasma / haemoconcentrate (1 / 2 or 1 / 3)
- platelets / haemoconcentrate (1 / 5).

In general, the objective of haemostatic resuscitation is to obtain the following levels:

- haemoglobin: 7–9 mg / dl
- platelets: 50–100 x $10^9$ / l.

### *Damage-control surgery*

Damage-control surgery is referred to as **brief surgical interventions**, whose sole objective is to obtain **rapid initial control of bleeding and contamination**, minimising the duration of the procedure and not causing any additional tissue injury until the patient is more stable. Among the main characteristics that define it are:

- The duration must be less than 1 hour.

It is performed in three successive phases:

1. **First phase**, in which a **brief first surgical procedure** (**<1 hour**) is performed, the aim of which is to stop bleeding and contamination.
2. **Second phase**, in which the **patient is stabilised by correcting abnormalities** regarding acidosis, hypothermia and coagulation.
3. **Third phase**, in which the **injuries are definitively and surgically corrected** in a procedure of conventional duration.

The main complications of damage containment surgery include:

- abdominal compartment syndrome
- sepsis
- multiple organ failure.

### Optimal surgical correction time

Determining the optimal time for surgical correction in poly-trauma patients is currently a source of discussion, and there is a significant lack of scientific literature to support the clinical approach to it. In human medicine there are clinical recommendations that provide clear guidelines. However, in veterinary medicine recommendations are available regarding only the management of surgery time in the case of diaphragmatic hernias. In this type of pathology, **delaying surgery for 24–48 hours** is suggested to allow adequate stabilisation of patients.

## Analgesia

The **treatment of pain**, both acute and chronic, should **always be a priority** in the management of critical and emergency patients, for obvious ethical reasons and to minimise the pathophysiological consequences, since it is widely understood **that pain considerably increases morbidity and mortality**. The administration of analgesia should never be delayed or avoided, regardless of the nature and severity of the pathology. A huge variety of pharmacological and non-pharmacological options are available capable of providing effective and safe pain management even in the most critical and unstable animals.

Unfortunately, in some cases the administration of analgesics is avoided due to the erroneous belief that pain suppression will hide or alter some of the physiological indicators warning that the patient is deteriorating (for example, respiratory rate, heart rate and blood pressure). Both in human medicine and veterinary medicine it has been shown that this is not only not the case but, to the contrary, **once adequate analgesia is achieved, any physiological change detected is certain to be solely due to the patient deteriorating**, and not the presence of pain. Likewise, sometimes the administration of analgesia tends to be avoided due to fear of the potential systemic effects of certain drugs in critically and haemodynamically unstable patients. The reality is that **the pathophysiological consequences of untreated pain are equally dangerous** for these types of patient.

### *Systemic response to pain*

The **systemic consequences of acute pain** are different from those of chronic pain.

#### *Acute pain*

Acute pain triggers a **neuroendocrine stress response** proportional to the intensity of pain. This causes **sympathetic activation** which leads to an increase in both the visceral sympathetic tone and catecholamine release by the adrenal medulla.

Most relevant systemic effects of acute pain.

- With regard to the cardiovascular system:
  - tachycardia
  - hypertension
  - myocardial irritability (arrhythmias).

- With regard to the respiratory system:
  - decreased tidal volume
  - decreased functional residual capacity
  - effects on coughing
  - changes in the elimination of secretions from the airways.

- With regard to the gastrointestinal tract:
  - appearance of **ileus**
  - increased gastric acid secretion that can cause **stress ulcers**
  - vomiting
  - constipation.

- Others:
  - urine retention
  - different degrees of **immunosuppression**.

#### *Chronic pain*

Patients suffering from chronic pain have a virtually non-existent or very attenuated neuroendocrine response. If it occurs, it is usually in very specific cases:

- patients with pain of a central origin associated with paraplegia
- patients with continuous peripheral nociceptive stimulation.

### *Importance of pain*

The physiological implications of pain are so important that today this is **considered the fifth vital constant in human patients**, and the American hospital accreditation guarantees not only the establishment of adequate pain treatment but also measures for its evaluation. In veterinary medicine, in 2003 the **American Animal Hospital Association included pain as a fourth vital constant** (**along with temperature, pulse and breathing**) and has demanded the introduction of effective pain assessment and evaluation measures in all those accredited by their credentials.

### *Pain assessment*

The recognition and evaluation of pain in animals remains difficult and problematic. In people, the standard for evaluation is based on self-identification and subsequent communication, but logically this is not possible for animals.

Evaluating pain in animals is problematic in that it requires an **external observer to identify and assess its degree**. This depends on the observer recognising and correctly interpreting signs of pain, which involve both behavioural and physiological responses.

In this regard, it should be stressed that administration of analgesia should never be withdrawn or avoided because the observer was not able to detect and evaluate the patient's pain. In cases of uncertainty, the guideline is **always to administer analgesia** and evaluate subsequent changes.

The most widely recognised and useful pain assessment scale for critical and emergency patients is the **Glasgow composite measure pain scale (GCMP)**, based on behaviour and developed to detect acute (post-surgical) pain in dogs. This is a questionnaire that should be completed by the observer while following a certain protocol. The latter includes the **evaluation of both evoked and spontaneous behaviour, interactions with the animal** and **a series of clinical observations**.

To simplify and reduce the time of completion for the evaluation, the short form of the Glasgow composite pain scale (CMPS-SF) was developed, which requires only a few minutes to complete. The CMPS-SF has been designed as a clinical decision instrument, intended only for canine patients with acute post-surgical pain (Box. 1.1). It includes 30 descriptors, distributed in six behavioural categories, ordered numerically based on the severity of pain associated with each of them. The observer is in charge of assigning the descriptor that best suits the status of the patient within each category. The numerical value obtained from the sum of the descriptors is the final result of the evaluation. The **maximum result for the six categories is 24 points** and, if **mobility cannot be evaluated, 20 points**. This final result has proved to be an extremely useful indicator of the patient's analgesic requirements. **Analgesic intervention is recommended as long as the result is greater than or equal to 6/24 or 5/20**. Since pain is a dynamic process and is not static, frequent evaluations are necessary. Finally, it should be emphasised that, whenever this scale is used, it is essential to perform the **evaluation systematically**, following the patient evaluation protocol meticulously as described by the questionnaire.

In the case of feline patients, a similar pain scale has been available since the end of 2014 developed by the same team from the veterinary faculty at the University of Glasgow. This is the revised GCMP for acute pain in cats (**rGCMPS-Feline**), which allows an assessment of pain of acute origin associated with various clinical situations in the feline patient (Box. 1.2). It consists of a questionnaire similar to the canine one, whose objective is the identification of pain and its quantification, so that it serves as a therapeutic decision-making instrument by creating a cut-off point at which clinical intervention is indicated. **In cats**, analgesic intervention is recommended whenever the result of the questionnaire reaches a **score greater than or equal to 4/16 points**.

## Short format of the Glasgow composite measure pain scale in dogs

Dog's name:

Case number: Date: Time:

Surgery Yes/No (*cross out as appropriate*)

Procedure or condition:

In the lists that appear in the following sections, circle the corresponding score and add all the scores to get the total score.

A. Watch the dog in its cage:

(I) How is the dog?

| | |
|---|---|
| Calm | 0 |
| Crying or groaning | 1 |
| Complaining | 2 |
| Howling | 3 |

(II)

| | |
|---|---|
| Ignores wounds or painful areas | 0 |
| Looking at the wound or the painful area | 1 |
| Licking the wound or painful area | 2 |

| | |
|---|---|
| Rubbing the wound or painful area | 3 |
| Biting the wound or painful area | 4 |

If there are fractures in the spine, pelvis or in more than one limb or if the dog needs help to move, skip section B and go to C.

*Mark the box if it is one of these cases and go to section C.*

B. Put a lead on the dog and guide it out of the cage.

(III) When the dog gets up/walks, how does it do it?

| | |
|---|---|
| Normally | 0 |
| Limping | 1 |
| Slowly or resists | 2 |
| Stiff and rigid | 3 |
| Does not want to move | 4 |

C. If there is a wound or have pain in any area, including the abdomen, gently press around the area leaving a distance of 5 cm.

(IV) What does the dog do?

| | |
|---|---|
| Nothing | 0 |
| Looks around | 1 |
| Moves away from the pain | 2 |
| Growls or protects the area | 3 |
| Tries to bite | 4 |
| Cries | 5 |

D. General state

(V) How is the dog?

| | |
|---|---|
| Cheerful and happy or cheerful and eager to play | 0 |
| Calm | 1 |
| Indifferent or not reacting to surroundings | 2 |
| Nervous, anxious or fearful | 3 |
| Dejected or does not react to stimuli | 4 |

(VI) How is the dog?

| | |
|---|---|
| Relaxed | 0 |
| Restless | 1 |
| Agitated | 2 |
| Hunched or tense | 3 |
| Rigid | 4 |

Total score (I + II + III + IV + V + VI):

## Guide for use of the short format of the Glasgow composite measure pain scale in dogs

The clinical veterinarian can use this composite, abbreviated score (CMPS-SF) to quickly and reliably measure pain and it has been designed as a decision-making tool in the case of dogs suffering from acute pain. 30 descriptive options are included within 6 behaviour categories, including mobility. Within each category the descriptors are classified numerically according to the severity of the associated pain and the person making the evaluation chooses the descriptor within each category that best fits the dog's behaviour/condition. It is important to perform the evaluation procedure exactly as described in the questionnaire carefully following the protocol. The pain score is the sum of the scores from each row. The maximum score for the 6 categories is 24, or 20 if mobility cannot be assessed. It has been shown that the total CMPS-SF score has been a useful indicator of the analgesic requirement and the recommended level for analgesic intervention is 6/24 or 5/20.

## Glasgow composite measure

### Pain scale in cats: cmps, felines

### *(Glasgow feline composite measure pain scale: cmps – feline)*

Select the most appropriate expression in each section and add the scores to calculate the total pain score which applies to the cat. If more than one expression is applicable, select the one with the highest score.

**Observe the cat in its cage:**

**How is the cat?**

***Question 1***

Silent/purring/meowing 0
Crying/growling/groaning 1

***Question 2***

Relaxed 0
Licking its lips 1
Restless/hiding at the back of the cage 2
Tense/crouched 3
Rigid/hunched 4

***Question 3***

Ignore wounds or painful areas 0
Pay attention to a wound 1

***Question 4***

a) Look at the following drawings. Circle the drawing that best represents the position of the cat's ears.

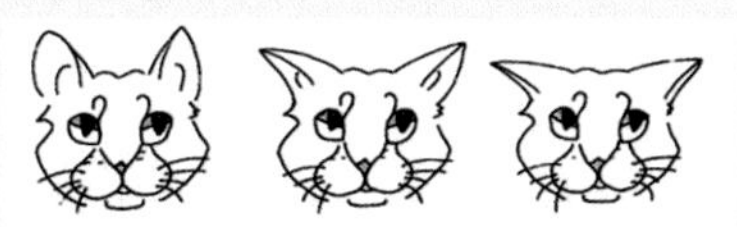

0 1 2

b) Look at the shape of the nose in the following drawings. Circle the drawing that most closely resembles the cat's nose.

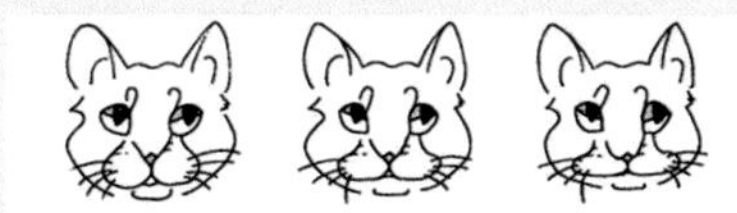

0 1 2

Approach the cage, call the cat by name and pet its back, from head to tail.

***Question 5***

How does it react?
Responds to attention 0
Does not react 1
Responds aggressively 2

If there are wounds or painful areas, gently press around the area leaving a distance of 5 cm. If there are no painful areas, apply similar pressure around the hind leg above the knee.

***Question 6***

How does it react?
Does nothing 0
Moves its tail/lowers its ears 1
Cries/snorts 2
Hisses 3
Bites/attacks 4

***Question 7***

Overall impression

How is the cat?

| | |
|---|---|
| Happy and content | 0 |
| Indifferent/quiet | 1 |
| Anxious/fearful | 2 |
| Listless | 3 |
| Depressed/irritable | 4 |
| Pain score: | 20 |

## Guidelines for use of the Glasgow composite

### Measure pain scale in cats

### *Guidance for use of the Glasgow feline composite measure pain scale (cmps – feline)*

The Glasgow Composite Scale for measuring feline pain (CMPS, felines), which can be applied quickly and reliably in a clinical setting, has been designed as a clinical decision-making tool for use in cats suffering from acute pain. It includes 28 descriptor options divided into 7 behavioural categories. Within each category, the descriptors are classified numerically according to the intensity of the pain and the person carrying out the assessment chooses the descriptor from each category that best corresponds to the cat's behaviour or condition. It is important that the assessment procedure be performed as described in the questionnaire, carefully following the protocol. The pain score is the sum of the classification scores. The maximum score for the 7 categories is 20. In felines the total CMPS score has been shown to be a useful indicator of the need for analgesia and the recommended level for analgesic intervention is 5/20.



### *Pharmacological interventions*

The term '**analgesia**' is usually defined as **the absence of pain perception**, although the clinical reality is different and, in the best-case scenario, only a decrease in the perception of pain is achieved (with the exception of the administration of local anaesthetic in locoregional blocks). **Pain may be of a different nature** depending on the pathophysiology associated with its development.

#### *Analgesic strategies*

In critical and emergency patients, pain is usually nociceptive in nature, **transmitted through the nociceptive pathway** and comprising four successive phases (transduction, transmission, modulation and perception; Figure 1.10). Therefore, with this type of pain **analgesia can be achieved by interrupting the said pathway** at one or more of the transmission points between the peripheral nociceptor and the cerebral cortex. In fact, the four phases can be pharmacologically altered, giving rise to what we normally call **multimodal analgesia** which, at the clinical level, consists of a **combination of various analgesic drugs** and/or different administration techniques to achieve this, by different mechanisms of action, and the nociceptive pathway is blocked simultaneously at multiple points. This strategy therefore depends on the **additive or synergistic action of the different analgesics** administered. Hence, it allows a reduction in the individual doses of each drug, thus limiting the severity of the side effects of each of them. Therefore, it can be concluded

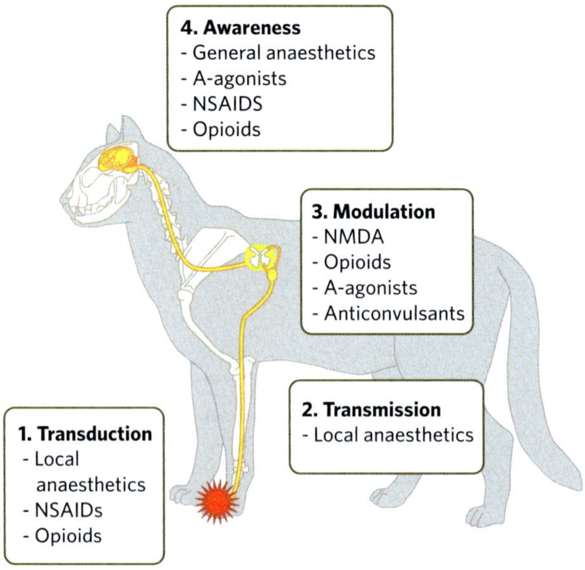


**Figure 1.10.** Nociceptive pathways.

that a multimodal strategy allows not only more effective but also **safer analgesic management**.

On the other hand, the concept of preventive analgesia is of great clinical relevance: today the selection of the analgesic is understood to be as important as the **time of administration**. Preventive analgesia is understood as being the application of multimodal analgesia techniques **prior (if possible) to the patient's exposure to the painful stimulus**. This avoids exposing the spinal cord to the continuous arrival of nociceptive afferent stimuli for too long, thus **minimising the development of central hypersensitivity**.

In summary, the recommended strategy for the analgesic management of critical and emergency patients is based on **multimodal and preventive analgesia techniques**.

### *Analgesic drugs*

From a pharmacological point of view, until relatively recently the drugs used in pain management were agents whose main pharmacological indication was analgesia only. These drugs are what we generally consider traditional analgesics and include three large groups:

- opioids
- NSAIDs
- local anaesthetics.

However, in recent decades the usefulness of other drugs whose main use is not necessarily analgesia has been discovered. These are adjuvant analgesics, and range from anticonvulsants to antidepressants.

In order to provide effective and safe analgesia in the most critical and unstable patients, a solid knowledge of the main characteristics of opioids, NSAIDs, local anaesthetics, n-methyl D-aspartate (NMDA) antagonists, α-2 agonists, bisphosphonates, tricyclic antidepressants and anticonvulsants is essential. Likewise, the analgesic protocol must always be designed individually to cover the specific needs of each patient, so detailed knowledge of the pathophysiology of pain associated with their condition is also essential.

Regarding non-pharmacological techniques on which to base pain management in critical and unstable patients, a series of simple modifications can be made to the daily nursing care plan (dry beds, empty bladder, eye lubrication, oral care, care of IV catheters, treatment of anxiety) and the environment (adaptation of lights to the circadian rhythm, owner visits etc.) that allow both the physical and emotional components of the complex phenomenon that is pain to be addressed.

#### Opioids

Opioids constitute the cornerstone of pain treatment in both human and veterinary patients. The most frequently used are:

- morphine
- methadone
- fentanyl
- buprenorphine
- pethidine
- butorphanol.

These constitute a group of versatile drugs, with a wide range of possibilities regarding their administration and clinical application. In fact, they are the **therapeutic option of choice** in many different clinical situations: from severe and acute trauma or surgical procedures to pathologies that lead to chronic pain and require long-term treatment. Lastly, it should be clear that these are narcotic drugs and that, therefore, they are **strictly regulated** in terms of prescription, storage and dispensing.

Their side effects are dose and drug dependent. In general, these include:

- **Bradycardia** (more or less severe, depending on agent and dose).
- **Respiratory depression** (more or less severe, depending on the agent and dose).
- **Histamine release** (pethidine and morphine, especially when administered IV).
- **Ileus** (morphine, especially).
- **Vomiting** (morphine, especially).
- **Abnormalities in thermoregulation**: in the dog, hypothermia and panting, in the cat, hyperthermia.
- **Dysphoria** (as a result of the diverse distribution and relationships of different opioid receptors in different brain regions). Factors that may predispose to the onset of excitation include the dose (high), the existence/absence of pain, the temperament of the animal, the route of administration as well as the agent itself.

All opioids mentioned here have two clinically vital advantages:

1. They are **potentially reversible** using a pure μ-receptor antagonist, such as naloxone, whose effects last for about 20–30 minutes, which allows the re-narcotisation phenomenon when used to reverse long-lasting opioids.
2. They are very **versatile regarding the format and route of administration**. In addition to conventional (IV), intramuscular (IM) or subcutaneous (SC)

bolus routes, constant-rate infusion (CRI), can be considered.

A clear example of versatility is **fentanyl**, which can be administered via different routes:

By **CRI**, the use of which has been studied for the control of pain in hospitalised patients, providing they are constantly monitored for detection and correction of the occurrence of respiratory depression.

**Transdermal**, through **patches**, although its effectiveness is unpredictable on many occasions (due to the existence of situations that alter absorption, such as the presence of hypovolaemia, hypothermia or obesity). This option is particularly interesting in patients who do not tolerate oral medication and need administration of opioids for a prolonged period of time. However, it should be remembered that with the use of transdermal patches, plasma fentanyl levels **do not reach therapeutic levels until 18–24 h after placement**, so provision of an alternative form of analgesia during this initial time is necessary.

Recently introduced to the market, the **depot form** makes use of a novel technology based on the deposition of the drug on the stratum corneum of the interscapular region, from which it is passively diffused into the systemic circulation over several days (minimum four). Its clinical use is not yet widespread, but initial results are very promising.

### Tramadol

It is a synthetic codeine analogue that exerts **agonist effects on μ-receptors**. However, since it is **not an opioid**, regulations regarding its prescription and storage are much more relaxed, making it a perfect option for pain management once the patient has been discharged and is at home. The main side effects include **sedation and sometimes dysphoria** (mainly in the cat), while respiratory depression and constipation are reduced compared to those observed with pure opioids. Although its **potency is only one tenth that of morphine**, its efficacy has been demonstrated both orally and parenterally. Its clinical use is very frequent, mainly due to the few side effects it causes.

### NSAIDs

The use of **NSAIDs** is frequent in situations where there is **mild or moderate pain** associated with inflammation, since these are drugs that have excellent **anti-inflammatory properties** and, therefore, are capable of providing analgesia. These anti-inflammatory mechanisms are capable of prolonging the plasma half-life of these drugs, since one of the properties of NSAIDs is that they are selectively stored in inflamed tissue. However, it should be remembered that they are **non-reversible agents** with a very low therapeutic index, so their use is strictly **contraindicated in certain cases**, especially in critical and emergency patients who may have haemodynamic abnormalities, in perfusion or coagulation, that include:

- Patients with hypovolaemia, hypotension, dehydration or shock.
- Patients with coagulopathies.
- Patients with ulcers or gastrointestinal lesions.
- Patients with liver or kidney failure.
- Patients that are pregnant or in breeding or lactation periods.
- Patients under 6 weeks of age.
- Patients that have already been treated with another NSAID or some type of corticosteroid.

### *Local anaesthetics*

Local anaesthetics administered **loco-regionally** are the only drugs **capable of completely blocking the transmission of pain** and, therefore, of producing complete analgesia in the desensitised area. They are extremely versatile and can be **administered via many different routes** such as via an epidural, through the application of transdermal patches, irrigation catheters, topically, interpleurally, by intracavitary inoculation and even IV. For example:

- **Proparacaine eye drops** for very quick desensitisation of the cornea (their effect is brief, lasting 15 min).
- Cream made of a eutectic mixture of 2.5% lidocaine and 2.5% prilocaine (**EMLA cream**) to minimise pain and discomfort when performing venepuncture procedures.
- **5% transdermal lidocaine patches** applied to the edge of wounds that present with allodynia phenomenon or focal areas of neuropathic pain. It has been shown that their analgesic effect is due to local action and not systemic absorption, and that these constitute a safe route of administration because there is minimal systemic absorption. Excellent results have been demonstrated.
- **Irrigation catheters**. These provide analgesia after very invasive surgeries where there are very large, extensive incisions. Local anaesthetics can be applied through them at different depths in the wound. If they are placed under sterile and aseptic conditions and fixed correctly, they usually do not present complications with regard to either their management or for the patient. The administration of local anaesthetics using these catheters achieves optimal levels of comfort for patients, and a considerable

decrease in the administration of systemic drugs during the most acute stages of pain. Administration of **local anaesthetics every 6–8 hours** depending on the drug is recommended (for example, *bupivacaine at 1–2 mg/kg*) with removal of the catheter after 48 hours of placement. Their use is of particular interest in clinically unstable patients, since they provide excellent-quality analgesia with virtually no systemic effects.

- The **interpleural pathway** can be used to provide thoracic analgesia after the placement of pleural drains, invasive thoracic surgeries or to manage the pain caused by different pleural pathologies. This strategy is particularly useful in patients with high analgesic requirements but who also need systemic stability. Local anaesthetics can be administered using pleural drainage tubes once the chest is drained at varying frequencies dependent on the chosen drug. The administration of *0.25% bupivacaine at 1 mg/kg/6h (after drainage)* is usually recommended. It should be noted that the analgesic action is not affected by the frequency of drainage that each patient requires clinically, that is, **analgesia lasts 6 hours** (in the case of bupivacaine) even if the chest is drained every hour.

## Lidocaine

**Lidocaine** is a local anaesthetic that can be administered both **locally and parenterally** to provide analgesia. When administered IV it has different effects, classically attributed to the blockade of both central and peripheral $Na^+$ channels:

- anti-arrhythmic effects
- analgesia (especially in pain of neuropathic origin)
- reduction of anaesthetic requirements (reduces the minimum alveolar concentration of inhaled anaesthetics).

One of the main limiting factors for the use of lidocaine is the risk of **systemic toxicity** (due to accidental overdose or greater individual sensitivity of a specific patient).

The use of **lidocaine in the cat is controversial**, and many authors advise against it due to the greater toxicity of local anaesthetics in this species. On the other hand, there is evidence in the scientific literature about its benefits in different clinical situations. Therefore, its use should not be completely ruled out although it should be limited in feline patients to those receiving treatment from appropriately qualified personnel (anaesthesiologist or emergency cardiac care specialist).

**In dogs, lidocaine has a very high safety margin** and is well tolerated.

Any **signs of systemic toxicity** should be identified immediately. **One of the first signs of toxicity is sedation**, if this occurs, the infusion rate must be reduced or stopped completely. Later on, the signs may become obvious as small **facial myoclonus, tremors and even seizures**. In addition to neurological effects, **cardiovascular toxicity** can occur, leading to bradyarrhythmias and even hypotension.

## *α-2 Adrenergic agents*

**Medetomidine and dexmedetomidine** are drugs used very frequently in practice for their sedative and muscle relaxant effects, but they also produce **excellent analgesia**. Therefore, these should be included in multimodal analgesia protocols in patients where their use is not contraindicated. For analgesic purposes, they are usually administered by CRI at low doses.

Their main side effects include:

- sedation
- peripheral vasoconstriction
- bradycardia
- polyuria
- increase in uterine tone
- hyperglycaemia.

Therefore, use with great caution in patients presenting with any of the following:

- Symptoms of **urinary obstruction**.
- **Pregnancy**.
- **Cardiovascular instability**: their main contraindication, since their haemodynamic effects can be clinically destabilising in very unstable critical patients. However, the doses necessary to produce analgesia are much lower than those needed to produce sedation, so adverse cardiovascular effects are noticeably more limited, which makes them a safe option in patients with stable cardiovascular function.

## *NMDA receptor blockers*

**Ketamine, magnesium and amantadine** have the ability to **block NMDA receptors**. These receptors are located post-synaptically in the central nervous system, both in the brain and spinal cord, and are **involved in the process of central hypersensitisation** (responsible for the chronification of pain and hyperalgesia). Therefore, all these agents are indicated for the prevention and treatment of conditions causing central hypersensitisation, which means they are of significant therapeutic interest for certain **critically ill or poly-trauma patients** at risk of suffering from this type of condition. On the other hand, they are an excellent option for the treatment of **somatic pain**, as is the case of burn injuries or bone fractures in poly-trauma patients.

The administration of a **ketamine bolus or a low-dose continuous infusion** is especially useful in the treatment of severe pain associated with possible central hypersensitivity, and for somatic pain in certain clinical situations such as poly-trauma or amputee patients experiencing phantom limb pain. Among its **main effects** are:

- **Relatively stable cardiovascular** function (although oxygen consumption increases).
- **Conservation of respiratory function** even when there is a certain degree of bronchodilation (despite an irregular respiratory pattern).
- **Increase in brain metabolism** (and, consequently, oxygen consumption, cerebral blood flow and intracranial pressure). However, recent studies attribute neuroprotective properties providing maintenance levels of exhaled $CO_2$ are guaranteed at values close to the lower physiological limit (30–35 mmHg).

This drug can be administered as part of a **multimodal analgesia protocol**, in **combination with opioids and/or lidocaine** (colloquially known as MLK infusion (morphine, lidocaine and ketamine)).

There are currently not a large number of studies documenting the use of amantadine in small animals, although some publications support its use within multimodal analgesia protocols for the treatment of **osteoarthrosis-associated pain and chronic pain in dogs**. Since its side effects are not very severe, it is another therapeutic alternative in critical patients.

### Anticonvulsants

In recent years, neuromodulatory drugs such as **gabapentin and pregabalin** have been introduced as therapeutic options, mainly because they are the treatment of choice for **neuropathic pain**. Their side effects are minimal and include **moderate sedation and mild ataxia of the hind end**. There are also studies that prove their safety even when administered to animals with renal insufficiency, so they are particularly useful in critically ill patients with neuropathic pain conditions.

**Gabapentin** is a drug widely used in human medicine for the treatment of neuropathic pain and pain associated with various surgical soft tissue procedures. Recommended administration guidelines include *doses of 10 mg/kg/8–12 h PO*, although in most cases it is common to have to adjust the dose to achieve the desired clinical effect without causing excessive sedation.

**Pregabalin** is considered the pharmacological successor to gabapentin, showing more favourable pharmacokinetics and **greater potency**. Its analgesic efficacy has been widely studied in human medicine, where it has proved effective in the treatment of neuropathic pain as well as in perioperative pain for various soft tissue surgical procedures. In animals, the only pharmacokinetic study available suggests an *administration regimen of 4 mg/kg/12 h PO in dogs*.

Table 1.7 lists the recommended dosages for the analgesic agents discussed above.

Table 1.7. Recommended doses for the main analgesics used in veterinary medicine.

| | Dose |
|---|---|
| Morphine | 0.1–0.5 mg/kg/4 h SC, IM, IV |
| Methadone | 0.1–0.3 mg/kg/4 h SC, IM, IV |
| Pethidine | – |
| Fentanyl | 0.3–0.7 mcg/kg/min |
| Remifentanil | Bolus: 3 mcg/kg IV<br>CRI: 0.1–0.3 mcg/kg/min |
| Buprenorphine | 10–20 mcg/kg/8 h SC, IM, IV |
| Butorphanol | 0.2–0.4 mg/kg/2 h SC, IM, IV |
| Tramadol | – |
| Intravenous lidocaine | Bolus: 0.5 mg/kg IV<br>CRI: 30–50 mcg/kg/min (dogs)<br>Attention to toxicity in cats |
| Lidocaine patch (5%) | – |
| Bupivacaine (0.25%) interpleural/catheter irrigation of wounds | 1 mg/kg/6 h<br>(through drainage or catheter wound irrigation) |
| Medetomidine | Bolus: 1 mcg/kg<br>CRI: 0.5–1.0 mcg/kg/h |
| Dexmedetomidine | Bolus: 0.25 mcg/kg<br>CRI: 0.25–0.5 mcg/kg/h |
| Ketamine | Bolus: 0.25 mg/kg IV<br>CRI: 10 mcg/kg/min IV |
| KLM | Morphine: 0.2 mg/kg/h<br>Lidocaine: 2 mg/kg/h<br>Ketamine: 2 mg/kg/h<br>For cats, do not include lidocaine |
| Amantadine | 3 mg/kg/24 h VO |
| Gabapentin | 10 mg/kg/8 h VO |
| Pregabalin | 4 mg/kg/12 h VO |

## Clinical recommendations for cardiopulmonary resuscitation (RECOVER 2012)

### Introduction

In recent decades, in human medicine there has been consistent, standardised development and training in cardiopulmonary resuscitation procedures (CPR). This has been possible thanks to the development of specific evidence-based recommendations derived from extensive literature reviews conducted by the International Liaison Committee on Resuscitation (ILCOR) for cardiopulmonary resuscitation.

In veterinary medicine, however, until recently there were no recommendations based on evidence that were comparable, only some recommendations extrapolated from humans published periodically by ILCOR. The absence of comprehensive and standardised training, together with the lack of consensus on the contents of these adapted recommendations, led to inconsistencies in the approach to veterinary CPR, probably to the detriment of patients.

That is why the main objective of the veterinary resuscitation evaluation campaign **RECOVER (reassessment campaign on veterinary resuscitation)** was to develop a set of **universal clinical recommendations** for the application of **CPR in dogs and cats** based on an extensive and systematic review of literature. The literature review was carried out throughout 2011 and, although there was an overlap of the literature examined by ILCOR and RECOVER, the scientific concepts were evaluated based on how applicable they are in canine and feline patients. This led to conclusions that were divergent in some areas. From the results of the evidence-evaluation process, a total of 101 clinical recommendations were developed and made available to members of the veterinary community for review over a period of four weeks. The result was used to modify and refine the recommendations, thus yielding the final set of agreed recommendations that were collected in a monograph in the *Journal of Veterinary Emergency and Critical Care* published in June 2012. In this final version, 101 recommendations were included that were divided into five domains:

1. preparedness and prevention
2. basic life support
3. advanced life support
4. monitoring
5. post cardiac arrest care.

This set of recommendations should be seen as a first step towards achieving a standard and **evidence-based approach to CPR in small animals**. As such, all veterinary health professionals should be aware of it and adopt its recommendations, exactly as the recommendations developed by ILCOR that are published every 5 years by the American Heart Association are adopted by the biomedical professionals responsible for emergency care. The ultimate goal of these recommendations is to provide a standard for the practice of veterinary CPR and thus **improve the survival prognosis** of dogs and cats suffering from cardiorespiratory arrest. In any case, as stated, the availability of recommendations is only the first step: the development of standardised training tools, evaluation of results, implementation of recommendations and scientific research aimed at solving the knowledge gaps identified are also necessary.

## *Preparedness and prevention*

The recommendations are based on the premise that resuscitation attempts which are organised, cohesive and led by a team that works well, that possesses knowledge and adheres to recommendations for evidence-based CPR should **improve CPR survival**. Therefore, these focus on the organisation and preparation of human resources and material equipment.

## *Equipment organisation and cognitive aids*

An **organised and efficient response** to the management of a medical or surgical crisis is always crucial. In this sense, the effects of **accessibility to the material needed for CPR** have been well studied in human medicine, and various studies have shown that inaccessibility to equipment and supplies is related to a delay in the start of CPR in up to 18% of cases. Therefore, the **location, content and replacement of resuscitation equipment** should always be standardised and regularly monitored. Likewise, the presence of cognitive aids such as **checklists, algorithms (Figure 1.11) and dosing tables (Table 1.8)** has been shown to improve compliance with CPR recommendations, providing that personnel have been trained to use these aids. The placement and high visibility of these tables and algorithms in the areas in which CPR is expected to occur, such as anaesthetic induction rooms or the emergency care area, is recommended.

## *CPR training*

Adherence to the recommendations for CPR can be guaranteed only if **staff receive standardised and effective training**, as well as regular opportunities to update their knowledge and skills. CPR requires the acquisition of both **cognitive** (correct performance of all the steps indicated in a fast and orderly manner) and **psychomotor** (performing chest compressions and ventilation) skills; therefore, effective CPR training must include both didactic components. Specifically, effective training options for psychomotor skills include the use of **high- and low-fidelity simulators** as well as visual and auditory feedback devices. Regardless of the technology

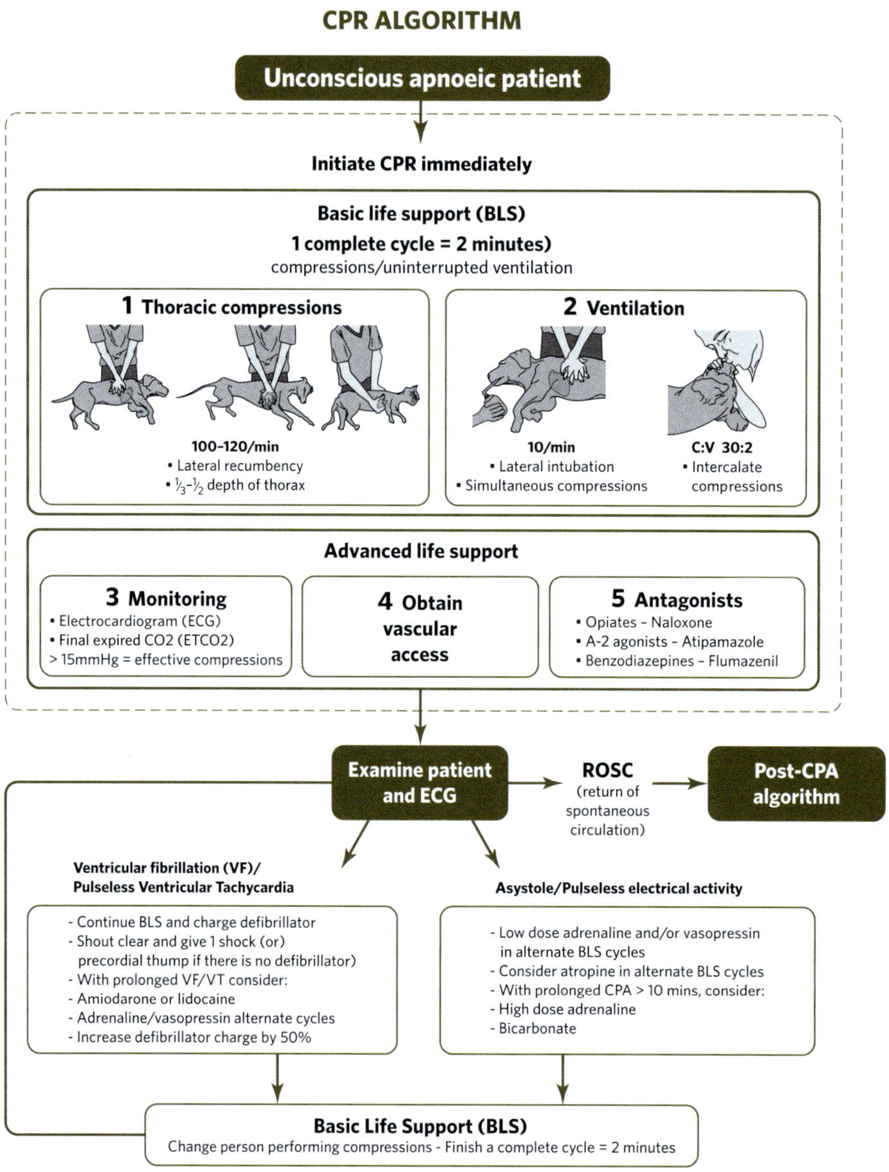


**Figure 1.11.** CPR algorithm.

used for training, regular six-monthly updating is recommended to refresh knowledge and minimise the loss of acquired skills. There is some evidence that validates the use of **simulation methodologies** as the most beneficial for reinforcing training. Logically, although high-fidelity simulators have a large number of advantages, the implementation of simple simulations every 3–6 months in low-fidelity dummies may be sufficient if it is the only option available.

On the other hand, **post-simulation debriefing** have been shown to play a crucial role in acquiring the knowledge posed. Therefore, the implementation of a structured evaluation at the end of training, and a session in which participants can review and criticise their own performance and that of the team as a whole, is recommended. During these discussions, participants should be encouraged to lead the debate and **identify the strengths and weaknesses** of the team for themselves. The presence and performance of a team member trained in facilitation techniques is very useful. Finally, it is particularly important to avoid accusations directed towards those who have shown lower or worse performance levels. The **discussion must be constructive, open and honest** and be focused at all times to seek opportunities for improvement and objective improvement of future CPR procedures.

## *Team dynamics*

With regard to the professional qualifications of the individual responsible for directing a CPR, extrapolation of data from human medicine confirms that both **veterinarians and veterinary nurses can be leaders** of the CPR team. Studies in human medicine did not identify any difference in the prognosis of patients resuscitated by teams led by emergency biomedical personnel with different

Table 1.8. Doses of emergency drugs (only the most commonly used are included) separated into categories based on their use, and showing their dose by volume previously calculated based on different body weights, to reduce calculation errors.

| | | Weight (kg) | 2.5 | 5 | 10 | 15 | 20 | 25 | 30 | 35 | 40 | 45 | 50 |
|---|---|---|---|---|---|---|---|---|---|---|---|---|---|
| | **Drug** | **Dose** | **ml** | **ml** | **ml** | **ml** | **ml** | **ml** | **ml** | **ml** | **ml** | **ml** | **ml** |
| | Adrenaline (1:1 000; 1 mg/ml) Low: alternate cycles | 0.01 mg/kg | 0.03 | 0.05 | 0.1 | 0.15 | 0.2 | 0.25 | 0.3 | 0.35 | 0.4 | 0.45 | 0.5 |
| Cardiopulmonary arrest | Adrenaline (1:1 000; 1 mg/ml) High: prolonged CPR | 0.1 mg/kg | 0.25 | 0.5 | 1 | 1.5 | 2 | 2.5 | 3 | 3.5 | 4 | 4.5 | 5 |
| | Atropine (1 mg/ml) | 0.04 mg/kg | 0.1 | 0.2 | 0.4 | 0.6 | 0.8 | 1 | 1.2 | 1.4 | 1.6 | 1.8 | 2 |
| Anti-arrhythmic | Vasopressin (20 U/ml) | 0.8 U/kg | 0.1 | 0.2 | 0.4 | 0.6 | 0.8 | 1 | 1.2 | 1.4 | 1.6 | 1.8 | 2 |
| | Amiodarone (50 mg/ml) | 5 mg/kg | 0.25 | 0.5 | 1 | 1.5 | 2 | 2.5 | 3 | 3.5 | 4 | 4.5 | 5 |
| | 2% Lidocaine (20 mg/ml) | 2 mg/kg | 0.25 | 0.5 | 1 | 1.5 | 2 | 2.5 | 3 | 3.5 | 4 | 4.5 | 5 |
| Reversal | Naloxone (0.4 mg/ml) | 0.04 mg/kg | 0.25 | 0.5 | 1 | 1.5 | 2 | 2.5 | 3 | 3.5 | 4 | 4.5 | 5 |
| | Flumazenil (0.1 mg/ml) | 0.01 mg/kg | 0.25 | 0.5 | 1 | 1.5 | 2 | 2.5 | 3 | 3.5 | 4 | 4.5 | 5 |
| | Atipamezole (5 mg/ml) | 0.1 mg/kg | 0.06 | 0.1 | 0.2 | 0.3 | 0.4 | 0.5 | 0.6 | 0.7 | 0.8 | 0.9 | 1 |
| Single-phase defibrillator | External defib. (J) | 4–6 J/kg | 10 | 20 | 40 | 60 | 80 | 100 | 120 | 140 | 160 | 180 | 200 |
| | Internal defib. (J) | 0.5–1.0 J/kg | 2 | 3 | 5 | 8 | 10 | 15 | 15 | 20 | 20 | 20 | 25 |

qualifications. There is ample evidence of the importance of training in **communication techniques and team dynamics**. Additionally, specific training in leadership techniques is recommended for those individuals potentially in a position to lead this emergency action. Among other responsibilities, the person in charge must **delegate tasks to team members** and enforce rules and procedures. The main leadership behaviours that can improve the performance of a CPR team include:

- **Sporadic refreshers** to ensure a mental model shared by the team.
- The **request for active input** from all team members to identify problems and obtain new ideas.
- The **delegation of specific tasks** to individual team members.

The implementation of a **closed-loop communication** model allows further improvement of joint actions. This provides **clear and targeted communication** to a specific individual to assign a task and minimises the possibility of confusion. This type of communication is obtained by issuing a **direct instruction addressed to a particular member of the team**, after which the **receiver repeats the order to the sender** to verify the accuracy of the message received. This simple technique has been shown to **significantly reduce medical errors**, especially in emergency situations, since it allows one to identify when an instruction has not been heard or was misunderstood.

## Monitoring of patients at risk of CPA

The **identification of at-risk patients** and early diagnosis of CPA are crucial to improving the survival prognosis of critical and emergency patients. Therefore, animals at risk of CPA should always be **monitored thoroughly and continuously**. Although there are no specific studies investigating the effects of pre-CPA monitoring on the prognosis, it is reasonable to recommend that **ECG and arterial pressure** should be monitored continuously through the use of Doppler or direct arterial pressure. Also, continuous **monitoring of $CO_2$ in exhaled air** ($EtCO_2$) is recommended in intubated patients at risk of CPA.

## Basic life support (BLS)

In veterinary CPR, BLS includes:

- recognition of CPA
- administration of thoracic compressions
- control of the airways
- ventilation.

It is essential for BLS to be implemented immediately after the diagnosis or suspicion of cardio-respiratory arrest (CRA). Most of these techniques can be performed by both professional and non-professional resuscitators. Numerous experimental studies in humans and animals have shown that the rapid implementation and quality of BLS have a direct relationship with the return of spontaneous circulation (ROSC) and survival of patients. Although in these recommendations BLS is studied independently of advanced life support (ALS) and monitoring, in clinical practice, BLS is carried out simultaneously with ALS and monitoring.

## Diagnosis of CPA

Early implementation of CPR in patients who have experienced a CPA is crucial for an improved prognosis, and therefore a **rapid initial assessment of airway, breathing and circulation** (**ABC**) is essential to rule out CPA in any unconscious and apnoeic patient. For this purpose, different monitoring techniques have been proposed.

**Pulse palpation** is frequently used by veterinarians as part of the initial examination of critical patients. Although there are no studies in veterinary medicine concerning this, many human studies have shown that it is an unreliable technique in regard to the diagnosis of CPA. Therefore, until studies in veterinary medicine are performed, the **use of pulse palpation as a diagnostic method for CPA is not recommended**. Immediately commencing CPR is advised in all animals in which there are problems identifying the pulse during the initial ABC.

Although Doppler blood pressure monitoring may be useful for early recognition of CPA, no study has investigated its usefulness as a diagnostic method for CPA. Given the time needed to place a sensor and achieve a signal, the **use of Doppler to validate a CPA diagnosis before starting CPR is not recommended in unconscious or apnoeic dogs and cats** (unless the sensor has been placed before CPA, as for example in the case of patients under general anaesthesia who already have Doppler sensors in place).

ECG monitoring is of great value during CPR as it allows the stop rhythm to be identified and ALS therapy to be guided. However, some rhythms may appear as perfusion rhythms despite the presence of CPA, and therefore their identification has the potential to delay initiation of BLS. Therefore, the **use of ECG as the sole diagnostic method for CPA in unconscious and apnoeic dogs and cats is not recommended**.

Finally, the diagnostic capacity of $EtCO_2$ has been analysed in recent decades, with the conclusion that the initial values of **$EtCO_2$ prove to be unreliable** for this purpose in different species. Therefore, the use of $EtCO_2$ values immediately post-intubation for the diagnosis of CPA in dogs and cats is not recommended.

### *Delay in commencing CPR*

**Rapid diagnosis of CPA is crucial**, since the negative effects of delayed initiation of BLS are significant and related to lower survival rates. In addition, **the risk of injury due to CPR in patients not in CPA is low**. Therefore, the immediate **initiation of CPR procedures is recommended in patients suspected of undergoing CPA**. In fact, when assessing unconscious apnoeic patients, a rapid evaluation of ABC that lasts no more than 5–10 seconds is recommended: if CPA is suspected then CPR should be started immediately.

### *Thoracic compressions*

Thoracic compressions should be **started as soon as possible** after diagnosis of CPA.

#### Patient position and placement of hands for thoracic compressions

In both the dogs and cat, it is advisable to perform **thoracic compressions in lateral recumbency** wherever possible. Experimental evidence shows that, in this position, greater ventricular pressure and aortic flow are generated, as well as a higher rate of ROSC. Both **left and right lateral recumbency are acceptable**. However, substantial **variations in the thoracic conformation of dogs and cats** suggest that a single, identical approach to performing thoracic compressions is not appropriate.

There are two theories that explain the mechanism by which external thoracic compression generates blood flow during CPR:

- **Cardiac pump theory**. Generation of blood flow is due to direct **compression of the ventricles**, either between the sternum and spine (in the case of patients in dorsal recumbency) or between the ribs (in the case of patients in lateral recumbency).
- **Thoracic pump theory**. Blood flow is generated as a result of the **increase in global intrathoracic pressure** that occurs in the patient's thorax during compressions. This means that during compression the aorta is compressed and the vena cava is collapsed, so that blood flow is directed outside of the thorax. Meanwhile, during elastic recovery of the thorax, subatmospheric intrathoracic pressure provides a pressure gradient that favours blood flow from the peripheries to the thorax.

Although the study of these theories is limited, it is believed that the predominant mechanism in each patient depends on the anatomical conformation of the thorax:

In most **medium-sized, large and giant dogs** with a rounded thorax, the thoracic pump mechanism is probably predominant. Therefore, performing compressions with the **hands on the widest region of the thorax**, thus allowing the maximum increase in intrathoracic pressure, is recommended (Figure 1.12).

In **dogs with a keel chest** (narrow or deep) such as Greyhounds, the cardiac pump theory is possibly the predominant one, so performing external chest compressions with the **hands located directly over the heart** is recommended (Figure 1.13).

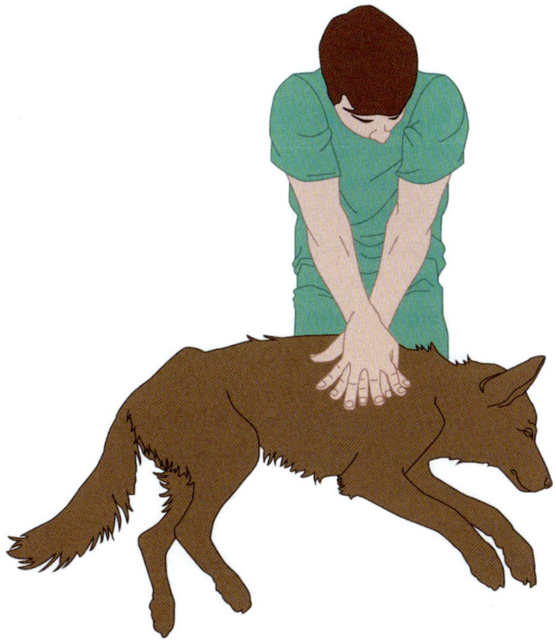

**Figure 1.12.** Cardiac massage in dogs with a rounded thorax.

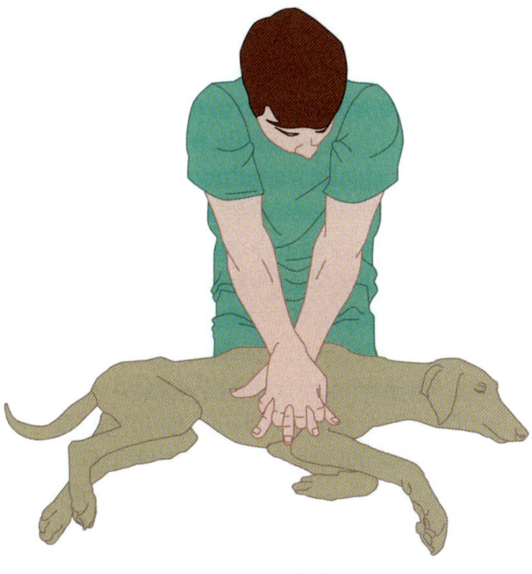

**Figure 1.13.** Cardiac massage in dogs with a keel chest.

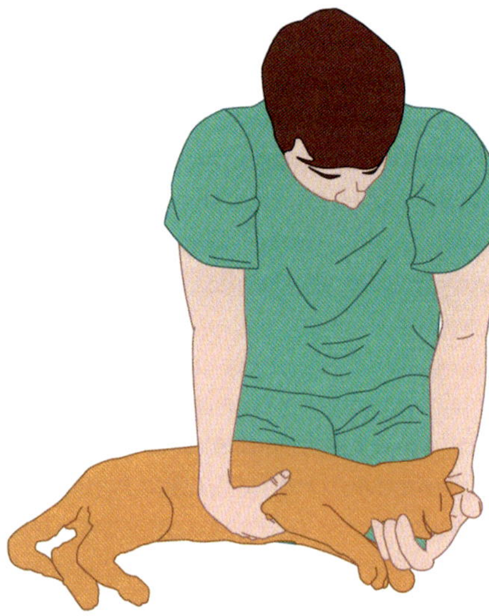

Figure 1.14. Cardiac massage in cats and small dogs.

In **dogs with a barrel-shaped chest**, such as the English Bulldog, thoracic compressions on the **sternum with the patient placed in dorsal recumbency** are recommended since the predominant mechanism is possibly explained by the cardiac pump theory.

**Cats and small dogs** tend to have greater elasticity in their chest wall, and hence the generation of blood flow can be explained by the heart pump theory. Therefore, thoracic compressions performed by placing the **fingers around the breastbone over the heart** (Figure 1.14) are recommended. This, therefore, is a circumferential compression rather than a lateral one.

#### Thoracic compression technique

A **compression frequency of 100–120/min** is recommended in dogs and cats: there is evidence that associates these speeds with higher rates of ROSC and survival. It is also advisable for the **depth of the compressions to reach 1/3–1/2 of the thoracic diameter**. Finally, the **complete recovery of the thoracic diameter** between compressions should be allowed, since various studies have shown a reduction in coronary and cerebral perfusion when complete elastic recovery is not allowed.

### *Ventilation*

Both hypoxia and hypercapnia reduce the chances of ROSC, so establishin**g a patent airway** and **implementing ventilation** are essential during CPR.

#### Ventilation technique for intubated patients

In dogs and cats with CPA, **rapid intubation in lateral recumbency** is recommended so that chest compressions do not have to be interrupted during the procedure. Once the endotracheal tube (ET) is properly positioned, it must be properly fixed to the maxilla or jaw so that it does not move. The endotracheal tube cuff should be inflated immediately afterwards, so that ventilation and chest compressions can be carried out simultaneously.

There are few data for small animals evaluating the optimal ventilation strategies for patients intubated during CPR, but some studies show that **high ventilation frequencies**, prolonged inspiration times and high tidal volumes cause an **increase in mean intrathoracic pressure**. This is associated with a decrease in venous return, as well as a reduction in cerebral and coronary perfusion, and ultimately with a **worse prognosis for survival**. Therefore, a **conservative ventilation strategy is recommended,** with a **respiratory rate of 10 inspirations/min, tidal volumes of 10 ml/kg and a short inspiratory time of 1 s**.

#### Checking endotracheal intubation

Verifying the **correct placement of the ET in the trachea** (and not in the oesophagus) is crucial. To assist in this **verification process, Et$CO_2$ monitoring** has been used, since $CO_2$ can be detected only if the ET is in the trachea. Therefore, the monitoring of Et$CO_2$ can be considered a complementary tool for the verification of correct endotracheal intubation provided it is used in association with direct visualisation, auscultation and observation of thoracic movements in CPA patients.

#### Ventilation technique for non-intubated patients

To achieve **mouth-to-snout breathing technique**, the resuscitator must hold the patient's mouth tightly closed, placing their mouth on the **patient's nostrils** so that a perfect seal is created with the muzzle, and then blowing into the nostrils. Although there are no studies investigating CPR in the non-intubated patient, limited evidence in other species suggests maintaining a compression:ventilation (C:V) ratio of at least 30:2. To achieve this goal, a series of 30 thoracic compressions should be performed at a frequency of 100–120/min, followed by a brief break from compressions, at which time **two breaths are quickly delivered, followed by another series of 30 compressions**.

## *CPR cycles*

Although there are no studies evaluating the synchrony of CPR cycles in veterinary patients, evidence in human medicine suggests that **chest compressions should be performed in cycles**:

- **Uninterrupted for 2 minutes** (if there are several resuscitators).

- Then 2 minutes with **brief interruptions every 30 compressions**, to provide two rapid breaths using the mouth-snout technique (if there is only one resuscitator or the animal is not intubated).

After each 2-minute cycle, the **person performing compressions should be replaced** to minimise the effects of muscle fatigue on the effectiveness of compressions.

### *Interposed abdominal compressions*

In dogs and cats in CPA, when there are personnel sufficiently trained available, the use of abdominal compressions interspersed with thoracic compressions is reasonable given that this technique increases venous return from the abdomen and improves cardiac output.

## *Advanced life support*

ALS encompasses all veterinary CPR manoeuvres performed from the beginning of BLS until ROSC is achieved. This includes:

- pharmacological therapy (vasopressors, positive inotropes, anticholinergics, electrolytes, correction of pH)
- fluid therapy
- early defibrillation.

### *Vasopressors and vagolytics*

Obtaining adequate coronary and cerebral perfusion pressures during CPR requires the central circulation to be as close as possible to physiological levels. However, it is known that even in the case when optimal chest compressions are provided, **only 25–30% of cardiac output is achieved**. Therefore, the administration of **vasopressors is essential to create a high peripheral resistance** capable of redirecting a greater proportion of the circulating volume to the central circulation and thus guarantee adequate coronary and cerebral perfusion pressures.

#### Epinephrine

**Epinephrine is a catecholamine**, which is a non-specific adrenergic agonist. Its use in CPR is due to its **$\alpha$-adrenergic activity** capable of generating a vasopressor effect. It also causes $\beta$1-adrenergic activity, giving rise to inotropic and chronotropic effects (which can be harmful due to the increase they cause in myocardial oxygen consumption, exacerbating myocardial ischaemia and predisposing to arrhythmias). **Early use of low doses (0.01 mg/kg IV) administered every 3–5 minutes** during CPR is recommended, while **high doses of epinephrine (0.1 mg/kg IV) should be considered only in prolonged CPR situations** (given that, although associated with an increase in the rates of ROSC, they have not been related to an increase in hospital discharge survival).

#### Vasopressin

The vasopressor effects of vasopressin are mediated by activation of the **peripheral V1 receptor located in vascular smooth muscle**. This mechanism of action is completely independent of the $\alpha$1 effects of epinephrine. In fact, unlike adrenergic receptors, V1 receptors remain sensitive even in an acidic pH, and their activation does not generate inotropic or chronotropic effects that might aggravate myocardial ischaemia. The **use of vasopressin (0.8 U/kg IV) can be considered as a substitute** or in combination with epinephrine every 3–5 minutes.

#### Atropine

**Atropine is a parasympatholytic agent** that has frequently been used in patients in CPA. **Routine use (0.04 mg/kg IV) during CPR** can be considered, as it may be useful in dogs and cats with asystole or pulseless electrical activity (PEA) associated with a **high vagal tone.**

#### Anti-arrhythmic drugs

The use of **anti-arrhythmic agents, such as amiodarone**, can be considered as adjuvant therapy in refractory cases of **ventricular fibrillation/ventricular tachycardia**, although **electrical defibrillation** is the recommended primary treatment for ventricular fibrillation/pulseless ventricular tachycardia. If amiodarone is not available, the **administration of lidocaine could be considered**.

Routine use of magnesium is not recommended for the treatment of cardiac arrhythmias during CPR, except for the treatment of torsades de pointes (long Q–T syndrome).

#### Reversal agents

Naloxone has been the only reversal agent evaluated for use in CPA. Although evidence of its beneficial effects is limited, available data suggest that, **in cases of recent opioid administration, the administration of naloxone** during CPR can be considered.

With respect to other reversal agents, there are no specific studies evaluating their use; nevertheless, their administration can be considered in patients who have received potentially reversible anaesthetic/sedative medications, since the potential risk associated with these drugs is low.

## *Electrolyte therapy*

### Calcium

**Hypocalcaemia is common in patients undergoing prolonged CPA**. However, most studies investigating the usefulness of calcium administration during CPR showed no effect, so the **routine use of calcium IV during CPR is not recommended**. On the other hand, there are no studies that have investigated the use of calcium in patients with documented hypocalcaemia during CPR. Given the importance of calcium in the contraction of skeletal and smooth muscle, its IV administration can be considered in patients with moderate to severe hypocalcaemia documented during CPR.

### Potassium

Hyperkalaemia frequently develops in patients in prolonged CPA, and its treatment with haemodialysis during CPR is associated with a better prognosis. Therefore, the treatment of hyperkalaemia documented during CPR is recommended, through the administration of medical treatments. There have also been reports of hypokalaemia associated with CPA, so the treatment of hypokalaemia documented during CPR can also be considered.

## *Other treatments*

### Corticosteroids

**Routine use of corticosteroids during CPR is not recommended**, due to the lack of satisfactory evidence about their potential beneficial effects and the known potential to cause negative side effects (especially in patients with reduced perfusion).

### Alkalinisation therapy

Severe acidaemia as a consequence of metabolic acidosis is common in patients in CPA, and this acid–base imbalance can have serious consequences. However, given the available evidence, **treatment with bicarbonate (1 mEq/kg of sodium bicarbonate)** can be considered in prolonged CPA situations (>10–15 min).

### Intratracheal drug administration

When available, the IV and intra-osseous routes are preferred over intratracheal administration for the administration of resuscitation drugs, since these are associated with higher rates of survival in CPA. However, the **use of the latter for the administration of epinephrine, vasopressin or atropine can be considered in animals in which IV or intra-osseous access is not possible**.

Information related to this type of administration is lacking (such as the most appropriate location within the trachea for drug delivery, the optimal dose, volume and type of diluent recommended). However, **drugs should be diluted in saline or sterile water** and should be **administered by a catheter longer than the ET tube**. An increase in the doses of drugs administered by this route has been recommended, but there is no scientific evidence that provides accurate data.

### Supplemental oxygen administration

The use of 100% inspired oxygen fractions ($FiO_2$) during CPR has been justified as a means of maximising arterial oxygen content in an effort to compensate for decreased cardiac output (25–35% of normal) during external thoracic compressions. However, the presence of **hyperoxia may be associated with high concentrations of oxygen free radicals, which could aggravate tissue damage during CPR**. Therefore, the use of 21% $FiO_2$ (ambient air) during CPR in dogs and cats can be considered providing arterial blood gas measurements can be performed to guide the maintenance of normal blood oxygenation. In the absence of blood-gas measurements, the use of 100% $FiO_2$ is reasonable since the risk of hypoxaemia is probably greater than that of hyperoxaemia.

## *IV fluids*

During the RECOVER initiative, a worksheet to evaluate the scientific literature available in this regard was not included. Therefore, the ILCOR fluid therapy worksheet was evaluated and some conclusions from the evaluation of these data were extrapolated. Some of these studies showed that the administration of fluids during CPR in normovolaemic animals was associated with a decrease in coronary perfusion pressure. Hence, routine administration of IV fluids in normovolaemic or hypervolaemic canine and feline patients during CPR is not recommended. However, the **administration of IV fluids in hypovolaemic patients seems reasonable**, since they probably benefit from the increase in circulating volume during CPR.

## *Defibrillation*

Sudden **cardiac arrest due to ventricular fibrillation (VF) is common in humans**, and much of the literature indicates that electric defibrillation is the most effective treatment to correct it. Since VF and ventricular tachycardia (VT) are the result of an abnormal rhythm that arises in groups of myocardial cells instead of pacemakers, the goal of electric defibrillation is to depolarise as many of these cells as possible, forcing them into a refractory period and therefore stopping their random electrical activity along with their uncoordinated mechanical activity. In this way, pacemakers can resume control (establishing a sinus rhythm) or the patient develops an asystole. It should be stressed that either of the two outcomes (sinus rhythm or asystole) is considered a satisfactory defibrillation. In the absence of an electric defibrillator, **mechanical defibrillation can be attempted by applying a precordial thump**, although the effectiveness of this procedure is probably poor.

### Electric defibrillation technique

The use of biphasic over single-phase defibrillators is recommended, using 4–6 J/kg with the monophasic defibrillator or 2–4 J/kg with the biphasic defibrillator. If the first discharge is unsuccessful in dogs and cats with pulseless VF/VT, it is reasonable to progressively increase defibrillation energy (for example, by 50%).

In order to maximise the current through the ventricles, the **paddles should be placed on opposite sides of the thorax**, approximately level with the costochondral junction and directly over the heart. To facilitate their use, the patient should preferably be placed in **dorsal recumbency** (the use of a plastic support can help achieve this). **Abundant defibrillator gel** or paste should be placed on the paddles to ensure better skin contact. If defibrillation patches are used, the hair from the area must be clipped prior to this to facilitate contact. Once the defibrillator is loaded, the operator must announce the intention to defibrillate by means of a warning like "**Clear!**", and visually confirm that no one is in contact with the patient or the table (including themselves). On the other hand, avoiding electric defibrillation if there is alcohol on the patient's hair is imperative, since the risk of ignition is high.

### Synchronisation of electric defibrillation

The optimal time to start defibrillation during CPR is determined by the time elapsed since the patient entered CPA. After perfusion is lost, the myocardium goes through three phases:

1. The electrical phase, during which there is minimal ischaemic damage (lasting 4 minutes).
2. The circulatory phase, during which reversible ischaemic changes occur (lasting 6 minutes).
3. The metabolic phase, during which potentially irreversible damage begins. This may require more advanced techniques, such as therapeutic hypothermia or cardiopulmonary bypass to achieve reversal.

Therefore, immediate defibrillation is only recommended if:

- In cases of CPA due to VF/VT without a pulse, lasting less than or up to 4 minutes.
- If VF is diagnosed once CPR has begun in the diagnostic period between cycles.

To the contrary, if the patient has been in VF/VT without a pulse for more than 4 minutes, finishing a BLS cycle of 2 minutes' duration is recommended before defibrillation.

### Precordial thump

This is a method of mechanical defibrillation that is achieved by **hitting the patient with the edge of the hand directly over the heart**. Recent studies have shown that this technique is of minimal efficacy in the treatment of VF. Therefore, a precordial thump should be considered only if there is no electric defibrillator available.

### *Open-chest CPR*

**Open-chest CPR has proved more effective than closed-chest CPR** in restoring ROSC. However, open-chest CPR requires significant resources not only in terms of staffing, with a team of professionals properly trained to carry out CPR, but also in order to offer advanced post-CPA supportive care. Therefore, immediately performing open-chest CPR routinely should only be considered in certain situations:

- tension pneumothorax
- pericardial effusion
- intra-operative cardiopulmonary arrest in cases of laparotomy or thoracotomy.

## Monitoring

The literature provides sufficient evidence to support the use of **ECG and EtCO$_2$ monitoring** in dogs and cats in CPA. If available, these should always be used early in any attempt at CPR.

### *Electrocardiography*

Although during chest compressions artefacts may be seen on the ECG, the information it provides is valuable. ECG evaluation is **recommended during the breaks between cycles**, since it allows an accurate diagnosis of the rhythm and can be used as a guide to ALS. ECG evaluation should be performed quickly and should not delay resumption of chest compressions between 2-minute cycles, which should never be interrupted to interpret the ECG.

In patients with VF, it is reasonable to perform a **rapid ECG evaluation** to determine whether VF has resolved immediately after defibrillation, but resumption of chest compressions should never be delayed.

### *Capnography*

EtCO$_2$ is a valuable instrument during CPR, given that it is an early indicator of ROSC and a measure of effectiveness of CPR, and potentially allows clinicians to adjust treatment to maximise perfusion during CPR. Constant minute ventilation should be maintained when capnography is used for these purposes, since $EtCO_2$ is affected by both pulmonary perfusion and minute ventilation. Sudden increases in $EtCO_2$ may occur with CPR during CPA, as when it is performed it generates a sharp increase in pulmonary flow. Finally, it is recognised that $EtCO_2$ values >15 mmHg during CPR are associated with a better prognosis for ROSC.

### *Other monitoring during CPR*

Other methods of haemodynamic monitoring including the following can be used during CPR:

#### Pulse palpation

Pulse palpations should not be considered a reliable diagnostic tool for CPA, and therefore interruption of chest compressions during CPR specifically to palpate the pulse is not recommended. However, identifying ROSC during breaks between cycles (providing it does not delay resuming compressions) is advisable. It is also recommended during thoracic compressions, although should be interpreted with caution since retrograde flow through the venous system could be mistakenly considered as an arterial pulse.

#### Detection of blood flow by Doppler

This should be interpreted with care, due to the possibility of motion artefacts or the detection of retrograde venous flow. The evaluation of pulsatile flow measured with Doppler may be useful during breaks between cycles, although it should not delay compressions being restarted.

#### Electrolyte levels

Monitoring is recommended because, in prolonged CPR situations, electrolyte abnormalities often occur. Knowing electrolyte levels helps guide treatment.

Blood-gas measurements of central venous blood or mixed venous blood should be taken to evaluate the effectiveness of CPR.

### *PCA care*

A high percentage of dogs and cats that survive CPA fail to survive to hospital discharge: Survival fluctuates between 2 and 10% despite the fact that the percentage for ROSC is 35–45%. ROSC can therefore be considered as an intermediate point in CPR. **Post-cardiac arrest (PCA) syndrome** is characterised by a combination of multi-organ failure, cardiogenic shock, brain injury due to anoxia and sequelae of pre-existing disease, and is very likely to be responsible for the high mortality of animals that manage to achieve ROSC. Therefore, the key to improving the prognosis of these patients is based on **optimising PCA care**. For this, complex clinical management is required since the objectives of such care vary with the course of the post-ROSC phase.

Initially, PCA care is focused on the **prevention of a repeat arrest** and, secondly, the prevention of the appearance of **subsequent systemic injuries** and the necessary rehabilitative care in each case. In short, PCA care should be considered as an essential part of CPA management and may be the necessary link for CPR to be successful.

#### Patient monitoring after ROSC

PCA monitoring should meet two objectives:

- Detect the impending recurrence of CPR.
- Guide treatment according to the clinical situation of each patient.

This should include, as a minimum:

- continuous ECG monitoring
- intermittent blood pressure monitoring
- evaluation of oxygenation and ventilation.

In addition, the following can be monitored:

- body temperature
- lactate concentrations in arterial blood
- blood glucose levels.

#### Haemodynamic optimisation strategies

The use of haemodynamic optimisation strategies can be one of the key procedures in the clinical management of patients who reach the PCA period. It is a treatment guided by objectives, among which the optimisation of the following is included:

- arterial blood pressure
- central venous pressure
- haematocrit
- lactate levels
- $ScvO_2$
- arterial oxygen saturation.

The use of this strategy guided by objectives **allows treatment to be adjusted to the individual needs of each animal**. To achieve these haemodynamic objectives in patients with persistent hypotension and/or cardiovascular instability, clinical interventions such as the use of vasopressors and/or positive inotropic support are recommended. On the other hand, the routine use of **large volumes of fluids is not recommended PCA, except in cases diagnosed with hypovolaemia**. In

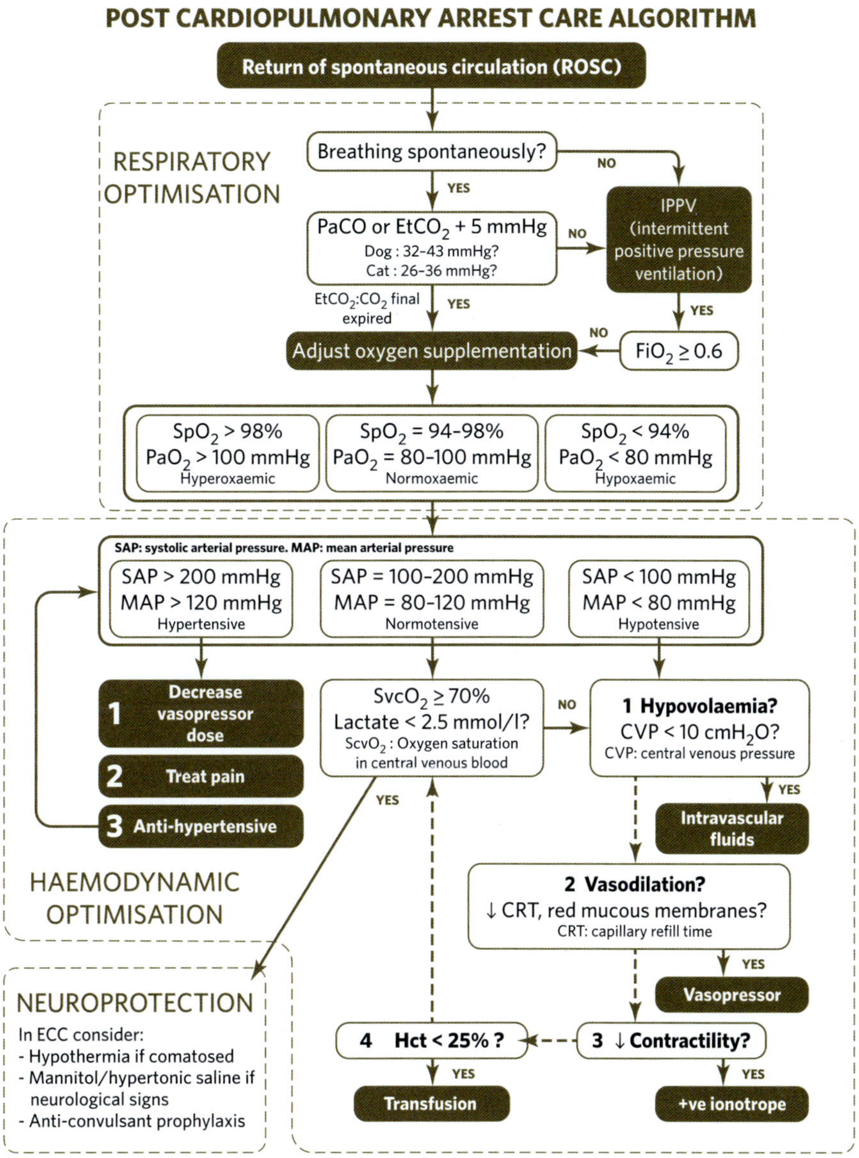


**Figure 1.15.** The CPA algorithm.

animals with evidence of congestive heart failure, fluid therapy should be avoided completely. To achieve cardiovascular optimisation from a clinical point of view, following the CPA care algorithm (Figure 1.15) is advised.

## Respiratory function control

Although data describing the effect on the prognosis of respiratory disturbances during the PCA period are scarce, ventilation affects a significant number of physiological processes that deserve special consideration in the context of PCA care. In fact, on the one hand correct ventilation constitutes the main way of eliminating $CO_2$ from the organism (fundamental to guaranteeing correct cerebrovascular reactivity to $CO_2$) while, on the other, the use of mechanical ventilation can have haemodynamic and/or pulmonary consequences, which are particularly harmful in already compromised patients. Therefore, the ventilatory strategy that is recommended for patients in the PCA period is based on **achieving normal $CO_2$ levels in the PCA period ($PaCO_2$ of 32–43 mmHg in dogs and 26–36 mmHg in cats)**. Serial $CO_2$ monitoring by capnography ($EtCO_2$ or arterial blood gas ($PaCO_2$) is recommended to ensure adequate ventilation.

Regarding mechanical ventilation, its routine use is not recommended in all patients' PCA, but only in those with diagnosed hypoventilation or hypoxaemia, as well as in those requiring high concentrations of inspired oxygen ($FiO_2$ >0.60) to maintain normoxaemia.

Finally, it is recommended that oxygen supplementation be adjusted in order to **achieve normoxaemia ($PaO_2$ = 80–100 mmHg, $SpO_2$ = 94–98%)**, avoiding hypoxemia (risk of tissue ischaemia) and hyperoxaemia (risk of oxygen free radical release) at all times.

## Hypothermia and overheating

The use of mild therapeutic hypothermia (MTH, central body temperature of 32–34 °C) in the PCA period is becoming increasingly common in human medicine. For its application in veterinary medicine, a number of aspects must be taken into account. First, the safe application of the principles of MTH requires the ability to perform advanced intensive care and mechanical ventilation as an essential prerequisite. Initiation of MTH can be considered in patients in a coma as soon as possible after ROSC, and its maintenance for 24–48 hours provided there is availability of mechanical ventilation and advanced intensive care. In cases where minimum resources are not available but patients have moderate hypothermia, it is reasonable to slow their reheating. In general, slow reheating with increments of 0.25–0.5 °C/h is recommended, avoiding reheating speeds >1 °C/h at all times.

## Pharmacological treatment

In veterinary medicine there are no studies in this regard, but in human medicine a series of pharmacological treatments have demonstrated neuroprotective and metabolic effects during PCA care.

## Corticosteroids

There is conflicting evidence in the literature regarding the usefulness of corticosteroids in providing neuroprotection in the PCA period. Routine administration is not recommended, since the evidence supporting the beneficial effects is limited and the potential for adverse effects is well known (especially in animals with hypoperfusion). However, the administration of *hydrocortisone (1 mg/kg followed by 1 mg/kg/6 h or an infusion of 0.15 mg/kg/h* may be considered, reducing the dose as soon as the patient's condition allows) for cats and dogs that they remain haemodynamically unstable despite the administration of fluids and ionotropics/vasopressors during PCA care.

## Hyperosmotic therapy

Cerebral oedema has been identified in human patients during the PCA period and is associated with a worse prognosis for survival. Therefore, the use of hypertonic saline or mannitol in dogs and cats with neurological signs indicative of cerebral oedema can be considered. However, the diuretic effects of mannitol must be taken into account and fluid therapy should be adjusted to prevent the development of hypovolaemia.

## Prophylactic anticonvulsants

Seizures and myoclonus occur in 5–15% of adult human patients during the PCA period, and in 40% of those who remain comatose after ROSC. Therefore, the prophylactic administration of barbiturates (phenobarbital) during the PCA period can be considered.

## Care in referral centres

Human literature suggests that ICUs led by ECC specialists achieve better survival outcomes. Therefore, it is reasonable to refer all veterinary patients requiring intensive care PPC to centres where they can receive care 24 hours per day, intensive monitoring and more sophisticated treatments.

# Bibliography

Beekley, A.C. (2008) Damage control resuscitation: a sensible approach to the exsanguinating surgical patient. *Critical Care Medicine* 36(7) (Suppl.).

Dutton, R.P., Mackenzie, C.F. and Scalea, T.M. (2002) Hypotensive resuscitation during active hemorrhage: impact on in-hospital mortality. *Journal of Trauma* 52(1), 141–146.

Dutton, R.P., McCunn, M. and Grissom, T.E. (2009) Anesthesia for trauma. In: Miller, R.D. *Miller's Anesthesia*, 7th edn. Churchill Livingstone, Philadelphia, PA.

Fletcher, D.J., Boller, M., Brainard, B.M., Haskins, S.C., Hopper, K., McMichael, M.A. et al. (2012) American College of Veterinary Medicine; Veterinary Emergency and Critical Care Society. RECOVER evidence and knowledge gap analysis on veterinary CPR. Part 7: Clinical guidelines. *Journal of Veterinary Emergency and Critical Care (San Antonio)* 22 (Suppl. 1), S102–S131.

Lisciandro, G.R. (2011) Abdominal and thoracic focused assessment with sonography for trauma, triage, and monitoring in small animals. *Journal of Veterinary Emergency and Critical Care (San Antonio)* 21(2), 104–122.

Palmer, L. and Martin, L. (2014) Traumatic coagulopathy. Part 2: Resuscitative strategies. *Journal of Veterinary Emergency and Critical Care (San Antonio)* 24(1), 75–92.

Peterson, N.W., Buote, N.J. and Barr, J.W. (2015) The impact of surgical timing and intervention on outcome in traumatized dogs and cats. *Journal of Veterinary Emergency and Critical Care (San Antonio)* 25(1), 63–75.

Rivers, E., Nguyen, B., Havstad, S., Ressler, J., Muzzin, A., Knoblich, B. et al. (2001) Early Goal-directed Therapy Collaborative Group. Early goal-directed therapy in the treatment of severe sepsis and septic shock. *New England Journal of Medicine* 345(19), 1368–1377.

Rockar, R.A., Drobatz, K.S. and Shofer, F.S. (1994) Development of a scoring system for the veterinary trauma patient. *Journal of Veterinary Emergency and Critical Care (San Antonio)* 4(2), 77–83.

Ruys, L.J., Gunning, M., Teske, E., Robben, J.H. and Sigrist, N.E. (2012) Evaluation of a veterinary triage list modified from a human five-point triage system in 485 dogs and cats. *Journal of Veterinary Emergency and Critical Care (San Antonio)* 22(3), 303–312.

Stillion, J.R. and Fletcher. D.J. (2012) Admission base excess as a predictor of transfusion requirement and mortality in dogs with blunt trauma: 52 cases (2007–2009). *Journal of Veterinary Emergency and Critical Care (San Antonio)* 22(5), 588–594. https://ahdc.vet.cornell.edu/sects/coag/clinical/transfu.cfm (accessed 24 February 2016).

## Test

1. **Which is the correct answer regarding the clinical signs of SIRS in the dog?**
   A) temperature <38°C
   B) heart rate <120 bpm
   C) respiratory rate <40 bpm
   D) leukocytes <18 000 GB/µl.
2. **The existence of an inappropriate vascular tone due to microcirculation dysfunction resulting in generalised vasodilation is called?**
   A) cardiogenic shock
   B) hypovolaemic shock
   C) obstructive shock
   D) distributive shock.
3. **Regarding acute traumatic coagulopathy (ATC), select the correct answer.**
   A) It is characterised by the early development of signs of hypercoagulability and hypofibrinolysis in the most immediate post-traumatic period.
   B) There is no method to identify ATC reliably and definitively.
   C) Identification of ATC is based solely on the existence of indices that suggest its presence, such as coagulation times which are 1.5 times faster than average times.
   D) Pharmacologically, its treatment can be based on the administration of vasopressor drugs.
4. **Regarding sympathomimetic drugs, select the correct answer.**
   A) Dopamine at high doses (10–20 µg/kg/min) exerts its action on dopamine receptors, leading to diuresis and increased blood flow in the kidney and digestive system.
   B) The main side effects of dobutamine may include tachycardia, arrhythmias and vasodilation.
   C) Norepinephrine is an agent with an indirect action, and its effectiveness can be limited by the occurrence of tachyphylaxis phenomena in the case of depletion of norepinephrine reserves in sympathetic terminals.
   D) Phenylephrine exerts its action on β1 receptors, causing an increase in myocardial contractility and heart rate.
5. **Regarding the pharmacological treatment of hypotension, select the correct answer.**
   A) In the presence of hypovolaemia, it is recommended to start with the administration of a potent vasoconstrictor (such as vasopressin).
   B) All available data are sourced from animal studies, so the clinical criteria derived from these are completely reliable.
   C) When hypotension continues even after the administration of vasopressors and there are signs of vasodilation, consider the administration of inotropic agents that allow a direct increase in myocardial contractility.
   D) When hypotension continues even after the administration of inotropes and there are signs of vasodilation, consider the administration of α-adrenergic agents that allow a direct increase in vascular tone and combat vasodilation.
6. **Regarding opioids. Which answer is incorrect?**
   A) Buprenorphine has a lower affinity for the µ-receptor than fentanyl.
   B) Pethidine does not cause vomiting.
   C) Methadone does not cause histamine release.
   D) Fentanyl causes severe respiratory depression.
7. **Regarding tramadol, which answer is incorrect?**
   A) It causes respiratory depression, although less than that caused by opioids.
   B) Its administration is contraindicated in epileptic patients.
   C) Part of its mechanism of action is based on the inhibition of the reuptake of norepinephrine and serotonin.
   D) It is not reversible.
8. **Regarding anticonvulsants (gabapentin and pregabalin), select the incorrect answer.**
   A) They imitate the physiological effects of the GABA neurotransmitter.
   B) Their side effects are rare and minimal (mild ataxia and sedation).
   C) Their administration is indicated for the treatment of neuropathic pain.
   D) Their mechanism of action is based on a blockade of the alpha-2-delta subunits of calcium channels.

**9. Regarding the diagnosis of cardiorespiratory arrest (CRA), select the incorrect answer.**
A) ECG analysis is not reliable since it is slow and may present artefacts.
B) Pulse evaluation has proven to be non-specific and insensitive.
C) Auscultation is a fast, ideal method.
D) In case of doubt, resuscitation procedures should always be initiated as no damage occurs even if there is no CRA.

**10. Indicate which answer is correct regarding cardiac massage.**
A) In the best-case scenario, the cardiac output generated is 75%.
B) Allowing the total expansion of the thorax is not necessary.
C) The depth of compression should be a minimum of ¾ parts of the total depth of the chest.
D) The compression frequency should be approximately 100–120 cpm.

**11. Regarding cardiac massage, select the incorrect answer.**
A) It must be performed in uninterrupted 2-minute cycles.
B) The compression ratio:relaxation of each compression should be 1:2.
C) To avoid compressor fatigue, it is advisable to perform a relay every 2 minutes at the end of each cycle.
D) Internal cardiac massage is the method of choice in the case of intraoperative arrests in animals with an open thorax or abdomen.

**12. Regarding the placement of the compressor's hands, indicate which answer is true?**
A) In a Greyhound, the hands should be placed on the widest part of the thorax (near the vertebrae), since the flow is generated by the thoracic pump theory.
B) In an English Bulldog, hands should be placed on the sternum with the patient in dorsal recumbency, since the flow is generated by the thoracic pump theory.
C) In a cat, the hands should be placed around the chest and compressions performed circumferentially, since the flow is generated by the cardiac pump theory.
D) In a German Shepherd, hands should be placed on the narrowest part of the thorax (near the sternum), since the flow is generated by the cardiac pump theory.

**13. In situations where cardiopulmonary resuscitation (CPR) is necessary, which of the following is necessary to verify the correct placement of the endotracheal tube?**
A) Check the presence of $CO_2$ using capnography.
B) Perform a direct visualisation with the help of a laryngoscope.
C) Auscultate bilateral respiratory sounds.
D) All of the above are correct.

**14. Regarding the 'B' of the basic life support phase, indicate which answer is correct.**
A) The recommended respiratory rate is 15–20 bpm.
B) Airway pressures should not exceed 40 cm $H_2O$.
C) High respiratory rates are not recommended since they decrease venous return.
D) All of the above are correct.

**15. Regarding CPR, indicate which is the correct answer.**
A) The use of doxapram is always indicated since it decreases the consumption of cerebral oxygen.
B) External cardiac massage should be paused for as long as it takes to be able to correctly evaluate the ECG.
C) The intratracheal (IT) administration of sodium bicarbonate is recommended, provided it is diluted in 10 ml of 0.9% NaCl and the dose is increased 2–2.5 times.
D) When performing CPR, epinephrine is used with the aim of achieving an increase in systemic vascular resistance that produces arteriolar vasoconstriction capable of guaranteeing better perfusion of vital organs.

**16. Regarding fluid therapy, select the correct answer.**
A) Sodium bicarbonate should always be administered concomitantly with lactated Ringer's.
B) The fluid of choice in patients with traumatic brain injury in which the blood–brain barrier could be damaged is lactated Ringer's.
C) After administration of 7.5% NaCl, monitoring of plasma Na levels and continuing administration of crystalloids is highly recommended.
D) The use of 10% Hetastarch is indicated in patients with kidney problems due to the decrease in COP, as well as in patients with coagulation disorders.

**Answers on page 56**

## Clinical case

**Signalment**: 3-year-old male castrated Newfoundland dog, weight 62 kg.
**Reason for consultation**: The owners take the dog to the practice on Friday night because when they arrive at the farm to spend the weekend there, they find the dog in lateral recumbency with an abnormal level of consciousness. The abdomen is clearly distended and the dog does not respond to stimuli. Since no one lives there during the week, it is unknown how long he has been in this state.
**Physical examination**: Pale mucous membranes and capillary refill time greater >3 s, weak and irregular pulse that does not always coincide with the heartbeat. Cold extremities. Altered state of consciousness. Heart rate: 140 bpm; tachypnoea with respiratory rate impossible to calculate due to the presence of gasping.
**Thoracic auscultation**: Cardiac and pulmonary auscultation within normal limits.
**Complete blood count and biochemistry**: Values within the reference ranges except for Hct 65%, PT 8.5 g/dl, K 2.4 mEq/l, alkaline phosphatase 328 U/l and glucose 52 mg/dl.

Arterial blood gas (with approximately 100% $O_2$): pH 7.1, $PaO_2$ 42 mmHg, PaCO– 28 mmHg, BE –18, $HCO_3$ 12, lactate 7.6 mmol/l.

1. **Based on the signalment and history, what is the most likely cause of this patient's condition?**
   A) pancreatitis
   B) urinary obstruction
   C) pleural effusion
   D) gastric dilatation and torsion.
2. **What is the first clinical procedure you should perform on this patient?**
   A) administration of 100% oxygen and peripheral vein catheterisation
   B) echocardiography and thoracic radiography
   C) abdominal radiography
   D) abdominal ultrasound.
3. **Once the presumptive diagnosis has been confirmed, what should the elective stabilisation treatment be?**
   A) administration of sodium bicarbonate
   B) recovery of intravascular volume by aggressive fluid therapy
   C) begin aggressive antibiotic therapy
   D) immediately begin a 25% albumin transfusion.
4. **What are the parameters used to monitor fluid therapy resuscitation?**
   A) lactate
   B) diuresis
   C) heart rate and blood pressure
   D) all of the above.
5. **Which type of analgesia is the most appropriate for this patient?**
   A) no pain relief
   B) continuous infusion of dexmedetomidine
   C) continuous infusion of ketamine
   D) methadone.
6. **What is the fluid therapy of choice for stabilisation of this patient?**
   A) 5% glucose in water
   B) 0.9% NaCl supplemented with 2.5% glucose
   C) Isofundin® supplemented with 2.5% glucose together with 10% HemoHes®
   D) fresh whole blood transfusion.

## Correct answers

### Test

| | | |
|---|---|---|
| 1. A | 7. D | 13. D |
| 2. D | 8. A | 14. C |
| 3. B | 9. C | 15. D |
| 4. B | 10. D | 16. C |
| 5. D | 11. B | |
| 6. A | 12. C | |

### Clinical case

1. D
2. A
3. B
4. D
5. D
6. C

# 2

# Oncology

Pachi Clemente Vicario

## Chapter summary



Cancer is recognised as the **most frequent cause of death in geriatric companion animals**. However, cancer as a whole includes more than **100 diseases** with different treatments and prognosis. Indeed, the approach to each cancer case varies depending on the histological type, location, degree of advancement at the time of diagnosis and the patient's species. Therefore when faced with an oncological patient **the first step is to determine**:

- A **definite diagnosis of the cancer type**, which is made via cytology, histopathology and/or molecular diagnostic tests.
- The **clinical stage of disease**.

This chapter aims to give a practical overview of a rational approach to the cancer patient as an individual. Also, with an understanding of cancer on a cellular level and how this affects the body as a whole, this enables the clinician to select the most appropriate diagnostic tests and make informed decisions about treatment options.

Chemotherapeutic drugs play an important part in the treatment of cancer. However, these drugs must be handled with great care and in an appropriate manner. For the practitioner in general practice, who doesn't handle such treatments regularly, this chapter is an invaluable aid to calculating dosages and becoming familiar with administering these medications in a manner that is safe for both the patient and staff.

### Key learning points

- Identifying markers of paraneoplastic disease.
- The role of molecular tests for the purpose of prognostication.
- Decision making when taking biopsy samples.
- Assessing a patient's suitability for chemotherapy.
- Understanding the use of multi-modal therapies.

## Diagnosis

The patient may be presented to the veterinarian because the owner has noticed the **presence of a mass**, but this is not always the case. Sometimes the tumour's presence is not obvious and remains asymptomatic until the oncological process is advanced, or the tumour may manifest itself with non-specific symptoms. The latter may occur because of the **tumour's physical presence** or the **release of substances that act at a distance to the mass** itself, causing so-called **paraneoplastic syndromes** (**PNS**). PNS are often the first sign of disease, so early recognition is vital in order to flag up the need for investigation.

In veterinary medicine the most frequent PNS signs include:

### *Endocrine changes*

#### *Hypercalcaemia*

The main cause of **hypercalcaemia in dogs is cancer**, especially lymphoma, mainly mediastinal, although it is also associated with other tumours. In general, it is caused by the **tumour producing substances related to parathyroid hormone** (**PTH**). The **symptoms are due to changes in renal function** and initially manifest as **polydipsia/polyuria**, which progresses to **renal failure**, so the presence of hypercalcaemia must be handled as an emergency.

#### *Hypoglycaemia*

**Insulinoma**, a beta-cell tumour, is the **most frequent cause of hypoglycaemia in dogs**, followed by other neoplasms such as hepatocellular carcinoma and intestinal tumours.

### *Haematological changes*

#### *Anaemia*

Cancer patients frequently present with anaemia, often due to chronic disease but less commonly with immune-mediated, ferropenic or micro-angiopathic disease. Although it can be associated with various types of cancer, **iron deficiency anaemia (microcytic, hypochromic) caused by chronic blood loss** is frequently associated with gastrointestinal tract tumours. Micro-angiopathic anaemia, characterised by haemolysis and the presence of schistocytes, is mostly related to **haemangiosarcoma**.

#### *Hypergammaglobulinaemia*

**Multiple myeloma**, a plasma cell tumour, can produce **monoclonal immunoglobulins** by altering the proteinogram and causing clinical signs of hyperviscosity, which include ataxia and seizures.

### *Bony changes*

#### *Hypertrophic osteopathy*

This alteration, characterised by the **proliferation of the periosteum in long bones**, is associated with both neoplastic and non-neoplastic diseases (Figure 2.1). Like PNS, it is mainly due to **primary or metastatic pulmonary tumours**. However, non-oncological diseases such as heartworm, heart disease, pneumonia, abscesses and foreign bodies – and gestation – have been linked to this change.

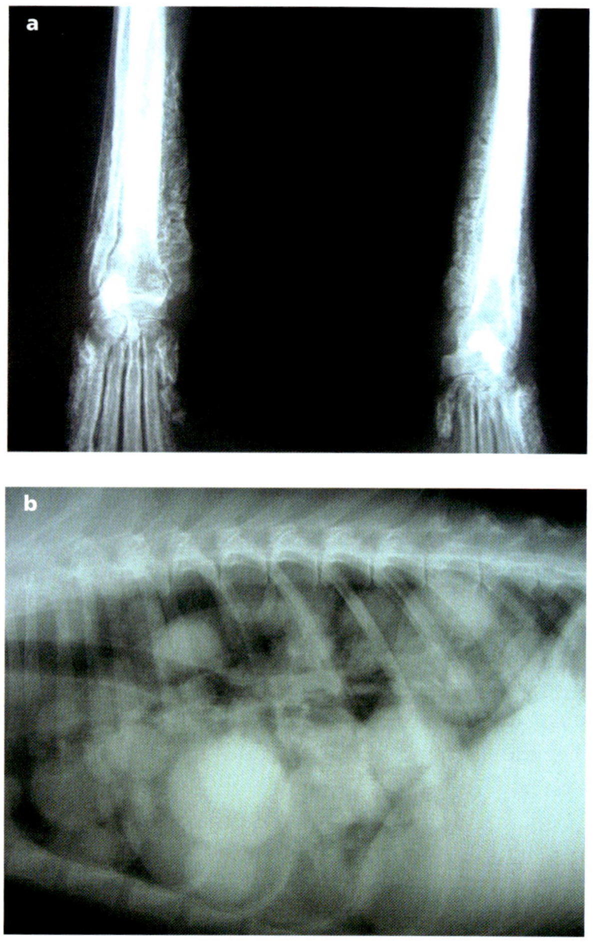


**Figure 2.1.** a, Hypertrophic osteopathy. b, Pulmonary tumours (origin of the hypertrophic osteopathy).

## Neurological changes

### Myasthenia gravis

This alteration to the neuromuscular junction is mainly caused by **thymoma in acquired cases**.

## Cytology

In cases in which the tumour is evident, **cytology may yield a diagnosis**. Although it does not replace histopathology, in many cases it can give a **quick and inexpensive answer**. It can be performed on masses, effusions, bone marrow or mucous membranes.

Although cytology is usually performed using aspiration, in highly vascularised tissues the sample is taken by pricking the mass with a fine needle, without aspiration, to try to avoid contamination with large amounts of blood that would hinder interpretation.

Cytology can either be interpreted in the clinic or sent to a veterinary clinical pathologist, depending on the experience of the clinician and the characteristics of the sample. The first distinction is between **an inflammatory and a neoplastic sample**. In cases where the sample has a mixed population, and as a result it is difficult to differentiate between neoplasia with secondary inflammation and inflammation with cell dysplasia, tissue biopsy is recommended.

If the sample is tissue, it is classified according to its origin:

- epithelial (Figure 2.2)
- mesenchymal (Figure 2.3)
- round cells (Figure 2.4).

**Signs of malignancy** should be sought once the cell type is established.

## Biopsy

When the results of **cytology are not definitive, a tissue biopsy is required**. This is indicated in all cases where the diagnosis changes either the prognosis (benign versus malignant) or the type of treatment

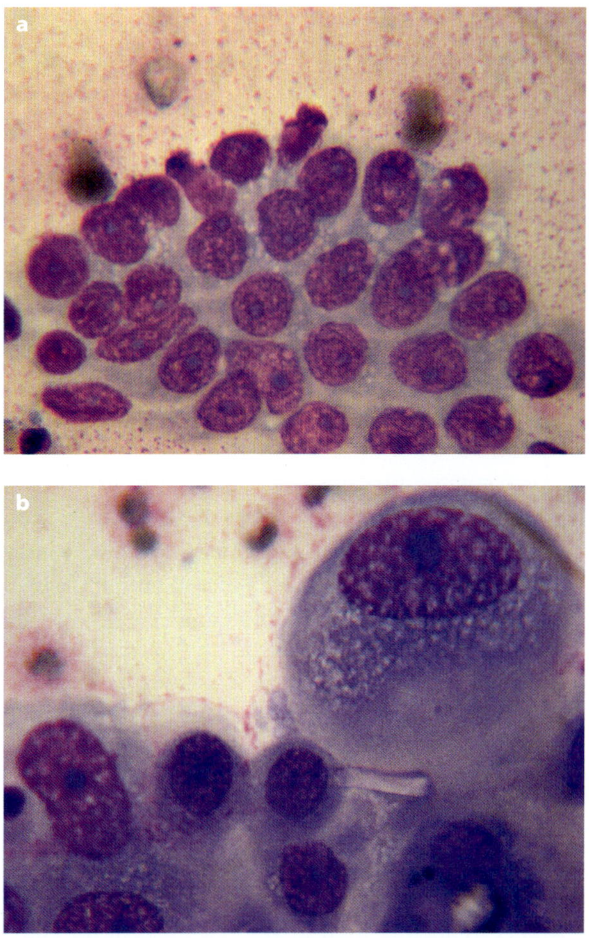

**Figure 2.2.** a, Population of glandular cells of epithelial origin, displaying no signs of malignancy – adenoma. b, Epithelial cells with marked differences in nucleus, nucleolar and cell size – carcinoma. Both samples originated from tumours in mammary tissue.

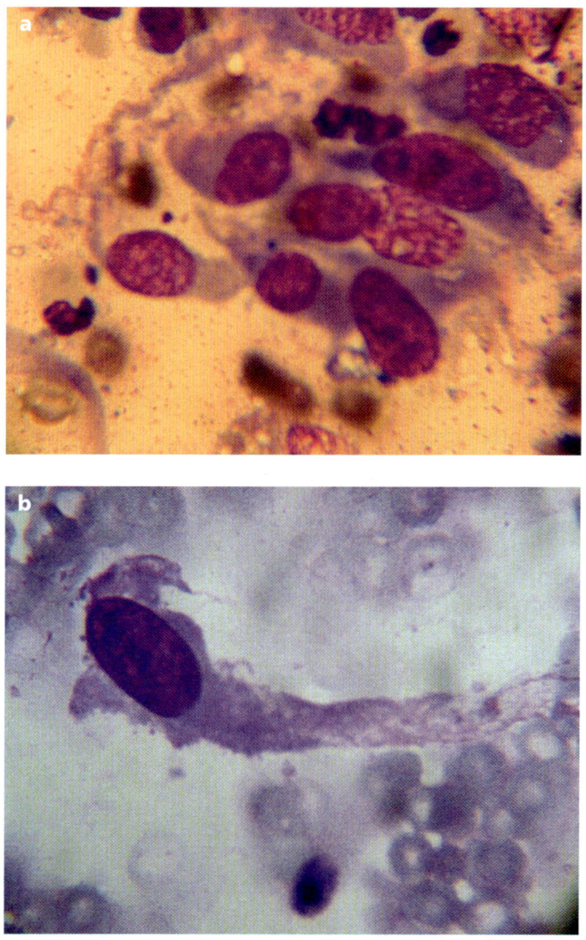

**Figure 2.3.** Aspirate showing mesenchymal cells. a, Fibrosarcoma. b, Splenic haemangiosarcoma.

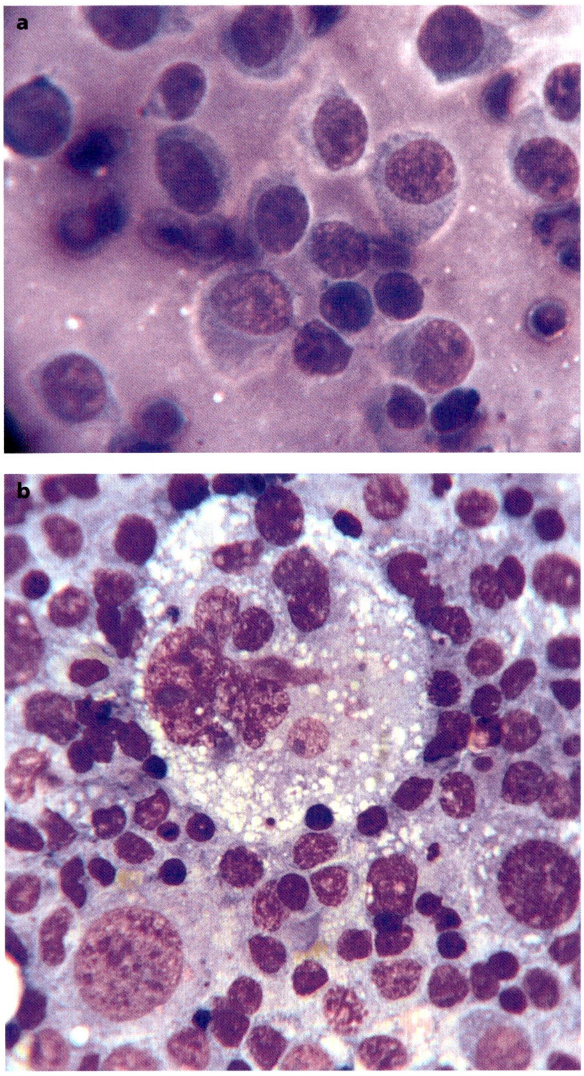


**Figure 2.4.** Round cell tumours. a, Histiocytoma. b, Same cell type but showing signs of malignancy – differences in nucleus and cell size, different numbers of nuclei and multinucleated cells. Histiocytic sarcoma.

(conservative versus aggressive surgery, surgery versus chemotherapy).

The most commonly used methods are:

- punch biopsy
- incision biopsy
- excision biopsy.

**Excisional biopsies** should be used only in cases where **treatment would not change** depending on the diagnosis (for example, benign skin tumours) or, in areas where the lesion has not been removed completely when taking the biopsy, a second surgery can be performed. These should not be used in areas where a second intervention may be compromised, such as the limbs.

In addition to the diagnosis, the biopsy should offer relevant information such as:

- The **histological grade**, for example, in:
  - Soft tissue sarcoma: high-grade sarcomas have a higher rate of metastasis.
  - Mast cell tumor: high-grade/III usually exhibits more aggressive behaviour.
  - Mammary gland carcinoma: where the prognosis varies depending on the histological grade.
- **Mitotic count**. If it is high, this reflects greater tumour activity and is associated with a worse prognosis.
- The presence of **vascular or lymphatic embolisation**. Indicates a risk of metastatic dissemination.
- The existence of **tumour cells in the borders of the excised tissue** (in excisional biopsies) indicates an incomplete resection and the potential need for additional treatments.

## *Molecular diagnosis*

In addition to cytology and histology, molecular diagnostic techniques are used more and more frequently in veterinary oncology. This is a process used to identify a disease by studying **molecules such as proteins or DNA** in a tissue or fluid, and is utilised in cancer patients for:

- diagnosis
- monitoring
- risk detection
- choice of treatment.

Knowledge of different types of cancer at the molecular level has allowed the development of diagnostic tests and/or specific treatments. Many of these are aimed at blocking the molecular mechanism of the disease which, in numerous instances, improves the prognosis.

To recognise proteins, **stains linked to antibodies against proteins** of interest can be used in biopsies, and this is called **immunohistochemistry**. However, fixing the sample with formalin affects certain proteins, sometimes limiting the usefulness of this technique.

## *Flow cytometry*

**Detection of different markers** that help to characterise the cell population of interest is possible using flow cytometry. These markers are generally identified by the letters **CD** (**Cluster of Differentiation**, differentiation groups) followed by a number (Table 2.1). The markers frequently used in veterinary oncology allow identification of haematopoietic precursor cells and different types of lymphocyte.

Its most frequent application in veterinary oncology is the **diagnosis of lymphoproliferative and**

Table 2.1. Differentiation groups.

| Marker | Cell type |
|---|---|
| CD34 | Undifferentiated haematopoietic precursors |
| CD45 | Leukocytes |
| CD20 | B cells |
| CD3 | T cells |
| CD5 | T cells |
| CD4 | Helper lymphocytes |
| CD8 | Cytotoxic lymphocytes |
| CD14 | Monocytes |

**haematological diseases**. It requires cells to be in suspension, and the **sample should be analysed in the first 24–48 hours**, which may limit its use on some occasions. After aspirating the sample from a lymph node, it is placed in a tube with a preservative and sent to the laboratory. In the case of leukaemia, blood can also be analysed.

The use of flow cytometry has not only allowed improvements in the diagnosis of lymphoproliferative diseases, but also for additional information about the prognosis of each type to be obtained. Observations based on flow cytometry have brought to light how **some breeds have higher incidences of certain immunophenotypes**.

In the case of **canine lymphoma**, the routine use of flow cytometry has contributed to the **characterisation of different types of lymphoma**, associated with very different prognoses. In initial studies it was seen that there was a group of T-cell lymphomas associated with a less aggressive clinical course, although it was not possible to identify a marker that would help in their diagnosis. More recently, studies describing this type of lymphoma have been published, characterised by an immunophenotype $CD4^+$ $CD45^-$, which is associated with an average survival of around 2 years, while that of $CD4^+$ $CD45^{++}$ is only 5 months.

**Chronic lymphoid leukaemia**. Cytometry has allowed identification of **different immunophenotypes**, which are associated with very **different prognoses**: from an average survival of less than a month in atypical phenotypes to more than 30 months in chronic lymphoid T-cell leukaemia ($CD3^+$ $CD8^+$).

The use of flow cytometry also **allows the extent of the disease to be established**. For example, in canine lymphomas, analysis with cytometry makes possible detection of disease in the bone marrow, peripheral blood or spleen, when it has not been identified by cytology. Although clinical stage V in lymphomas has traditionally been associated with a worse prognosis, this is not the case in low-grade lymphomas, with an average survival of 21 months for stages I–IV and 26 months for stage V.

In addition, it can be used to **establish whether complete remission has been achieved** at a molecular level after chemotherapy, which is associated with a better prognosis, and to predict clinical relapses of lymphomas, although this type of monitoring is still in the research phase. The potential use of specific immunotherapy for B- or T-cell lymphomas (for example, using anti-CD20 antibodies) is another reason for identification of the specific immunophenotype of these diseases.

A group of tumours where flow cytometry may have an advantage over immunohistochemistry is **histiocytic tumours**. Many of the markers used to characterise the different clinical presentations, with different prognoses and treatments, can **be detected only in fresh (such as cytometry samples) or frozen tissue**, and not in samples already fixed in formaldehyde.

## Polymerase chain reaction

Techniques based on the polymerase chain reaction (PCR) consist of the **amplification of a particular DNA fragment**, and have several applications in veterinary oncology:

- Identification of **monoclonal lymphoid populations** (mostly neoplastic) **versus polyclonal** (inflammatory or infectious), amplifying the genes that code for lymphocyte antigen receptors.
- Detection of **certain mutations important regarding the prognosis** and treatment of the patient (*KIT* mutations in mastocytomas and gastrointestinal stromal tumours).
- Evaluation of the **risk of side effects during chemotherapy** (assessing the presence of mutation in the p-glycoprotein in at-risk breeds).

## Combination of techniques

The information provided by each technique is **different and complementary**, and the use of several may be necessary for a definitive diagnosis – for example, in morphologically similar diseases such as feline inflammatory bowel disease and low-grade intestinal lymphoma. The use of immunohistochemistry in biopsies helps to differentiate whether lymphocytes are from a single population (B or T) or a mixture of both. The cloning technique **PARR (PCR for Antigen Receptor Rearrangement)** provides information about the **clonality of lymphocytes** (if they express the same or different antigen receptors). It is important to remember that, even though if in immunohistochemistry there is a uniform population of lymphocytes (for example T lymphocytes), they may be different in terms of their antigen receptors, which would indicate inflammatory disease. In a study of feline intestinal disease, the diagnosis was altered in 25% of cases (from inflammatory to lymphoma) after immunohistochemistry was performed. When analysed using both immunohistochemistry and PARR, 50% of cases diagnosed by biopsy as inflammatory were found to be lymphoma.

Another example is **KIT expression**, which can be assessed by **immunohistochemistry**, but this technique does not report on the presence or absence of mutations in the receptor, it simply indicates **whether the cell has the receptor or not**. The presence of a *KIT* mutation produces an activation of the receptor by phosphorylation, and it is **important in predicting the response to treatment** when KIT inhibitors are used. In the case of toceranib phosphate, between 60 and 91% of mastocytomas with an exon 11 *KIT* mutation respond to treatment, compared with a response of 27–31% of cases without mutation. Similar findings occur when comparing masitinib to a placebo. If there is an exon 11 mutation, survival is significantly greater when treated with masitinib, whereas in mastocytomas without mutation, there was no significant difference between cases treated with masitinib and those treated with placebo.

Of the gastrointestinal stromal tumours which express KIT, just under half have mutations in the gene. This illustrates the difference between the presence of the receptor (as detected by immunohistochemistry) and activation or mutation of that receptor. Thus, immunohistochemistry helps diagnose these tumours (differentiating them from intestinal leiomyosarcomas that do not express KIT), whilst the presence of mutation helps predict the response to KIT inhibitors.

The presence of mutations in tumour tissue can be used not only to predict the response to targeted therapies, but also as a diagnostic method. In humans, the V600E mutation in the *BRAF* gene is common in different tumours. Recently it has been described in 80% of dogs with prostate carcinoma, and in about 70% of transitional cell bladder carcinomas. In those that have a bladder tumour, the presence of mutation can be analysed in urine samples without the need for biopsy or cytology.

In addition to tumour tissue mutations, the patient may also have mutations that make them more sensitive to chemotherapy and cause greater toxicity. In some breeds (e.g. Collie) the mutation in the gene encoding the p-glycoprotein, important in the metabolism and distribution of various drugs, including cytotoxic ones, is present in more than half of cases. It is important to know whether the animal has the mutation and, if so, whether it is homozygous or heterozygous, in order to adjust the treatment dose and avoid adverse effects.

Thus, for the diagnosis of the disease and detection of mutations both in the tumour and in the patient, molecular diagnosis has more and more applications and uses in veterinary oncology.

## Clinical staging

In order to offer the most complete clinical information, once the histological, cytological or molecular diagnosis has been obtained, the **clinical stage must be established** – that is, **the extent of the primary tumour and metastatic disease (if present)**, and to evaluate the **general condition of the patient**. With these data, prognostic information and therapeutic alternatives can be offered for each case and, later on, the response to treatment can be assessed.

As a rule, the Tumour, Node, Metastasis (TNM) system is used to assess the cancer's clinical stage, and this evaluates:

- **primary tumour**
- **lymph nodes**
- **presence or absence of distant metastasis**.

To correctly establish the clinical stage, a **knowledge of the biological behaviour** of the different tumours is important – for example, that mastocytomas metastasise to the liver and spleen but not to the lungs.

On physical examination, the primary tumour is measured and regional nodes are evaluated.

The size of the primary tumour, which should be measured using a Vernier calliper, and its location provide prognostic information. For example, canine oral melanoma <2 cm has a survival time of 3 years in 54% of cases if it is located in the rostral jaw or caudal maxilla, but in 12% if it is located in another area.

Another important factor is the invasion of adjacent tissues. Thyroid carcinomas often invade blood vessels, the larynx and the trachea, making surgical treatment impossible.

Advanced imaging tests (CT and MRI) offer important information about the tumour, of both the primary lesion and potential metastases. CT is especially useful in investigation of the margins of a tumour before surgery or to plan radiotherapy treatments, while MRI is the technique of choice for central nervous system tumours. To avoid errors, it is important that these tests are interpreted by diagnostic imaging specialists.

Due to the low sensitivity in relation to the size of lymph nodes and presence of neoplasia, **these should be aspirated even if they are normal in size**, to recognise those that have metastases (Figure 2.5). It

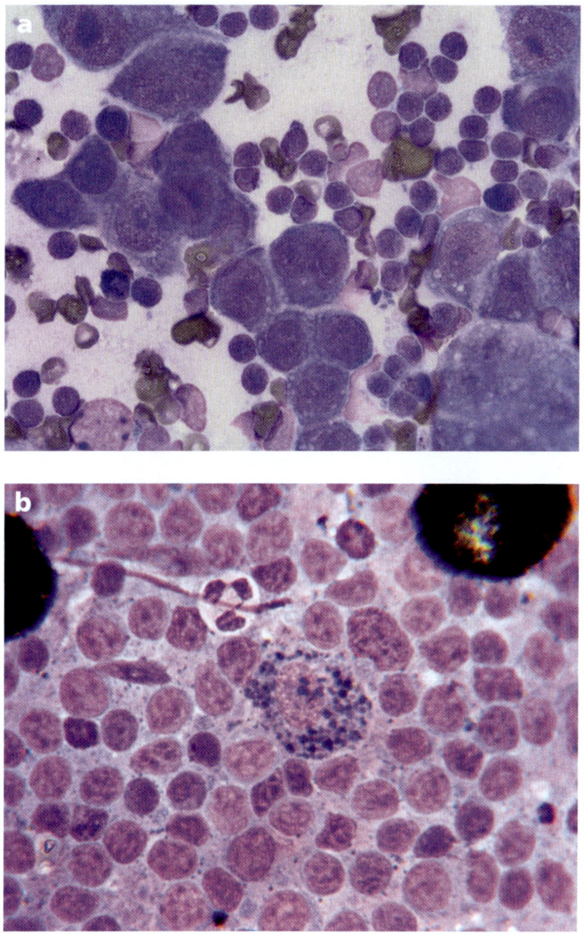


Figure 2.5. Lymph node cytology. a, With metastasis from a carcinoma. b, With metastasis from a melanoma.

is important to have a **knowledge of normal lymphatic drainage**, since it is not always the lymph node closest to the lesion. For example, the skin of the hip, tail and perineal area drains into lymph nodes that are located in the abdominal cavity, so abdominal ultrasound is necessary for their location and aspiration.

In some cases, the presence of certain cells in lymph nodes indicates the existence of metastases because these would not normally be there (for example, epithelial cells). In others, it is more difficult to differentiate between metastatic lesions and normal lymph nodes (for example, if there are mast cells).

In the case of mastocytomas, five groups have been proposed depending on the lymph node:

- normal
- reactive
- with possible metastasis
- with probable metastasis
- with certain metastasis.

Only the **last two are associated with lower survival**. The proposed cytological criteria for these are:

- **Probable metastasis**: at least one slide with >3 foci of 2–3 aggregated mast cells and/or 2 foci of >3 mast cells.
- **Certain metastasis**: presence of poorly differentiated cell aggregates, with pleomorphism, anisocytosis or anisokaryosis and/or >5 aggregates of >3 mast cells (Figure 2.6).

The presence of pulmonary metastases is evaluated by three thoracic radiographs:

- right lateral
- left lateral
- ventrodorsal.

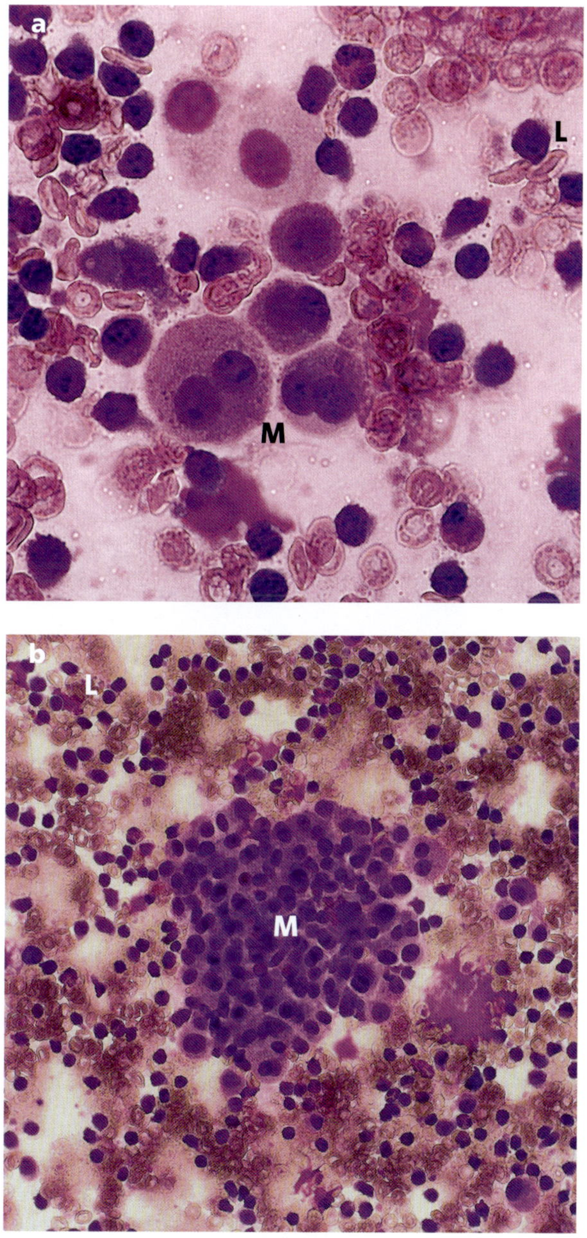


Figure 2.6a,b. Sample from a lymph node with abundant small lymphocytes (L) and mast cell aggregates (M), some of which are binucleate with anisocytosis and anisokaryosis.

**Abdominal metastases are examined using ultrasound**. Abdominal ultrasound mainly detects lesions in the liver and spleen, although it should be noted that non-neoplastic pathologies can cause **images similar to metastases**:

- **Hyperplastic nodules**, both in the liver and spleen, can be seen as hypoechoic lesions with a diameter of 0.5 cm to several centimetres.
- **Myelolipomas** are nodular echoic lesions, ranging from several millimetres to several centimetres in size, formed by cells with lipids and haematopoietic cells.
- **Extramedullary haematopoiesis** appears similar to hyperplastic nodules, such as hypoechoic nodules that can be seen in both liver and spleen.

Some of these conditions are frequent in older dogs, and therefore if during ultrasound examination there is evidence of this type of **lesion, an aspirate should be obtained** for cytology before assuming they are metastases (Figure 2.7).

In addition to the lungs and abdomen, some **tumours may metastasise to the bone** – for example, osteosarcoma (Figure 2.8) and certain carcinomas.

Once the tumour type and its reach are known, the possibilities of **treatment, cost and prognosis can be calculated**. Knowing the clinical stage at the time of diagnosis also provides a reference for assessment of response to treatment and tumour progression.

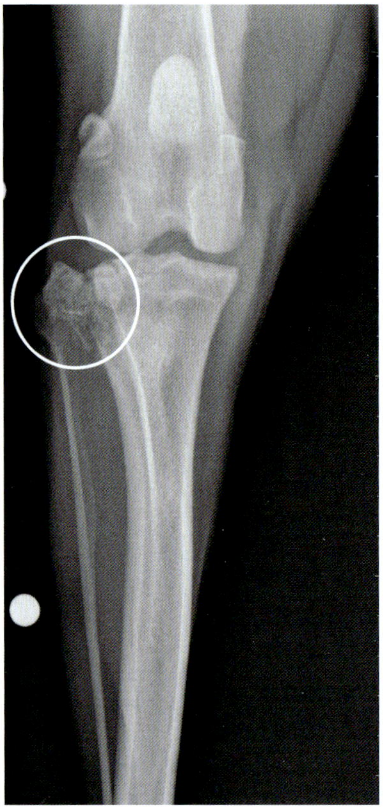

Figure 2.8. Pathological fracture (circled) in canine stifle joint secondary to metastasis from osteosarcoma of the forelimb.

The clinical staging of mammary tumours, lymphomas and soft tissue sarcomas is summarised in Textbox 2.1.

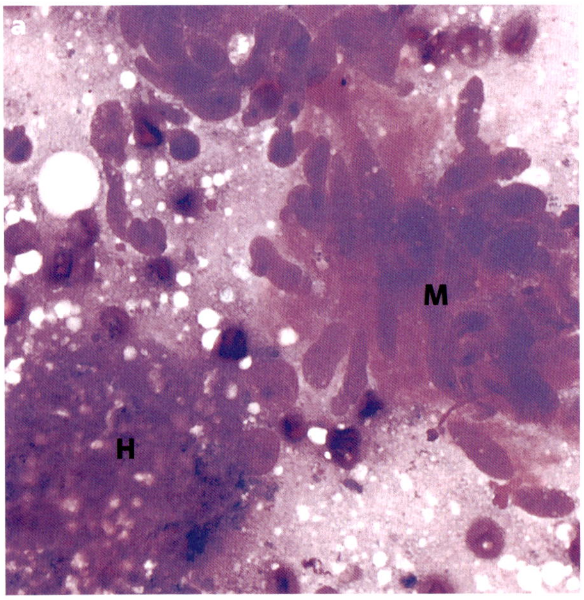


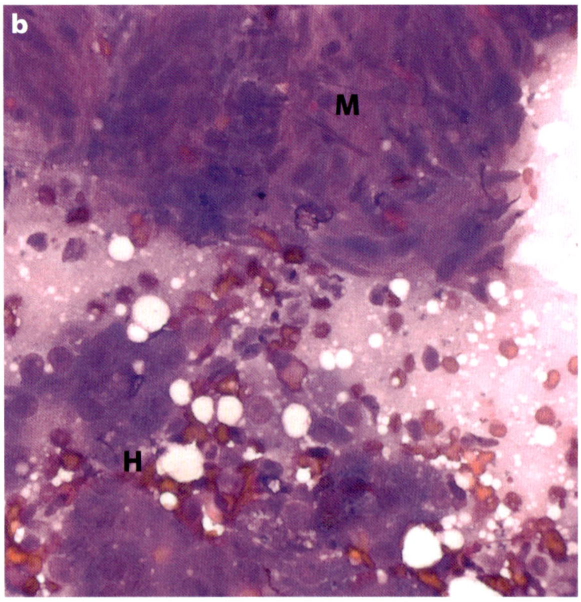


Figure 2.7a,b. Liver aspirates showing hepatocytes (H) and mesenchymal cells (M) with an oval nucleus and the presence of an extracellular matrix: hepatic metastasis of a sarcoma.

## Textbox 2.1. Clinical staging of mammary tumours, lymphomas and soft tissue sarcomas

### Clinical stages of mammary tumours

#### *Dog*

***T Primary tumour***

T1: <3 cm maximum diameter
T2: 3–5 cm maximum diameter
T3: >5 cm maximum diameter

***N Regional lymph nodes***

N0: Without metastasis (histology or FNA)
N1: With metastasis (histology or FNA)

***M Distant metastases***

M0: No evidence of distant metastasis
M1: Distant metastasis

***Clinical stages***

| | | |
|---|---|---|
| **I:** T1 | N0 | M0 |
| **II:** T2 | N0 | M0 |
| **III:** T3 | N0 | M0 |
| **IV:** Any T | N1 | M0 |
| **V:** Any T | Any N | M1 |

#### *Cat*

***T Primary tumour***

T1: <2 cm maximum diameter
T2: 2–3 cm maximum diameter
T3: >3 cm maximum diameter

***N Regional lymph nodes***

N0: Without metastasis (histology or FNA)
N1: With metastasis (histology or FNA)

***M Distant metastases***

M0: No evidence of distant metastasis
M1: Distant metastasis

***Clinical stages***

| | | |
|---|---|---|
| **I:** T1 | N0 | M0 |
| **II:** T2 | N0 | M0 |
| **III:** T1,2 | N1 | M0 |
| **IV:** T3 | N0, N1 | M0 |
| **V:** Any T | Any N | M1 |

### Clinical stages of lymphoma (World Health Organization)

#### *Anatomical location*

A: generalised
B: digestive
C: thymus
D: skin
E: leukaemia (true*)
F: others (including solitary kidney tumours).

#### *Stage (includes anatomical location)*

**I:** condition limited to a single lymph node or lymphoid tissue of a single organ
**II:** condition affecting several lymph nodes in a region
**III:** generalised involvement of lymph nodes
**IV:** hepatic and/or splenic involvement (with or without stage III disease)
**V:** condition affecting bone marrow, blood and/or other organs (with or without disease in stages I to IV)

* only blood and bone marrow affected.

***Sub-stage***

**a:** without clinical signs
**b:** with clinical signs.

## Clinical stages of soft tissue sarcomas in dogs

### *T Primary tumour*

T1: <5 cm maximum diameter
- T1a: superficial
- T1b: deep

T2: >5 cm maximum diameter
- T2a: superficial
- T2b: deep tumour.

| Stage | Tumor | Node | Metastasis | Grade |
|---|---|---|---|---|
| I | Any T | N0 | M0 | I–II |
| II | T1a-1b, T2a | N0 | M0 | III |
| III | T2b | N0 | M0 | III |
| IV | Any T | N1 | M0 | I–III |
| V | Any T | Any N | M1 | I–III |

### *N Lymph node*

- N0: no lymph node metastasis
- N1: with lymph node metastasis.

### *M Distant metastases*

- M0: without distant metastasis
- M1: with distant metastasis.

Once the diagnosis and clinical stage have been established, treatment options should be discussed with the owner:

- For **localised tumours, surgery** offers the best option to control the tumour.
- In **systemic or metastatic tumours, chemotherapy or tyrosine kinase** inhibitors may be needed.
- Access to techniques such as **radiotherapy or electrochemotherapy** offers new possibilities for oncological treatment.

## Oncological surgery

### *Introduction*

The type and degree of tumour strongly influence the choice of appropriate surgical method. The **first surgery represents the best chance of a cure** and, if not successful, it can compromise local control of the local disease and even survival. So ideally a diagnosis should be made before an excisional surgical biopsy.

To achieve complete resection of the tumour, a knowledge of its **margins** and whether or not there are **metastases** is important, and therefore **clinical staging** of the patient should be performed prior to surgery as indicated above.

After surgery, in order to determine whether additional treatments are needed, histology is crucial to **check that resection is complete**. When resection is incomplete, the possibility of alternative treatments should be considered rather than waiting for recurrences or metastasis.

With the information obtained from biopsy and the pre-surgical clinical stage, together with good technique, surgery is the treatment that gives the highest cure rate in cancer patients. It is important to consult with a specialist before ruling out surgical treatment, even in advanced cases. Even when cure is not possible, **palliative surgery can provide relief from symptoms** and it is the clinician's obligation to inform the owner of the different options, including referral of the case to a specialist.

In older patients, **other conditions that may affect the decision** about treatment and survival time should be taken into account – for example, amputation due to osteosarcoma in an animal with osteoarthritis in the other limbs. Equally, an animal should not be denied treatment purely due to age.

Although techniques unique to oncological surgery have been described, such as mandibulectomies or maxillectomies, resection of the nasal plane, etc., the current trend is to **operate on small tumours** rather than performing large-scale surgeries on advanced tumours, which are frequently difficult to control. More surgery does not mean better surgery, as has been demonstrated in human and canine mammary tumours, where results obtained are similar using aggressive or conservative surgeries. It should also be remembered that surgery is no longer the only possible treatment for a tumour, and **multidisciplinary treatment is essential in many cases**. A clear example of this is canine osteosarcoma, where surgical treatment does not influence survival and chemotherapy does. In surgeries that affect the morphology of the animal, it is important to inform the owner about the appearance it will have after the procedure, if possible showing examples of the results of similar surgeries (Figure 2.9).

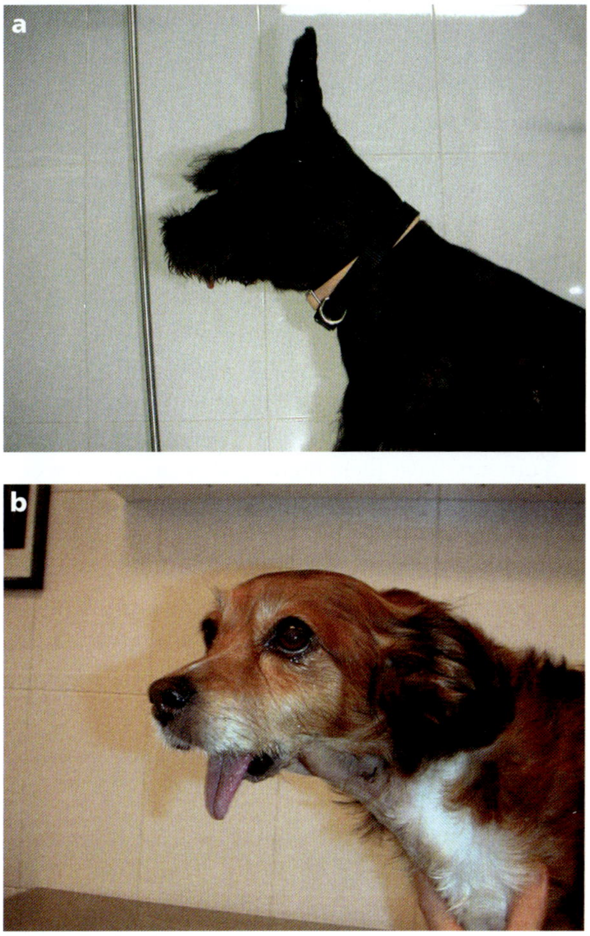

Figure 2.9. Appearance of two dogs following a rostral mandibulectomy, due to melanoma (a) and fibrosarcoma (b).

## Principles

The first step is to define the goal of surgery. It can be performed to:

- Determine the type and extent of a tumour (diagnostic).
- Alleviate clinical signs and increase quality of life (palliative).
- Try to excise the tumour completely (curative).

Occasionally:

- Treat complications of chemotherapy, such as ulcer due to extravasation.
- Implant a catheter for nutrition.
- Administer cytotoxic drugs.

## Diagnostic surgery

When performing a biopsy, the site should be carefully chosen so it does not hinder future cancer treatment. **The site of the biopsy should be able to be resected with the tumour**. All techniques have uses, advantages and disadvantages.

Excisional biopsy should be used in cases where treatment will not be affected by the particular type of tumour (for example, benign skin tumours) or in those in which a second intervention is possible (for example, if there is incomplete removal of the tumour). It should not be the first choice in areas where a second intervention is not possible, such as the distal parts of the extremities.

Biopsy complications:

- absence of diagnosis
- wound infection
- compromised surgical resection due to poor choice of biopsy site.

## Palliative surgery

This is an attempt to **improve the patient's quality of life**, but not necessarily to extend it. The expected morbidity, together with the increase in quality trying to be achieved, should be considered, so that the technique opted for is not worse than the disease. A difficult decision for a cancer surgeon is to know when not to operate.

It may be indicated in fistulised, infected mammary tumours, or to control pain in dogs with a pathological fracture of an osteosarcoma, even if it has been decided not to use adjuvant chemotherapy.

## Curative surgery

Curative surgery aims to try to **resect the tumour completely**, during the first surgery. If this is not achieved, more aggressive procedures and surgeries that involve greater complications may be needed in the future.

In tumours in which an incomplete resection is expected and additional treatment with radiotherapy is needed, the use of vascular clips is recommended to limit the surgical field and plan radiotherapy treatment (Figure 2.10).

## Surgery with special applications

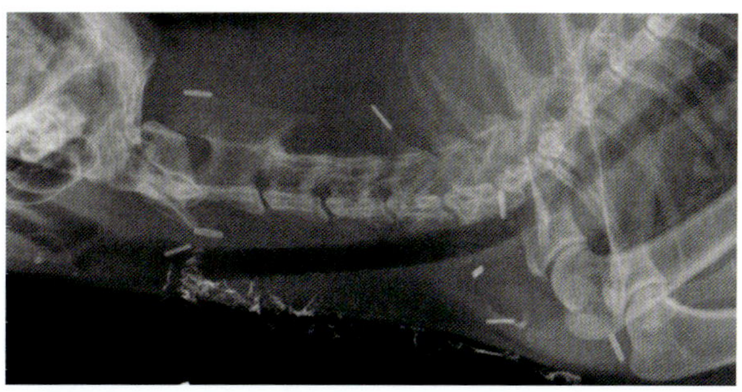

Figure 2.10. Vascular clips used to delineate the surgical field after removal of a melanoma.

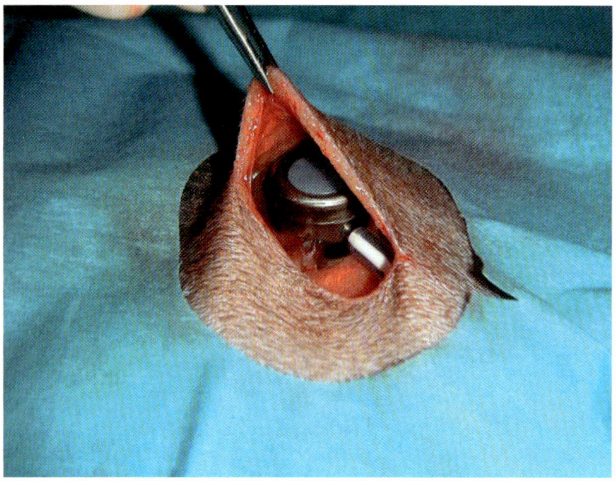

**Figure 2.11.** Pleural drainage tube, with a permanent portal surgically implanted into subcutaneous tissue. Using this portal, pleural effusion can be drained and intra-cavitary chemotherapy administered.

This group includes procedures aimed at implanting reservoirs (to achieve permanent venous access or to drain fluid from body cavities), and brachytherapy application systems (especially in cases of sarcoma) (Figure 2.11).

## Chemotherapy

### *Guidelines*

Chemotherapy is indicated in the following cases:

- **Haematological tumours sensitive to chemotherapy**: for example, canine lymphoma which, untreated, has a predicted survival time of 6–8 weeks and, treated with chemotherapy, of about one year.
- As **adjunctive treatment after localised treatments**: surgery or radiotherapy to prevent local recurrence or to delay the development of metastases – for example, in haemangiosarcoma, osteosarcoma, certain carcinomas and high-grade mastocytomas. In osteosarcoma, survival time with surgery is tripled when chemotherapy is added.
- As a **preoperative treatment** to try to decrease the size of the tumour (neoadjuvant chemotherapy).
- As a **palliative treatment** in metastatic or inoperable disease.

### *Cell cycle and tumour kinetics*

To understand the mechanism of action and effect of chemotherapy on normal and tumour tissues, it is necessary to have some knowledge of **cell and tumour kinetics**. In general, normal and tumour cells follow a similar cycle that includes four phases:

- Phase G1. **Enzymes** necessary for DNA synthesis are produced.
- Phase S. **DNA** is synthesised.
- Phase G2. **Proteins** are synthesised.
- Phase M. **Mitosis** occurs.

After mitosis, the cell may **start the cycle again**, either with a new division or entering a resting phase (G0). The mitotic count measures the percentage of dividing cells in a tissue (normal or tumoral). Since **chemotherapy primarily affects dividing cells**, tissues with a high mitotic count are more sensitive to chemotherapy than those with a low mitotic rate (Figure 2.12).

Tumours have their **highest mitotic count when they are too small to be detected** by means of imaging or physical examination, and this **rate decreases as tumour size increases**, and therefore tumours **respond better to chemotherapy when they are small**. There are exceptions such as lymphomas, which maintain a very high rate of cell division and, despite the large size

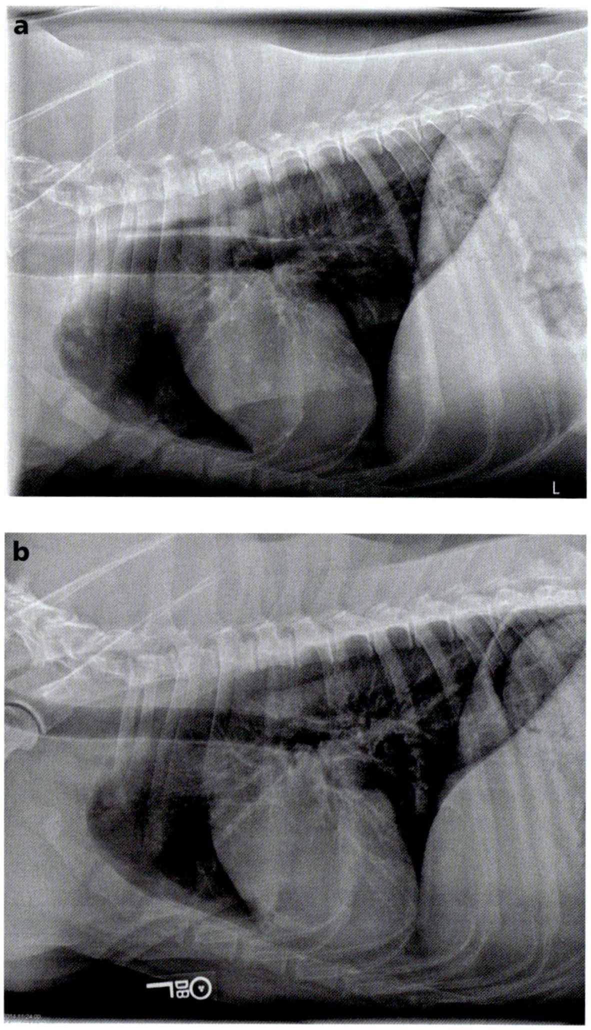

**Figure 2.12.** Radiographs from a dog with a high-grade soft tissue sarcoma, with pulmonary metastasis before chemotherapy (a) and after chemotherapy, in complete remission (b).

of the lymph nodes at the time of diagnosis, respond very well to chemotherapy. In general, the only normal tissues having a high mitotic index are the epithelium of the intestinal villi and the bone marrow, which explains why these tissues are sensitive to chemotherapy.

The **effects of chemotherapy follow logarithmic kinetics** – that is, they **kill a percentage of cells** rather than a constant number. Doses are usually given at regular intervals, determined by the **time needed by normal tissue** (gastrointestinal and bone marrow) **to recover**, but tumour cells that survive each dose proliferate between treatment sessions. As it has a **dose-dependent effect**, if the dose is decreased the effectiveness of the treatment against the tumour decreases, the side effects decrease and the same occurs if the interval between doses is increased. A reduction by 20% of the dose can mean a 50% decrease in efficacy. It is therefore important to adjust the dose as much as possible, without reducing it if not essential, and to stick to the timeframes established in the protocols.

## Dosification of medications

Dosages of cytotoxic drugs are generally **calculated using an estimate of the body surface area**, which is assumed to be proportional to the metabolism of the animal. However, this system can produce overdoses in small animals.

In general, **combinations of drugs have been shown to be more effective** than the use of just one (exceptions to this are vincristine in transmissible venereal tumour and carboplatin in osteosarcoma). These combinations should follow some basic rules:

- Use drugs that have shown efficacy against the tumour separately.
- Use drugs with different mechanisms of action.
- Do not use drugs with overlapping toxicities.
- Use the maximum tolerated dose, as often as possible.
- Use drugs whose mechanisms of action and possible interactions are known.

## General treatment principles

Although the general indications of chemotherapy have already been mentioned, a number of **factors must be taken into account** when deciding on treatment with chemotherapy.

### Factors related to the patient

A **general evaluation of the patient** (age, presence or absence of systemic diseases, functional changes, etc.) directly influences the choice of treatment for a particular tumour. For example, although amputation (plus chemotherapy) is the treatment of choice in dogs with osteosarcoma, it may not be an option in animals with osteoarthrosis or neurological deficits in other extremities.

### Factors related to the owner

Attitude to treatment, tolerance of side effects, availability for necessary visits to the practice and the cost of treatments should be discussed with the owner.

### Factors related to the disease

The main objective is to cure the disease, but when chemotherapy is used (without surgery) this is rarely achieved. If the chances of cure are low, the **goal is to maintain a good quality of life** and try to achieve remission of the tumour. Different clinical stages of the same tumour (for example, the presence or absence of metastatic disease) require different approaches to treatment but, in general, early diagnosis and treatment increase the chances of cure.

## Complications and side effects

As mentioned, **chemotherapy affects dividing cells** but it does so in a **non-selective manner**, so normal tissues in the body with a high rate of dividing cells are also affected. In fact, the chemotherapeutic dosage is limited by the tolerance of the normal tissues that are affected (digestive and bone marrow). It is important to explain to the owner what effects may appear and to what extent.

### Gastrointestinal alterations

Gastrointestinal effects during chemotherapy treatments (anorexia, vomiting and diarrhoea) are usually mild or moderate, and respond to symptomatic treatment.

With an awareness of the effects of the drugs used, the appearance of side effects should be anticipated:

- Cisplatin produces vomiting immediately, so **preventive anti-emetics** should always be administered.
- Doxorubicin takes 3–4 days to produce digestive effects, whose intensity decreases with administration of **maropitant**, so its administration is therefore recommended whenever this cytostatic is administered.

### Bone marrow involvement

Another tissue affected by chemotherapy is the **bone marrow**, in which toxicity can also be foreseen with knowledge of the physiology of blood cells.

**Neutrophils** have a transition time in bone marrow, since they are generated until they are released into peripheral blood, already mature, at approximately 6 days, and their half-life in blood is only a few hours. If production is interrupted due to chemotherapy, those stored in the marrow will continue to be released so that their **lowest level (nadir) will occur 6–7 days after chemotherapy administration**. Due to their longer half-life, platelets present their nadir 10 days after treatment. Effects on erythrocytes will be seen 3 months after treatment.

Generally, the number of neutrophils is what limits the chemotherapeutic dose that can be used but monitoring of platelet levels is also important. Anaemia secondary to chemotherapy that requires changes in the doses of the drugs is rarely seen.

It is also necessary to be aware of the specific side effects of each drug to try to prevent them or, if necessary, treat them as soon as they occur. The most common are:

- cystitis with cyclophosphamide
- cardiotoxicity with doxorubicin
- dermatitis or necrosis due to extravasation of vincristine (Figure 2.13) or doxorubicin.

## Supportive treatment

In many cases the goal of chemotherapy is to **achieve tumour remission** while maintaining a **good quality of life**. To do this it is essential to use treatments to avoid or reduce the side effects of cytotoxic drugs, which can directly affect the quality of the patient's life – for example:

- **Anti-emetics** in cases where there is nausea or vomiting (or preventatively, when they are expected).
- **Stomach protectants** when corticosteroids are administered.
- **Antibiotics in myelosuppressive protocols**, since the prophylactic use of antibiotics decreases the number and severity of infections secondary to chemotherapeutically induced neutropenia.

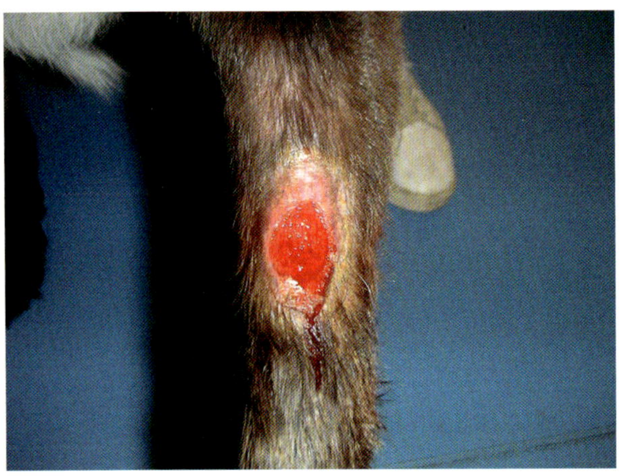

**Figure 2.13.** Ulcer secondary to vincristine extravasation.

## Molecular therapy

Increasing knowledge of the molecular pathways of tumour cells has allowed the development of specific drugs for molecular changes present in tumour cells.

**Protein kinases** are fundamental proteins in the transduction signal of normal cells. Normally, these are activated in the presence of specific growth factors **favouring cell proliferation**. In some tumours, due to a mutation, these **protein kinases are activated autonomously** (without the need for growth factor), producing an **uncontrolled proliferation** of tumoral tissue. Similar to what has previously been mentioned with regard to cyclooxygenase, the mere expression of these proteins does not mean that the tumour depends on them for growth, nor that inhibitors will be effective.

In veterinary oncology, **KIT is the receptor** about which most is known. At the end of the 1990s, Dr Cheryl London described how some mastocytomas had mutations that kept the receptor active and showed that the **KIT inhibitor toceranib (Palladia®)** was more effective in cases where the tumour was mutated than in those where it was not, which led to the approval of toceranib for use in mast cell tumours. Similar findings showed that efficacy of the other inhibitor approved for veterinary use, **masitinib (Masivet®)**, depended on the presence of a KIT mutation.

**In addition to mast cells, KIT is present in other cells**, which explains some of the side effects of using these inhibitors. In the **intestine**, cells of Cajal, which act as a pacemaker when regulating intestinal motility, express KIT normally and their function can be affected with the use of inhibitors. Thus, **gastrointestinal side effects**, from decreased appetite to vomiting or diarrhoea, are the most frequent with these medications. Precisely because of the presence of KIT receptors in the cells of Cajal, tumours that originate from them, the so-called gastrointestinal stromal tumours, can be treated with KIT inhibitors.

Other cells where KIT is found normally include **melanocytes and haematopoietic precursors** (in fact, the KIT growth factor is the growth factor for stem cells, stem cell factor, SCF). In veterinary medicine, however, it is not common for melanomas to have a *KIT* mutation, so the use of KIT inhibitors has not been shown to be **beneficial in cases of canine melanoma**.

Currently the recommended **dose of toceranib is 2.5–3 mg/kg three times a week (Monday, Wednesday and Friday)**, as this achieves therapeutic levels and decreases the side effects described with the dose indicated on the instruction leaflet for the medication *(3.25 mg/kg every 48 hours)*. The most frequently observed **side effects at doses of 2.5–2.8 mg/kg** were:

- digestive:
  - anorexia
  - vomiting
  - diarrhoea
- neutropenia (low-grade)
- increase in arterial blood pressure
- proteinuria.

It is necessary to monitor these parameters during treatment.

**Toceranib phosphate** has also shown efficacy in tumours not related to mast cells:

- anal sac carcinoma
- thyroid carcinoma
- nasal cavity carcinoma.

For the first two above, the treatment of choice is **surgery** and, for the latter, **radiotherapy**, but if it is **not possible or the patient has metastases, toceranib** can be used as a last resort. The responses obtained in these cases vary from complete remission to stabilisation of disease, through partial remission (Figure 2.14). In most cases the mechanism that explains the response to treatment is not known, but a percentage of these tumours has active (phosphorylated) receptors that are inhibited by toceranib, which may explain its efficacy.

Likewise, clinical trials conducted in dogs with **osteosarcoma or haemangiosarcoma** have shown that, after completing the usual treatment (surgery and carboplatin in osteosarcoma, surgery and doxorubicin in haemangiosarcoma), the use of **toceranib does not improve survival**. In both cases, studies looked at whether toceranib prolonged disease-free time (from initial treatment until the disease progressed) or survival if used as maintenance therapy. In neither of the two trials was it evident that this drug improved the parameters studied.

Recently, research has begun into **the use of toceranib combined with other cytotoxic drugs** such as vinblastine, lomustine and doxorubicin. A common finding in these studies is the need to **decrease the dose of intravenous drugs**, with neutropenia as the limiting side effect.

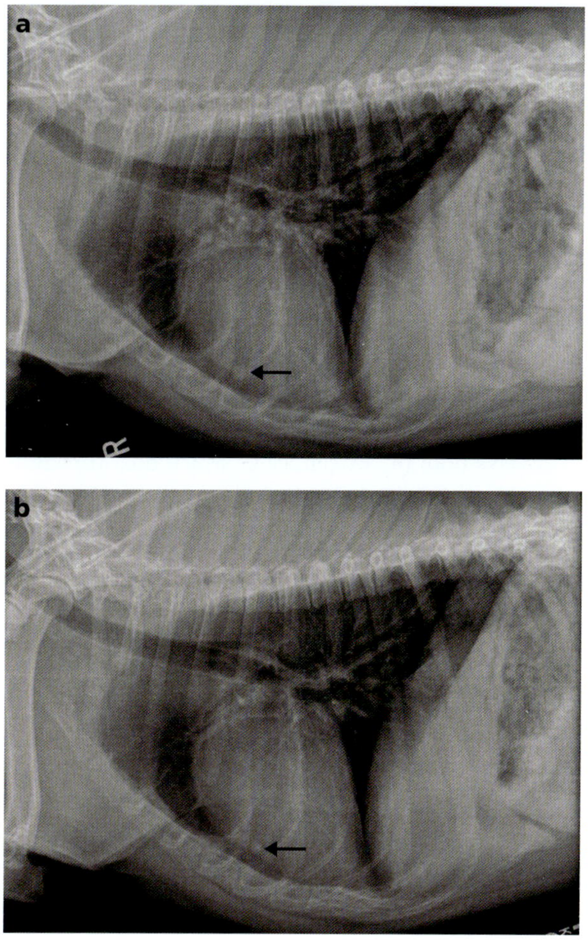


**Figure 2.14.** Pulmonary metastasis in a bitch with anal gland carcinoma. a, At the time of diagnosis. b, 11 months later, in partial remission.

## *Safe handling of cytotoxic drugs*

Continuous exposure to cytotoxic drugs can **pose a risk to the staff that handle them**. If there is someone on the clinical team who may be pregnant, it is important that they **avoid contact with these medications (and the faeces and urine of patients treated with them)**. Therefore, it is important to follow a series of recommendations when handling these treatments.

Ideally, chemotherapy should be prepared in a **vertical laminar flow cabinet** and with a closed system. A closed system and personal protective equipment should be used to prepare and administer chemotherapy. Capsules should never be split, as their content is not distributed evenly and also dust is released that could be inhaled.

All chemotherapy material (drip kits, syringes, absorbent pads, etc.) must be disposed of in **specific containers for cytotoxic agents**.

A knowledge of the drugs and their effects is necessary, and also an individualised assessment of each case to optimise results, from both clinical aspects and owner satisfaction.

Communication by the veterinarian with the owners, their participation in the treatment and monitoring of the animal and the continuous follow-up of each case improve evolution in veterinary oncology patients, so that on many occasions tumours are seen as simply another chronic disease.

## Administration protocols

### Doxorubicin protocol (Table 2.2)

**Administer doxorubicin only if the animal is clinically well**. In case of fever, lack of appetite, vomiting or diarrhoea, do not administer chemotherapy. If, after the previous dose, the animal experienced vomiting, diarrhoea or serious side effects, consider reducing the dose. Consulting a veterinary oncologist is recommended.

Always note the extremity in which doxorubicin is administered.

Textbox 2.2 gives detailed instructions on doxorubicin administration.

### CHOP protocol (Wisconsin-Madison 25; Table 2.3)

**CHOP** is the acronym for a chemotherapy regimen used in the treatment of non-Hodgkin lymphoma. **CHOP** consists of **C**yclophosphamide, **H**ydroxydaunorubicin, **O**ncovin and **P**rednisone.

**Administer only if the patient is clinically well**. In case of fever, lack of appetite, vomiting or diarrhoea, do not administer chemotherapy. If after the previous dose the animal has experienced vomiting, diarrhoea or serious side effects, consider reducing the dose. Consulting a veterinary oncologist is recommended.

Always note the extremity in which vincristine and doxorubicin are administered.

### Carboplatin protocol for dogs (Table 2.4)

**Administer only if the patient is clinically well**. In case of fever, lack of appetite, vomiting or diarrhoea, chemotherapy should be delayed. If after the previous dose the animal experienced vomiting, diarrhoea or serious side effects, consider reducing the dose. Consulting a veterinary oncologist is recommended.

## Radiotherapy

In human oncology, a large proportion of patients **receive radiotherapy as part of their multimodal treatment**. Although in veterinary medicine access to these techniques has been more limited, it is increasingly common for these facilities at specialist veterinary referral centres. It is usually used to **treat nasal cavity or central nervous system tumours**, where radiotherapy is the main or only treatment, and tumours such as soft tissue sarcomas, which may be

Table 2.2. Doxorubicin protocol.

| Day(s) | Date | kg | Body surface area ($m^2$) | Medication | Total dose | Observations: toxicity, vein used |
|---|---|---|---|---|---|---|
| 1 | | | | Complete blood count<br>Doxorubicin 30 mg/$m^2$ IV*<br>Maropitant 1 mg/kg IV | | |
| 2–4 | | | | Maropitant 2 mg/kg VO | | |
| 7 | Perform blood count to check for neutropenia** | | | | | |
| 21 | | | | Complete blood count***<br>Doxorubicin 30 mg/$m^2$ IV*<br>Maropitant 1 mg/kg IV | | |
| 22–24 | | | | Maropitant 2 mg/kg VO | | |
| 42 | | | | Complete blood count<br>Doxorubicin 30 mg/$m^2$ IV*<br>Maropitant 1 mg/kg IV | | |
| 43–45 | | | | Maropitant 2 mg/kg VO | | |
| 63 | | | | Complete blood count<br>Doxorubicin 30 mg/$m^2$ IV*<br>Maropitant 1 mg/kg IV | | |
| 64–66 | | | | Maropitant 2 mg/kg VO | | |

Before administering further doses, consult a veterinary oncologist about the risk of cardiotoxicity.
* For dogs <15 kg, use 1 mg/kg.
** If neutropenia is evident one week after the first dose, consider administering prophylactic antibiotic. Consulting a veterinary oncologist is recommended.
*** Check neutrophils and platelets. If < 1.500 neutrophils/ul or 50,000 platelets/ul, delay chemotherapy administration and consult a veterinary oncologist.

## Textbox 2.2. Instructions for doxorubicin administration

**Doxorubicin should be administered intravenously**. Any extravasation can produce severe side effects. To avoid these, it should be administered only if there is complete certainty that the intravenous catheter works perfectly. The use of gloves and protective material is essential. **Pregnant women should not administer chemotherapy**.

1. Clip and clean the area where the **intravenous catheter** will be inserted.
2. Use the **longest possible catheter** for the patient to be treated.
3. Place the catheter and secure it. If it does not enter without resistance on the first attempt and it is necessary to redirect several times, use another vein.
4. Once placed and fixed, **administer a saline bolus (1 ml/kg) with a syringe**. If there is resistance or signs of extravasation, rule out that route. Aspirate and see whether blood comes out, to check that the path is permeable.
5. The use of **closed chemotherapy delivery systems** is recommended to minimise exposure to cytostatic drugs (Figure 2.15). In this way, if the patient moves, the intravenous catheter is less likely to move.

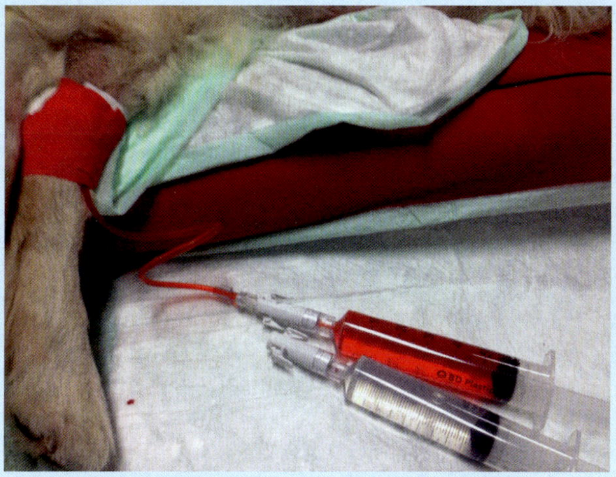

**Figure 2.15.** Cap with injection point and butterfly for administration of doxorubicin.

6. Once fixed and the permeability has been checked several times (blood comes out when aspirating, saline goes in without any resistance and without extravasation at the end of the catheter), **doxorubicin administration** can be started.
7. **Check the dose** that has been prescribed for the patient (usually this is 30 mg/m$^2$ for dogs >15 kg and 1 mg/kg for those <15 kg). If the patient is a breed that is at **high risk of MDR mutation (Collie, Australian cattle dog or Shetland sheepdog), do not administer doxorubicin** and consult a veterinary oncologist.
8. **Dilute each mg of doxorubicin in 2 ml of saline**.
9. **Administer the dose over 30 minutes**, regularly checking that blood comes out when suctioning and that it goes in without resistance. In the author's practice, manual administration is used without infusion pumps. Although some pump models are sensitive to an increase in infusion pressure, others may initially continue with the infusion even if the catheter has been moved.
10. Although the use of **antihistamines** is not necessary before treatment is started, if signs of an anaphylactic reaction (pruritus, facial oedema, cutaneous erythema, wheals, vomiting or diarrhoea) are observed, administration should be paused and **diphenhydramine (3–4 mg/kg IM) and/or dexamethasone (0.1 mg/kg IV) administered** and, once the reaction has calmed down, the infusion should be continued at a slower rate.
11. Upon completion of the treatment, the **circuit should be cleaned with saline** and the catheter removed and discarded along with other cytotoxic residues, in the appropriate container.

Table 2.3. CHOP protocol.

| Week | Date | kg | Sc ($m^2$) | K | Medication | Total dose | Observations: toxicity |
|---|---|---|---|---|---|---|---|
| 1 | | | | | Vincristine 0.5–0.7 mg/$m^2$ IV<br>Prednisone 2 mg/kg SID VO* | | |
| 2 | | | | | Cyclophosphamide 200–250 mg/$m^2$ VO**<br>Prednisone 1.5 mg/kg BID VO | | |
| 3 | | | | | Vincristine 0.5–0.7 mg/$m^2$ IV<br>Prednisone 1 mg/kg BID VO | | |
| 4 | | | | | Doxorubicin 30 mg/$m^2$ IV***<br>Prednisone 0.5 mg/kg BID VO<br>Maropitant 1 mg/kg IV | | |
| Maropitant 2 mg/kg VO on days 2–4 after doxorubicin | | | | | | | |
| 6 | | | | | Vincristine 0.5–0.7 mg/$m^2$ IV | | |
| 7 | | | | | Cyclophosphamide 200–250 mg/$m^2$ VO** | | |
| 8 | | | | | Vincristine 0.5–0.7 mg/$m^2$ IV | | |
| 9 | | | | | Doxorubicin 30 mg/$m^2$ IV***<br>Maropitant 1 mg/kg IV | | |
| Maropitant 2 mg/kg PO on days 2–4 after doxorubicin | | | | | | | |
| 11 | | | | | Vincristine 0.5-–0.7 mg/$m^2$ IV | | |
| 13 | | | | | Cyclophosphamide 200–250 mg/$m^2$ VO** | | |
| 15 | | | | | Vincristine 0.5–0.7 mg/$m^2$ IV | | |
| 17 | | | | | Doxorubicin 30 mg/$m^2$ IV***<br>Maropitant 1 mg/kg IV | | |
| Maropitant 2 mg/kg VO on days 2–4 after doxorubicin | | | | | | | |
| 19 | | | | | Vincristine 0.5–0.7 mg/$m^2$ IV | | |
| 21 | | | | | Cyclophosphamide 200–250 mg/$m^2$ VO** | | |
| 23 | | | | | Vincristine 0.5–0.7 mg/$m^2$ IV | | |
| 25 | | | | | Doxorubicin 30 mg/$m^2$ IV***<br>Maropitant 1 mg/kg IV | | |
| Maropitant 2 mg/kg VO on days 2–4 after doxorubicin | | | | | | | |

* While administering corticosteroids, add omeprazole once a day, in the morning, after fasting.
** Adjust to a whole number of tablets (cannot be split) and divide the total dose over two days to reduce the incidence of sterile haemorrhagic cystitis. If it develops despite this, change from cyclophosphamide to chlorambucil (Leukeran, 2 mg) at a dose of 1.4 mg/kg VO.
*** If the dog weighs <15 kg, the doxorubicin dose should be 1 mg/kg IV.

treated treated with surgery and adjuvant radiotherapy to achieve better control.

Depending on **the purpose of the treatment**, radiotherapy is either **definitive** (or with curative intention) or **palliative**. The former tries to control the tumour in the long term, while the latter focuses on trying to reduce the symptoms associated with the tumour, such as the pain caused by the tumour affecting the bone.

The **mechanism of action** of radiotherapy is due to **DNA damage**, which occurs when ionising radiation pulls electrons from their orbit around the atom. This atom can directly hit the DNA molecule damaging it (**direct damage**) or hit water molecules producing OH radicals, which in turn damage DNA (**indirect damage**).

As with chemotherapy, the impact of treatment on normal tissues, close to the irradiated tumour, is a limiting factor. To minimise these side effects, two strategies can be used.

The most frequent is **fractionation of the total dose**. This maximises effects on tumoral tissue and minimises side effects on normal tissues. This is because normal tissue has a greater ability to repair non-lethal cell damage than tumoral tissue.

In certain locations, such as for pituitary tumours, modern radiotherapy equipment can administer a **high dose of radiation focused** on the tumour, which does not affect surrounding tissues, without the need to fractionate treatment.

**Effects of radiation therapy on healthy tissues can be acute or chronic**, depending on the type of treatment used and the tissue affected.

Table 2.4. Carboplatin protocol for dogs.

| Day | Date | Kg | Sc ($m^2$) | Medication | Total dose | Observations: toxicity, vein used |
|---|---|---|---|---|---|---|
| 1 | | | | Complete blood count, BUN and creatinine<br>Carboplatin 300 mg/$m^2$ IV*<br>Maropitant 1 mg/kg IV | | |
| 2–4 | | | | Maropitant 2 mg/kg VO | | |
| 10 | | | | Perform blood count to check for neutropenia** | | |
| 21 | | | | Complete blood count, BUN and creatinine***<br>Carboplatin 300 mg/$m^2$ IV*<br>Maropitant 1 mg/kg IV | | |
| 22–24 | | | | Maropitant 2 mg/kg VO | | |
| 42 | | | | Complete blood count, BUN and creatinine***<br>Carboplatin 300 mg/$m^2$ IV*<br>Maropitant 1 mg/kg IV | | |
| 43–45 | | | | Maropitant 2 mg/kg PO | | |
| 63 | | | | Evaluate response<br>Complete blood count, BUN and creatinine***<br>Carboplatin 300 mg/$m^2$ IV*<br>Maropitant 1 mg/kg IV | | |
| 64–66 | | | | Maropitant 2 mg/kg VO | | |

For osteosarcoma:
Perform thoracic radiographs (3 views) every 3 months.
Do not administer metronomic chemotherapy during the follow-up.
Consult with an oncologist when metastases are detected.
* Administer intravenously, diluted in saline over about 10 minutes.
** If there is neutropenia one week after the first dose, consider administering prophylactic antibiotic.
Consulting a veterinary oncologist is recommended.
*** Check neutrophils and platelets. If <1500 neutrophils/μl or 50,000 platelets/u μl, delay chemotherapy administration and consult a veterinary oncologist. If there is an increase in BUN or creatinine, consult a veterinary oncologist before administration.

Tissues with a **high tissue turnover rate** (skin and mucous membranes) show **acute side effects** with definitive treatments (fractionated) and, although these can be a nuisance for the patient, they have a limited duration and resolve within a few weeks of having completed treatment. Acute side effects include, among others, various degrees of:

- dry and moist dermatitis (Figure 2.16)
- mucositis
- conjunctivitis
- colitis.

**Chronic effects are more frequent with palliative treatments**, affect tissues with a slower growth rate (such as bone or connective tissue) and take months or years to appear. However, once they occur, they are permanent. These may include:

- alopecia and changes in hair colour (Figure 2.17)
- fibrosis
- bone necrosis
- fistula formation.

In order to administer the maximum dose to tumour tissue and the minimum possible to the surrounding tissues, these tissues should be delineated and a treatment plan established. For the most advanced planning, CT images are used and the animal should be placed in the same position for administration of the different fractions. Positioning systems can be vacuum mattresses or those that combine dental moulds with thermoplastic masks, which hold the patient in the same position as the planning CT is performed (identifying the tumour and the risk tissues around it) and for each of the treatment fractions (Figure 2.18).

With these treatments a survival time of up to 2 years can be achieved for nasal tumours, although the response to treatment depends on the clinical stage:

- Stage I, 23 months
- Stage IV, around 6 months.

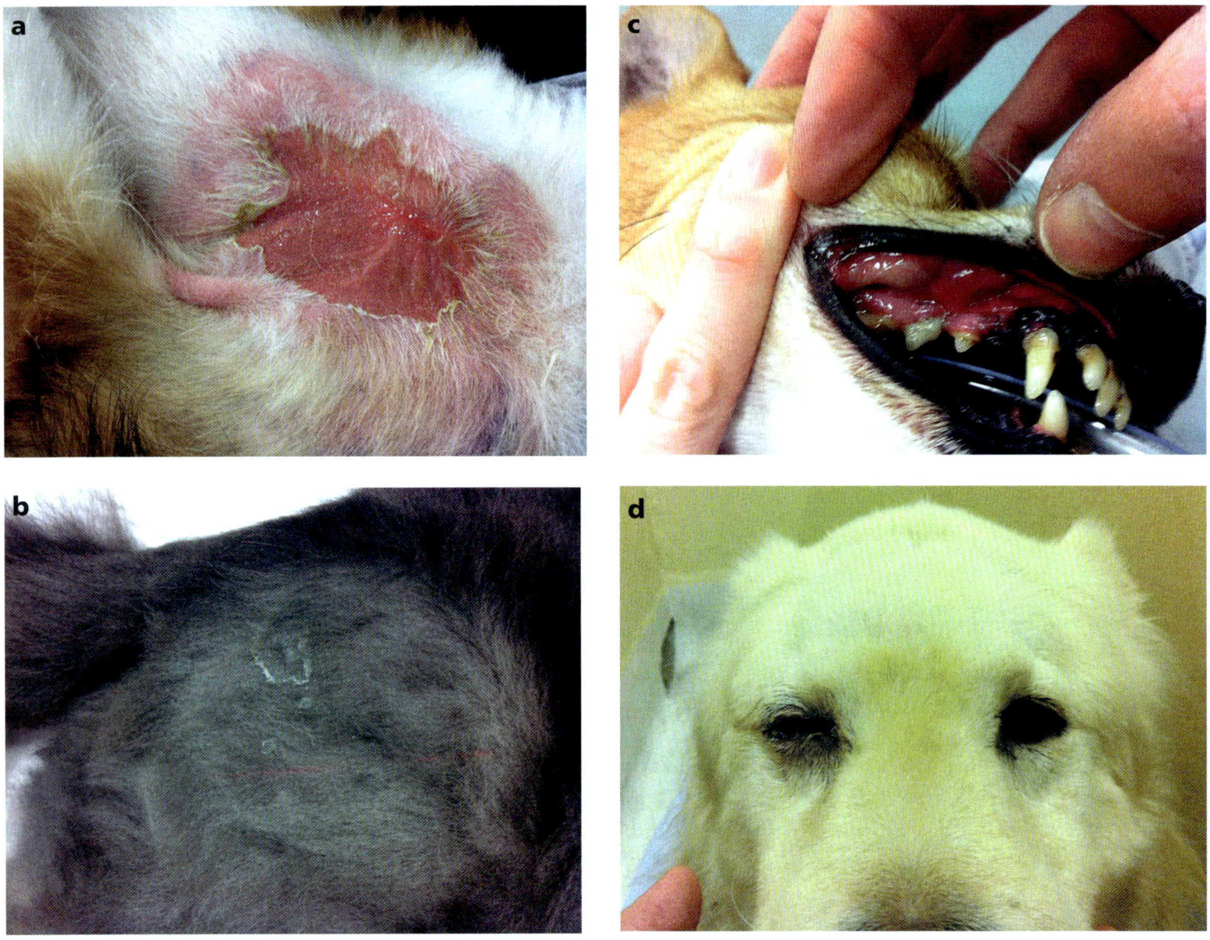

**Figure 2.16.** a, Moist dermatitis in a dog treated for sarcoma. b, Dry dermatitis in a cat treated for sarcoma. c, Mucositis in a dog with a tumour of the nasal cavity. d, Conjunctivitis in a dog with a frontal sinus carcinoma. All of these lesions occurred during fractionated treatment.

Similarly, in meningiomas treated with radiotherapy, the average survival time is around 2 years compared to 2 months when not treated with radiotherapy and only symptomatic treatments are used. In the case of feline sarcomas, where the main problem is the high rate of local recurrence, the use of radiation therapy after surgery can achieve a 40-month survival time when protocols with curative intent are used.

## New treatments

New treatment tools are being developed, such as **electrochemotherapy** (Figure 2.19). This combines the **administration of chemotherapy**, either intravenously or intra-tumourally, with the application of **local electrical stimuli** that increase the permeability of tumoural cells to cytotoxic agents. The use of these techniques has achieved a lasting remission of more than **80% of squamous cell carcinomas in cats**. New studies also show its efficacy in mastocytomas, both in those that are non-operable and those that have been incompletely removed, and it is being researched in different types of tumour where surgical resection is not straightforward, radiotherapy is not viable and where they do not respond to medical treatments.

## Management of common canine tumours

### *Multicentric lymphoma*

#### *Clinical signs*

Multicentric lymphoma is a **common type of cancer in dogs**. It is called multicentric because it **affects multiple lymph nod**es (clinical stages I, II or III), may also affect the **liver** and/or **spleen** (stage IV) and, in some cases, the **bone marrow** (stage V).

#### *Treatment*

This type of cancer **responds well to medical treatment**, but treatment depends on several factors:

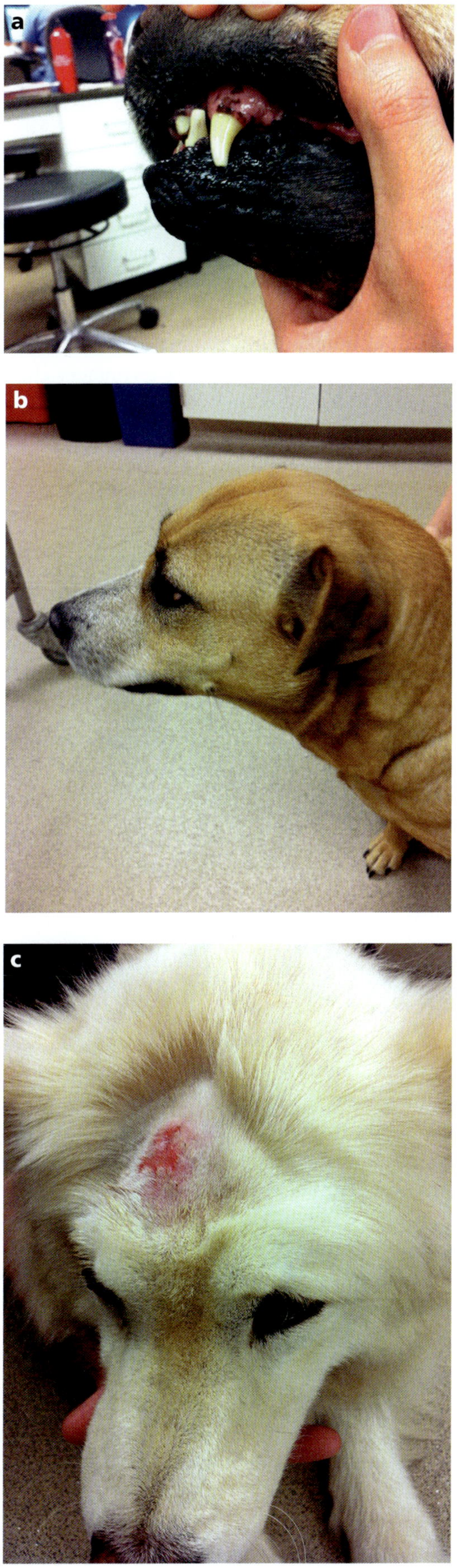

**Figure 2.17.** a, Alopecia and hyperpigmentation. b, Leukotrichia. c, Fistula secondary to osteonecrosis of the cranium.

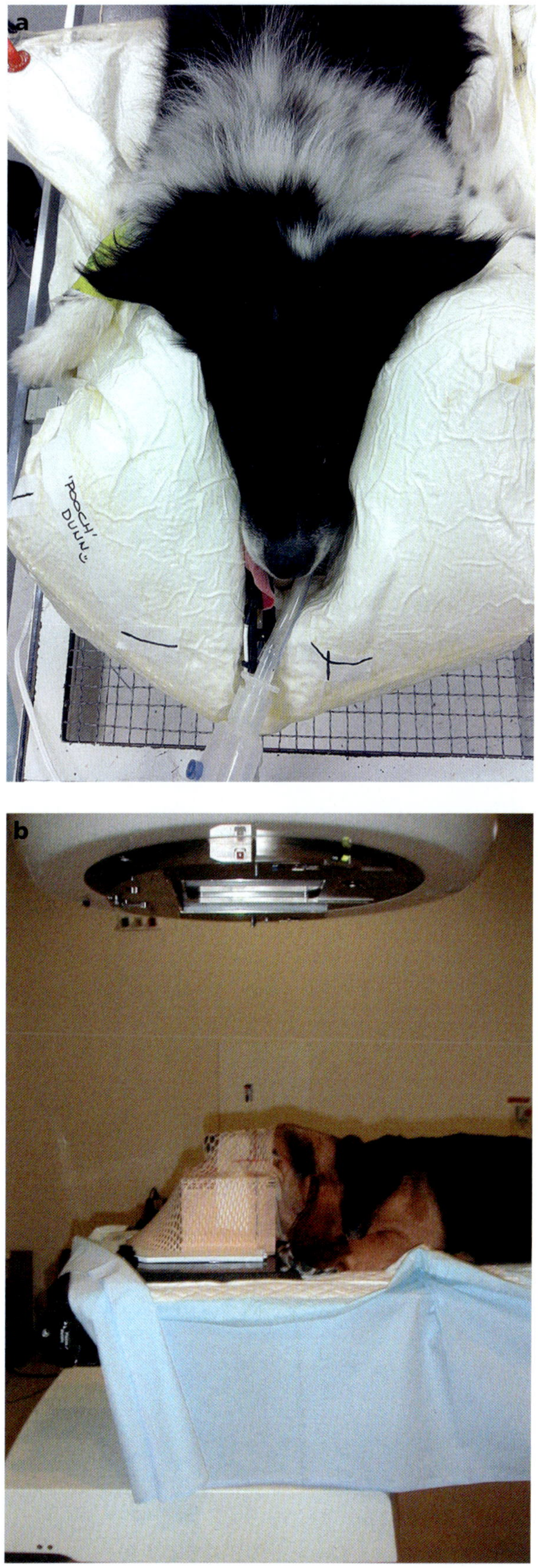

**Figure 2.18.** Dog positioned on a vacuum mattress (a), dog positioned with a system that combines a dental mould with a thermoplastic chamber (b). Both have marks (lines and crosses) that are positioned with laser equipment, so that the position of the system, mattress or mask is the same for each treatment.

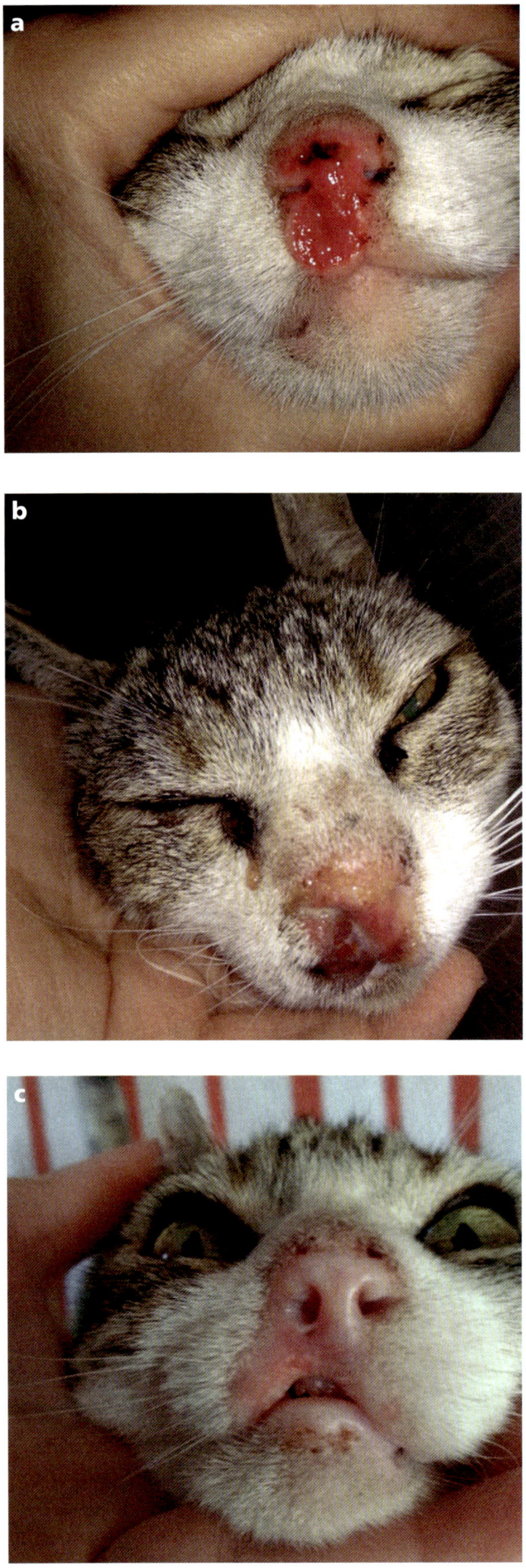


**Figure 2.19.** Cat with squamous cell carcinoma, before (a), seven days after (b) and 30 days after (c) the treatment with electrochemotherapy.

## Immunophenotype (B or T cells)

When treated with doxorubicin, >**80% of B-cell lymphomas respond** with complete remission, while **only half of T-cell lymphomas** respond to this drug and <20% achieve complete remission.

## Grade (high or low)

Treatment varies depending on the grade, so an **accurate diagnosis is important** to determine the appropriate prognosis and treatment. For the diagnosis of 5–30% of all low-grade lymphomas, additional tests are necessary, such as **biopsy with immunohistochemistry or flow cytometry**. The use of these techniques changes the initial diagnosis in up to 20% of cases. **Intravenous chemotherapy protocols are recommended for high grades**, and **oral chemotherapy is recommended for low grades**.

## Treatment of high-grade lymphoma

High-grade lymphoma is treated with protocols that combine several drugs.

## CHOP protocol

See above for the constituent parts of the CHOP protocol. With this protocol, which is **administered over 19–25 weeks**, about **80–95% of cases go into remission** and the **average survival time is 10–12 months** (about 20–25% of cases treated can live for more than two years). This regime, once completed, **does not need maintenance therapy**. The response rate and duration of remission are higher for B- than T-cell lymphomas.

## COP Protocol

The COP protocol, unlike the CHOP, does not include doxorubicin, **lasts 6–12 weeks** and offers a good response rate but, in general, the remission time is usually shorter than with the CHOP protocol. In addition, **COP requires administration of maintenance treatment** orally after the induction phase.

## Treatment of low-grade lymphoma

Low-grade lymphomas are treated differently and have a better prognosis. In these cases, treatment is **oral and consists of corticoids and chlorambucil**.

Most dogs tolerate chemotherapy well, and it is rare (<5% of cases) that a patient will suffer serious complications (requiring hospitalisation). Normally during treatment, quality of life is similar to that before diagnosis.

**Certain breeds** (Collie, Shetland sheepdog, long-haired Whippet and Australian cattle dog, among others) may have a **mutation that makes them more sensitive to chemotherapy**. The frequency of this mutation depends on the breed, and varies from 60–70% in Collies to 20–25% in Australian cattle dogs. In these cases, changes to the type of chemotherapy administered may be necessary and it is advisable to consult with a veterinary oncologist before starting treatment.

**T-cell lymphomas** may benefit from the **inclusion of lomustine** in the protocol and, in the case of cutaneous lymphomas, the inclusion of lomustine is recommended.

### *Prognosis*

Without treatment, there is a poor prognosis: in about two months the cancer progresses to the point where the animal's quality of life is poor.

Most dogs with **high-grade B-cell lymphoma respond well to treatment**, and complete remission can be achieved in most cases. Complete remission means the disappearance of symptoms caused by the tumour, but it does not mean the tumour is cured. On average, dogs treated with chemotherapy live for about a year.

**High-grade T-cell lymphomas respond to a lesser extent**, and sometimes only partial remission is achieved with an average survival time of about 5–9 months.

**Low-grade lymphoma has a much better prognosis**, with an average survival of 4 years.

## *Splenic lymphoma*

### *Clinical signs*

A minority of dogs present with **lymphoma located in the spleen** (most with a single nodule, measuring several centimetres, and the remainder with diffuse splenomegaly).

### *Diagnosis*

In most cases the lymphoma is a **casual finding** during examination for other problems (most have **no associated symptoms**), and lymphoma diagnosis is by histopathology after removal of the spleen due to splenomegaly or the presence of a nodule.

Occasionally, **peripheral lymph nodes** may also be affected with splenic lymphomas but this is not common.

To establish the type of lymphoma, an **immunophenotype test** (flow cytometry of an aspirate from a lymph node or spleen) or a sample for histopathology (lymph node or spleen) is necessary.

Removal of the spleen has been carried out occasionally in dogs with lymphoma, for histological diagnosis, to decrease tumour volume or to prevent the risk of splenic rupture in cases of severe splenomegaly.

### *Prognosis*

The prognosis is worse when the disease is not restricted solely to the spleen.

**Splenic T-cell lymphomas have a poor prognosis** and the expected survival time is only a few weeks to months.

Of the lymphomas found in the spleen there are two B-cell types, which are associated with a better prognosis and show a favourable progression after removal of the spleen.

## *Mediastinal lymphoma*

### *Clinical signs*

**Mediastinal lymphoma is unusual** (around 5% of lymphomas in dogs) and is located in the cranial mediastinal lymph nodes (in the thorax), without peripheral adenopathy.

### *Treatment*

The goal of treatment is to **reduce tumour size and pleural effusion or hypercalcaemia** if present and improve quality of life.

### *Prognosis*

About **10–40% of these lymphomas present with hypercalcaemia** as a paraneoplastic syndrome, which is considered a poor prognostic factor because it can lead to **renal failure**. These types of lymphoma usually affect T cells.

The prognosis for this type of lymphoma depends on the response to treatment and the progression of hypercalcaemia.

With treatment the **average survival time is around 9 months**, because T-cell lymphomas do not respond as well as B-cell lymphomas.

## *Cutaneous lymphoma*

### *Clinical signs*

Cutaneous lymphoma can present with both **single and multiple lesions**, and usually affects T cells. It can produce **skin lesions** (**epitheliotropic**) or affect the deep and **subcutaneous dermis** (**non-epitheliotropic**). The lesions vary from nodules or plaques, to ulcers, exfoliative dermatitis or alopecia.

## *Mast cell tumor*

### *Epidemiology*

Mast cell tumor is the most frequently diagnosed malignant tumour affecting the skin and subcutaneous tissue in the dog.

### *Diagnosis*

The biological behaviour is very variable. To try to predict aggressiveness and the prognosis, and to make treatment decisions, different factors are considered, including:

- histological grade (I–III or high–low)
- mitotic count
- clinical stage
- clinical factors such as rapid growth.

If there is no previous biopsy reporting the histological grade, to some extent cytology can be used to predict the degree of malignancy. The presence of >3 multinucleated cells (in 1000 mast cells) has a sensitivity of >80% for the diagnosis of high-grade mast cells.

A recent paper proposed the use of cytology to predict histological grade, looking for the presence of poorly granulated cells or that at least two of the following criteria were fulfilled: mitotic figures, bi- or multinucleated cells, nuclear pleomorphism or >50% anisokaryosis. With these criteria, when compared with histopathology, a sensitivity of 88% for diagnosis of high-grade tumours was obtained. The expected survival time was similar when using histological and cytological grades.

### *Treatment and prognosis*

**Surgery is the treatment of choice** for tumours without distant metastases that can be removed. In low-grade tumours with no negative prognostic signs, surgery may be the only treatment necessary. Depending on the factors discussed above, additional treatments may be required.

Due to their location, some tumours cannot be removed completely without affecting the normal function of the area (for example, those present over a joint).

In the case of an **incompletely excised grade II mast cell tumor,** if no additional treatments are used the **risk of recurrence is 23%** which, on average, occurs about 5 years after the first procedure. The proportion of mastocytomas that recur increases as time passes: 17% at 1 year post-treatment, 22% at 2 years and 33% at 3 years.

In a study of 40 incompletely resected grade II mastocytomas where no other treatment was administered, the local recurrence was 16% in tumours located in the perineal region (after two and a half years) and 8% in other areas of the body. In this study, 37% of the animals developed new mastocytomas in other areas.

In cases of incomplete excision, a **second intervention or the use of radiotherapy** can be assessed. In a study of 70 tumours, the recurrence rate was 38% in the group without any additional treatment compared to 13% in cases that received additional surgery and 8% in those treated with radiotherapy. In addition to reducing the risk of recurrence, these additional treatments meant that recurrence took longer, with a difference from 2 years in the control group to 6–8 years in the group that received additional surgery or radiotherapy.

An alternative is **electrochemotherapy** (a technique used after the **administration of intravenous chemotherapy, where electrical stimuli are applied to the area of the tumour or the scar**, leaving the cells in the treated area more amenable to chemotherapy). This technique consists of a single treatment that is administered under general anaesthesia. In a recent study of 51 dogs with mast cell tumor, 14 were treated after incomplete surgery, 13 of 14 (93%) were in complete remission (without signs of recurrence) for an average of 4 years, and in only one case (7%) was recurrence noted.

In dogs with **multiple mast cell tumor** the only factor associated with poor prognosis was that some of the tumours were grade III (or high grade within the new classification system). In low-grade tumours, whether excision was complete or not did not affect prognosis.

At the time of diagnosis, 18–30% of dogs with mast cell tumor have metastases in regional lymph nodes and 4–7% have distant metastases, although this can be as high as 19%. It is rare to see distant metastasis without it being present in a lymph node.

The risk of metastasis depends on the histological grade of the tumour:

- 6% in grade I
- 16% in grade II
- 49% in grade III.

If the new two-grade classification proposed by Kiupel in 2011, is used, the rate of metastasis is:

- 15% for low-grade mast cell tumor
- 30% for high-grade mast cell tumor.

In **high-grade or grade III tumours**, or with negative prognostic factors, a **complete clinical staging** is recommended prior to treatment. The following are considered to be negative factors:

- mitotic count ≥5
- rapid growth
- recurrence after previous surgery
- presence of systemic signs such as anorexia, vomiting or melaena.

To establish the clinical stage, the **lymph node is usually assessed using cytology**. Five groups have been proposed:

- normal lymph node
- reactive lymph node
- possible metastasis
- probable metastasis
- certain metastasis.

Only the last two were associated with lower survival; the proposed cytological criteria for these are:

- **Probable metastasis**: at least one slide with more than 3 foci of 2–3 aggregated mast cells and/or 2 foci of >3 mast cells.
- **Certain metastasis**: presence of poorly differentiated cell aggregates, with pleomorphism, anisocytosis or anisokaryosis and/or more >5 aggregates of >3 mast cells.

These groups were associated with a mean survival of 2.9 years (range 0.4–4.1) and 0.8 years (0.4–1.9), respectively (compared to 5.2 years of survival for the group with possible metastases).

A study on sentinel nodes **found that metastases in nodes that were not the closest to the tumour** (for example, prescapular ganglion metastasis in two dogs with tumour in the ear, which had no submandibular lymph node metastasis), emphasising the importance of **evaluating the sentinel node**. However, lymphatic drainage of the different areas of skin is described in the dog and, for example, lymphatic drainage of the auricular area is to the prescapular lymph node (and not to the submandibular). Some of the **lymph nodes that drain the skin of the hind limb are located in the abdomen**. It is therefore important to have a sound knowledge of the anatomy of the lymphatic system in order to be able to take samples from the appropriate lymph node.

If the **lymph node is evaluated using histopathology**, the classification also uses the presence of **aggregates of at least 3 mast cells to classify it as positive for early metastasis**, compared to the complete invasion of the lymph node by tumour cells. The mean survival time for cases with metastasis (early or complete) was 2.2 years compared with cases without lymph node metastasis, which had a survival time of 5 years. However, not all dogs received the same treatment and some were treated with surgery only, others with surgery and chemotherapy (several protocols) or surgery and radiotherapy.

The next step in establishing the clinical stage is to **assess the presence of distant metastases**. More than 30% of high-risk cases (grade II with aggressive behaviour, or grade III) have distant metastases (liver or spleen) at the time of diagnosis. Although part of the diagnostic work-up includes abdominal ultrasound, this technique has a low sensitivity since the presence of abnormalities on ultrasound (enlargement, modified echogenicity, nodular lesions or heterogeneous parenchyma) can be found in the liver or spleen without metastasis of the mast cell tumor. On the other hand, organs with metastases may have a normal appearance on ultrasound. The **recommendation is to perform spleen/liver aspirates** for cytology, regardless of the ultrasound appearance of these organs. The presence of mast cell aggregates or atypical mastocyte cells is indicative of metastasis. Another factor to consider is the presence of a high number of mast cells, and although the normal number in the spleen is not established and may be more difficult to interpret, in liver aspirates there should not be more than one mast cell per 100 hepatocytes under normal conditions.

In the case of grade II mastocytomas, survival at one year is similar with and without lymph node metastasis (88% of dogs with metastasis and 93% without), but this difference increases with time to 90% of dogs still alive four years later when metastases are not present, compared to 66% if they were present on diagnosis. **Removing the metastatic lymph node as part of treatment improves survival**, and 88% of the dogs remained alive at four years, similar to those without metastases, according to a study published in 2014.

Miller and his team reviewed cases of grade II and III mastocytomas with metastases present at the time of diagnosis, and observed that the presence of metastasis is a factor that causes a worse prognosis, with an average survival time of around seven months (both for metastasis in lymph nodes and distant metastasis), compared to those without metastasis, with an average survival time of about 2 years. In cases with metastases, survival time was improved if the primary tumour was removed, even if incompletely, and treated medically with vinblastine/prednisone or masitinib (9 months on average), than if chemotherapy is used without removal of the primary tumour (3 months), regardless of whether the metastasis was in lymph nodes or distant.

The **treatment of undifferentiated mastocytomas or those with distant metastases** is not easy and, in general, it is considered that **combinations of drugs are more effective** than monotherapy. **Corticosteroids, vinblastine, tyrosine kinase inhibitors (masitinib or toceranib), lomustine or combinations of some of these are the most commonly**

**used drugs**. A randomized study that compared the response rate to toceranib or vinblastine found that is about 50% for both drugs, and interestingly the presence of *kit* mutation does not predict the response to toceranib. The response rate can be increased up to 90% when both drugs are used in combination, but it is necessary to decrease the dosage of vinblastine to 1,6 mg/m$^2$ given every other week. When this combination is used, the median survival time depends on the clinical stage, being better for cases with lymph node metastasis that for those with distant (liver, spleen) metastasis. Lomustine can be used as well for high grade mast cell tumor, with median survival times of 30 months; however, there are some side effects associated to this drug like neutropenia (67%) and elevations in ALT (60%).

In the case of macroscopic disease, treatment with diphenhydramine and omeprazole to reduce the side effects of histamine release is recommended.

## Canine mammary carcinomas

### Prognosis and treatment

The **prognosis of malignant mammary tumours depends on the histological grade**. In general, half of tumours are benign and half malignant. There are up to 20 different histological types of the latter but, as far as prognosis is concerned, these are grouped according to **three degrees of malignancy: I, II and III (or low, medium and high)**.

When treated with surgery only, low-grade (I) malignant tumours do not present with local recurrence or metastasis during the following 2 years. Among medium-grade (II) tumours, recurrence or metastasis occurs in about 16% which, on average, occurs at 27 months after diagnosis with an average survival time of 32 months. In high-grade (III), almost 60% of cases develop local relapses or metastasis. The average time for the development of these new lesions (local or distant metastasis) is 7 months – that is, of the cases that relapse or develop metastasis, half do so in <7 months and half in <7 months. The average survival time is 20 months.

Traditionally, there has been **controversy about the benefit of neutering when mammary tumours are removed**. Although neutering in females with benign tumours has been shown to reduce the risk of new lesions, it has not been proven whether this is the case for malignant tumours. A study published in December 2015 showed that it is only beneficial in some cases: grade II malignant tumours, those that express oestrogen receptors (special staining is necessary to identify these) and those that contain high levels of oestradiol (>35 pg/ml) in blood at the time of diagnosis. As the degree and expression of oestrogens can only be established after surgery, **analysis of oestradiol in blood is recommended to assess whether to perform ovariohysterectomy at the same time as removing mammary tumours**.

As more than **half of grade III carcinomas relapse** or develop metastasis, it is recommended that these be **treated with chemotherapy** to reduce this risk and increase disease-free time. What is not proven so far is the effectiveness of different chemotherapy protocols. **Doxorubicin and mitoxantrone** have been used in some cases, but there are no published data on their efficacy. Doxorubicin can cause digestive side effects (decreased appetite, vomiting and diarrhoea) and a decrease in the number of white blood cells. Digestive effects can be prevented by using medications that have been shown to be effective in reducing the risk and intensity of vomiting associated with chemotherapy. Most patients treated with doxorubicin do not experience severe side effects and, if they have any, they respond well to supportive treatment with <5% needing to be seen urgently for side effects.

Sometimes less aggressive protocols are also recommended, such as the administration of low doses of chemotherapy, with consistent oral administration. These protocols, termed **metronomic chemotherapy**, use anti-inflammatory medications that can have effects on the tumour and the blood vessels supplying it, combined with low-dose chemotherapy, but there is no evidence yet of its efficacy.

In summary, although it is thought that in grade III carcinomas chemotherapy is beneficial for the animal, which protocol and to what extent it improves the disease-free interval or survival have not yet been published.

## Bibliography

Book, A.P., Fidel, J., Wills, T., Bryan, J., Sellon, R. and Mattoon, J. (2011) Correlation of ultrasound findings, liver and spleen cytology, and prognosis in the clinical staging of high metastatic risk canine mast cell tumors. *Veterinary Radiology and Ultrasound* 52(5), 548–554.

Hay, J.K. and Larson, V.S. (2019) Lomustine (CCNU) and prednisone chemotherapy for high-grade completely excised canine mast cell tumors. *Canadian Veterinary Journal* 60(12), 1326–1330.

Krick, E.L., Billings, A.P., Shofer, F.S., Watanabe, S. and Sorenmo, K.U. (2009) Cytological lymph node evaluation in dogs with mast cell tumours: association with grade and survival. *Veterinary and Comparative Oncology* 7(2), 130–138.

Masserdotti. C. (2013) Proportion of mast cells in normal canine hepatic cytologic specimens: comparison of 2 staining methods. *Veterinary Clinical Pathology* 42(4). 522–525.

Olsen, J.A., Thomson, M., O'Connell, K. and Wyatt. K. (2018) Combination vinblastine, prednisolone and toceranib phosphate for treatment of grade II and III mast cell tumours in dogs. *Veterinary Medicine and Science* 4(3), 237–251.

Scarpa, F., Sabattini, S. and Bettini, G. (2014) Cytological grading of canine cutaneous mast cell tumours. *Veterinary and Comparative Oncology*. Available at: https://doi:10.1111/vco.12090.

Stefanello, D., Buracco, P. Sabattini, S. et al. (2015) Comparison of 2- and 3-category histologic grading systems for predicting the presence of metastasis at the time of initial evaluation in dogs with cutaneous mast cell tumors: 386 cases (2009–2014). *Journal of the American Veterinary Medical Association* 246(7), 765–769.

Stefanello, D., Valenti, P., Faverzani, S. et al. (2009) Ultrasound-guided cytology of spleen and liver: a prognostic tool in canine cutaneous mast cell tumor. *Journal of Veterinary Internal Medicine* 23(5), 1051–1057.

Suami, H., Yamashita, S., Soto-Miranda, M.A. and Chang, D.W. (2013) Lymphatic territories (lymphosomes) in a canine: an animal model for investigation of postoperative lymphatic alterations. PLOS ONE 8(7): e69222. https://doi.org/10.1371/journal.pone.0069222.

Thamm, D.H., Vail, D.M. and Vail, D. (2007) Aftershocks of cancer chemotherapy: managing adverse effects. *Journal of the American Animal Hospital Association* (43), 1–7.

Weishaar, K.M., Thamm, D.H., Worley, D.R. and Kamstock, D.A. (2014) Correlation of nodal mast cells with clinical outcome in dogs with mast cell tumour and a proposed classification system for the evaluation of node metastasis. *Journal of Comparative Pathology* August, 1–10.

Weishaar, K.M., Ehrhart, E.J., Avery, A.C., et al. (2018) c-Kit mutation and localization status as response predictors in mast cell tumors in dogs treated with prednisone and toceranib or vinblastine. *Journal of Veterinary Internal Medicine* 32(1), 394–405.

Worley, D.R. (2012) Incorporation of sentinel lymph node mapping in dogs with mast cell tumours: 20 consecutive procedures. *Veterinary and Comparative Oncology* 12(3), 215–226.

## Test

1. **A dog with multiple mastocytomas comes in to the practice for consultation. The prognosis depends on:**
   A) the number of lesions
   B) the size of the lesions
   C) the histological grade
   D) the breed of the dog.
2. **The risk of metastasis with mast cell tumor is:**
   A) generally, very low
   B) up to 50% in grade III tumours
   C) 6% in grade III tumours
   D) 16% in grade III tumours.
3. **A non-spayed dog with a mammary tumour that on cytology has marked criteria of malignancy is admitted. Blood oestradiol is measured, and it is 40 pg/ul. With these results, what would be your recommendation?**
   A) Perform an ovariohysterectomy with removal of the tumour.
   B) Do not perform an ovariohysterectomy with the removal of the tumour.
   C) Remove the tumour and, depending on the grade, recommend a posterior ovariohysterectomy.
   D) Repeat the test because the result is not possible.
4. **The histological grade of malignancy of canine mammary tumours is prognostic and it is known that, in cases of grade III treated with surgery only, recurrence/metastasis develops in what percentage of cases?**
   A) <10
   B) 10–25
   C) 25–50
   D) >50%.
5. **Which of the following lymphomas carries the best prognosis?**
   A) high-grade T-cell lymphoma
   B) diffuse large B-cell lymphoma
   C) splenic T-cell lymphoma
   D) low-grade T-cell lymphoma.

**6. Which of these breeds is at a higher risk of having an MDR mutation (making it more sensitive to the side effects of chemotherapy)?**

A) Collie
B) Old English sheepdog
C) Border collie
D) Chihuahua.

**7. Lymphoma is diagnosed in a Golden retriever and flow cytometry is performed on a ganglion aspirate; the result is CD4++ CD45–. With these results, the average survival time for this case is:**

A) 5 months
B) 9 months
C) 12 months
D) 20 months.

**8. After surgery for an intestinal mass, the histopathological diagnosis is leiomyosarcoma. The laboratory offers the possibility of performing immunohistochemistry with an additional cost to be able to diagnose which of the following?**

A) C-KIT to identify leiomyoma.
B) C-KIT to identify a gastrointestinal stromal tumour.
C) Vimentin to identify leiomyoma.
D) Cytokeratin to diagnose a gastrointestinal stromal tumour.

**9. For which of these tumours should the pathology report include the histological grade?**

A) mast cell tumor
B) mammary carcinoma
C) soft tissue sarcoma
D) all of the above.

**10. In feline digestive lymphoma, maximum sensitivity is obtained by:**

A) the combination of histopathology, immunohistochemistry and clonality tests
B) clonality tests
C) the combination of histopathology with immunohistochemistry
D) cytology.

**11. The use of toceranib phosphate has shown efficacy and can therefore be recommended for what?**

A) To increase disease-free interval after amputation and carboplatin chemotherapy in dogs with osteosarcoma.
B) To increase disease-free time after splenectomy and chemotherapy with doxorubicin in dogs with haemangiosarcoma.
C) In cases of anal sac carcinoma with pulmonary metastases.
D) All of the above.

**12. A West Highland white terrier is going to be treated with doxorubicin. The protocol is?**

A) doxorubicin 1 mg/kg and maropitant 1 mg/kg IV
B) doxorubicin 30 mg/m$^2$ and maropitant 1 mg/kg IV
C) doxorubicin 1 mg/kg
D) doxorubicin 30 mg/m$^2$.

**13. In a dog with lymphoma, cyclophosphamide is administered using 50 mg tablets. The total corresponding dose is between 75 and 100 mg, and therefore which of the following should be prescribed:**

A) one and a half tablets in one dose
B) one tablet and 24 hours later half a tablet
C) one tablet and 24 hours later another
D) two tablets in one dose.

**14. Given the possibility of using radiation therapy to treat the tumour, the owner asks about the possibility and duration of side effects. You explain that:**

A) With the definitive treatment it is common to see acute side effects during the treatment, but their duration is limited.
B) With palliative treatments, acute side effects are less frequent and chronic effects are more likely.
C) Chronic side effects, if they appear, do so after several months, but are permanent.
D) All the above is correct.

**15. The survival prognosis for clinical stage I unilateral nasal tumours treated with radiotherapy is:**

A) <6 months
B) around 2 years
C) 1 year
D) >5 years.

**16. A bitch with a mammary tumour is presented for consultation and assessment of whether it can take part in a clinical trial. The tumour is 2 cm at its widest diameter, the cytology shows tumour cells in the regional lymph node and no distant metastasis are observed. The clinical stage is:**

A) I
B) II
C) III
D) IV.

## Clinical case 1

Braco, a 10-year-old uncastrated male, Weimaraner, comes to the practice because he has a subcutaneous lump in the salivary gland area. After the physical examination the veterinarian treating him performs a fine-needle aspiration and sends it to the laboratory. The results were as follows:

'A high number of round cells, with moderate anisocytosis, which show a cytoplasm occupied by variable quantities of purple granules are observed. The cells present some anisokaryosis and mitosis is not seen. Very few bi-nucleate cells are observed. There are also a high number of eosinophils and small lymphocytes, and occasional plasma cells. Cytology is consistent with a mast cell tumor and the presence of lymphocytes may suggest that it is developing in a lymph node (metastasis). A biopsy is needed to confirm this.'

**1. With this result, explain why or why you would not carry out each of the following options:**

A) Take a biopsy as recommended by the laboratory, under anaesthesia.
B) Remove the mast cell tumor with a 2 cm margin.
C) Start treatment with prednisone and a tyrosine kinase inhibitor.
D) Perform a detailed physical examination to look for the primary tumour.
E) Perform thoracic radiography.
F) Perform an abdominal ultrasound.
G) If there are changes on ultrasound, aspirate the spleen.
H) Aspirate the spleen independently of the appearance on ultrasound.
I) If there are changes on ultrasound, aspirate the liver.
J) Aspirate the liver independently of the appearance on ultrasound.

**2. In a physical examination, a 1 cm nodule is detected on the lip which, according to the owner, has been there for more than 1 year without causing any problems. However, an aspirate is taken and cytology shows a population of round cells with purple granules in the cytoplasm. With this information, can you offer the owner a diagnosis?**

**3. Eventually, a decision was taken to perform a 2 mm punch biopsy of the primary tumour and liver and spleen aspirates under sedation. The results indicate that the primary tumour is a grade II mast cell tumor according to the Patnaik classification, but of a low grade according to the Kiupel system. Liver cytology shows hepatocytes and fewer than 1 mast cell per 100 hepatocytes. Mast cells are not seen in the spleen. What prognosis and treatment options can now be offered to the owner?**

## Clinical case 2

1. Given the suspicion of a metastatic mast cell tumor, the recommendation is to seek, through a detailed physical examination and a thorough clinical history (masses removed previously), the primary tumour (option D), in order to evaluate the histological grade and the clinical stage before beginning treatment. Options A–C are incorrect. In order to establish the clinical stage, evaluation of whether there are distant metastasis present is necessary, by cytology of the liver and spleen, regardless of the ultrasound appearance (options F, H and J). The risk of pulmonary metastasis in the case of mast cell tumor is minimal. There may be metastases in organs that look normal or alternatively, ultrasound changes in the liver or spleen may be due to problems unrelated to the metastases (options E, G and I are incorrect).
2. At this point it has been established that the dog has a mast cell tumor on its lip with metastasis in the lymph node, but this is not enough to give a prognosis because this depends on the histological grade of the primary tumour and the presence of distant metastases.
3. Mastocytomas in the nose area show a more aggressive clinical picture than in other locations, with up to 58% associated with lymph node metastases at the time of diagnosis. Although the presence of metastasis is associated with a worse prognosis, the histological grade is also important and dogs with grade I or II mast cell tumor had an average survival of almost 5 years, superior to those with grade III, with an average survival of <10 months (Gieger JVIM, 2003). In the case of grade II mast cell tumor, the survival time per year is similar with and without metastasis in the lymph node (88% of surviving dogs with metastasis and 93% without), but this difference increases over time to 90% surviving for 4 years when they did not have metastasis at the time of diagnosis, compared to 66% with metastasis. Removing the metastatic lymph node as part of treatment improves survival, and 88% of dogs remain alive 4 years later, similar to those without metastasis (Baginski JAAHA, 2014). Thus, the recommendation for this case would be to remove the primary tumour and the metastatic lymph node, and then consider medical treatment.

## Correct answers

### Test

| | | | |
|---|---|---|---|
| 1. C | 5. D | 9. D | 13. C |
| 2. B | 6. A | 10. A | 14. D |
| 3. A | 7. D | 11. C | 15. B |
| 4. D | 8. B | 12. A | 16. D |

# Endocrine Disorders

3

Dolores Pérez Alenza

## Chapter summary



Disorders of the endocrine system represent a range of conditions resulting from an **imbalance of endocrine hormone** production. Endocrine disorders can arise as a result of an **underproduction** of hormone such as in canine hypothyroidism, or **overproduction** such as in feline hyperthyroidism. Indeed these examples illustrate how different species show a tendency towards different types of endocrine diseases.

It is vital the clinician fully understands the **diagnosis** and **management** of endocrine disease. This can be challenging, given the **vague nature of the presentation**, and **lack of specificity** of some tests. Of course, not all endocrine diseases are life-threatening, but good management makes a real and positive impact on the patient's quality of life, while for other endocrine diseases poor management results in shortened life expectancy (diabetes mellitus) or even acute fatality (hypoadrenocorticism or eclampsia).

Many of the symptoms of endocrine disorders are general, such as weight gain or loss, lethargy, polydipsia and polyuria. For this reason, endocrine disorders may appear on the **differential diagnosis list** for many commonly occurring presentations in practice.

While the clinician may have a high index of suspicion for a particular endocrine disease, confirming the diagnosis can be tricky. Often there are several different **test protocols** available, each having pros and cons with regards to **specificity and sensitivity**. Choosing the most worthwhile and accurate test makes the difference between a firm or unreliable diagnosis.

This chapter on endocrine disorders reviews the aetiopathology, clinical signs, diagnosis, and treatment of many endocrine diseases, providing a **practical guide** for the clinician faced with a tricky case in practice.

## Key learning points

- Know the **specificity and sensitivity** of various tests for the diagnosis of hyperadrenocorticism, and which test is most appropriate in different circumstances.
- The **management** of diabetes mellitus, from the selection of insulin type, to monitoring, dose adjustment, and diet.
- Managing the more **complex diabetic**, including rescue treatment for ketoacidosis and coping with **insulin resistance**.

- The **hypercalcaemic or hypocalcaemic** patient: understanding the aetiology and how to go about correcting the issues.
- Feel equipped to work up cases of hypoadrenocorticism, diabetes insipidus, pituitary dwarfism, and insulinoma.

## Adrenal diseases

### *Canine hyperadrenocorticism*

#### *Definition*

Hyperadrenocorticism (HAC) or Cushing's disease is a syndrome of symptoms arising from an excess of cortisol in the body; it can be of pituitary or adrenal origin, or iatrogenic due to prolonged corticosteroid administration.

Table 3.1. Hyperadrenocorticism: findings from clinical history and physical examination.

| Clinical history | Physical examination |
|---|---|
| Polyuria, polydipsia | Endocrine alopecia |
| Polyphagia | Skin atrophy |
| Abdominal distention | Comedones |
| Endocrine alopecia | Calcinosis cutis |
| Weakness | Hyperpigmentation |
| Lethargy | Abdominal distention |
| Calcinosis cutis | Hepatomegaly |
| Hyperpigmentation | Muscular weakness |
| Neurological symptoms: | Fragile skin |
| – Stupor | Testicular atrophy |
| – Ataxia | Dyspnoea |
| – Circular movements | |
| – Disorientated movements | |
| – Behavioural changes | |
| Dyspnoea/respiratory distress | |

#### *Epidemiology*

Hyperadrenocorticism is common in adult dogs aged 6 years or over, with the average age at diagnosis being 10 years.

Certain breeds have a predisposition to HAC, including the Poodle, Dachshund, German Shepherd, Beagle, Labrador Retriever, Boxer, and terriers.

In general, **pituitary hyperadrenocorticism** is seen more frequently in **small dogs** (<20 kg), whereas **adrenal hyperadrenocorticism** tends to occur in **larger dogs** (>20 kg). In addition, female dogs are at greater risk of developing adrenal HAC than males.

#### *Clinical signs*

HAC is typified by a gradual, slow progression of clinical signs.

The most common symptoms (Table 3.1) present in 85–90% of cases are:

- polydipsia
- polyuria
- polyphagia
- endocrine alopecia
- abdominal distention
- weakness.

#### *Diagnosis*

Dogs with HAC usually show some clinical signs. In the absence of appropriate symptoms, positive tests should be questioned as a possible stress response.

##### Blood tests

Screening blood tests often show moderate erythrocytosis and hypercoagulability, along with a stress leucogram (mature leucocytosis, neutrophilia, lymphopenia, and eosinopenia).

The most frequent changes on biochemistry are raised levels of alkaline phosphatase (ALP; 95% of cases), alanine aminotransferase (ALT), and cholesterol (75% of cases). Moderate hyperglycaemia, hyperlipidaemia, hypertriglyceridaemia, and low blood urea nitrogen may also be present.

##### Urinalysis

In 85% of cases urine specific gravity is less than 1.013. This dilute urine means urinary tract infections are common, occurring in around 50% of cases, so urinary culture is advisable. In addition, 10% of cases have glycosuria secondary to the presence of diabetes mellitus.

A **urine cortisol/creatinine ratio** can be useful to rule out HAC as a diagnosis. An overnight urine sample should be collected in a non-stressful environment, such as at home. Normal values make HAC unlikely; conversely the presence of cortisol does not confirm HAC but suggests it as a differential diagnosis.

##### Abdominal ultrasound

Abdominal ultrasound is useful for diagnosis of hyperadrenocorticism, especially of adrenal origin. A scan provides information about the size and echogenicity of the adrenal glands (whose size is also influenced by breed and age) and facilitates evaluation of other organs such as the liver and kidneys.

Ultrasound is the most widely used test to **differentiate** hyperadrenocorticism of **pituitary or adrenal origin.** In general, adrenal glands of normal or increased size (maximum diameter of lobes >0.6–0.75 cm) suggest

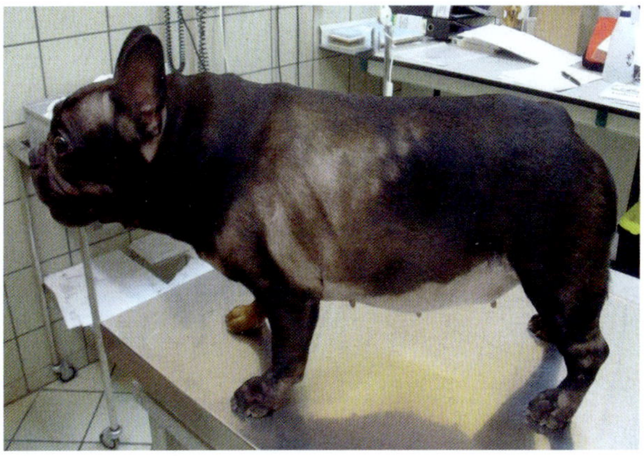

**Figure 3.1.** A 12-year-old female French Bulldog with HAC showing signs of pyoderma and endocrine alopecia.

the presence of pituitary HAC in patients with a compatible clinical picture.

This enlargement of the adrenal glands is due to the **pituitary gland** releasing high levels of adrenocorticotrophic hormone (ACTH), which stimulates the adrenal glands to produce cortisol. This size increase is usually **symmetrical**, with both adrenal glands affected. However, the absence of adrenal enlargement does not rule out HAC.

**Adrenal-based** disease is due to a functional tumour. The latter manufactures excessive cortisol, which has a negative feedback effect on the opposite adrenal gland. Thus adrenal tissue, with the exception of the tumour, is **atrophied**. Ultrasound can be used to evaluate the adrenal mass, invasion of adjacent structures, the presence of metastasis, and atrophy of the contralateral gland.

## Other tests

In dogs with pituitary HAC and central neurological symptoms, magnetic resonance imaging (MRI) or computed tomography (CT) should be used to visualize the pituitary lesion. Pituitary HAC is most commonly caused by a tumour (pituitary adenoma) which enlarges slowly.

**Blood pressure** should also be measured in parallel, since 30–40% of dogs with HAC are hypertensive at the time of diagnosis.

## Adrenocortical function tests

After establishing a clinical diagnosis, the origin of the disease (adrenal vs. pituitary) should be determined.

The general consensus for the diagnosis of canine HAC is that hormonal tests should always be interpreted in the light of relevant clinical signs, since no test is 100% sensitive and specific. In other words, if an animal does not present with compatible symptoms, or presents with other decompensated diseases, performing diagnostic tests or treatment is neither recommended nor reliable.

If a diagnostic test is negative in a patient where there are clinical signs of HAC, another of the available screening tests should be performed.

It should be remembered that the current reference ranges were established in the 1970s and 80s. Since cases are now detected earlier, often in the initial stages,

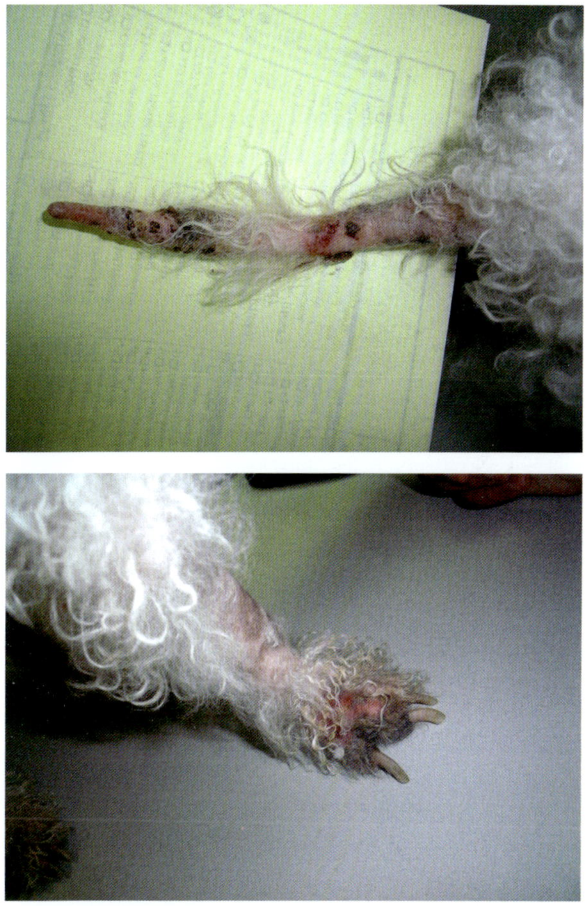

**Figures 3.2 and 3.3.** Bacterial pyoderma affecting the tail and interdigital spaces in a female Poodle with pituitary HAC.

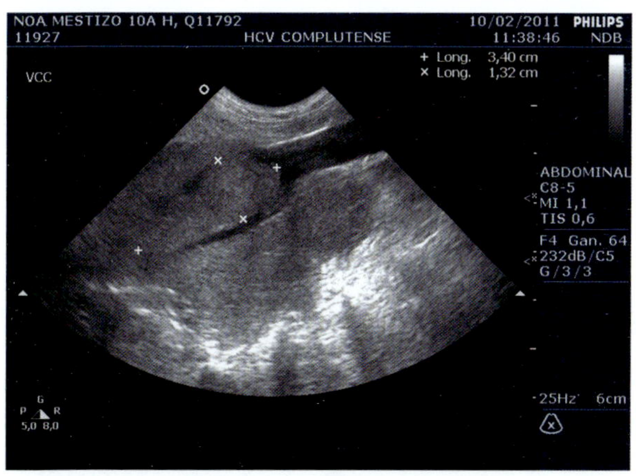


**Figure 3.4.** Abdominal ultrasound. A thrombus in the caudal vena cava in a dog suffering from adrenal Cushing's disease. Image courtesy of the diagnostic imaging service at the Hospital Clínico Veterinario Universidad Complutense (HCVC).

these cut-off points should probably be re-evaluated. Also, cortisol concentrations vary depending on the laboratory and technique used; therefore each laboratory should establish its own reference ranges.

There are several drugs that interfere with the measurement of cortisol. It is recommended that a minimum interval of 24 hours should elapse between the last dose of steroids and a cortisol assay. However, even this period does not eliminate the possibility of hypothalamic–pituitary–adrenal axis suppression, the duration of which is difficult to predict.

### *Low dose dexamethasone suppression test (LDDST)*

The LDDST is a useful way to confirm a diagnosis of HAC. This involves determining plasma cortisol before, at 4 hours, and then 8 hours after administration of dexamethasone (IM or IV) 0.01–0.05 mg/kg.

More than 90% of dogs with HAC have a cortisol concentration at 8 hours of 0.9 μg/dl (Figure 3.5). Therefore, the test has a very high sensitivity (85–100%). However, many dogs with non-adrenal diseases can produce results compatible with HAC, so the test has a low specificity (44–73%).

Occasionally, this test can also differentiate the type of HAC: if the cortisol at 4 hours is <1.0 μg/dl or <50% of the basal cortisol and at 8 hours it is ≥1.4 μg/dl, this is compatible with pituitary HAC rather than adrenal HAC.

It should be noted that phenobarbital accelerates the metabolism of dexamethasone, so the test can give false results in patients treated with phenobarbital.

### *ACTH stimulation test*

This is done by determining cortisol before and 1 or 2 hours after administering 5 μg/kg (or 0.25 mg/dog) of synthetic ACTH (Synacthen® IV or IM, Nuvacthen depot® IM). A post-ACTH cortisol level >19 μg/dl (reference values according to the laboratory) is considered

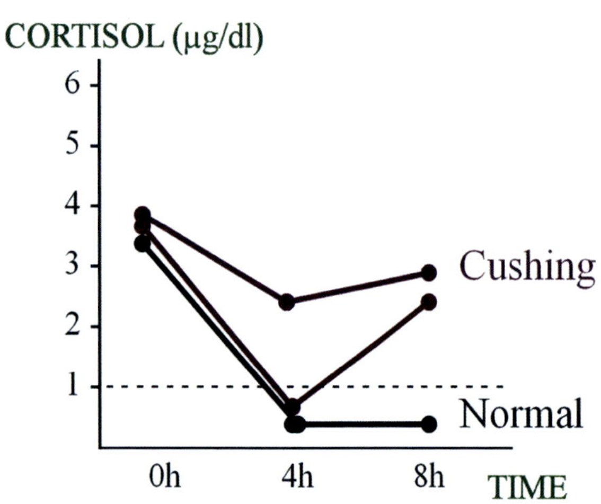


**Figure 3.5.** Low dose dexamethasone suppression test.

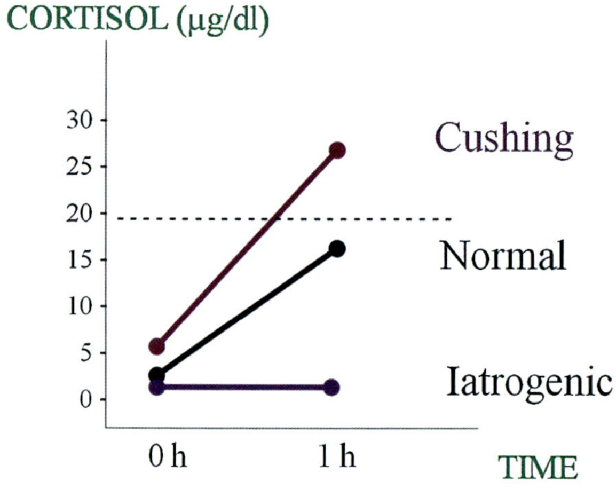


**Figure 3.6.** ACTH stimulation test.

compatible with HAC (Figure 3.6). However, 20% of dogs with HAC produce normal values.

This test has a **lower sensitivity** (57–95%) than the LDDST although its specificity is higher (86–93%). It is, however, one of the recommended methods for monitoring patients on treatment with trilostane and the only method that differentiates between spontaneous and iatrogenic HAC.

### *Urine cortisol/creatinine ratio*

This is considered a screening test, where a normal result rules out HAC as a diagnosis. It measures the relationship between cortisol and creatinine concentrations (which is relatively consistent) in urine samples after 8 hours (first urine sample in the morning).

In animals with HAC, the ratio is high (cut-off value established by the laboratory). It is a **very sensitive** test (>95%), but not very specific, since many dogs with other diseases (diabetes mellitus, pyometra, and hypercalcaemia) can give pathological results.

### *High dose dexamethasone suppression test (HDDST)*

This test helps determine whether HAC is of pituitary or adrenal origin. The HDDST requires the determination of plasma cortisol before and 8 hours after the administration of 0.1–1 mg/kg dexamethasone IV or IM.

- If at 8 hours plasma cortisol is <1.4 μg/dl or <50% of the basal level, the HAC is suppressible and is of pituitary origin.
- If at 8 hours it is >1.4 μg/dl or >50% of basal cortisol, it is not possible to differentiate between different types of HAC and another test should be used (endogenous ACTH levels).

### *Determination of endogenous ACTH levels*

This is the test of choice to establish the origin of the HAC, especially in dogs that do not show suppression with dexamethasone at high doses. However, it is not a routine technique; the plasma sample requires careful handling and rapid freezing, plus the test is expensive.

ACTH values are:

- normal: 10–100 pg/ml
- pituitary HAC: 45–450 pg/ml
- adrenal HAC: <20 pg/ml.

*Combination of the urinary cortisol/creatinine ratio with oral dexamethasone suppression*

This requires the collection of three urine samples over three consecutive days.

On **Day 1,** a reference reading is established.

On **Day 2** after collection of the urine sample, 0.1–1 mg/kg dexamethasone is given by mouth every 8 hours.

The mean of Days 1 and 2 indicates whether the results are compatible with HAC.

The sample from **Day 3** indicates whether the HAC can be suppressed or not.

- A value less than 50% of the first value indicates pituitary origin.
- A value greater than 50% of the first value indicates adrenal origin.

This test is quite sensitive, but not very specific, since other causes of polydipsia/polyuria can give rise to false positive results.

### Treatment

There are currently several treatment options: the choice of treatment (Table 3.2) should be made depending on the patient and the type of HAC. Other factors that must be taken into consideration when choosing the treatment are: efficacy, side effects, the condition of the patient, the availability of treatment, the owner's willingness to collaborate, cost, and the veterinarian's experience with the medication.

Most patients with **pituitary HAC** are treated with **trilostane**, although in some cases mitotane may be used as an alternative. Other options such as selegiline, cabergoline, or retinoic acid are not used frequently because of the lack of studies that demonstrate their efficacy and safety. There is also the possibility of surgical treatment (hypophysectomy), but this procedure is not readily available. In dogs with large invasive pituitary tumours, cobalt radiation treatment may be beneficial.

Regardless of the treatment method chosen, treatment is expensive and requires **lifelong, periodic monitoring** and a high level of owner dedication. When conditions are optimal, a satisfactory response can be achieved in most patients.

Table 3.2. Treatments for non-hepatic diseases that can cause elevation of liver enzymes.

| Treatments |
|---|
| **Medications that inhibit the synthesis of adrenal hormones** |
| Trilostane |
| Ketoconazole |
| **Medications that cause necrosis of the adrenal cortex** |
| Mitotane |
| Trilostane (occasionally) |
| **Medications that inhibit the synthesis of ACTH** |
| Selegiline |
| Cabergoline |
| Retinoic acid |
| **Surgery** |
| Adrenalectomy |
| Hypophysectomy |
| **Radiotherapy** |
| Cobalt radiation |

In some cases treatment may be postponed, for example in those patients with few symptoms, of advanced age, or with other severe non-adrenal disease.

## Medical treatment of pituitary hyperadrenocorticism

*Trilostane*

Trilostane is a steroid hormone analogue that competitively inhibits the enzyme 3-β-hydroxysteroid dehydrogenase. It thereby decreases the levels of adrenal and gonadal steroid hormones, including cortisol and aldosterone. This inhibition is reversible, reaching its maximum level between 2 and 6 hours, and usually ending 8–12 hours after oral administration.

Initial studies used high doses of trilostane to treat canine HAC; however, subsequent reports agree that treatment should be started at a low dose and progressively adjusted as indicated on follow-up. The necessary dose varies between patients according to their size, breed (large breeds require a relatively lower dose), severity of the clinical picture, and concurrent diseases.

Trilostane is marketed for the treatment of canine HAC as Vetoryl® in 10, 30, and 60 mg capsules. It can be administered every 12 or 24 hours. Once the patient is stable, periodic reviews should be undertaken to monitor and adjust the dose in each case, since overdose risks inducing hypoadrenocorticism.

### *Trilostane: once-daily dosing*

The initial dose is 2 mg/kg/d, which should be adapted in subsequent check-ups. Once-daily dosing is recommended by the manufacturer and often most convenient for the owner. However, between 10 and 30% of dogs do not show a good response with once-daily administration due to trilostane's short duration of effect.

Symptoms should improve in the first 10 days of treatment, especially polyuria, polydipsia, and activity levels. The polyphagia may take longer to resolve. Skin problems and abdominal distension need between 2 and 4 months to resolve; in some cases, dermatological signs may get slightly worse in the first weeks of treatment.

Monitoring check-ups take place:

- 7–10 days after starting treatment
- after 1 month
- 3 months later
- and thereafter every 3 months.

**Monitoring** includes assessment of the clinical picture, a complete blood count, biochemistry (with electrolytes), and measurement of cortisol levels. The biochemistry allows verification that the liver enzymes are going down and glucose is maintained at normal levels, as well as evaluating possible overdosing with trilostane.

In cases of overdose, azotaemia and hyperkalaemia are usually observed. Traditionally an ACTH stimulation test was performed coinciding with the point of maximum efficacy of trilostane, around 2 to 6 hours (4 hours) after the tablet has been administered. However, as an alternative to the ACTH test, the manufacturer now recommends a pre-pill blood cortisol test as appropriate to detect overdose in non-stressed animals, although not all members of the scientific community agree with this recommendation.

**Dose adjustments** should be made in line with clinical signs and the results of an ACTH stimulation or blood cortisol test.

- The dose should be **maintained** if there is clinical improvement and cortisol pre- or post-ACTH is **2–6 μg/dl** (50–200 nmol/l).
- The dose should be **increased** if symptoms persist and pre- or post-ACTH cortisol is **>7 μg/dl** (200 nmol/l).
- The dose should be **reduced** if symptoms improve but the cortisol before or after ACTH is **<2 μg/dl** (50 nmol/l), or if there are symptoms of Addison's disease.

Twice-daily dosing should be instituted if there is a poor clinical response despite adequate cortisol levels (suggested by pre- and post-ACTH cortisol levels between 2 and 6 μg/dl [50–200 nmol/l]).

After each dose change the patient should be **re-evaluated 2 to 4 weeks later**. Once good control is achieved, re-evaluation is recommended every 3 months for life.

### *Trilostane administered every 12 hours*

**Advantages:**

- effective in practically all patients
- requires a lower total daily dose
- survival rate slightly higher than in dogs treated once daily
- similar or superior efficacy to the 24-hour protocol
- steadier state blood cortisol levels than with once-daily dosing.

**Disadvantages:**

- owner co-operation essential to achieve regular twice-daily dosing.

The initial dose is 2 mg/kg/d, divided into two doses, while some studies recommend even lower initial doses (1 mg/kg/d). The average long-term daily dose for good control of the disease is 8 mg/kg/d.

**Monitoring** check-ups are the same as those described for administration every 24 hours. An ACTH stimulation test 2–6 hours after trilostane administration is recommended, although it can also be performed 8–12 hours afterwards. If it is performed after 8–12 hours, cortisol levels between 2 and 10 μg/dl indicate good control of the condition. Alternatively, measuring pre-trilostane cortisol levels (in non-stressed animals) helps decision making, especially with regards to overdosage.

### *Dose adjustments should be performed in a similar manner to the protocol described for once-daily administration. The ideal dose for any given patient may remain stable or vary with time.*

**Side effects** such as depression, anorexia, vomiting, diarrhoea, and weight loss may occur if excessive reduction of cortisol and aldosterone levels are caused by overdosing with trilostane. This risk of hypocortisolism highlights the importance of regular check-ups even when the animal is clinically well, since the symptoms associated with hypocortisolaemia are highly variable.

There have been reports of prolonged hypocortisolism during treatment with trilostane due to necrosis of the adrenal cortex. This necrosis is probably secondary to the presence of excessive levels of ACTH, although the factors behind it are still unknown.

In contrast to mitotane, there have been no reports of severe liver toxicity or neurological side effects associated with trilostane.

### *Mitotane*

Mitotane (o,p'-DDD) causes selective necrosis of the adrenal cortex, thereby reducing cortisol production. For years it has been the treatment of choice for dogs with HAC, although at present it is used very rarely, and then mainly for economic reasons since in large breeds it can be cheaper.

To promote its absorption and reduce gastrointestinal toxicity, administration with food is recommended, in two to three doses.

There are two treatment protocols, the selective and the complete destruction protocols.

#### *A: Selective destruction protocol*

This consists of two phases, the induction phase and the maintenance phase:

**1. Induction phase.** The initial dose is 30 to 50 mg/kg/d, divided into two doses, for 7 to 10 days. This phase ends after 10 days, or when a decrease in appetite is seen or side effects appear secondary to the medication; 25% of cases present with lethargy, vomiting, anorexia, weakness, diarrhoea, or ataxia, although in most cases the clinical signs are mild and due to a rapid decrease in cortisol levels. If these side effects occur, in addition to ceasing treatment with mitotane, a glucocorticoid should be administered.

With ACTH stimulation the values of cortisol before and after ACTH administration should be between 1 and 5 μg/dl.

If cortisol levels are low (<1 μg/dl), mitotane should be discontinued and glucocorticoids should be administered (prednisone 0.2–0.5 mg/kg/d) and progressively reduced, and an ACTH stimulation test should be performed.

If cortisol levels are high (>5 μg/dl), mitotane should be continued and the stimulation with ACTH repeated at intervals of 5 to 10 days, until cortisol levels of 1–5 μg/dl are achieved.

**2. Maintenance phase.** The maintenance dose is 30–50 mg/kg weekly divided into two or three doses. If toxicity occurs during maintenance, mitotane should be discontinued and a glucocorticoid administered. Iatrogenic hypoadrenocorticism develops in 5% of dogs.

An ACTH stimulation test should be repeated after 1 month, 3 months, and every 6 months:

If cortisol is high (5–10 μg/dl), the maintenance dose should be increased by 25–50%.

If cortisol is very high (>10 μg/dl), an induction protocol should be started.

#### *B: Complete destruction protocol*

This consists of administering a dose of 50–75 mg/kg/d for 25 days. A glucocorticoid (prednisone 0.4 mg/kg/day or hydrocortisone at 2 mg/kg/d for 3 weeks, and subsequently 0.2 mg/kg/day) and a mineralocorticoid (fludrocortisone 0.01 mg/kg) should be administered after the third day of treatment.

Side effects are similar to those described in the selective destruction protocol.

An ACTH stimulation test is recommended every 3–6 months to monitor possible recovery of the adrenal cortex.

This protocol may be more economical in the long term than the selective destruction protocol; however, the owner needs to administer glucocorticoids and mineralocorticoids daily.

### *L-deprenyl (selegiline)*

In approximately 30% of dogs with pituitary HAC, the origin of the disease is an excessive secretion of ACTH from the intermediate part of the pituitary, probably associated with a dopamine deficit.

L-deprenyl is a selective inhibitor of monoamine oxidase B, which restores the central levels of dopamine, normalizing the release of ACTH. The efficacy of this treatment is around 25%, with the main advantage being its low toxicity.

### *Cabergoline*

Cabergoline can act on the pituitary gland to reduce the release of ACTH. In the only study published on the treatment of canine HAC with cabergoline, doses of 0.07 mg/kg/week caused a decrease in ACTH concentration, urinary cortisol/creatinine ratio, and the size of the tumour in 42% of the dogs.

### *Retinoic acid*

The efficacy of retinoic acid in 22 dogs with pituitary HAC was evaluated and a clinical improvement demonstrated in all patients, as well as a reduction in the ACTH concentration, urinary cortisol/creatinine ratio, and the size of the pituitary adenoma. No side effects have been reported. More clinical studies are necessary.

### *Ketoconazole*

Ketoconazole inhibits several enzyme systems in the adrenal gland, reducing the synthesis of cortisol. The initial dose, which is adjusted at subsequent check-ups, is 5 mg/kg every 12 hours for 7 days. The goal is to achieve cortisol levels before and after the administration of ACTH of 1–5 μg/dl. If there is an exaggerated response to ACTH, the dose of ketoconazole may be increased to 15 mg/kg administered twice daily.

The efficacy of ketoconazole in dogs with HAC is 30–50% and the most common side effects are gastrointestinal symptoms (vomiting, diarrhoea, anorexia) resulting directly from the drug or associated with hypocortisolaemia.

### Radiotherapy

Radiation therapy may be useful in cases of HAC caused by a pituitary macroadenoma, especially in patients with neurological symptoms.

Cobalt 60 radiation is the most widely used radiotherapy treatment, although gamma-knife or stereotactic radiotherapies are better alternatives. In general, the total radiation dose is divided into fractions over 4 to 6 weeks.

Dogs with mild neurological signs and smaller tumours (<2 cm) have a better prognosis than those with severe neurological deficits and large tumours (>2.5 cm). In most cases the radiation has a minimal effect on the secretory capacity of the tumour, so the animals continue to need medical treatment for the HAC.

### Surgical treatment

Pituitary HAC can be treated by performing a hypophysectomy; a favourable response is obtained in more than 85% of cases. Associated complications are transient hypernatraemia, transient decrease in the production of tears, diabetes insipidus, and hypothyroidism, and recurrence occurs in approximately 15% of dogs that have been treated. At present its availability is limited.

### Treatment of adrenal hyperadrenocorticism

Adrenalectomy can be a curative treatment and is therefore considered the treatment of choice. However, the perioperative mortality of this surgery is high (20–35%) and many owners opt for medical treatment to avoid taking this risk. Medical treatment is also recommended in adrenal tumours with metastasis or which are locally invasive.

#### *Adrenalectomy*

Adrenalectomy is the treatment of choice for dogs with small adenomas or adrenal carcinomas, because if it is performed successfully, it can completely cure the condition. It requires a treatment protocol before and after surgery that includes the administration of glucocorticoids, heparin, and plasma, and inpatient monitoring.

#### *Mitotane*

Mitotane is used to destroy all the adrenal tumour tissue. The complete destruction protocol is normally used. The objective is to obtain low or undetectable cortisol levels (<1.0 μg/dl).

The selective destruction protocol is also an option, using higher doses (induction dose of 50–75 mg/kg/d for 10–14 days and maintenance doses of up to 100 and 200 mg/kg per week). Dose adjustments are based on ACTH stimulation.

When side effects appear (anorexia, weakness) mitotane administration should be discontinued and treatment with prednisone continued until the animal is re-evaluated and an ACTH stimulation test is performed. If electrolyte concentrations are normal but cortisol is undetectable or low, the daily dose of prednisone should be increased to 0.4 mg/kg/d. If clinical signs reappear when mitotane is reintroduced again, they are a direct consequence of the mitotane administration.

#### *Trilostane*

Trilostane is also effective for the resolution of clinical signs related to chronic hypercortisolaemia. It can be used initially to control hypercortisolaemia and improve the clinical and analytical status of the patient. However, trilostane does not act on adrenal neoplasia, so the prognosis depends on the malignancy, the degree of local invasion, and the presence of metastases from adrenal neoplasia.

The average survival of dogs with adrenal HAC is similar in dogs treated with mitotane, trilostane, or by adrenalectomy, so trilostane can be considered as a long-term alternative when adrenalectomy is not an option.

#### *Tyrosine kinase inhibitors*

The use of tyrosine kinase inhibitors (toceranib) has been proposed as treatment in adrenal cortex carcinomas, although studies are needed to support its efficacy.

## Canine hypoadrenocorticism

### *Aetiopathogenesis*

Canine hypoadrenocorticism (Addison's disease) typically occurs due to an atrophy or immune-mediated destruction of the adrenal cortex, leading to an insufficiency of mineralocorticoid and glucocorticoid production.

### *Epidemiology*

This condition mainly affects young adult dogs of average age 4 to 5 years, ranging from 1 month to 16 years old.

It is more common in females than males. Dogs with a breed predisposition are the Great Dane, Rottweiler, Portuguese Water Dog, Giant Poodle, West Highland White Terrier, and Wheaten Terrier.

## *Clinical signs*

There are two types of hypoadrenocorticism, classified according to their presentation.

- **Classic presentation:** This is the most common and associated with both mineralocorticoid and glucocorticoid deficiency (hypocortisolism and electrolyte alterations).
- **Atypical presentation:** Characterized by a hypocortisolaemia but with the presence of aldosterone and therefore normal electrolytes.

The **clinical picture is non-specific** and includes lethargy, weakness, loss of appetite, and vomiting. The symptoms can be mild to severe, with a waxing and waning time course. As the symptoms become more severe, the development of a hypovolaemic shock (an Addisonian crisis) can be fatal.

As this is a rare disease with a non-specific clinical picture, hypoadrenocorticism is probably underdiagnosed. However, some clinical signs are characteristic, including:

- episodic bouts of the disease
- aggravation due to stress
- bradycardia despite being dehydrated or in shock
- excellent, transient response to non-specific treatments such as hospitalization and fluid therapy.

## *Diagnosis*

### Radiological and ultrasonographic findings

Due to hypovolaemia a number of changes may be evident, such as:

- a decrease in cardiac size (microcardia)
- hypoperfusion of the cranial lobar pulmonary artery
- hypoperfusion of the caudal cava vein
- decreased liver size.

Ultrasonographically, if the left adrenal gland has a thickness of less than 3.2 cm, this is compatible with the disease.

### Electrocardiographical findings

In the presence of bradycardia or severe hyperkalaemia ($K^+$ >6.5 mEq/l), an electrocardiograph (ECG) should be performed, since the changes in cardiac conduction can be lethal. Typical ECG findings include bradycardia, an absence of P waves, prolongation of the QRS complex, a decrease in the amplitude of the R wave, an increase in the amplitude of the T wave, or prolongation of the PR interval.

### Laboratory findings

Mild or moderate normocytic, normochromic, non-regenerative anaemia can be observed. The absence of a stress leucogram (mild leucocytosis, lymphopenia, eosinopenia, monocytosis) in a sick patient should raise suspicion of hypoadrenocorticism.

Typical biochemical changes are:

- hyperkalaemia
- hyponatraemia
- hypochloraemia
- azotaemia, usually prerenal and usually resolves after adequate fluid replacement
- acidosis
- hypercalcaemia.

However, some patients have normal electrolyte levels. Urinalysis often shows a urine density of less than 1.030 even in the presence of azotaemia.

### ACTH stimulation test

This is the test of choice to confirm the presence of hypoadrenocorticism. Cortisol levels before and after ACTH administration are low (<2 μg/dl). The protocol is the same as that described for hyperadrenocorticism.

### Basal cortisol

A baseline cortisol value >2 μg/dl practically rules out the disease.

### Endogenous cortisol/ACTH ratio

Recently the cortisol/ACTH ratio has been identified as being a valid means of diagnosing the disease: in dogs with Addison's it is significantly low.

## *Treatment*

### Treatment of the Addisonian crisis

The main goals of treatment are to:

- correct blood volume (Figure 3.7)
- correct hypotension
- correct electrolyte imbalances
- correct the azotaemia
- correct the hypoglycaemia.

The most common cause of death during an Addisonian crisis is **hypovolaemic shock**. Therefore, the urgent administration of intravenous fluids is essential and potentially life-saving.

The volume of fluids to be administered in 24 hours is calculated based on the percentage dehydration

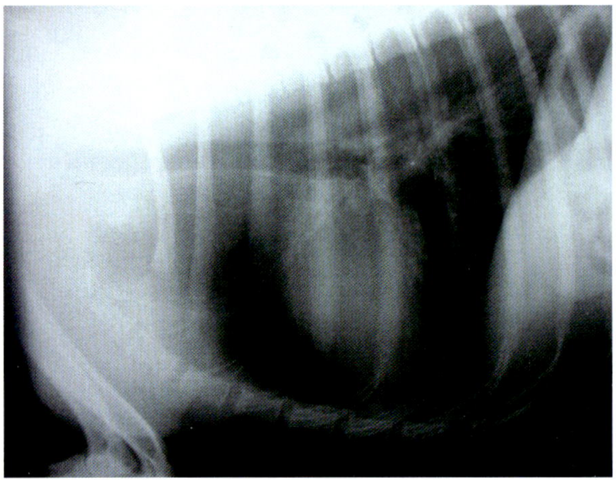

**Figure 3.7.** Thoracic radiograph showing hypovolaemia in a patient with Addison's disease. Image courtesy of the diagnostic imaging service at the HCVC.

and additional losses such as polyuria, vomiting, and diarrhoea.

1. Initially, a large volume is administered: for example, 40–80 ml/kg/h during the first 2 hours.
2. Subsequently, 90–120 ml/kg over 24 hours.

The most suitable fluid is **0.9% saline solution (0.9% NaCl)**, since it allows blood volume and electrolyte alterations to be corrected. Where hypoglycaemia is present, 50% glucose should be added to produce a 5% dextrose solution.

If the animal is in anuric or oliguric in the first few hours of treatment, the volume of fluids should be checked and if this is correct and the anuria persists, dopamine should be administered.

As a glucocorticoid supplement, dexamethasone sodium phosphate at a dose of 0.5 mg/kg IV is recommended, since it does not interfere with the analysis of cortisol levels when performing ACTH stimulation tests. Subsequently, 0.05–0.1 mg/kg/8–12 h IV can be administered. If the ACTH stimulation test has already been performed, other glucocorticoids such as methylprednisolone sodium succinate (1–2 mg/kg/6 h IV), hemisuccinate, or hydrocortisone phosphate (2–4 mg/kg/8 h IV) can be used. Another alternative is sodium succinate hydrocortisone at doses of 0.5–0.625 mg/kg/h IV, via a drip.

Currently, there are no fast-acting parenteral mineralocorticoids available. Fluid therapy is sufficient to correct hypovolaemia, hyponatraemia, and hyperkalaemia. From the moment the animal begins to eat, mineralocorticoids should be administered orally (fludrocortisone).

Acidosis is usually moderate and resolves with emergency treatment. However, if serious acidosis is present (the concentration of serum bicarbonate is less than 12 mEq/l), a solution of bicarbonate should be administered. The amount to be administered can be calculated using the following formula:

$$\text{Deficit (mEq/l)} = \text{Weight (kg)} \times 0.3 \times \text{Base deficit}$$

The base deficit is calculated by subtracting the venous $CO_2$ concentration of the patient from the normal $CO_2$ venous concentration (22 mEq/l). In severely affected animals, it is assumed there is a base deficit of 10 mEq/l.

If the animal has severe hyperkalaemia (>8.5 mEq/l) that does not resolve, 4–10 ml/kg of a 10% glucose solution can be administered over 30 to 60 minutes along with regular (crystalline) insulin at a dose of 0.06–0.125 IU/kg. Another option is to administer a calcium gluconate solution at a dose of 0.5–1.0 mg/kg over 10–20 minutes, which protects the myocardium from the effects of hyperkalaemia.

## Maintenance therapy

This consists of a mineralocorticoid supplementation for life, usually with glucocorticoids. The response to treatment and the prognosis are excellent.

### *Mineralocorticoids*

There are two alternatives: oral therapy with fludrocortisone or injections of desoxycorticosterone pivalate (DOCP).

**Fludrocortisone** is administered at an initial dose of 0.01–0.02 mg/kg/d divided into two doses, adjusted according to clinical response and measurement of urea and electrolytes (sodium and potassium). Initially, the electrolytes are monitored weekly until their normalization and, subsequently, monthly and semi-annual reviews are carried out. Most dogs need between 0.02 and 0.03 mg/kg/d.

The DOCP (Zycortal® injection) is started at a dose of 2.2 mg/kg IM or SC every 4 weeks and is reviewed weekly until the minimum effective dose is reached. Most dogs require the medication every 3 to 4 weeks. It is very effective and has no adverse effects.

### *Glucocorticoids*

Treatment with glucocorticoids (prednisone 0.2 mg/kg/d or hydrocortisone 0.5–1.0 mg/kg/d) is initially added to mineralocorticoid therapy. Because fludrocortisone has some glucocorticoid activity, glucocorticoid dose can be progressively decreased until it is removed indefinitely in 50% of dogs. However, administration of glucocorticoids during periods of stress (e.g. trips to the veterinary surgery) are recommended.

On the other hand, if the animal has to be fasted for more than 12 hours (surgery, gastroenteritis), an injectable glucocorticoid or DOCP should be administered to replace oral medication.

## Thyroid diseases

### *Canine hypothyroidism*

#### *Epidemiology*

Hypothyroidism usually affects dogs of medium or large size. The majority are middle-aged (4–10 years old) and there is no sex predisposition.

#### *Clinical signs*

The classic clinical signs are multisystemic and include:

- lethargy (Figure 3.8)
- weakness
- exercise intolerance
- weight gain
- intolerance to cold.

The severity of the symptoms is variable; in fact, some cases remain practically asymptomatic.

Most hypothyroid dogs have **dermatological symptoms**: a dry, dull coat, seborrhoea, alopecia on their body, a 'rat-like' tail, comedones, hyperpigmentation, and pyoderma (Figure 3.9). Myxoedema may appear due to accumulation of glycosaminoglycans in the dermis, which gives animals a tragic facial expression.

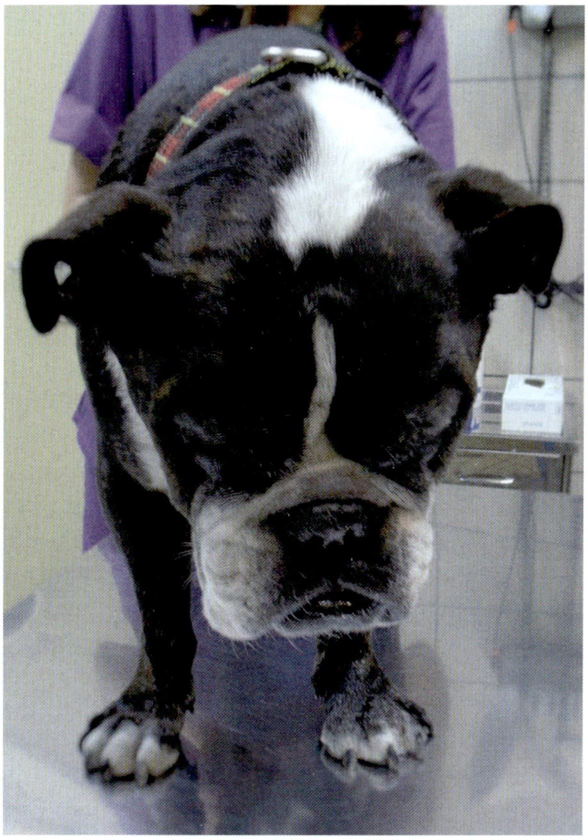

**Figure 3.8.** Weakness and lethargy in a 9-year-old male Boxer with hypothyroidism.

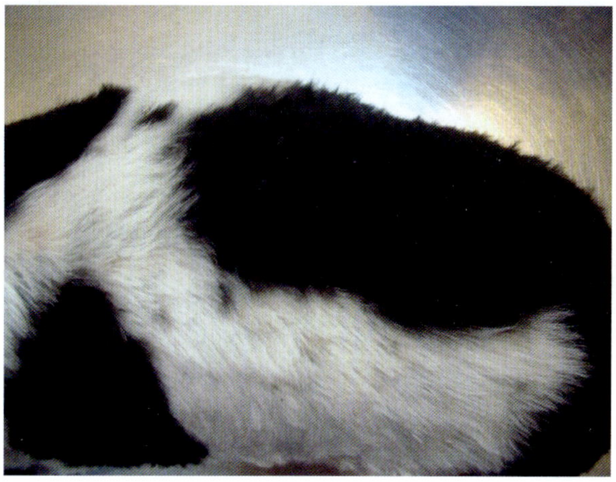

**Figure 3.9.** Seborrhoea and matted hair in a 5-year-old female American Cocker Spaniel with hypothyroidism.

Other less frequent signs are galactorrhoea and clinical signs similar to those of acromegaly, such as increased jaw size, increased interdental spaces, and megaoesophagus (Figure 3.10).

Some hypothyroid dogs show both central and peripheral **neurological changes**. The central signs (decreased consciousness, seizures) are probably due to changes in the blood–brain barrier and are usually reversible. Sometimes there are other signs, also reversible, such as vestibular disease, laryngeal paralysis, facial paralysis, proprioceptive deficits, and lower motor neuron signs.

Although it is rare, myxoedema coma can occur, typified by severe generalized weakness, stupor, and bradycardia. This condition requires the intravenous administration of thyroxine at 5 μg/kg/12 h.

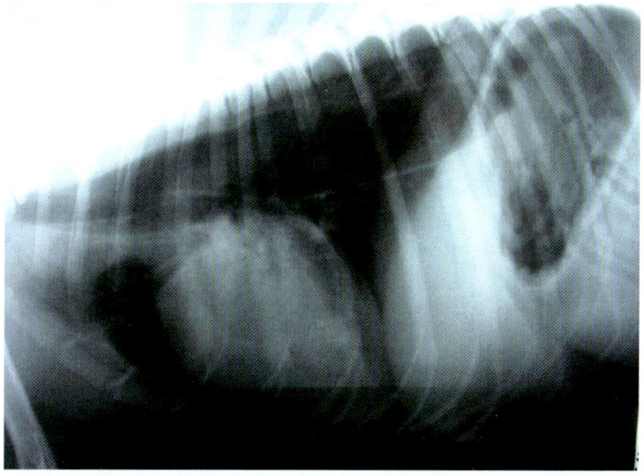

**Figure 3.10.** Megaoesophagus in a 4-year-old female Labrador with hypothyroidism. Image courtesy of the diagnostic imaging service at the HCVC.

### *Diagnosis*

The diagnosis of canine hypothyroidism should be based on the joint interpretation of a clinical examination and thyroid function tests.

The complete blood count, biochemistry, and urinalysis are useful tests to support a clinical suspicion of hypothyroidism and rule out other concurrent diseases. One third of hypothyroid dogs have mild, non-regenerative, normocytic, normochromic anaemia.

On blood biochemistry, hypercholesterolaemia and hypertriglyceridaemia are frequent, although occasionally elevations of serum levels of creatine kinase, lactate dehydrogenase (LDH), aspartate aminotransferase (AST), ALT, and ALP are observed.

#### Thyroid function tests

No test has an efficacy of 100% so it is advisable to use a combination of hormonal tests, which are interpreted in conjunction with the clinical picture. It should be remembered that false positives may occur in the presence of concurrent diseases of moderate severity or the polymedicated patient (especially with anticonvulsants, sulphonamides, corticosteroids.)

#### Total thyroxine (T4)

Total T4 has a high sensitivity, since 90% of hypothyroid dogs have low concentrations; however, some hypothyroid dogs do have normal levels of T4.

The basal plasma concentration of T4, or circulating total thyroxine in the blood, corresponds to the fraction of free circulating hormone (0.1%) and hormone circulating in association with proteins.

The main limitation of T4 is its **low specificity**: 30% of sick dogs have low levels of T4, a condition known as sick euthyroid syndrome. The greater the severity of the disease, the more likely T4 levels are to be low, with 60% of seriously ill dogs having low T4. On the other hand, many medications such as glucocorticoids, sulphonamides, anticonvulsants, and non-steroidal anti-inflammatory drugs (NSAIDs) can lower T4 concentrations in euthyroid dogs, and some breeds such as Greyhounds have T4 concentrations below the canine reference range.

There are several methods for measuring T4 concentrations in the dog, such as radioimmunoassay, chemiluminescence, and enzyme-linked immunosorbent assay (ELISA). They are all reliable, although reference ranges can vary.

If there is a high suspicion of hypothyroidism, concentrations of other hormones including thyroid stimulating hormone (TSH) must be determined to confirm the diagnosis and reduce the possibility of a false positive result.

#### Total triiodothyronine (T3)

The serum concentration of T3 remains normal in many hypothyroid dogs, so this hormone is generally not recommended for making a diagnosis.

#### TSH stimulation test

For many years this was the test of choice for the diagnosis of canine hypothyroidism. However, its limited availability, high cost, and the potential anaphylactic reactions mean it is now rarely used.

In general, this test is only indicated when the results of total T4, TSH, and free T4 tests are unclear, or when there are concurrent diseases or medications that interfere with the results for thyroid hormones.

Recombinant human TSH (rhTSH) can be used. The recommended dose is 50–100 μg/dog, although when there are concurrent diseases or the animal is receiving medication, 150 μg is recommended. Total T4 levels should be determined before and 6 hours after the IV administration of rhTSH (Thyrogen®). A total T4 concentration greater than 40 nmol/l at 6 hours or an increase in T4 levels of more than 20 nmol/l rules out hypothyroidism.

#### Free thyroxine (FT4)

This reflects the amount of T4 that circulates freely (not bound to proteins) and is available to enter the cells. There are three methods for its detection:

- equilibrium dialysis – reference method for the determination of FT4
- radioimmunoassay
- chemiluminescence.

The sensitivity of FT4 for hypothyroidism detection is high (98%), especially in hypothyroid dogs with anti-T4 antibodies, as these do not affect its measurement. FT4 concentrations decrease with concurrent diseases to a lesser extent than T4 concentrations. Even so, 20% of sick euthyroid dogs have low levels of FT4.

#### Endogenous TSH

The majority (>95%) of hypothyroid dogs have primary hypothyroidism and should therefore have high levels of TSH. However, the concentration of TSH is normal in 20–40% of hypothyroid dogs, since over time the pituitary gland loses the ability to respond to low T4 concentrations. Due to the low sensitivity of TSH (60–80%), a normal value in a dog with clinical signs compatible with hypothyroidism does not rule out a diagnosis of hypothyroidism.

On the other hand, the majority (90%) of sick euthyroid dogs have normal TSH levels. A low T4 together with a high TSH confirm the diagnosis of hypothyroidism, while the probability of finding this combination among dogs with euthyroid disease is less than 2%.

### Anti-thyroid antibodies

The presence of anti-thyroid antibodies (anti-thyroglobulin [TGAA], anti-T4, or anti-T3) in a hypothyroid dog suggests lymphocytic thyroiditis. However, it is not very useful for the diagnosis of hypothyroidism. Not all dogs with thyroiditis are hypothyroid or progress towards hypothyroidism. At a 1-year follow-up of euthyroid dogs with high levels of antibodies, approximately 20% of them had developed hypothyroidism, 60% were still euthyroid TGAA positive, and 20% were euthyroid TGAA negative.

## *Diagnostic imaging*

### Ultrasound of the thyroid

Euthyroid dogs have a homogeneous, isoechogenic or hyperechogenic thyroid parenchyma compared to surrounding tissue. However, hypothyroid dogs have a more heterogeneous and hypoechogenic parenchyma, a significantly smaller sized thyroid gland and a more irregular thyroid capsule. In addition, the thyroid volume continues to decrease during treatment with levothyroxine.

### Thyroid scintigraphy

Stable pertechnetate or 99mTcO4 is selectively concentrated in the thyroid and salivary glands. Recently it has been shown to be useful for differentiating between hypothyroid and sick euthyroid animals. The main drawback is the limited availability of this test.

## *Treatment and monitoring*

The treatment of choice is synthetic levothyroxine, from human medicine (Eutirox®) or preferably from veterinary medicine (Leventa®, Canitroid®). Owners should be warned that the doses for dogs are much higher than for people: 10–15 µg/kg twice a day; in large dogs, the lower to middle part of this range is used because the upper part can be excessive in more than 20% of dogs.

The half-life in plasma is 12 to 16 hours, and the maximum concentration is reached between 4 and 8 hours after oral administration. At 4 weeks, the clinical response and total T4 concentration 4 hours after administration of the medication is evaluated, and must be at the higher limit of the normal range or even slightly elevated (2.5–5 µg/dl).

- If it is below or around the normal low limit (1–2.5 µg/dl), the dose of levothyroxine should be increased by 25%.
- If total T4 concentrations are very high, the dose should be decreased by 25–50% especially if there is polyuria and polydipsia, weight loss, panting, excitability, and tachycardia.

The response to treatment is satisfactory in most cases. Apathy, weakness, and lethargy resolve within 1–2 weeks, but resolution of dermatological problems can take several months. Only neurological symptoms have a very variable range of responsiveness and can respond well, partially, or not at all.

## *Feline hyperthyroidism*

### *Epidemiology*

In many countries (USA, UK, Germany, Holland), hyperthyroidism is the most frequently occurring feline endocrinopathy. In countries such as Spain, its incidence seems to be lower, although it has increased in the last 10 years, with studies that indicate a 10% incidence in geriatric cats.

Feline hyperthyroidism affects middle- to old-aged animals (between 4 and 22 years old; average age 13 years), although it tends to occur in **geriatric cats** (95% of cases are older than 9 years of age). There is no breed or sex predisposition.

## *Aetiology*

The aetiology is multifactorial. The following factors influence the condition.

- **Genetic** (mutations in the gene that encodes the TSH receptor).
- **Environmental** (polybrominated diphenyl ethers [PBDE], the use of sand).
- **Dietetic** (frequent consumption of wet canned food, especially easy-to-open foods and certain flavours such as fish, liver, and gizzards). The iodine content of commercial diets may be involved in the pathogenesis of the disease: commercial cat diets contain very variable amounts of iodine, sometimes excessive or deficient for a cat's needs.

The most frequent pathology is a functional adenomatous hyperplasia of the thyroid gland. It has been described that over time hyperplasia can transform into a malignant neoplasm. Functional thyroid carcinoma is responsible in only 2% of cases.

### *Clinical signs*

The clinical picture depends on the stage of the disease at the time of diagnosis. Currently this condition is often diagnosed in the early stages, so the clinical signs are milder than those described years ago.

**Weight loss** is the most frequent symptom (90% of cases). Other common symptoms (between 25 and 50% of cases) are polyphagia, polyuria/polydipsia, hyperactivity, and vomiting.

Other symptoms of thyrotoxicosis are less frequent and include diarrhoea, decrease or loss of appetite, muscle weakness, polypnoea, behavioural alterations (vocalization), increased faecal volume, lethargy, and searching for cold areas.

Development of the clinical signs is progressive and, at the start, it is not normally obvious to the owner that the animal has a problem, as animals usually eat and drink well and are more active.

The most important finding upon clinical examination is an enlargement of the thyroid gland, which may be bilateral (70%) or unilateral (30%). In more than 80% of hyperthyroid cats one or both thyroid glands can be detected. It has been described that the size of the gland, observed by palpation, is related to T4 levels (Figure 3.11).

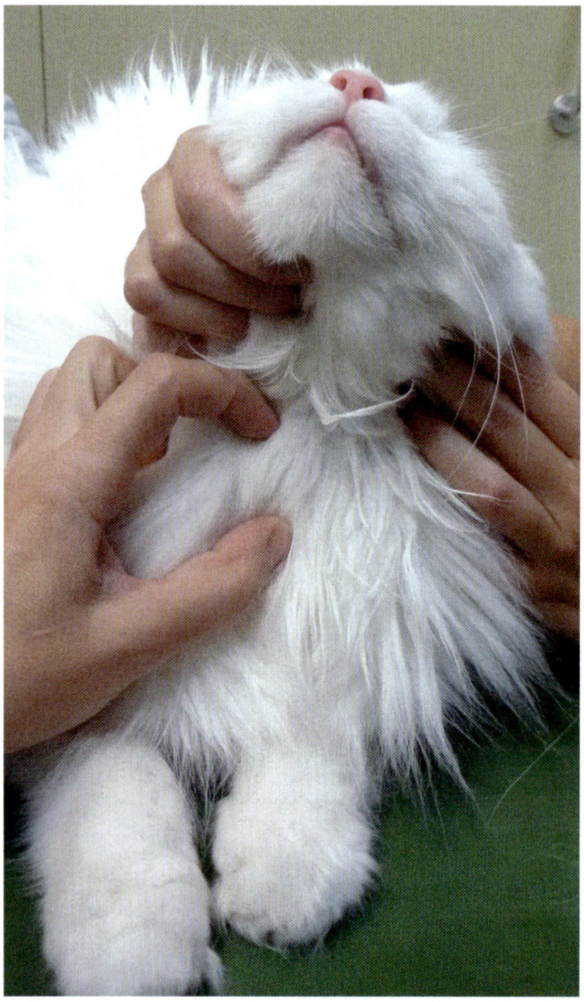

**Figure 3.11.** Increase in size in the thyroid gland in a 10-year-old male Common European cat with hyperthyroidism.

Other frequent findings on physical examination, in 40 to 65% of cases, are wasting, poor coat quality, heart murmurs, and tachycardia. In less than 15% of cases the following symptoms can also be seen: gallop rhythm, hyperkinesia, aggressiveness, coat changes, onychogryphosis, alopecia, heart failure, and ventral flexion of the neck.

## *Diagnosis*

### Laboratory tests

There is a mild to moderate polycythaemia in approximately 50% of cases. Leucocytosis with mature neutrophilia, eosinopenia, and lymphopenia is relatively common (20 to 40%) in these animals and probably reflects a stress response caused by excess thyroid hormones.

The most frequent changes (between 50 and 85%) are the increased serum concentrations of ALT, LDH, ALP, and AST. Between 20 and 40% of hyperthyroid cats have concurrent renal failure.

Urinalysis and renal function tests are essential. Chronic kidney disease is a common condition in elderly cats and, although associated with hyperthyroidism, it is not caused by the hyperthyroid state. Measurement of urine specific gravity is useful to distinguish prerenal azotaemia from primary renal disease, and urinalysis aids detection of concurrent diseases such as diabetes mellitus or urinary tract infections.

### Diagnostic imaging

#### *Radiology*

The most common radiological finding is cardiomegaly of variable degrees, which is present in approximately 30–50% of hyperthyroid cats. Radiological findings associated with congestive heart failure (pulmonary oedema, pleural effusion, pericardial effusion) occur less frequently (<10%).

#### *Ultrasound*

Ultrasound examination of the thyroid is a very useful diagnostic tool. On ultrasound, nodular thyroid lesions are well defined and surrounded by parenchyma with a normal appearance. In some cases, changes affect the entire thyroid lobe. The thyroid gland can appear considerably enlarged and tubular in shape.

**Thyroid carcinomas** (2% of cases) are seen on ultrasound as large, non-homogeneous masses, with irregular margins and a lesser echogenicity than normal thyroid tissue. Ultrasound is also useful to evaluate whether there is invasion of adjacent structures and of cervical lymph nodes.

### Hormonal diagnosis: diagnostic confirmation

#### *Total T4 concentration*

A total T4 level above the normal range in a cat with symptoms consistent with hyperthyroidism confirms diagnosis of the disease in 90% of cases. It is also very specific (barely any false positives in sick euthyroid cats). The main diagnostic challenge is the confirmation of hyperthyroidism in cats with 'hidden hyperthyroidism', that is, hyperthyroid cats with total T4 concentrations within normal limits (2–10% of cases).

#### *Total T3 concentration*

Only between 70 and 75% of hyperthyroid cats have high T3 concentrations, so measurement of T3 does not offer advantages over the single measurement of total T4.

#### *Endogenous feline TSH*

TSH levels can be measured using the canine TSH test to rule out feline hyperthyroidism.

- TSH >0.07 μg/l practically rules out the disease.
- TSH <0.03 μg/dl has a diagnostic sensitivity of 98%.

TSH is especially useful if it is measured together with levels of free T4 and total T4, which increases its specificity from 69 to 99%.

#### *T4 suppression test*

This consists of measuring total T4 levels before and after oral administration of a 3-day course of synthetic sodium liothyronine. Post-suppression T4 concentrations differ between cats with mild hyperthyroidism and healthy or sick euthyroid cats. The test is effective in diagnosing occult hyperthyroidism and is not very expensive; however, it needs several days for results to be obtained, and its effectiveness depends on oral administration of the medication, so it is not often used.

#### *Free T4 using dialysis and/or chemiluminescence technique*

Equilibrium dialysis is considered the most reliable assessment of free T4 and is especially useful in hyperthyroid cats with concurrent diseases in which the total T4 concentration remains at the normal high limit. However, the determination of free T4 should not be used as the sole diagnostic criterion, since some euthyroid cats with concurrent diseases may present with high concentrations of free T4.

## *Treatment*

Feline hyperthyroidism can be treated in four ways:

- medical treatment (anti-thyroid drugs)
- surgical thyroidectomy
- radioactive iodine (I-131)
- dietary treatment.

The choice of treatment in each case depends mainly on:

- the age of the cat
- the presence of associated cardiovascular changes
- the presence of concurrent pathologies (e.g. renal failure)
- the availability of nuclear medicine
- cost factors
- behavioural and environmental factors (such as the cat being aggressive or living in a multi-cat household).

When the clinical signs of hyperthyroidism are very mild, or if the cat has advanced concurrent diseases (e.g. kidney disease), treatment can be postponed. In the case of renal failure, a relative hyperthyroidism is beneficial since it increases glomerular filtration. However, if the decision is made to treat these patients, medical treatment is preferable, as its effects are reversible, especially in very old animals or where the anaesthetic risk is high.

### Medical treatment

Anti-thyroid medications are useful in the short term to stabilize the patient in preparation for thyroidectomy and in the long term as the sole treatment for hyperthyroidism.

Medical treatment decreases the synthesis of thyroid hormones but does not destroy hyperfunctional thyroid tissue. Some side effects seen include vomiting, anorexia, lethargy, or haematological alterations.

#### *Methimazole (Tirodril®, Felimazol®)*

This is the medical treatment of choice. It is administered orally, but also marketed as a gel for topical administration. Likewise, carbimazole can be used, which is metabolized to methimazole.

The goal of treatment is to maintain T4 levels in the low to normal range. The initial dose of methimazole is 1.5 to 2.5 mg/12 h (total dose/animal). After 2 or 3 weeks the concentration of T4 should be assessed; if T4 levels have not decreased, the dose is increased by 1.5 mg every 2 or 3 weeks. Some cats require up to 20 mg to control hyperthyroidism.

Most side effects occur during the first 3 months of treatment. In the long term, the minimum effective dose should be used to maintain the concentration of T4 between 1 and 2.5 μg/dl (13–30 nmol/l); in most cases, this dose is 7.5 to 10 mg/d. The occurrence of vomiting, diarrhoea, and lethargy are frequent (15%), but they are transient and do not prevent the continuation of treatment. Other more serious problems (occurring in less than 3% of cats treated with methimazole) include agranulocytosis, thrombocytopenia, haemorrhage, liver disease, and facial skin reactions.

### *Ipodate*

Ipodate is an organic iodinated agent that is used as a cholecystographic contrast medium. It rapidly reduces the concentration of T3, and only partially reduces the concentration of T4; however, it is very rarely used.

The initial dose is 50 mg/kg/12 h, and this is progressively increased up to 100 mg/kg/12 h. Approximately 70% of hyperthyroid cats, especially those with mild hyperthyroidism, respond well. In all animals the concentration of T4 remains high and no side effects are observed.

## Surgical treatment

Thyroidectomy is an effective treatment as long as clinical state and cardiovascular functionality are good, especially in cases where only one thyroid lobe is affected.

It is essential to stabilize cats ahead of surgery by administering methimazole, in order to achieve a euthyroid state 2 to 3 weeks before the intervention. A β-adrenergic antagonist, propranolol at 2.5–5 mg/kg/8 h, may also be used in animals in which anti-thyroid medication is not sufficient to normalize the heart rate. This medication prevents the appearance of intraoperative ventricular arrhythmias, frequent in hyperthyroid cats that have not been prepared preoperatively.

In 30% of hyperthyroid cats only one gland is affected, so unilateral thyroidectomy is curative, easy and does not run the risk of iatrogenic hypoparathyroidism. However, in **70%** of hyperthyroid cats both glands are hyperfunctional and a **bilateral thyroidectomy** is necessary. In these cases, conservation of at least one of the four parathyroid glands is necessary. Preoperative thyroid scintigraphy is useful to determine if one or both thyroid glands are affected, since 15% of hyperfunctional thyroid glands have a normal macroscopic appearance.

There are several surgical techniques.

- Original extracapsular technique: this can cause postoperative hypocalcaemia.
- Intracapsular technique, associated with a greater number of recurrences of hyperthyroidism.
- Modified intra- or extracapsular techniques are currently recommended.

If a bilateral thyroidectomy is performed, cats should be checked to monitor the following.

- **Hypocalcaemia** caused by hypoparathyroidism, which usually appears between 1 and 4 days after the procedure. If tremors, involuntary contractions of the limbs, and convulsions appear, treatment with vitamin D and calcium should be instituted.
- **Hypothyroidism**, which is usually transient if the thyroidectomy was unilateral, but may be permanent after bilateral surgery. The day after or 2 days after surgery supplementary thyroid hormones (levothyroxine 0.1–0.2 mg) should be administered; this can be stopped several months later, since the thyroid tissue remaining around the parathyroid glands is usually enough to maintain euthyroidism.
- **Recurrence of hyperthyroidism**: the concentration of T4 should be measured every 6–12 months for monitoring purposes.

## Radioactive iodine

This treatment has no side effects, is effective, and does not require anaesthesia, so it is undoubtedly the treatment of choice. However, renal function should be carefully assessed beforehand, to identify cases vulnerable to renal decompensation.

A single dose of subcutaneous radioactive iodine is sufficient to achieve a state of euthyroidism in most hyperthyroid cats. The dose used varies between 2 and 6 mCi depending on the size of the thyroid gland on palpation, the severity of the clinical signs, and the concentration of T4.

With this treatment, T4 concentrations are reduced to normal limits in 98% of cats and, in some cases, below the reference range. Clinical hypothyroidism occurs in approximately 2% of these cats and 2.5% suffer from recurrences of hyperthyroidism. The main drawback of this treatment is its limited availability.

### *Dietary treatment*

For the synthesis of thyroid hormones, a continuous supply of iodine in the diet is necessary, and therefore a reduction in iodine ingestion can cause a decrease in the levels of thyroid hormones.

It has been demonstrated that feeding a diet with a very reduced amount of iodine (0.47 ppm, in dry matter) to hyperthyroid cats results in the normalization of T4 levels after 9 weeks in 80% of cases, and that reducing the iodine content of the diet even further (0.17 ppm, in dry matter) means a euthyroid state can be achieved in all cases. These same authors have shown that a diet with an iodine content of 0.32 ppm or less is an effective and economical treatment in cats with hyperthyroidism.

This is therefore an alternative treatment option already available in Europe, which is safe and effective, ideal for cats without concurrent diseases or with mild, compensated diseases. It requires strict compliance with the diet and periodic reviews, where T4 levels and renal function are evaluated, among other parameters.

However, dietary management can be difficult in multi-cat households, where the patient has access to other foods. Also, all other sources of iodine must be avoided or the treatment is negated, and this can include substances as varied as plant potting compost and certain medications.

## Parathyroid diseases

### *Hypercalcaemia and hyperparathyroidism*

Calcium homeostasis within the body is maintained thanks to the combined action of two hormones.

- **Parathyroid hormone** (PTH), is responsible for promoting the absorption, reabsorption, and excretion of calcium.
- **Calcitonin** inhibits bone resorption and intestinal resorption of calcium and enhances calciuresis.
- 1,25 dihydroxycholecalciferol

#### *Aetiology*

##### Primary hyperparathyroidism

This is characterized by an excess of PTH due to an adenoma, hyperplasia, or carcinoma of the parathyroid glands.

It is uncommon in the dog and rare in the cat. The secretion of PTH is autonomous and does not depend on calcium levels; that is, PTH secretion does not become blocked despite hypercalcaemia.

##### Secondary hyperparathyroidism

Secondary hyperparathyroidism is more common than primary hyperparathyroidism. It occurs when the parathyroid glands are affected due to an imbalance in calcium and phosphorus levels. This is typically produced by chronic renal failure (secondary renal hyperparathyroidism) or nutritional alterations (secondary nutritional hyperparathyroidism).

When renal function is impaired, renal excretion of phosphorus is inadequate and phosphorus levels begin to increase. In the body, levels of calcium and phosphorus are kept in equilibrium, so that if phosphorus levels increase, calcium levels decrease and vice versa.

Therefore, in **chronic renal failure**, initially calcium levels decrease in response to excess phosphorus, causing hyperplasia of the parathyroid glands and release of PTH in an attempt to keep calcium levels within normal limits. In addition, in cases of chronic renal failure renal synthesis of vitamin D is lower, which further reduces calcium levels. However, although most dogs and cats with chronic renal failure have secondary hyperparathyroidism, total calcium plasma levels may be low, normal, or elevated.

**Secondary nutritional hyperparathyroidism** occurs due to the chronic feeding of diets deficient in calcium or vitamin D content, or with excessive phosphorus content; for example, diets exclusively based on meat. This nutritional imbalance gives rise to calcium levels slightly lower than normal, so that the parathyroid glands become hyperplasic and secrete an excess of PTH.

#### *Epidemiology*

Primary hyperparathyroidism affects elderly animals, with an average age of 11 years (4–17 years). There is no sex predisposition and although it is observed more frequently in certain breeds such as the Keeshond, Labrador Retriever, German Shepherd, or Golden Retriever, a clear breed predisposition has not been proven.

#### *Clinical signs*

In primary hyperparathyroidism, all symptoms are secondary to the presence of hypercalcaemia. Initially, the symptoms are mild and include polydipsia, polyuria, and lower urinary tract disorders (urinary incontinence, dysuria, stranguria, haematuria). Clinical signs related to the lower urinary tract may be secondary to urinary tract infections, urinary stones, or both. Bladder stones are usually calcium oxalate or calcium phosphate, favoured by hypercalciuria and metabolic renal acidosis that give rise to an alkaline urine.

Other less common symptoms are weakness, exercise intolerance, and decreased appetite and even anorexia, vomiting, and constipation. Neurological alterations can occur secondary to hypercalcaemia, for example, decreased consciousness, obtundation, or coma.

##### Physical examination

In primary hyperparathyroidism the physical examination is usually normal. In secondary hyperparathyroidism due to renal failure, animals may present with:

- weakness
- uraemic smell
- ulcers and/or pale mucous membranes (especially oral)
- dehydration.

## *Differential diagnoses*

In most dogs and cats with hypercalcaemia the cause is not hyperparathyroidism but other conditions such as:

- neoplasms (dog)
- idiopathic (cat)
- poisonings.

Therefore, on the physical examination, special attention should be paid to examination of palpable lymph nodes and the perianal region, since lymphoma and carcinoma of the anal sacs are two of the most frequent causes of tumour-related hypercalcaemia in dogs.

## *Diagnosis: laboratory findings*

### Complete blood count

In contrast to other causes of hypercalcaemia, such as neoplasms or renal failure (which are associated with anaemia, leucocytosis, or leucopenia), there are not usually any changes in dogs or cats with hyperparathyroidism.

### Blood biochemistry

#### *Hypercalcaemia*

The plasma concentration of total calcium in healthy dogs is 8.5–11.5 mg/dl; in dogs with primary hyperparathyroidism, the mean concentration is 14 mg/dl (range 12–23 mg/dl).

Plasma calcium or total calcium (CaT) is formed of three fractions.

- **Ionized** or free (56%). This is the active fraction.
- **Chelated** or combined with other compounds (phosphate, bicarbonate, etc.; 10%).
- **Bound to proteins** (34%). Acts as a reservoir. If albumin and globulin levels are altered, total calcium levels are also altered, without the biologically active calcium fraction being affected.

In a patient whose total calcium level is elevated (or decreased), it is necessary to measure the **ionized calcium** level, since this more truly reflects the actual calcaemia.

To correct for the effect of the albumin level on the total calcium level, the following formula can be used:

Total corrected calcium = total calcium (mg/dl) − albumin (g/dl) + 3.5

However, it is still advisable to determine the level of **ionized calcium**, since it has been shown that this formula does not accurately reflect the calcaemia of the patient. Relying on the total calcium level tends to overestimate hypercalcaemia and minimize hypocalcaemia, especially in the cat. Also, the total calcium level can be altered by laboratory errors such as haemolysis and haemoconcentration, while lipaemia causes false elevation.

**Sampling technique** is also very important, because it can have an impact on the final result. Changes are anticipated if sampling is done postprandially, placed in tubes containing EDTA anticoagulant, left in the tube for several hours, or is contaminated (e.g. with chalk).

To determine the ionized calcium level, the blood sample must be obtained in a vacutainer tube without anticoagulant, be handled with caution, and in the most anaerobic conditions possible. Although reference values should be established by each laboratory, the normal ionized calcium range is usually between 1.1 and 1.4 mmol/l.

#### *Hypophosphataemia*

Serum phosphorus levels are usually low or within the normal to low range (<4 mg/dl). This is due to the effect of PTH on the kidney, which causes an excessive loss of phosphorus at a tubular level.

Phosphorus levels should always be interpreted along with calcium levels. The presence of hypophosphataemia, together with hypercalcaemia or even with normal high levels of calcium, is indicative of hyperparathyroidism or hypercalcaemia caused by tumours. If there is hyperphosphataemia and hypercalcaemia, it is most likely that the hypercalcaemia is due to other causes (not primary hyperparathyroidism).

#### *Other biochemical alterations*

Urea and creatinine levels are usually normal in animals with primary hyperparathyroidism. However, chronic untreated hyperparathyroidism (due to chronic hypercalcaemia) can cause kidney damage resulting in azotaemia. Some animals with hyperparathyroidism have mild to moderately elevated levels of ALP, while ALT levels are usually normal.

### Urinalysis

In 40% of cases, hypercalcaemia results in a reduced urinary specific gravity (<1.012). Other frequent findings include haematuria, pyuria, bacteriuria, and crystalluria.

### Differential diagnoses of hypercalcaemia

The causes of hypercalcaemia in the dog and in the cat are many and varied. Table 3.3 describes the biochemical features that identify the most frequent causes of hypercalcaemia.

Table 3.3. Biochemistry keys for establishing the cause of hypercalcaemia in dogs and cats.

| | Total calcium | Ionized calcium | Corrected calcium | Phosphorus | PTH |
|---|---|---|---|---|---|
| Primary hyperparathyroidism | ↑ | ↑ | N↑ | ↓ or N | ↑ or N |
| Nutritional hyperparathyroidism | N↓ | N↓ | N↓ | N↑ | ↑ |
| Renal hyperparathyroidism | N↓ ↑ | N↓ | N | ↑ or N | ↑ |
| Hypercalcaemia humoral tumour (lymphoma) | ↑ | ↑ | ↑ or N | ↓ or N | ↓ or N |
| Hypercalcaemia local tumour (osteolytic) | ↑ | ↑ | ↑ or N | N↑ | ↓ or N |
| Hypervitaminosis D | ↑ | ↑ | ↑ | ↑ or N | ↓ |
| Hypoadrenocorticism | ↑ | ↑ | ↑ | ↑ or N | ↓ or N |
| Idiopathic (cat) | ↑ | ↑ | ↑ | N↑ | ↓ or N |
| Dehydration | ↑ | N↑ | ↑ or N | N↑ | N↓ |
| Hyperthyroidism (cat) | ↑ | ↑ | ↑ | N↑ | ↑ or N↓ |

*Note*: N, normal; N↑, value around the upper limit of the normal range; N↓, value around the lower limit; PTH, parathyroid hormone.

## Radiology

For cats and dogs with hypercalcaemia, radiographic studies of the chest are essential (at least two lateral views). This is because neoplastic causes of hypercalcaemia, for example, mediastinal lymphoma, may become evident.

## Ultrasound

In dogs with primary hyperparathyroidism, the size of the mass (adenomas and parathyroid carcinomas) is variable (2–23 mm in diameter), although most measure more than 4 mm. In comparison with the surrounding thyroid tissue, these masses are usually round or oval, well defined, and hypoechoic or anechoic. In addition, in dogs, there may be changes to the thyroid gland which are visible on ultrasound.

An abdominal ultrasound should be performed in all patients with hypercalcaemia. This is to evaluate the echogenicity and size of the liver and spleen, and to detect the possible presence of abdominal masses (neoplasms), lymphadenopathies, or urolithiasis (throughout the urinary tract).

## Computed tomography

Where there is suspicion of hypercalcaemia secondary to a neoplastic process, CT imaging is the technique of choice to detect the underlying neoplasm.

## Diagnostic confirmation of hyperparathyroidism

A definitive diagnosis is made by histology of the parathyroid mass/masses after surgical removal. However, a tentative diagnosis can be made by determining the serum levels of PTH and parathyroid hormone-like protein (PTHrP).

PTH levels in normal dogs and cats are between 2 and 13 pmol/l, while the majority of dogs with primary or secondary hyperparathyroidism have PTH levels above 13 pmol/l.

The most sensitive measurement of PTH is whole PTH, but not all laboratories offer it. However, assessment of PTHrP is less complicated, and in dogs with primary or secondary hyperparathyroidism PTHrP levels are less than 0.2 pmol/l. When the origin of hypercalcaemia is a tumour, or is due to an increase in osteolytic activity, PTHrP levels are high.

### *Treatment*

## Treatment of hyperparathyroidism

Where there is a suspicion of primary hyperparathyroidism, the treatment of choice is exploratory neck surgery and removal of the parathyroid mass or masses.

One of the two thyroid lobes and their associated parathyroid glands should always be preserved. This is to avoid the development of permanent hypoparathyroidism and hypothyroidism after the procedure.

After the removal of a parathyroid lobe, calcium levels should be monitored from the first week onwards. In dogs with high presurgical levels of calcium (>14 mg/dl) or chronic hypercalcaemia, a hormonal supplement with vitamin D can be administered. The latter is given 12 hours after surgery as a preventative measure, for up to 2 weeks, depending on calcium levels.

There are various **vitamin D supplements** which can be used, mainly in the form of vitamin D3 or cholecalciferol (always marketed together with calcium) or calcitriol (Rocaltrol® 0.25 and 0.50 µg) at doses of 0.02 to 0.06 µg/kg/d.

Heat or ethanol ablation of the hyperfunctional parathyroid lobes under ultrasound guidance has also been described, and is reported to be effective in 85% of cases, with side effects in 11% of the animals treated.

## Treatment of hypercalcaemia

The treatment of hypercalcaemia depends on many factors, with the objectives being to increase urinary calcium excretion and reduce bone resorption.

Emergency stabilization of hypercalcaemia is required when:

- the symptoms are severe
- there is rapid onset hypercalcaemia, e.g. rodenticide poisoning
- calcium levels are severely raised (>14mg/dl), especially when phosphorus levels are also raised.

Emergency treatment is based on:

- rehydration with intravenous saline solution
- administration of diuretics (furosemide)
- administration of glucocorticoids, but only if a definitive diagnosis has been made.

If the hypercalcaemia persists despite this therapy, then substances that inhibit osteoclast activity and slow down bone resorption can be used. Typically these are IV bisphosphonates such as pamidronate.

Management of chronic hypercalcaemia can be performed with the administration of oral glucocorticoids (prednisone or dexamethasone).

Table 3.4 describes the doses and the administration schedule of the medications recommended for treatment of hypercalcaemia in dogs and cats.

In cases of **feline idiopathic** hypercalcaemia, emergency treatment is not usually necessary. This is because, although ionized calcium (CaI) levels can be very high, levels of total calcium (CaT) are not usually higher than 13 mg/dl, and so the clinical picture is usually mild or moderate.

In these cases, the first step is to attempt correction of the hypercalcaemia with a **diet rich in fibre**. This reduces intestinal absorption of calcium by decreasing intestinal transit time, even when the diet is supplemented with extra calcium. If there is no response to this type of diet, a renal diet can be administered, which contains reduced levels of calcium and phosphorus and is alkalizing. As an alternative, homemade diets with reduced calcium content or canned food can be used. It should be recognized that maintenance diets are usually acidifying, and therefore increase the availability of CaI, facilitating intestinal absorption and increasing bone resorption.

In cats that do not respond to dietary treatment alone, **oral treatment with corticosteroids** can be attempted (Table 3.4), monitoring CaI levels at 15 days and 1 month after implementation, reducing the initial dose until the minimum effective dose is reached. Cats on treatment should be checked every 3 months. It has been reported that prednisone may increase the risk of oxalate stone formation, while prednisolone does not increase this risk.

Table 3.4. Treatment options in patients with hypercalcaemia.

| | Dose | Frequency | Route of administration | Comments |
|---|---|---|---|---|
| Saline solution (NaCl 0.9%) | 100–125 ml/kg/d | | IV | Care if hypertension |
| Furosemide | 5 mg/kg/h | | Continuous IV infusion | Hypercalcaemia that does not respond to fluid therapy |
| Furosemide | 2–4 mg/kg | BID or TID | IV, SC, or PO | If continuous infusion is not possible |
| Prednisone | 1.0–2.2 mg/kg | BID | PO, IV, or SC | Hypercalcaemia that does not respond to fluid therapy or fluids. Only if lymphoma has been ruled out |
| Prednisone | 5 mg | BID | PO | In feline idiopathic hypercalcaemia, up to 10 mg BID can be given |
| Dexamethasone | 0.1–0.22 mg/kg | BID | PO, IV, or SC | Hypercalcaemia that does not respond to fluid therapy or fluids. Only if lymphoma has been ruled out |
| Calcitonin | 4–6 IU/kg | BID or TID | SC | Failure of other treatments |
| Disodium pamidronate | 1.3–2.0 mg/kg | Once | IV over 20 minutes | Dilute in physiological saline |
| Sodium bicarbonate | 1–4 mEq/kg | According to effect | Slow IV | For hypercalcaemic crisis |

*Note*: BID, twice daily; TID, three times per day; IV, intravenous; PO, by mouth; SC, subcutaneous.

If idiopathic hypercalcaemia reappears or does not respond to corticosteroids, PO administration of bisphosphonates is possible. Typically, this is alendronate (Fosamax®), at doses of 10 to 30 mg per week. In human medicine, oesophagitis and oesophageal stenosis have been described with the use of this medication. Therefore it is recommended to wipe butter over the cat's lips and give a little water with a syringe after its administration, to ensure that the pill does not stay in the oesophagus. If alendronate is used, levels of CaI should be checked at 15 days, 1 month, and then every 3 months.

## *Hypocalcaemia and hypoparathyroidism*

### *Epidemiology*

Hypocalcaemia is rare in small animals. Although the age range of animals that present with hypocalcaemia is very wide, between 6 months and 13 years, it has a greater incidence in middle-aged female animals.

### *Aetiology*

Measurement of PTH concentrations enables the causes of hypocalcaemia to be differentiated into those that are PTH dependent and those that are independent of PTH.

### *PTH-dependent hypocalcaemia*

When hypocalcaemia is caused by low levels of PTH, this is due to hypoparathyroidism, either primary or secondary.

#### Spontaneous primary hypoparathyroidism

This occurs in dogs and cats as a result of immune-mediated destruction (probably a lymphocytic parathyroiditis) or idiopathic destruction of the parathyroid glands.

It is a rare disease and in common with many **immune-mediated processes** usually affects middle-aged bitches. The **Poodle** is one of the breeds with the greatest predisposition.

In cats, it can occur at very early ages as a result of agenesis of the parathyroid glands. Affected cats are usually young adults, but there is no sex predisposition.

Other causes of primary hypoparathyroidism are destruction of the glands by trauma or tumours in the neck region.

#### Primary iatrogenic hypoparathyroidism

This may occur as a result of bilateral thyroidectomy, as a treatment for hyperthyroidism. The PTH concentration is low or normal to low, which reflects an inappropriate response of the parathyroid glands to correct hypocalcaemia. Phosphorus is generally elevated as a result of decreased renal excretion.

#### Other causes of PTH-dependent hypoparathyroidism

When an animal has hypercalcaemia, the parathyroid glands respond by decreasing production of PTH. This is a crucial mechanism of calcium homeostasis. However, if calcium levels are persistently raised for long periods of time (weeks or months) the parathyroids undergo progressive atrophy and their capacity to produce PTH decreases.

Should it then become possible to correct the underlying cause of the hypercalcaemia, the atrophied parathyroids may not be able to respond appropriately. Thus, blood calcium concentrations should subsequently be monitored, in case the patient develops hypocalcaemia.

### *Hypocalcaemia independent of PTH*

Hypocalcaemia not dependent on PTH can be caused by two mechanisms.

### *Redistribution of calcium*

This may be due to eclampsia or calcium chelation.

**Eclampsia:** Pregnant females allocate large amounts of calcium to foetal development and, subsequently, to lactation. Generally, these calcium losses are compensated for by calcium homeostasis mechanisms which aim to maintain blood levels. However, in some females this compensation is not sufficient, and they develop hypocalcaemia (**postpartum tetany** or eclampsia).

**Calcium chelation:** Hypocalcaemia by chelation of ionized calcium can occur with substances such as citrate (after a transfusion) and oxalate (in ethylene glycol poisoning).

### *Deficiency of calcium or vitamin D intake*

This may be due to malnutrition or pancreatitis.

In the face of chronic hypocalcaemia (for reasons other than a PTH deficit), the parathyroid glands produce increased amounts of PTH to correct it. This is known as secondary hyperparathyroidism. This response to an alteration of mineral homeostasis can be caused by:

- lack of calcium intake
- excessive intake of phosphates
- accumulation of phosphate due to a decrease in renal excretion (kidney disease).

High levels of PTH have a positive effect to normalize low levels of ionized calcium. But when they are chronically high, this can cause negative effects such as bone demineralization. The magnitude of the elevation of PTH varies depending on the type of secondary hyperparathyroidism and, in general, is inversely proportional to the concentration of ionized calcium.

Higher PTH values (>100 pmol/l) are more frequently associated with secondary hyperparathyroidism than with primary hyperparathyroidism.

### Clinical signs

Animals with mild hypocalcaemia (total calcium 7.0–8.5 mg/dl) generally do not present with symptoms of hypocalcaemia. Indeed, if this mild hypocalcaemia is secondary to another disease, the clinical signs vary depending on that primary problem (e.g. kidney disease, pancreatitis, malabsorption syndrome, hypoalbuminaemia, etc.).

When the hypocalcaemia is **moderate or severe** (total calcium <7.0 mg/dl), episodic signs appear that can be triggered or aggravated by exercise or stressful situations. These symptoms include weakness, tremors, panting, nervousness, partial or generalized seizures, muscle spasms, decreased appetite, vomiting, diarrhoea, cardiac arrhythmias, cataracts, and fever.

**Eclampsia** or hypocalcaemia related to gestation or lactation in bitches usually appears 4 to 6 weeks after delivery. This presents with the classic symptoms of hypocalcaemia (tremors, muscle spasms, seizures, etc.). Occasionally, it starts at the beginning of lactation or even at the end of pregnancy. In cats, however, the predominant symptoms of hypocalcaemia are anorexia and lethargy.

On physical examination, neuromuscular symptoms may be evident if calcium concentrations are **very low** (moderate or severe hypocalcaemia) at the time of examination. Animals with chronic hypocalcaemia tend to be thin because of chronic appetite loss. On ocular examination, there may be bilateral cataracts that appear as multiple subcapsular punctate opacities.

### Diagnosis: laboratory tests

Routine screening tests should be carried out, including a complete blood count, biochemistry, and urinalysis. This helps identify or rule out some causes of hypocalcaemia (such as renal failure or hypoproteinaemia) and establish a diagnostic plan.

Whenever calcaemia is evaluated, total calcium levels should be measured, with the calcium corrected according to albumin and phosphorus levels. In patients with changes in total calcium, measurement of ionized calcium should also be included, which best reflects actual calcaemia. Table 3.5 shows the biochemical keys to detecting the main causes of hypocalcaemia.

### Treatment

The treatment protocol for hypocalcaemia depends on its magnitude and the patient's clinical presentation.

- Severe hypocalcaemia and symptomatology: treat with **calcium IV.**
- Mild and asymptomatic hypocalcaemia: treat with calcium supplements and **vitamin D PO**.

There are several calcium salts available, but the amount of usable calcium is different in each of them (Table 3.6). There are also three types of vitamin D, which differ in the dose needed to reach normocalcaemia. Calcitriol is normally used as it is the most effective in terms of duration of action and maximum effect.

#### Emergency treatment

*Calcium*

In the face of symptomatic hypocalcaemia, calcium gluconate 10% solution should be administered intravenously, at a dose of 5–15 mg/kg over 10–30 minutes, which works out at 0.5–1.5 ml/kg. Generally, calcium gluconate is used because, unlike calcium chloride, it

Table 3.5. Analytical keys to the main causes of hypocalcaemia.

| | Total calcium | Ionized calcium | Albumin | Corrected calcium | Phosphorus | PTH |
|---|---|---|---|---|---|---|
| Primary hypoparathyroidism | ↓ | ↓ | N | ↓ | N↑ | N↓ |
| Eclampsia | ↓ | ↓ | N | ↓ | ↓ | ↑mild, N |
| Hypoalbuminaemia | ↓ | N↓ | ↓ | N | N | N↑ |
| Phosphate enema | ↓ | ↓ | N | ↓ | ↑ | ↑ |
| Anti-freeze poisoning | ↓ | ↓ | N | ↓ | N↑ | ↑ |
| Paraneoplastic | ↓ | ↓ | N | ↓ | ↓ | N↑ |
| Sepsis/intensive care | N↓ | ↓ | N | N↓ | N↑ | N↑ |

*Note*: N, normal; N↑, value around the upper limit of the normal range; N↓, value around the lower limit; PTH, parathyroid hormone.

Table 3.6. Treatment of hypocalcaemia.

| | Supplements | Format | Available calcium | Dose | Observations |
|---|---|---|---|---|---|
| Parenteral calcium | 10% calcium | Gluconate solution | 9.3 | Slow IV until effect 0.5–1.5 ml/kg IV | Stop if bradycardia or shortened QT intervals are observed |
| | | | mg Ca/ml | 5–15 mg/kg/h IV | To maintain normocalcaemia<br>Avoid administering SC calcium salts, as these can cause skin necrosis and mineralization |
| | 10% calcium chloride | Solution | 27.2 mg Ca/ml | 5–15 mg/kg/h IV | Irritant on perivascular administration |
| Oral calcium | Calcium carbonate | Tablets, sachets | 40% | 25–50 mg/kg/d | Most frequent format |
| | Calcium lactate | 325, 650 mg/tablet | 13% | 25–50 mg/kg/d | |
| | Calcium chloride | Powdered | 27.2% | 25–50 mg/kg/d | Can cause gastric irritation |
| | Calcium gluconate | Wide variety | 10% | 25–50 mg/kg/d | |
| Vitamin D | Vitamin $D_3$ (calcitriol) | | | Initial: 5–20 ng/kg/d for 3–4 days<br>Maintenance: 2.5–6.0 ng/kg/d | Maximum effect in 1–4 days Resolution of toxicity in 2–7 days |
| | Vitamin $D_2$ (ergocalciferol) | | | Initial: 4000–6000 U/kg/d<br>Maintenance: 1000–2000 U/kg every 1–7 days | Maximum effect in 5–21 days<br>Resolution of toxicity in 1–18 days |
| | Dihydrotachysterol | | | Initial: 0.02–0.03 mg/kg/d<br>Maintenance: 0.01–0.02mg/kg/24–48 h | Maximum effect at 1–7 days<br>Resolution of toxicity in 1–3 weeks |

does not produce irritation if administered outside the vein. The recommended dose of calcium gluconate is between 1.0 and 1.5 ml/kg (Table 3.6). It is advisable to monitor an electrocardiogram during administration: if bradycardia or shortening of the QT interval appears, the administration of calcium should be reduced or paused.

Once the emergency situation is stabilized and until oral vitamin D takes effect, calcium can be added to fluid therapy at a dose of 60–90 mg/kg/d. When calcium is added to the serum, **0.9% saline** is always used because calcium can precipitate in bicarbonate, lactate, or acetate-containing solutions.

Calcaemia should be **monitored once or twice a day** until normocalcaemia is achieved. If calcium levels cannot be intensively monitored, 10% calcium gluconate diluted 1:1 with saline can be administered subcutaneously to minimize pain and possible tissue damage (0.25–0.5 ml/kg every 8 hours).

To avoid hypocalcaemia, calcium and vitamin D should be administered as soon as the animal can tolerate oral medication and parenteral calcium administration withdrawn 2–3 days after oral medication commences. Oral calcium supplements that provide 50–100 mg/kg/d of available calcium, a dose that will be divided into 2–4 daily administrations, should be prescribed.

### *Vitamin D*

Vitamin D should also be administered alongside treatment with an oral calcium supplement. Of the three types available (Table 3.6), the most recommendable product is calcitriol, because it normalizes calcaemia faster and, in the case of hypercalcaemia due to overdose, the effect also disappears more quickly.

The initial dose of calcitriol (Rocaltrol®) is 2.5–6.0 ng/kg/d (0.025–0.06 μg/kg/d), and this is adjusted according to calcaemia. When oral treatment is commenced it is advisable to monitor calcium levels daily over a number of days until it is firmly in the normal to low range.

### Maintenance therapy

This consists of the permanent administration of vitamin D (calcitriol) along with an adequate intake of calcium as a supplement or in the diet. The objective is to maintain the calcium concentration between 8.0 and 9.5 mg/dl, to avoid signs of hypocalcaemia and to prevent potential side effects of hypercalcaemia (hypercalciuria, nephrocalcinosis, and renal failure).

#### *Calcium*

Initially a supplement that provides about 25 mg/kg/d of available calcium should be used, and then the dose gradually decreased until calcium comes from the diet alone (balanced commercial diet). Regardless of whether long-term calcium supplements are used or not, the daily intake of calcium should be kept constant to avoid large variations in calcaemia.

#### *Vitamin D*

Calcium monitoring should be weekly for 2–3 weeks, then monthly for 2–3 months, and subsequently every 3 months. The dose of vitamin D (calcitriol) should be adjusted up or down by 20% if necessary, based on the measured blood calcium concentrations. The efficacy of treatment may decrease if changes are made in the diet.

Hypercalcaemia due to vitamin D overdose is a frequent complication, so owners should be taught to recognize signs of hypercalcaemia (polyuria, polydipsia, anorexia). If hypercalcaemia is severe, diuretics and furosemide should be administered until serum calcium levels are normalized, and subsequent doses of vitamin D should be reduced.

Hyperthyroid cats may suffer transient hypocalcaemia after bilateral thyroidectomy. The recovery of the parathyroid glands can occur weeks or months after surgery, so after 2–3 months of treatment a gradual reduction of the vitamin D dose can be started while monitoring the levels of calcium every week.

### Treatment of non-PTH-dependent hypocalcaemia

The treatment of non-PTH-dependent hypocalcaemia consists of correcting hypocalcaemia by means of calcium and vitamin D supplementation and, whenever possible, treating the triggering cause such as malabsorption syndrome, pancreatitis, or malnutrition.

## Diseases of the endocrine pancreas

The two diseases of the endocrine pancreas with the greatest clinical relevance are diabetes mellitus and insulinoma.

## *Diabetes mellitus*

### *Definition*

Diabetes mellitus is an endocrine disease where the body's ability to produce or respond to insulin is impaired, as characterized by persistent hyperglycaemia.

### *Epidemiology*

Canine diabetes affects middle- to advanced-aged dogs (average age 8 years) and is more frequent in females, largely as a consequence of insulin resistance in dioestrus. The breeds with the greatest predisposition to diabetes mellitus are the Cairn Terrier, Poodle, Miniature Schnauzer, Dachshund, and Beagle.

Feline diabetes affects **middle- to advanced-aged cats**. It is more frequent in **males**, especially those which are castrated and obese. There is a breed predisposition in Burmese cats.

### *Aetiopathogenesis*

There are several types of diabetes.

- **Insulin dependent or Type I diabetes** is caused by the destruction of pancreatic β cells and is characterized by an inability to produce insulin. It is the most frequent type in the dog.
- **Type II diabetes** may or may not be insulin dependent. It is characterized by hyperglycaemia and insulin resistance, but some capacity for insulin secretion is preserved and in some cases the condition may be reversible. It is common in cats and humans, but very rare in the dog.
- **Type III or secondary diabetes** is caused by diseases such as pancreatitis, hyperadrenocorticism, or acromegaly or by administration of medications such as glucocorticoids or progestogens. Secondary diabetes can be reversible after correction of the triggering factor, especially in the cat.

### *Clinical signs*

In the uncomplicated form the patient shows signs of diabetes, but not of decompensation. Generally these cases can be treated at home.

In the complicated form (diabetic ketoacidosis) the animal presents a severe clinical picture with dehydration, vomiting, and anorexia. This is due to ketosis and ketoacidosis, with the presence of high levels of ketone bodies in the blood and urine, and requires emergency treatment.

Long-term complications can include peripheral neuropathy and cataracts (Figures 3.12 and 3.13).

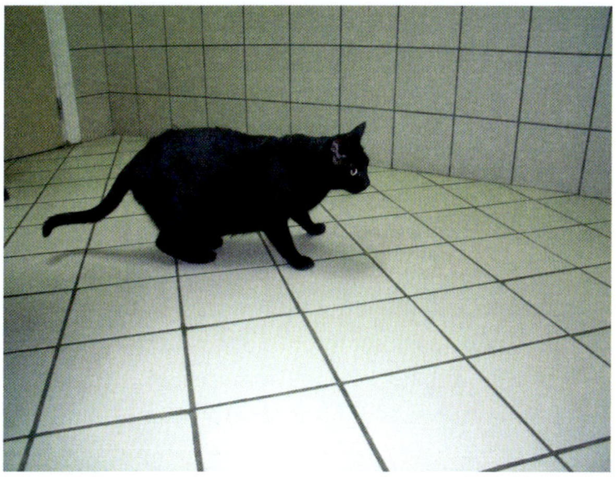

**Figure 3.12.** Wide-based stance due to diabetic neuropathy in a Common European male cat which has been suffering from diabetes mellitus for 8 months.

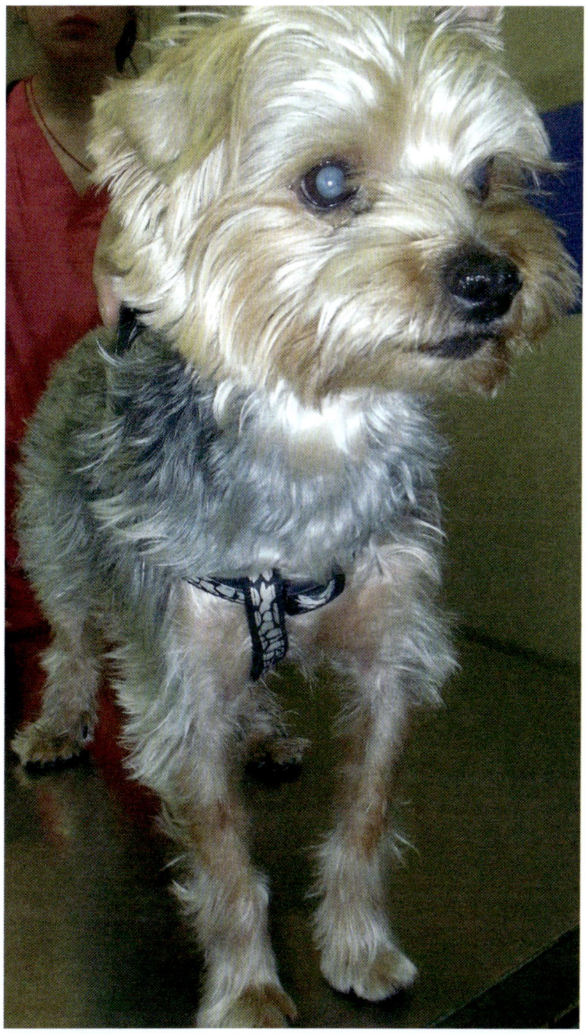

**Figure 3.13.** Cataracts in a female Yorkshire Terrier cross with diabetes mellitus.

## Diagnosis

Diagnosis is straightforward in most cases. The diagnosis is confirmed by the presence of persistent hyperglycaemia and glucosuria in a dog or cat with classic symptoms of diabetes such as polyuria, polydipsia, and weight loss.

However, there are cats in which it can be difficult to differentiate an incipient diabetes from a stress hyperglycaemia (usually due to concurrent diseases). In these cases, measurement of fructosamine levels, a complete history and physical examination, and a follow-up urine test from a home (unstressed) sample, will aid diagnosis.

## Treatment

In both the dog and the cat, treatment objectives are:

- resolution of the clinical signs
- avoid long-term complications such as peripheral neuropathy in the cat, or cataracts in the dog
- control risk factors (obesity, neutering in females)
- avoid hypoglycaemia.

An additional objective, particularly in newly diagnosed cats, is remission of the disease, which can potentially occur in a large number of cases (80%).

To achieve these objectives, several key aspects must be addressed:

- diet and exercise
- communication with the owner
- administration of insulin
- control of concurrent problems
- disease monitoring.

## Treatment of feline diabetes

### Diet and exercise

It has been shown that cats which live exclusively indoors, without other cats, lead a less active life and are predisposed to obesity and diabetes. In cats, the amount of exercise can be increased by dividing the daily food into small amounts and placing it in different parts of the house.

Feeding a specialized diet can help maintain an ideal body weight and minimize postprandial hyperglycaemia. There are several options available.

#### *Diets with high fibre content*

The classic diets for the management of diabetes have a high fibre content, which decreases the speed of glucose absorption and reduces insulin demand. However, fibre-rich diets are currently only recommended for diabetic cats with concurrent diseases that respond to fibre (constipation) or where a high protein diet is contraindicated, such as cases of renal insufficiency.

Commercial diets (dry or moist) with a high fibre content tend to be calorie restricted and may be useful for promoting weight loss in diabetic cats. However, if the diabetic cat is already below the ideal weight, these diets are not recommended initially. A diet with a higher caloric content and less fibre is preferable.

### *Low carbohydrate, high protein diet*

For over a decade, it has been shown that the most suitable diet for the treatment of feline diabetes is food low in carbohydrates and high in protein. The low carbohydrate content helps control hyperglycaemia, so that insulin requirements are reduced compared to a normal diet, and the protein helps maintain muscle mass.

The benefits of these diets are most evident in cats diagnosed early, which retain a greater capacity for insulin secretion. This type of feeding increases the probability of remission of diabetes by up to 30–50%. In cats with long-term diabetes, remission is less likely; even so, following these guidelines favours the regulation of the condition. When switching to this type of diet, the recommendation is to reduce the dose of insulin by 25–50%.

Diets low in carbohydrates and rich in protein are also recommended in diabetic cats with a normal or low weight, since weight loss or gain can be controlled by governing the cat's intake.

## Oral hypoglycaemic agents

Oral hypoglycaemic agents (e.g. sulphonyl ureas) reduce glucose levels by several mechanisms:

- stimulating pancreatic insulin secretion
- improving carbohydrate transport in muscle and adipose tissue
- reducing the release of glucose in the liver.

Some cats with uncomplicated diabetes mellitus, or type II diabetes caused by obesity and with an absence of ketone bodies, can be satisfactorily controlled by dietary treatment and oral hypoglycaemic agents alone. However, the use of oral hypoglycaemic agents is **not recommended** in the medium to long term, since this protocol can favour formation of amyloid deposits in the pancreas.

### *Glipizide*

This is the most commonly used sulphonyl urea in the cat. However, glipizide is no longer recommended. A dose of 0.25–0.5 mg/kg is administered, up to a maximum of 5 mg/12 h. It may cause side effects such as vomiting and anorexia, hypoglycaemia, and jaundice. The efficacy of the treatment is low (40%).

Home monitoring of blood glucose levels and ketone bodies in the urine is advisable.

- If hyperglycaemia decreases progressively, the dose of glipizide should be adjusted.
- If animals are normo- or hypoglycaemic, treatment should be paused.
- If hyperglycaemia reappears, glipizide should be administered at a dose lower than the initial dose.
- If the patient does not respond and symptoms persist, or they develop ketoacidosis or side effects, treatment should be stopped and insulin prescribed.

## Insulin

It is advisable to start treatment with insulin as soon as possible, since it increases the chances of remission in cats with reversible diabetes (type II or secondary).

There are different types of insulin with varying durations of action.

- **Regular insulin** has the fastest, shortest, and most powerful action. It is used for ketoacidosis. It can be administered IM or IV.
- **Intermediate-acting insulins** (NPH or slow) have a longer action (4–14 hours).
- **Long-acting insulins**, which include insulin analogues (glargine and detemir) or protamine zinc insulin (PZI).

Currently, the most commonly used insulins for the management of feline diabetes are slow-acting **porcine insulin** (Caninsulin®; MSD Animal Health), the **human insulin analogue** glargine (Lantus®) and the **human insulin PZI** (ProZinc®; Boehringer), designed with the aim of achieving a prolonged and predictable absorption rate.

The American Animal Hospital Association (AAHA) recommendations on the management of diabetes indicate that the insulins for veterinary use and therefore of first choice are, in **diabetic dogs, Caninsulin®**, and in **cats, Caninsulin® or ProZinc®**. However, glargine in cats and detemir in dogs have been shown to have an adequate duration of action.

### *Caninsulin®*

Treatment of uncomplicated feline diabetes can be started with a low carbohydrate/high protein diet, and with a low dose of slow-acting insulin (Caninsulin®, 1 IU/cat/12 h in cats of <4 kg and 1.5–2 IU/12 h in cats >4 kg). To avoid the development of hypoglycaemia, a conservative dose of insulin should be used initially, and the dose progressively adapted to the needs of the animal.

An important part of the treatment is to teach the owner:

- correct handling of insulin
- subcutaneous injection technique
- reading urine strips to measure glucose and ketone bodies in urine
- identification and treatment of hypoglycaemic episodes.

It is useful to remember that Caninsulin® is available at 40 IU/ml, while human insulins are all 100 IU/ml, so confusion should be avoided and U100 syringes should not be used to calculate U40 units of Caninsulin®.

#### *Insulin glargine (Lantus®)*
In newly diagnosed cases, some authors recommend beginning treatment with insulin glargine (Lantus®) but AAHA guidelines and the prescription cascade recommend PZI and Caninsulin® first. This is a synthetic analogue of human insulin with a very acidic pH (pH = 4), which after subcutaneous injection (where the pH is relatively neutral) causes microprecipitates that give rise to a slow and relatively continuous absorption. This insulin should not be diluted because the rate of absorption is altered. In normal cats its action lasts about 23 hours. Starting doses of 0.25 IU/kg/12 h are recommended. A greater proportion of remissions have been described with this insulin than with others (lente insulin, PZI).

#### *Detemir (Levemir®)*
This is a new insulin analogue biologically designed to achieve a slow and continuous absorption, in this case at a neutral pH. In humans, a prolonged and more predictable absorption is achieved than with other long-acting insulins. In cats, more studies are needed.

## *Treatment of canine diabetes*
### Diet and exercise
Exercise in diabetic dogs should be constant and moderate. Its duration and intensity should be similar every day, avoiding intense exercise around the peak of action of insulin to reduce the risk of hypoglycaemia.

Diets with a **high fibre and low fat** content favour the management of **canine diabetes** since they delay the absorption of glucose and contribute to weight loss in obese animals. However, high fibre, low calorie diets are not appropriate for cachectic diabetic dogs.

Feeding schedules should be based around when insulin is administered, and the dog should eat every time insulin is given. In addition, the owner should be warned that if the dog does not eat, then only one third of the insulin dose should be administered to avoid hypoglycaemia.

### Neutering
In the case of diabetic bitches, once the diagnosis has been confirmed and the disease stabilized, ovariohysterectomy is recommended. Unneutered females are very difficult to regulate in the long term because their insulin needs are very variable. Ovariohysterectomy should be performed immediately if diabetes emerges during dioestrus (luteal phase of the oestrous cycle), since there is a possibility that the need for insulin administration after surgery will disappear (remission of diabetes).

### Insulin
The use of intermediate-acting (slow) insulin at a dose of 0.2–0.5 IU/kg/12 h is generally recommended. It is preferable to start with a conservative dose (Caninsulin® 0.2–0.3 IU/kg/12 h) in order to prevent the onset of hypoglycaemia. This type of insulin is the

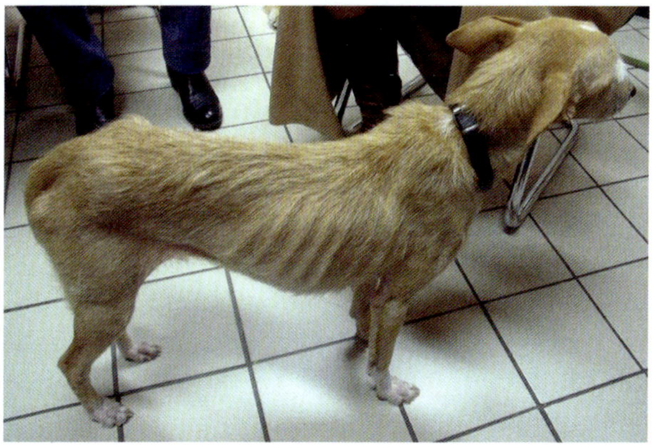

**Figure 3.14.** Body condition score of 3/9 in a 3-year-old mixed breed male dog with poorly controlled diabetes mellitus.

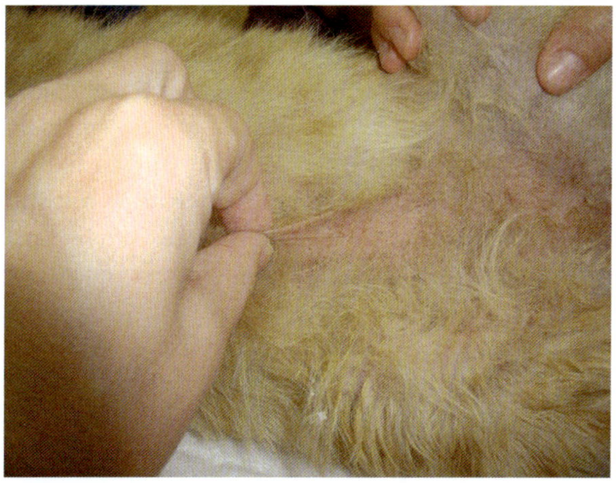

**Figure 3.15.** Thin skin and endocrine alopecia in an 11-year-old male cat with iatrogenic Cushing's disease and diabetes mellitus.

first choice in dogs, since porcine insulin is identical to canine insulin.

Some studies indicate that the high potency of the detemir insulin analogue in the dog (Levemir®), at a dose of 0.1–0.2 IU/12 h, makes it suitable for use in cases in where good control of the disease is not obtained with Caninsulin®.

### Oral hypoglycaemic agents

These are not recommended, since most diabetic dogs have a complete inability to synthesize insulin.

## *Monitoring feline and canine diabetes*

The ideal place to measure and regulate diabetes is the animal's usual environment. Initial home monitoring includes evaluation of the clinical response (decreased polyuria and polydipsia and increased activity) and measurement of glucose and ketones in the urine. During the first few weeks, glucose and ketones in the urine should be monitored at least once a day.

In addition, these animals should be assessed every 1 to 2 weeks in a consultation. By making small adjustments to the initial insulin dose, adequate glycaemic control is achieved. The veterinarian should adjust the dose depending on glycosuria and the clinical response. However, a blood glucose curve is also needed during the first month of treatment. In other words, the animal is reviewed every week, but a blood glucose curve is not obtained at each of these visits. However, this is controversial and some specialists advise that the insulin dose should not be adjusted based on urine glucose because of the risk of the Somogyi effect causing misleading readings.

A dose of insulin should be maintained for 4 to 5 days before considering whether it is adequate. If treatment is started with a **low dose of insulin (0.2 IU/kg)**, an increase of 10–25% will almost always be necessary. In most dogs, adequate control is achieved with an insulin dose of 0.5–1.0 IU/kg. Control can be achieved in some cats with very low doses of insulin; and also, in cats, diabetes can be transient and go into remission.

If the clinical signs of diabetes improve in an animal, control of the disease should be checked by measuring blood glucose (preferably 6–8 h post insulin) and fructosamine. To check that the insulin dose and quantity of food are adequate, a blood glucose curve should be carried out. Subsequently, monthly check-ups are needed and, when good control of the disease is achieved, check-ups should be every 3 months during the first year after diagnosis. The frequency of check-ups can then be reduced to every 4–6 months.

If clinical signs persist and blood glucose (nadir >150 mg/dl in dog, >170 mg/dl in cat; or throughout the day >200 mg/dl dog, >250 mg/dl cat) and fructosamine levels (>400 mmol/l) indicate poor control of the disease, it is essential to perform a **glucose curve**, since this is the only method that can distinguish between different causes of poor regulation.

### Glucose curve

A glucose curve determines blood glucose every 2 hours for 12 hours, maintaining the usual diet and insulin injections. The first curve should be done at the clinic and the owner should take the usual food ration and insulin and feed the animal in the presence of the veterinarian. Subsequently, the client can be trained to obtain a blood sample to determine blood glucose and perform the curves at home.

Interpretation of the glucose curve involves evaluating the following.

- The effectiveness of insulin: its ability to lower blood glucose (difference between maximum and minimum glucose >100 mg/dl). If the insulin is not effective, it may be due to poor handling or injection technique, insufficient dosage, poor insulin absorption, or insulin resistance (Figure 3.16).
- The **glucose nadir** is the **lowest blood glucose level** on the curve. It is important for determining the dose of insulin (Table 3.7). The normal values for the glucose nadir are: 90–150 mg/dl in the dog and 110–170 mg/dl in the cat.
- If the glucose nadir is below 90 mg/dl, there is a risk of rebound hyperglycaemia (**Somogyi effect**) as a consequence of hypoglycaemia (Figure 3.17). If this happens, the insulin dose should be reduced and control restarted at a conservative dose. If the glucose nadir remains above 150/170 mg/dl, the dose of insulin should be increased.
- The **duration of action** of insulin is the time that elapses from injection until the blood glucose rises again above 200–250 mg/dl. Blood glucose levels

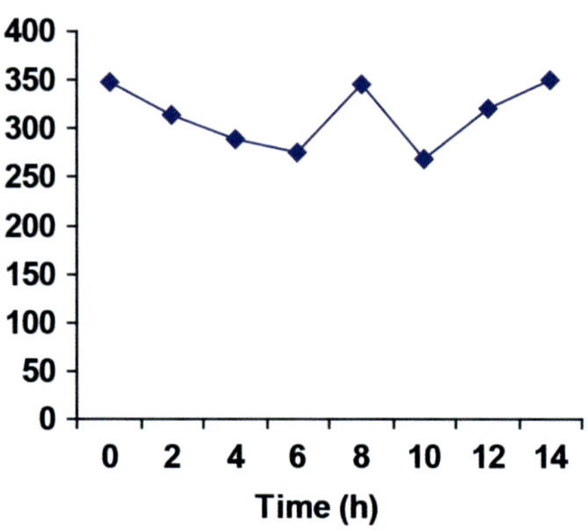


**Figure 3.16.** Insulin resistance (2 IU/kg/12 h Caninsulin®), caused by dioestrus in an 8-year-old female Husky.

Table 3.7. Changes to insulin dose depending on results of the glucose curve.

| Dog<br>Nadir (mg/dl) | Adjust the dose | Cat<br>Nadir (mg/dl) | Adjust the dose |
|---|---|---|---|
| <55 | Lower 50% | <60 | Lower 50% |
| 55–90 | Lower 20% | 60–110 | Lower 20% |
| 90–150 | Do not change | 110–170 | Do not change |
| >150 | Increase | >170 | Increase |
| **Glucose<br>0 h (mg/dl)** | **Adjust the dose** | **Glucose<br>0 h (mg/dl)** | **Adjust the dose** |
| <180 | Lower 25% | <180 | Lower 25% |

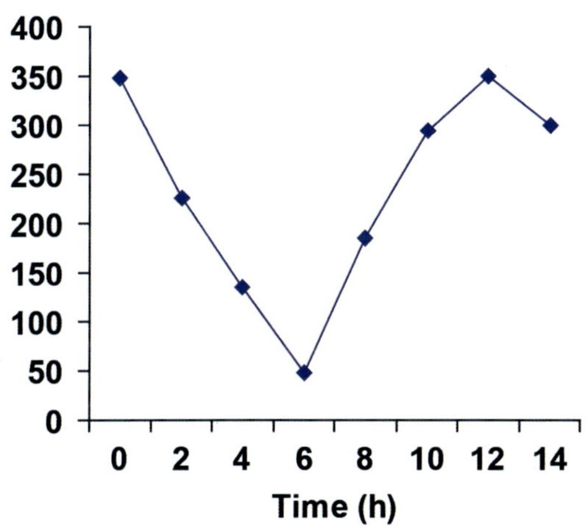


**Figure 3.17.** Somogyi effect (1 IU/kg/12 h Caninsulin®) in a castrated male Common European cat.

should remain between 90 and 200–250 mg/dl for at least 80–90% of the interval between insulin injections.

The results of the glucose curve can be affected by stress and lack of appetite. Stress hormones have an antagonistic effect to the action of insulin that can be confused with insulin resistance. A loss of appetite can also result in an underestimation of the patient's insulin needs.

Therefore, glucose curves must be interpreted with caution since there is often a wide variability in results of curves carried out over two consecutive days in the same animal and in the same conditions. Even so, the glucose curve is the only method available to diagnose insulin overdose, short insulin duration, and insulin resistance.

## Insulin resistance

### Definition

Insulin resistance is defined as when a diabetic patient requires very high doses of insulin (>1.5 IU/kg per dose) to control diabetes.

When using intermediate or long-acting insulins, the majority of diabetic dogs and cats are well regulated with doses of less than 1.5 IU/kg/12 h. If it is necessary to administer more than 1.5–2 IU/kg/12 h to obtain good control of the disease (without polydipsia, polyuria, polyphagia, or weight loss, and with blood glucose levels below 250–300 mg/dl throughout the day), there is insulin resistance.

Insulin resistance is one of the factors predisposing animals to developing diabetes mellitus and, in turn, in diabetic patients, it is a frequent cause of poor control of the disease.

### Aetiopathogenesis

Insulin resistance prevents insulin from acting as it should. It can be caused by several mechanisms.

- **Hormones** that interact with insulin receptors, such as growth hormone (GH) and glucocorticoids. In dogs, the most frequent cause of diabetes mellitus is insulin resistance provoked by **progestogens** (luteal phase or administration of progestins) or **glucocorticoids** (hyperadrenocorticism or by oral, cutaneous, or topical administration).
- **Concurrent diseases** that cause chronic release of stress hormones. In diabetic animals, any concurrent disease which is moderate or severe leads to an increase in **stress hormones** (cortisol, glucagon, epinephrine, and GH), whose effects are antagonistic to those of insulin.
- **Resistance at the receptor** and post-receptor level, as occurs in obesity (very common in the cat). In most cases, insulin resistance is a consequence of one of the following diseases or concurrent processes:
  - dioestrus (dog)
  - obesity (cat)
  - infections (oral, urinary, genital-pyometra)
  - administration of progestogens and/or glucocorticoids
  - hyperadrenocorticism
  - renal insufficiency

  - pancreatitis
  - cardiopathies
  - hepatopathies
  - neoplasms
  - acromegaly (excess of growth hormone)
  - hypothyroidism (dog)
  - hyperthyroidism (cat).
- **Loss of insulin activity** before binding to the receptor, usually due to the presence of anti-insulin antibodies. **Obesity**, mainly in the cat and to a lesser extent in the dog, causes resistance by decreasing the number of insulin receptors and altering their functionality, reducing their affinity for insulin and producing post-receptor defects.

### *Diagnosis*

Of all the concurrent diseases, bacterial infections are the most frequently occurring. Indeed, diabetes mellitus predisposes to infection by altering both cellular and humoral immunity. Urinalysis and culture are recommended in all dogs and cats that do not respond well to treatment, since a large number have a urinary infection, even when urinalysis is apparently normal.

On physical examination, signs of diseases that can cause insulin resistance, such as hyperadrenocorticism, should be noted. Treatment of diabetes should be commenced and then adrenal function tests performed when diabetes is relatively well regulated, to avoid false positives in adrenal function tests.

**Pancreatitis** is common in both dogs and cats with diabetes. In dogs, the signs can be mild to severe and include anorexia, vomiting, diarrhoea, tachypnoea, and abdominal pain. Although these symptoms can occur in cats, many feline patients only manifest lethargy and decreased appetite, so the absence of vomiting or abdominal pain does not rule out pancreatitis. When there is a suspicion of pancreatitis, the patient should be evaluated by performing a complete blood count, biochemistry, pancreatic tests (pancreatic lipase immunoreactivity; PLI), and abdominal ultrasound.

Another problem that can cause severe insulin resistance in cats is **acromegaly**, which mainly affects male geriatric cats. This condition is characterized by an increase in body size, especially in the head and extremities. In addition, the number of skin folds may increase and laryngeal stridor is common. Organomegaly (heart, kidneys, etc.) and osteoarthritis can be detected radiologically. Recently, it has been reported that feline acromegaly is not as uncommon as once thought, since one in four diabetic cats is affected.

Acromegaly is caused by an increase in the production of **growth hormone** due to the presence of a GH-producing **pituitary tumour**. The diagnosis is confirmed by demonstrating high plasma levels (>1000 nmol/l) of GH or insulin-like growth factor-1 (IGF-1). An MRI is needed to confirm the presence of pituitary neoplasia.

In elderly cats, hyperthyroidism is one of the diseases that causes insulin resistance.

If no cause of insulin resistance is found, the origin may be in the production of **anti-insulin antibodies**; this occurs more frequently with insulin of bovine or human origin. Anti-insulin antibodies interfere with the determination of plasma insulin and can (falsely) elevate its levels even 24 hours after administration (when the activity of the administered insulin has already disappeared).

### *Treatment*

Until the cause of the resistance is known, high doses of insulin are necessary to maintain control of the diabetes mellitus. However, once the cause has been diagnosed and treated, the dose of insulin should be lowered. This is to reduce the risk of hypoglycaemia, since resistance will disappear once the cause has been successfully treated.

For bitches in dioestrus, **ovariohysterectomy** should be performed once the patient is stable, hydrated, and electrolytes are normalized, even before there is good control of the disease. During the first week after ovariohysterectomy, progesterone and growth hormone levels fall to normal levels. During this time intensive follow-up is recommended, to identify and prevent the onset of symptomatic hypoglycaemia.

In obese animals, feeding a **hypocaloric diet** and increasing their physical exercise helps decrease resistance and therefore reduce insulin needs. It is advisable to reassess patients every 15 days to adjust the dose of insulin and amount of food fed, as weight loss occurs.

Secondary resistance due to **bacterial infections** disappears once infections begin to resolve, usually after 2 or 3 weeks of antibiotic treatment.

The duration of the insulin resistance caused by diseases such as neuropathies, hepatopathies, or pancreatitis depends on the partial or total resolution of these pathologies.

In cases of hyperadrenocorticism, insulin resistance decreases as cortisolaemia is normalized and, consequently, insulin needs also tend to diminish.

The definitive **treatment for acromegaly is hypophysectomy** or pituitary radiotherapy. Therefore, most cases are not treated effectively and require high doses of insulin over prolonged periods of time (>15 IU/12 h total dose per animal). The only medical treatment that is effective is pasireotide (Signifor®), a synthetic somatostatin analogue that decreases the synthesis of growth hormone, but it is very expensive. Other analogues, such as octreotide (Sandostatin®), are less effective.

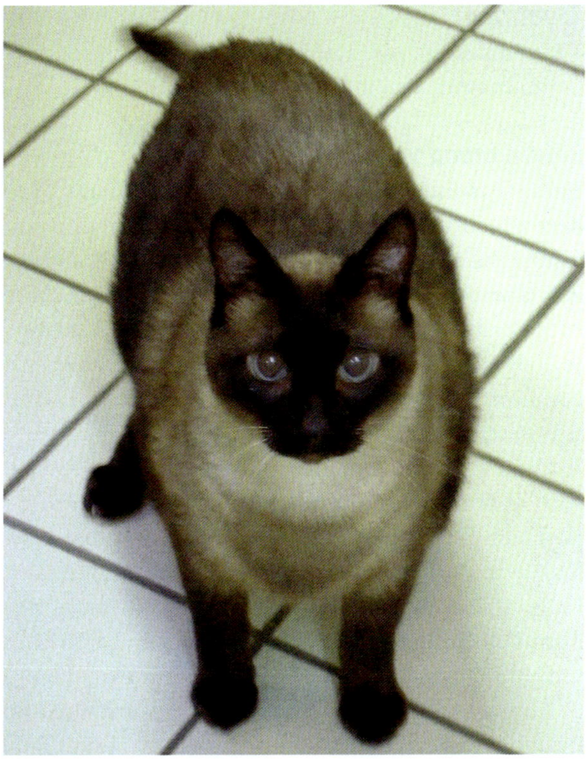

**Figure 3.18.** Body condition score of 8/9 in a male Siamese cat with type II diabetes.

## Diabetic ketoacidosis

### Definition

Diabetic ketoacidosis (DKA) is a serious complication of diabetes mellitus. It is characterized by the presence of hyperglycaemia, metabolic acidosis, ketonaemia, dehydration, and electrolyte losses.

In the diabetic cat, another serious complication is the **hyperosmolar hyperglycaemic state** (also called hyperosmolar hyperglycaemic non-ketotic coma). This is less frequent than DKA and is characterized by severe hyperglycaemia and plasma hyperosmolarity, but with the absence of ketoacidosis and ketonuria. Its treatment is similar to that of ketoacidosis.

### Aetiopathogenesis

Ketoacidosis may arise in animals with:

- undiagnosed diabetes mellitus
- inadequate control of the disease
- concurrent diseases
- excess hormones that cause insulin resistance (glucocorticoids, progestogens).

This complication is characterized by an absolute deficiency of insulin that induces the activation of **lipolysis to produce energy**. As a result of lipolysis, ketone bodies (acetoacetate, βß-hydroxybutyrate, and acetone) are produced and accumulate. The stimulation of lipolysis is usually accompanied by the presence of diabetogenic hormones (epinephrine, glucagon, cortisol, and growth hormone), stress, and fasting.

### Clinical signs

The vast majority of ketoacidotic animals constitute an emergency: they are usually dehydrated, acidotic, and in a hyperosmolar state. Clinical signs such as lethargy, weakness, anorexia, and vomiting present depending on the severity of the acidosis and concurrent disease.

The initial symptoms are the classic signs of diabetes mellitus: polydipsia, polyuria, polyphagia, and weight loss. But, as the levels of ketone bodies increase in the body, other symptoms such as lethargy, anorexia, vomiting, and weakness appear. The clinical picture can be complicated by secondary symptoms due to a concurrent or triggering process (e.g. infections, dioestrus, or pancreatitis).

In advanced cases, animals can present with **severe depression** of the central nervous system (stupor), even coma, although more often they are in a diminished state of consciousness, with dehydration, hypothermia, tachypnoea, a weak pulse, and marked general weakness (Figure 3.19).

### Diagnosis

Diagnosis seeks to identify DKA and the cause that triggered it. It is essential to perform a complete diagnostic work-up, complete blood count, and biochemical profile including amylase and lipase, urinalysis and culture, thoracic and abdominal radiographs, and, depending on the clinical history and the findings on physical examination, abdominal and cardiac ultrasound.

#### Routine laboratory tests

*Haemogram*

In 30% of cats with ketoacidosis, moderate anaemia with the presence of Heinz bodies may occur.

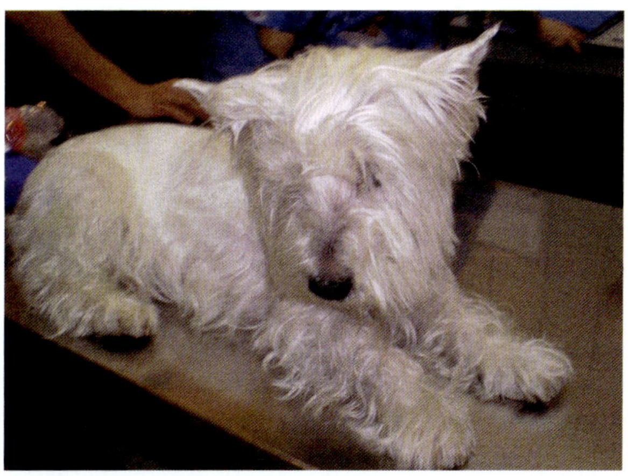

**Figure 3.19.** Weakness and reduced consciousness due to diabetic ketoacidosis in a male West Highland White Terrier.

Leucocytosis is also common, secondary to concurrent infections.

### *Biochemical profile*

The biochemistry profile is usually characterized by:

- **hyperglycaemia** oscillating between values close to normal and extreme values (in the case of coma)
- elevation of **liver enzymes** (ALT, ALP)
- **hypercholesterolaemia** and hypertriglyceridaemia
- **electrolyte alterations** (hyponatraemia, hypokalaemia, hypochloraemia).

Secondary metabolic acidosis due to the excess of ketone bodies is a serious complication in 40% of cases.

To confirm glucosuria and ketonuria, reagent strips (Keto-diastix®, Ketostix®, Diabur®, Clinistix®) are used to detect glucose and, semiquantitatively, two ketone bodies: acetoacetate and acetone. β-hydroxybutyrate (β-OHB), which is produced in greater quantities, is not detected with these strips. Hydrogen peroxide can be added, which transforms the β-OHB in urine into acetoacetic and acetic acid, but very high amounts of β-OHB need to be present for it to be detected. Some glucometers quantitatively measure the levels of β-OHB in whole blood.

### *Urinalysis*

Urinalysis should always be performed and shows:

- marked glycosuria
- ketonuria to variable degrees
- proteinuria to variable degrees.

## Other diagnostic tests

Correct diagnosis of the pathologies associated with DKA is essential to establish an appropriate treatment plan for both diseases. These pathologies include bacterial infections, pancreatitis, renal failure, heart failure, Cushing's syndrome, and neoplasms.

In an animal with DKA there should always be a high suspicion of recurrent infections. The latter most commonly affect the urinary tract, oral cavity, or skin.

One of the most frequent causes of mortality in dogs with DKA is necrotizing pancreatitis. The values of canine/feline lipase and ultrasound data are used to confirm suspicions of pancreatitis.

Whenever oliguria or anuria is present in the first hours of treatment, concurrent renal failure should be suspected. This is because glomerulosclerosis may develop, which initially presents with proteinuria and polyuria and, as renal failure progresses, with oliguria and anuria.

### *Treatment*

The steps to follow in treatment of diabetic ketoacidosis are summarized in Table 3.8.

## Return blood volume to normal

These patients are dehydrated, hypovolaemic, and have a reduced cardiac output and so the first step is to restore their blood volume levels. Most are hypotensive and oliguric, so expansion of the intravascular space is the primary objective. Furthermore, fluid therapy reduces glucose levels and osmolarity, improves renal perfusion, and decreases the effect of continuous secretion of stress hormones.

Initially, the fluid of choice is an isotonic crystalloid such as **sodium chloride (0.9% NaCl)**, PlasmaLiye or Isofundin, at a moderate rate, so as not to cause cerebral oedema. This fluid therapy is preferable to lactated Ringers, since renal elimination of the latter worsens the loss of electrolytes (sodium and potassium); however, lactated Ringers can also be used initially.

The volume of fluid therapy is calculated based on the fluid replacement needs over a 24-hour period; 80% of this total volume is administered in the first 8–10 hours.

Initially 60–100 ml/kg/24 h should be administered, equating to 1.5 to 2 times the maintenance needs. Subsequently, fluids should be adjusted according to hydration, urine production, and the severity of azotaemia.

After the initial 24–48 hours, when the blood glucose reaches 250 mg/dl, the fluid can be changed to Plasma-Lyte® or Isofundin® crystalloids, which allow adequate replacement of electrolytes while avoiding hypernatraemia, they can also be administered at the beginning of therapy.

During fluid therapy, it is advisable to monitor the patient for signs of:

- over hydration with pulmonary oedema due to excess fluid
- insufficient fluid administration, leading to tissue hypoperfusion and hypoxia, as indicated by a worsening of prerenal azotaemia and an increased risk of renal failure.

The following variables must also be monitored:

- state of awareness
- heart rate
- pulse
- mucous membrane colour
- capillary refill time
- skin turgidity
- cardiac and pulmonary auscultation

Table 3.8. Treatment guidelines in dogs and cats with diabetic ketoacidosis.

| Objective | | Treatment | Type | Rate, dose, and route |
|---|---|---|---|---|
| **Return blood volume and electrolyte levels to normal** | | Fluid therapy | Sodium chloride 0.9% | Dehydration × weight (kg) × 10 + (50–75 ml/kg) IV |
| | | | When blood glucose is 250–300 mg/dl: 2.5–5% dextrose solution in 0.9% NaCl IV | |
| | | | Potassium chloride | 20–80 mEq/l fluid according to K+ plasma IV |
| | | | Monopotassium phosphate | 0.01 to 0.12 mmol phosphate/kg/h IV |
| **Reduce blood glucose** | | Insulin | Regular | Initial: 0.2 IU/kg IM<br>Maintenance: 0.1 IU/kg/h IM<br>Initial: 0.05–0.1 IU/kg/h IV in continuous infusion in 0.9% NaCl<br>When blood glucose is 250–300 mg/dl: 0.1–0.5 IU/kg/6–8 h SC |
| **Only correct acidosis** if bicarbonate ≤11 Eq/l or pH <7.3 | | Bicarbonate | Sodium bicarbonate | mEq = weight (kg) × 0.4 × [12 – patient bicarbonate] × 0.5 slow IV over 1–2 hours |
| **Treat concurrent disease** | Infections | Antibiotics | Cephalosporin<br>Amoxicillin clavulanate | 22 mg/kg/8 h IV<br>12–20 mg/kg/12 h IV |
| | Renal failure | Forced diuresis | | |
| | Oliguria | Diuretics | Mannitol | 0.5 g/kg IV (10–20 min), 1 mg/kg/min IV continuous infusion |
| | | | Furosemide | 0.1–1 mg/kg/h IV continuous infusion |
| | | | Dopamine | 0.5–3 µg/kg/min IV |
| | Pancreatitis | Fasting 24 h<br>Highly digestible low fat diet<br>Analgesia<br>Anti-H2/Antiemetics | Buprenorphine | 0.005–0.015 mg/kg IV |
| | Dioestrus/ pyometra | Ovariohysterectomy | | |

- urine production: if during the initial phase of treatment there is not a minimum production of 1 to 2 ml of urine/kg/h, fluid therapy should be reviewed and diuresis should be increased with diuretics (mannitol)
- weight
- the arterial and venous pressures, if possible.

## Normalization of electrolytes

The second step in the treatment of DKA is the correction of electrolyte imbalances, especially potassium and phosphorus.

### *Hypokalaemia*

Hypokalaemia is the most frequent electrolyte disturbance. However, serum potassium levels do not always reflect the body's reserve since they may be falsely normal or even elevated due to hypovolaemia and lower renal excretion, acidosis (passage of potassium from the intracellular space to the extracellular space), insulin deficiency, serum hypertonicity, and protein catabolism.

Therefore, during treatment potassium levels should be carefully evaluated, since **potassium levels may fall**, especially once rehydration occurs. This is due to the correction of acidosis, and the passage of potassium and glucose into the intracellular space, as a result of exogenous insulin and urine losses.

Depending on serum potassium levels, potassium supplementation should be administered using potassium chloride (KCl; 2M vials = 2 mEq/ml) as indicated in Table 3.8.

Subsequent adjustments are made taking plasma levels into account, evaluating levels every 6 to 8 hours until the animal is stable. Electrocardiographic monitoring is also useful, observing the presence of signs of hypokalaemia (depression of T waves and ST segments, prolonged QT intervals, supraventricular and ventricular arrhythmias) or hyperkalaemia (peaked T waves, flat P waves, prolonged PR and QRS intervals, lower amplitude R waves, bradycardia, ventricular arrhythmias, complete cardiac block). However, this assessment is orientative, so measurement of potassium concentrations is also recommended.

### *Hypophosphataemia*

Hypophosphataemia is present in around 92% of feline hyperosmolar/ketoacidotic cases at first presentation. However, in dogs it is a rare finding, at least in the early stages.

Hypophosphataemia is linked to the severity and duration of diabetes and concurrent diseases. In addition, after treatment with insulin and the correction of acidosis, a severe decrease in phosphorus levels can occur within 24 hours, due to an existing chronic deficiency which was not previously reflected in serum levels.

If signs appear such as weakness, ataxia, tremors, muscular weakness, myocardial changes, respiratory failure, or haemolysis, and providing that the phosphorus level is <1.5 mg/dl, then potassium phosphate (0.01–0.12 mmol/kg/h) should be added to fluids. Two to four administrations at this dosage every 6 hours should raise serum phosphorus levels above 2.5 mg/dl.

In cases where there is anaemia, congestive heart failure, pneumonia, and other types of hypoxaemia, treatment with phosphorus is especially beneficial since it improves red blood cell levels of 2,3-diphosphoglycerate and therefore cellular oxygenation.

Phosphorus should not be administered in animals with hypercalcaemia, hyperphosphataemia, or oliguria.

### *Hypocalcaemia*

The presence of hypocalcaemia has been described in 18–76% of cats with DKA, although it is usually moderate hypocalcaemia and not accompanied by clinical signs.

## Correction of acidosis

Severe metabolic acidosis (pH <7) must be corrected as it has multiple consequences, including:

- inhibiting the action of insulin
- favouring the generation of cardiac arrhythmias
- generating hypotension
- depressing the central nervous and respiratory systems
- predisposing to acute renal tubular necrosis
- predisposing to intestinal ischaemia
- causing anorexia, nausea, and vomiting.

In general, initial administration of bicarbonate in all cases is not advised, because it can aggravate the existing hypokalaemia, decrease the release of tissue oxygen, and lead to sodium overload and rebound alkalosis.

Thus, if the concentration of plasma bicarbonate is 12 mEq/l or higher, administration of bicarbonate is not advisable: acidosis will be corrected with insulin and fluid therapy.

If the level of bicarbonate in blood is less than 11 mEq/l, acidosis should be corrected with caution, in order not to abruptly alter the pH of cerebrospinal fluid. For this, commercial solutions of 1 molar $NaHCO_3$ (at 8.4%, 1 mEq/ml) and also solutions at 1/6 molar (at 1.4%, 1 mEq/6 ml) should be used. Administration should be slow over 1–2 hours, and never in a bolus.

If plasma bicarbonate levels are unknown, 1 to 5 mEq/kg of bicarbonate can be administered depending on the severity of the acidosis.

## Reduce blood glucose levels

The insulin used should be fast acting, that is, regular crystalline (Actrapid®, Humulina Regular®, Humaplus Regular®); the alternatives (NPH, slow, ultra-slow) should only be used when the animal is compensated and can eat.

Hyperglycaemia should resolve after 4–10 hours, depending on previous blood glucose levels and the protocol used; while in the dog, ketosis takes 12 to 48 hours to resolve, and in the cat, ketonuria and acidosis take an average of 43 hours to disappear. However, the doses of insulin needed to block lipolysis are less than those needed to reduce blood glucose, so if blood glucose levels are going down, ketogenesis is already blocked.

Recently, the use of the insulin analogue lispro has been described in a continuous intravenous infusion protocol at a dose of 0.09 IU/kg/h in dogs with ketoacidosis.

There are several protocols depending on the route of administration (IM, IV, or SC) and the dose used. Traditionally, large doses of insulin were used; however, at lower doses reduction in blood glucose is more gradual and there are fewer episodes of hypoglycaemia and iatrogenic hypokalaemia. Therefore, administration of low doses of insulin is currently recommended. **Intramuscular** administration can be used, since the subcutaneous absorption of insulin in a dehydrated animal is difficult to predict, or continuous intravenous administration (the plasma half-life of insulin administered in a bolus is 6 minutes).

Blood glucose measurements should be taken every hour and the ideal drop is 50 to 100 mg/dl per hour. Even if blood glucose falls to the appropriate level (250–300 mg/dl), insulin administration should be continued, otherwise lipolysis and the production of ketone bodies will continue.

To avoid the development of **cerebral oedema**, blood glucose should be maintained above 250 mg/dl for the first 4–6 hours. When plasma glucose reaches 250 mg/dl, a solution containing 2.5% dextrose (10 ml/h) should be added to the fluid therapy.

#### *Slow IM administration protocol with low starting doses*

This is one of the most widely used protocols. It starts with low doses (0.2 IU/kg) and continues with injections of 0.1 IU/kg/h until a blood glucose level of 200–250 mg/dl is achieved. Subsequently, insulin should be administered SC (every 6–8 h) or IM (every 4–6 h) at a dose of 0.1–0.5 IU/kg depending on blood glucose levels, provided that the animal is already hydrated.

#### *Continuous low dose IV administration protocol*

Low doses are considered to be between 0.05 and 0.1 IU/kg/h. These can be prepared by adding 2.2 IU/kg (dog) or 1.1 IU/kg (cat) to 250 ml of a 0.9% NaCl solution administered at a rate of 10 ml/h, with an infusion pump, using a separate route from the fluid therapy (and in a different fluid). Since insulin adheres to plastic, passing 50 ml of the fluid containing insulin through the tube to saturate receptors prior to administration is recommended.

When the blood glucose reaches 250 mg/dl, IV administration can be stopped and IM or SC administration can be used, or the continuous infusion can be continued adding dextrose to the fluid. This protocol is preferable when fluid therapy is necessary for more than a day (e.g. pancreatitis, other causes of vomiting).

#### *Combined IM and SC management protocol*

This should be started with a high (0.025–0.5 IU/kg) IM dose (1 or 2 doses every 4 hours) followed by intermittent doses SC every 6–8 hours. The drawback is that a sudden drop in blood glucose and thus an increased risk of hypoglycaemia can occur. Currently, this protocol is used much less commonly than the previous two.

### Treatment of the triggering cause

At the start of hospitalization, routine administration of broad-spectrum bactericidal antibiotics is recommended (if culture and antibiogram are performed, the antibiotic should be modified according to the results).

If pancreatitis is diagnosed, fluid therapy should be continued for 72 hours, adding analgesia, anti-H2, and antiemetics, and oral feeding should be suspended. Subsequently, the patient should be fed a low fat, easily digestible diet.

In case of renal failure, if oliguria or anuria persists after checking the whole system, diuretics (mannitol and/or dopamine) should be used. Initially, mannitol can be administered in a bolus (0.5 g/kg) IV for 10–20 minutes and the effect assessed after half an hour.

- If there is urine production, a constant infusion of mannitol should be started at a dose of 1 mg/kg/min using a separate route from the fluid therapy.
- If there is no urine production, a continuous infusion of furosemide (0.1–1 mg/kg/h) and dopamine (2–5 μg/kg/min) should be administered.

### *Prognosis*

The prognosis is poor. Approximately 30% of hospitalized animals die during the first few days, usually due to concurrent diseases, mainly renal failure and pancreatitis. Mortality also occurs due to the persistence of severe acidosis and the development of complications such as cerebral oedema or hypokalaemia during emergency treatment.

## *Insulinoma*

Insulinomas are functional neoplasms of the β cells of the pancreatic islets, which secrete excessive amounts of insulin. In addition, they can produce other hormones such as somatostatin, glucagon, serotonin, gastrin, and pancreatic polypeptide.

### *Epidemiology*

The average age of affected dogs is 10 years. There is no sex predisposition. Although insulinomas can occur in any breed, they have been described more frequently in the Poodle, Boxer, Fox Terrier, German Shepherd, and Irish Setter.

In cats they are extremely rare, but have been described in some very old animals.

### *Clinical signs*

Symptoms can be intermittent or persistent, and usually appear when blood glucose is less than 40 mg/dl. This is due to a lack of glucose in the central nervous system and the presence of circulating catecholamines.

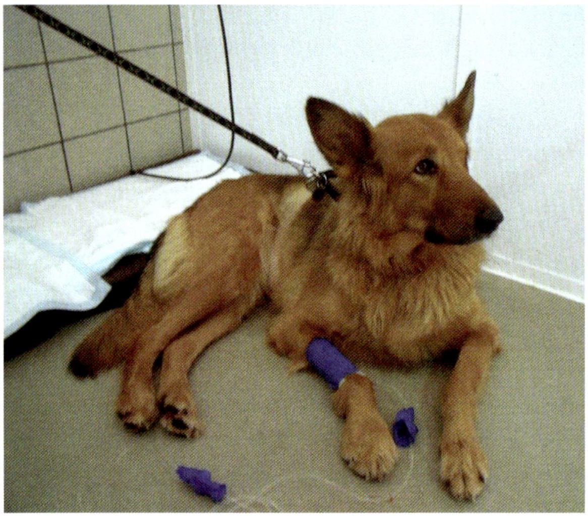

Figure 3.20. Weakness due to hypoglycaemia in a female Belgian Shepherd cross with an insulinoma.

These patients may present with:

- seizures (60%)
- weakness (45%; Figure 3.20)
- collapse (25%)
- ataxia (25%).

Less frequent symptoms include lethargy, blindness, polydipsia, polyuria, polyphagia, weight gain, diarrhoea, syncope, head tilting, and anorexia.

Symptoms are usually associated with fasting, excitement, and exercise. Paradoxically, symptoms can also occur 2 to 6 hours after eating, due to an increase in postprandial blood glucose that stimulates insulin secretion.

In a dog or cat with an insulinoma the disease should be staged so as to facilitate an appropriate treatment plan and guide the prognosis.

The clinical stages in dogs with insulinomas are as follows.

- Stage I: pancreatic nodule only, <2 cm.
- Stage II: pancreatic nodule only, >2 cm.
- Stage III: regional lymph node metastasis, pancreatic nodule of any size.
- Stage IV: distant metastasis, for example in the liver.

## Diagnosis

### Laboratory tests

In an animal with serum insulin levels >20 μU/ml and glucose <60 mg/dl, and the associated symptoms, the most likely diagnosis is insulinoma. Insulin concentrations should be evaluated in the same sample in which hypoglycaemia has been detected. With other causes of hypoglycaemia, when blood glucose is low, insulin levels should be low or towards the lower limit of the normal range.

Insulin and glucose levels can be evaluated by calculating quotients, for example:

$$\text{Serum insulin } (\mu\text{U/ml}) \times 100 \;/\; \text{Serum glucose } (\text{mg/dl}) = 30$$

A value of this quotient >30 is compatible with the diagnosis of an insulin-secreting tumour. In general, the absolute glucose and insulin values are measured and not the quotients.

### Diagnostic confirmation

After demonstrating hyperinsulinaemia in the presence of hypoglycaemia, the next step is to identify a pancreatic mass using abdominal ultrasound, CT, MRI, or exploratory laparotomy. Generally, insulinomas are malignant tumours and half the dogs that suffer from them have metastases by the time of diagnosis, almost always in the intra-abdominal ganglia, the liver, the mesentery, and the omentum.

### Diagnostic imaging

Insulinomas are usually small, so the radiological study of the abdomen and chest is often normal. These tumours do not usually metastasize to the lung.

In 35–56% of cases ultrasound is effective for detecting pancreatic masses. There may be false positives and false negatives.

The sensitivity increases if CT or contrast CT is performed.

#### *Surgical exploration*

Surgical exploration allows identification of the pancreatic mass, evaluation of adjacent organs and, finally, removal of the tumour.

## Treatment

### Surgery

If the tumour is resectable in its entirety, the animal's glucose levels should return to normal after surgery. If it is not, or if there are metastases, it can be considered a palliative surgery that will at least reduce the symptomatology and improve the response to medical treatment.

Surgery is not recommended in very old animals or with metastases in other organs; in these cases medical treatment is preferred.

### Medical treatment

Until surgery can be performed, hypoglycaemic crises should be avoided by means of diet and glucocorticoids.

Before and during surgery, fluid therapy should be administered using a 2.5 or 5% dextrose solution to maintain blood glucose above 40 mg/dl.

The **medical treatment is palliative** and is used when surgery is not an option or symptoms recur. The goal is to reduce the frequency and severity of symptoms. Food should be rich in proteins, fats, and complex carbohydrates, to prevent an abrupt rise in postprandial glucose and thus avoid a massive release of insulin. Animals with insulinoma should eat three to six times a day.

Treatment with **glucocorticoids** should begin when the diet no longer prevents hypoglycaemic crises. The initial regimen is prednisone at 0.25 mg/kg/12 h and the dose should be increased depending on the symptoms. When there is poor control with a dose of 0.5 mg/kg/12 h, other treatments should be considered to avoid iatrogenic hyperadrenocorticism.

**Diazoxide** is used when there is not a good response to diet or glucocorticoids. It inhibits the secretion of insulin, stimulates hepatic gluconeogenesis and glycogenolysis, and inhibits the uptake of glucose at a cellular level, leading to hyperglycaemia.

The initial dose of diazoxide should be 10 mg/kg/d and the maximum dose should not be more than 60 mg/kg/d, divided into two doses in both cases. The most common adverse side effects are vomiting and anorexia, although other less frequent side effects may occur such as hyperglycaemia, bone marrow suppression, diarrhoea, or tachycardia. Another limitation of diazoxide is its limited availability and its expense.

An analogue of somatostatin, octreotide (Sandostatin®, 10–20 µg/kg/8–12 h SC), has also been used as a palliative treatment for hypoglycaemia, since it inhibits the release of insulin. Its efficacy is variable, and some patients do not respond. Recently, the somatostatin analogue pasireotide has been described as being useful in these patients.

Streptozotocin is a cytotoxic drug for pancreatic cells, both normal and malignant. It can be used as the only treatment in inoperable cases, or it can be administered after surgery in dogs with a poor prognosis, to avoid recurrence. In dogs, it can cause acute renal failure if it is used as an intravenous bolus without adequate fluid therapy. Therefore, the following protocol for the administration of this drug has been described, in order to minimize toxicity.

1. Previous diuresis with saline (18 ml/kg/h) for 3 hours.
2. Streptozotocin infusion (500 mg/m$^2$) diluted in the volume corresponding to 18 ml/kg/h for 2 hours. And at the same time, butorphanol (0.4 mg/kg IM), as an antiemetic.
3. Subsequent diuresis with saline at 18 ml/kg/h for 2 hours.

Note that 10–15% of dogs can develop diabetes mellitus with this medication.

It has been reported that β cell tumours may respond to treatment with tyrosine kinase inhibitors such as toceranib. Studies are needed to prove its efficacy.

#### *Prognosis*

In the long term, prognosis is reserved or poor given the high probability of metastases. The prognosis depends on the treatment used and the tumour grade.

- Dogs with stage I insulinoma have a longer disease-free time after surgery (without hypoglycaemia for an average of 14 months).
- The survival period for stage II and III dogs (12–18 months) is higher than that for stage IV dogs (6 months). Younger dogs have a shorter survival period.

Dogs undergoing surgical treatment (with or without subsequent medical treatment) live longer than those treated only medically. In one study, the average survival of 26 surgically treated dogs was 381 days while the survival of 13 medically treated dogs was 70 days. Another study showed that dogs which have normal blood glucose after surgery survive longer (435 days) than hypoglycaemic dogs (215 days).

## Pituitary diseases

### *Acromegaly*

#### *Definition*

Acromegaly is characterized by a chronic excess of growth hormone or somatotropin (GH), which leads to overgrowth of connective and bony tissues and viscera.

#### *Epidemiology*

It is an unusual disease in the cat (although recent reports suggest that its frequency may be higher than previously believed) and extremely rare in the dog.

In dogs, the incidence is higher in females, and in cats, it is higher in males.

#### *Aetiopathogenesis*

In the cat, the excessive secretion of GH comes from a pituitary tumour.

In the dog, the most frequent cause is the production of GH in the mammary gland induced by endogenous progesterone or by exogenous progestogens. Pituitary neoplasia can also cause acromegaly in the dog, although it is rare.

### *Clinical signs*

The most frequent symptoms are:

- increase in weight and body size
- growth of soft tissues and skin
- increase in the size of abdominal organs (liver, spleen, kidneys)
- increase in size of the face
- increase in the size of distal extremities
- inferior prognathism
- increase in size of interdental spaces
- multiple arthropathies.

The anabolic effect of excess GH on the soft tissues can produce respiratory symptoms, such as respiratory stridor, panting, intolerance to exercise, or fatigue, which are frequent in the dog and less evident in the cat.

On the other hand, GH causes a **strong resistance to insulin**, which is why most acromegalic animals suffer from diabetes that is very difficult to control. They require large amounts of insulin (>2 IU/kg weight) to achieve good control of the disease; occasionally, extremely high doses (10 IU/kg) are not effective at reducing hyperglycaemia. The most frequent symptoms are polydipsia, polyuria, polyphagia, and weight gain.

### *Diagnosis*

Internal organs can be assessed through the use of radiology and ultrasound, since cardiomegaly, hepatomegaly, nephromegaly, splenomegaly, and adrenomegaly are common.

#### Diagnostic confirmation

The diagnosis of GH hypersecretion in small animals is not made by measuring the concentration of GH. Firstly, because this test is not available in veterinary laboratories and secondly, because it is secreted in a pulsatile manner, which reduces the sensitivity of the test. Indeed, some animals with acromegaly occasionally have normal concentrations of GH.

It has been known for years that the measurement of insulin-like growth factor 1 (IGF-1) is useful for diagnosing acromegaly. This test is usually available in veterinary laboratories.

In the cat, diagnosis should be confirmed by performing an MRI or CT of the head, to visualize the pituitary tumour.

### *Treatment*

#### Treatment of canine acromegaly

This consists of eliminating treatment with progestogens and, if the patient is an unneutered female, performing an ovariohysterectomy. This helps to progressively reduce GH levels and reverse most of the symptoms.

Diabetes can remain despite the resolution of acromegaly, since there may be an irreversible exhaustion of pancreatic function.

#### Treatment of feline acromegaly

Treatment is aimed at treating the pituitary tumour. There are several therapeutic options.

- Cobalt therapy.
- **Pituitary gland excision**.
- **Medical treatment.** This uses a somatostatin analogue, octreotide (Sandostatin®), which lowers GH concentrations, but is generally not effective in the long term because of its short duration of action; in addition, it is expensive. Recently is has been shown that pasireotide (Signifor®) is effective in cats at doses of 0.03 mg/kg/12 h SC. Until a reduction in GH levels occurs or the elimination of the pituitary tumour, these cats need large doses of insulin.

### *Prognosis*

In the dog the prognosis is good, as long as the source of progesterone is eliminated. In the cat it is guarded, with a survival time from 4 to 42 months.

## *Pituitary dwarfism*

### *Definition*

Pituitary dwarfism is a congenital disorder that results in a growth hormone deficiency, sometimes accompanied by a deficit of other pituitary hormones (TSH and prolactin). Generally, ACTH secretion is maintained.

### *Epidemiology*

It is observed more frequently in the German Shepherd, as a type of simple recessive autosomal hereditary alteration. It can also affect other breeds such as the Weimaraner, Spitz, or Toy Pinscher.

It is poorly documented in the cat.

### *Clinical signs*

The owners of these dogs usually visit the veterinarian when the animals are between 2 and 5 months old. The owners may see a delay in growth compared to littermates and a soft and woolly coat. There is retention of the lanugo (secondary coat) and no primary hair develops (Figure 3.21). The lanugo falls out easily and progressive alopecia develops on the trunk, although it does not usually affect the extremities or the head. The skin shows progressive hyperpigmentation and desquamation. Secondary bacterial infections are very common.

Initially, pituitary dwarfs are active and alert animals; however, later on, at around 2 to 3 years old, they become progressively less active due to the development of secondary hypothyroidism.

## *Differential diagnoses*

To confirm the diagnosis, other causes of delayed growth must be ruled out. These include endocrine and non-endocrine causes.

**Endocrine:**

- juvenile hypothyroidism, which gives rise to disproportionate dwarfism and is the most important differential diagnosis
- juvenile diabetes mellitus
- iatrogenic hyperadrenocorticism
- hypoadrenocorticism.

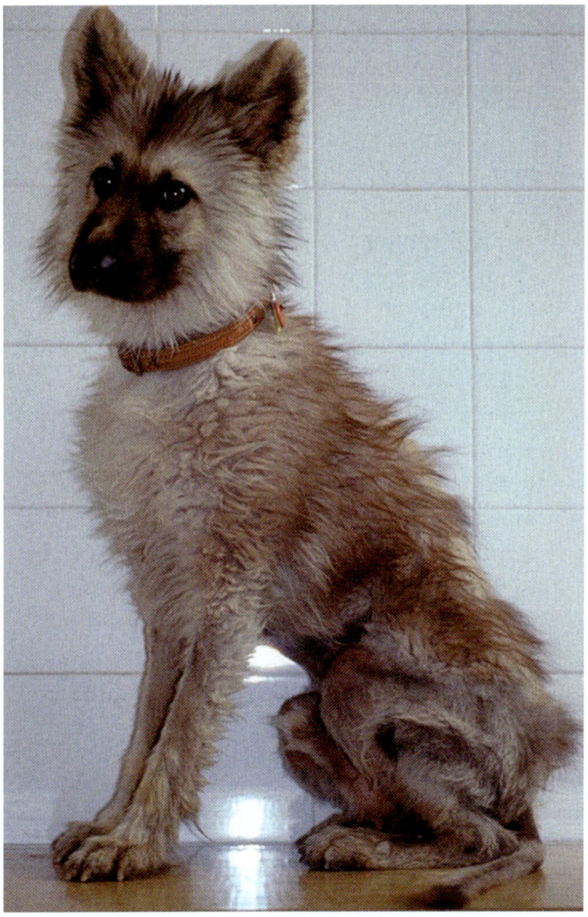

**Figure 3.21.** Endocrine alopecia and delayed growth in a 9-month-old male German Shepherd with pituitary dwarfism.

**Non-endocrine:**

- malnutrition
- gastrointestinal diseases
- liver disease (e.g. a portosystemic shunt)
- kidney disease
- cardiac failure
- bone diseases.

## *Clinical signs*

After 2 months of age, growth slows down, although normal body proportions are maintained. The epiphyses of the long bones are slow to close, the fontanelles remain open longer, and the appearance of the teeth is delayed.

## *Diagnosis*

The blood and biochemical tests in these patients are usually normal, although in some cases azotaemia may be present. GH deficiency can cause poor development of the renal glomeruli. In addition, renal function may be impaired due to a decrease in glomerular filtration as a consequence of both GH and thyroid hormone deficiencies.

Many animals with pituitary dwarfism have low plasma concentrations of total T4 and free T4 but, instead of this being associated with high TSH concentrations (as expected in an adult dog with primary hypothyroidism), this is around the normal lower limit, due to the reduced secretion of TSH in these dogs.

Currently, measurement of plasma levels of IGF-1 is used to indirectly reflect GH values; these fluctuate to a lesser extent and the test is available in veterinary laboratories. It has been found that levels of IGF-1 in pituitary dwarfs are significantly lower than normal. Otherwise, the value of IGF-1 depends on the breed and is higher in large breeds. Generally, in pituitary dwarfs it is <50 ng/ml.

## *Treatment*

In the dog, the use of certain progestogens (medroxyprogesterone) induces the production of GH in the mammary gland. A dose of medroxyprogesterone of 2.5–5.0 mg/kg/d SC is used every 3 weeks with up to six doses, and subsequently, depending on the response, one dose every 6 weeks. Animals should be checked weekly, as there can be side effects (acromegaly, diabetes mellitus). Its efficacy is variable, but there is always an increase in body weight, growth of adult hair, and an improvement of skin problems. Not only is there a clinical improvement, but also a large increase in IGF-1 and GH concentrations, without exceeding the normal upper limit.

It has been shown that proligestone may be useful in the treatment of this disease, although more studies are needed to confirm its efficacy.

Treatment with GH (bovine, porcine, or human) is expensive and can cause problems such as insulin resistance. Doses of 0.1 to 0.3 IU/kg SC have been used three times a week over 4 to 6 weeks. This treatment is not currently recommended.

### *Prognosis*

The long-term prognosis for German Shepherds with pituitary dwarfism without treatment is reserved. At the age of 3 to 5 years, they tend to lose weight and their coat, and become apathetic. These changes may be related to a progressive reduction of pituitary function, with growth of pituitary cysts and/or renal failure. At this age, or even before, many owners opt for euthanasia.

## *Diabetes insipidus*

### *Definition*

Diabetes insipidus causes intense polyuria and polydipsia, with hyposthenuric urine (urine density <1.008). Despite the polyuria, these animals do not become dehydrated while they have access to water; however, they run the serious risk of dehydration when denied access to fluid.

### *Aetiology*

The cause of diabetes insipidus may be insufficient secretion of antidiuretic hormone (ADH) in central diabetes insipidus, or a problem with ADH receptors in renal tubular cells (nephrogenic diabetes insipidus). The absence of ADH or a response to ADH prevents the reabsorption of water in the distal tubules and renal collectors, causing polyuria.

Renal insensitivity to ADH or nephrogenic diabetes insipidus may occur as a result of a primary or secondary renal problem.

#### Primary nephrogenic diabetes insipidus

Primary nephrogenic diabetes insipidus is rare and consists of a structural or functional renal defect that prevents the renal response to ADH. It usually manifests when the dog or cat is 2 to 3 months old.

#### Secondary nephrogenic diabetes insipidus

Secondary nephrogenic diabetes insipidus can occur due to progressive renal disease or other processes that affect the renal response to ADH, such as hypercalcaemia, hyperadrenocorticism, pyelonephritis, and endotoxins in animals with pyometra.

#### Central diabetes insipidus

In central diabetes insipidus, urine density is usually less than 1.008, although there are other causes of polyuria/polydipsia such as pyometra or Cushing's syndrome that can also present with urine with this degree of hyposthenuria.

Central diabetes insipidus occurs in animals with damage to the neurohypophysial system that may be of congenital origin, such as a malformation, or of traumatic, neoplastic, inflammatory, or idiopathic origin. Tumours that can cause diabetes insipidus are adenomas and pituitary chromophobe adenocarcinomas, craniopharyngiomas and mammary tumour metastases, lymphoma, melanoma, and pancreatic carcinoma. In many patients, the cause is unknown, although in geriatric dogs the most common cause is a pituitary tumour.

### *Clinical signs*

The clinical signs are those of extreme polydipsia and polyuria.

### *Diagnosis*

In the first instance, more common causes of polydipsia and polyuria should be ruled out. When diabetes insipidus is suspected, there is a range of diagnostic tests to choose from. In addition, it is advisable to differentiate between central and nephrogenic diabetes insipidus.

The options for establishing a diagnosis are as follows.

- **Water deprivation test.** This is **not recommended** because the sudden withdrawal of access to water risks acute dehydration.
- **Modified water deprivation test**. Withdrawal of water is carried out progressively; even so, this is not recommended if the animal has azotaemia, dehydration, hypercalcaemia, or any systemic disease.
- **Measurement of ADH concentrations**. This involves the administration of a vasopressin analogue (desmopressin or DDAVP) orally or conjunctivally (Minirin® 0.1 and 0.2 mg tablets or intranasal drops). The oral dose for a 20 kg dog is 0.1 mg every 8 hours, while the intranasal preparation is generally used in dogs and cats, applying 1 to 4 drops to the conjunctival sac once or twice a day. After administration of the vasopressin analogue commences, water intake and urine production are monitored: the absence of a response is compatible with nephrogenic diabetes insipidus. Animals with central diabetes insipidus manifest a rapid and evident response of the symptoms.

- **Measurement of plasma and urinary osmolarity**. In animals with central diabetes insipidus, serum osmolarity is higher than urine osmolarity, whereas in animals with psychogenic polydipsia (the most important differential diagnosis in these cases), serum osmolarity is low.

### Treatment

Once the appropriate response is reached, the dose of vasopressin analogue is decreased until the minimum effective dose for long-term treatment is established.

## Bibliography

### Hyperadrenocorticism

Arenas, C., Melián, C., and Pérez-Alenza, M.D. (2014) Long-term survival of dogs with adrenal-dependent hyperadrenocorticism: a comparison between mitotane and twice daily trilostane treatment. *Journal of Veterinary Internal Medicine* 28(2), 473–480.

Arenas, C., Melián, C., and Pérez-Alenza, M.D. (2013) Evaluation of 2 trilostane protocols for the treatment of canine pituitary-dependenthyperadrenocorticism: twice daily versus once daily. *Journal of Veterinary Internal Medicine* 27(6), 1478–1485.

Behrend, E.N., Kooistra, H.S., Nelson, R., Reusch, C.E., and Scott-Moncrieff, J.C. (2013) Diagnosis of spontaneous canine hyperadrenocorticism: 2012 ACVIM consensus statement (small animal). *Journal of Veterinary Internal Medicine* 27(6), 1292–1304.

Bonadio, C.M., Feldman, E.C., Cohen, T.A., and Kass, P.H. (2014) Comparison of adrenocorticotropic hormone stimulation test results started 2 versus 4 hours after trilostane administration in dogs with naturally occurring hyperadrenocorticism. *Journal of Veterinary Internal Medicine* 28(4), 1239–1243.

Clemente, M., De Andrés, P.J., Arenas, C., Melián, C., Morales, M., and Pérez-Alenza, M.D. (2007) Comparison of non-selective adrenocorticolysis with mitotane or trilostane for the treatment of dogs with pituitary-dependent hyperadrenocorticism. *Veterinary Record* 161(24), 805–809.

Feldman, E.C. and Kass, P.H. (2012) Trilostane dose versus body weight in the treatment of naturally occurring pituitary-dependent hyperadrenocorticismin dogs. *Journal of Veterinary Internal Medicine* 26(4), 1078–1080.

Feldman, E.C. (2011) Evaluation of twice-daily lower-dose trilostane treatment administered orally in dogs with naturally occurring hyperadrenocorticism. *Journal of the American Veterinary Medical Association* 238(11), 1441–1451.

Griebsch, C., Lehnert, C., Williams, G.J., Failing, K., and Neiger, R. (2014) Effect of trilostane on hormone and serum electrolyte concentrations in dogs with pituitary-dependent hyperadrenocorticism. *Journal of Veterinary Internal Medicine* 28(1), 160–165.

Pérez-Alenza, M.D., Arenas, C., López, M.L., and Melián C. (2006) Long-term efficacy of trilostane administered twice daily in dogs with pituitary dependent hyperadrenocorticism. *Journal of the American Animal Hospital Association* 42, 269–276.

Reusch, C.E., Sieber-Ruckstuhl, N., Wenger, M., Lutz, H., Perren, A., and Pospischil, A. (2007) Histological evaluation of the adrenal glands of seven dogs with hyperadrenocorticism treated with trilostane. *Veterinary Record* 160(7), 219–224.

Rose, L., Dunn, M.E., and Bédard, C. (2013) Effect of canine hyperadrenocorticism on coagulation parameters. *Journal of Veterinary Internal Medicine* 27(1), 207–211.

### Canine hypoadrenocorticism

Boretti, F.S., Meyer, F., Burkhardt, W.A., Riond, B., Hofmann-Lehmann, R., Reusch, C.E., and Sieber-Ruckstuhl, N.S. (2015) Evaluation of the cortisol-to-ACTH ratio in dogs with hypoadrenocorticism, dogs with diseases mimicking hypoadrenocorticism and in healthy dogs. *Journal of Veterinary Internal Medicine* 29(5), 1335–1341.

Klein, S.C. and Peterson, M.E. (2010) Canine hypoadrenocorticism: part I. *The Canadian Veterinary Journal* 51(1), 63–69.

Klein, S.C. and Peterson, M.E. (2010) Canine hypoadrenocorticism: part II. *The Canadian Veterinary Journal* 51(2), 179–184.

Lennon, E.M., Boyle, T.E., Hutchins, R.G., Friedenthal, A., Correa, M.T., Bissett, S.A., Moses, L.S., Papich, M.G., and Birkenheuer, A.J. (2007) Use of basal serum or plasma cortisol concentrations to rule out a diagnosis of hypoadrenocorticism in dogs: 123 cases (2000–2005). *Journal of the American Veterinary Medical Association* 231(3), 413–416.

Thompson, A.L., Scott-Moncrieff, J.C., and Anderson, J.D. (2007) Comparison of classic hypoadrenocorticism with glucocorticoid-deficient hypoadrenocorticism in dogs: 46 cases (1985–2005). *Journal of the American Veterinary Medical Association* 230(8), 1190–1194.

Van Lanen, K. and Sande, A. (2014) Canine hypoadrenocorticism: pathogenesis, diagnosis, and treatment. *Topics in Companion Animal Medicine* 29(4), 88–95.

Wenger, M., Mueller, C., Kook, P.H., and Reusch, C.E. (2010) Ultrasonographic evaluation of adrenal glands in dogs with primary hypoadrenocorticism or mimicking diseases. *Veterinary Record* 167(6), 207–210.

### Canine hypothyroidism

Diaz-Espiñeira, M.M., Mol, J.A., van den Ingh, T.S., van der Vlugt-Meijer, R.H., Rijnberk, A., and Kooistra, H.S. (2008) Functional and morphological changes in the adenohypophysis of dogs with induced primary hypothyroidism: Loss of TSH hypersecretion, hypersomatotropism, hypoprolactinemia, and pituitary enlargement with transdifferentiation. *Domestic Animal Endocrinology* 35(1), 98–111.

Diaz Espiñeira, M.M., Mol, J.A., Peeters, M.E., Pollak, Y.W., Iversen, L., van Dijk, J.E., Rijnberk, A., and Kooistra, H.S. (2007) Assessment of thyroid function in dogs with low plasma thyroxine concentration. *Journal of Veterinary Internal Medicine* 21(1), 25–32.

Gottschalk, J., Einspanier, A., Ungemach, F.R., and Abraham, G. (2011) Influence of topical dexamethasone applications on insulin, glucose, thyroid hormone and cortisol levels in dogs. *Research in Veterinary Science* 90(3), 491–497.

Kantrowitz, L.B., Peterson, M.E., Melián, C., and Nichols, R. (2001) Serum total thyroxine, total triiodothyronine, free thyroxine, and thyrotropin concentrations in dogs with nonthyroidal disease. *Journal of the American Veterinary Medical Association* 219, 765–769.

Pancotto, T., Rossmeisl, J.H., Panciera, D.L., and Zimmerman, K.L. (2010) Blood-brain-barrier disruption in chronic canine hypothyroidism. *Veterinary Clinical Pathology* 39(4), 485–493.

Peterson, M.E., Melián, C., and Nichols, C.E. (1997) Measurement of serum total thyroxine, triiodothyroxine, free thyroxine, and thyrotropin concentrations for diagnosis of hypothyroidism in dogs. *Journal of the American Veterinary Medical Association* 211, 1396–1402.

Randolph, J.F., Lamb, S.V., Cheraskin, J.L., Schanbacher, B.J., Salerno, V.J., Mack, K.M., Scarlett, J.M., and Place, N.J. (2015) Free thyroxine concentrations by equilibrium dialysis and chemiluminescent immunoassays in 13 hypothyroid dogs positive for thyroglobulin antibody. *Journal of Veterinary Internal Medicine* 29(3), 877–881.

van Dijl, I.C., Le Traon, G., van de Meulengraaf, B.D., Burgaud, S., Horspool, L.J., and Kooistra, H.S. (2014) Pharmacokinetics of total thyroxine after repeated oral administration of levothyroxine solution and its clinical efficacy in hypothyroid dogs. *Journal of Veterinary Internal Medicine* 28(4), 1229–1234.

## Feline hyperthroidism

Boretti, F.S., Sieber-Ruckstuhl, N.S., Schäfer, S., Gerber, B., Baumgartner, C., Riond, B., Hofmann-Lehmann, R., and Reusch, C.E. (2014) Transdermal application of methimazole in hyperthyroid cats: a long-term follow-up study. *Journal of Feline Medicine and Surgery* 16(6), 453–459.

Daminet, S., Kooistra, H.S., Fracassi, F., Graham, P.A., Hibbert, A., Lloret, A., Mooney, C.T., Neiger, R., Rosenberg, D., Syme, H.M., Villard, I., and Williams, G. (2014) Best practice for the pharmacological management of hyperthyroid cats with antithyroid drugs. *The Journal of Small Animal Practice* 55(1), 4–13.

Edinboro, C.H., Scott-Moncrieff, J.C., and Glickman, L.T. (2010) Feline hyperthyroidism: potential relationship with iodine supplement requirements of commercial cat foods. *Journal of Feline Medicine and Surgery* 12(9), 672–679.

Hui, T.Y., Bruyette, D.S., Moore, G.E., and Scott-Moncrieff, J.C. (2015) Effect of feeding an iodine-restricted diet in cats with spontaneous hyperthyroidism. *Journal of Veterinary Internal Medicine* 29(4), 1063–1068.

Kooistra, H.S. (2014) Feline hyperthyroidism: a common disorder with unknown pathogenesis. *Veterinary Record* 175(18), 456–457.

Milner, R.J., Channell, C.D., Levy, J.K., and Schaer, M. (2006) Survival times for cats with hyperthyroidism treated with iodine 131, methimazole, or both: 167 cases (1996–2003). *Journal of the American Veterinary Medical Association* 228, 559–563.

Peterson, M.E. and Broome, M.R. (2015) Thyroid scintigraphy findings in 2096 cats with hyperthyroidism. *Veterinary Radiology and Ultrasound* 56(1), 84–95.

Peterson, M.E., Kintzer, P.P., and Hurvitz, A.I. (1988) Methimazole treatment of 262 cats with hyperthyroidism. *Journal of Veterinary Internal Medicine* 2, 150–157.

Peterson, M.E., Guterl, J.N., Nichols, R., and Rishniw, M. (2015) Evaluation of serum thyroid-stimulating hormone concentration as a diagnostic test for hyperthyroidism in cats. *Journal of Veterinary Internal Medicine* 29(5), 1327–1334.

Peterson, M.E., Broome, M.R., and Rishniw, M. (2016) Prevalence and degree of thyroid pathology in hyperthyroid cats increases with disease duration: a cross-sectional analysis of 2096 cats referred for radioiodine therapy. *Journal of Feline Medicine and Surgery* 18(2), 92–103.

Sartor, L.L., Trepanier, L.A., Kroll, M.M., Rodan, I., and Challoner, L. (2004) Efficacy and safety of transdermal methimazole in the treatment of cats with hyperthyroidism. *Journal of Veterinary Internal Medicine* 18, 651–655.

Vaske, H.H., Schermerhorn, T., and Grauer, G.F. (2016) Effects of feline hyperthyroidism on kidney function: a review. *Journal of Feline Medicine and Surgery* 18(2), 55–59.

Wedekind, K.J., Blumer, M.E., Huntington, C.E., Spate, V., and Morris, J.S. (2010) The feline iodine requirement is lower than the 2006 NRC recommended allowance. *Journal of Animal Physiology and Animal Nutrition* 94, 537–539.

Williams, T.L., Peak, K.J., Brodbelt, D., Elliott, J., and Syme, H.M. (2010) Survival and the development of azotemia after treatment of hyperthyroid cats. *Journal of Veterinary Internal Medicine* 24, 863–869.

Williams, T.L., Elliott, J., and Syme, H.M. (2013) Renin-angiotensin-aldosterone system activity in hyperthyroid cats with and without concurrent hypertension. *Journal of Veterinary Internal Medicine* 27(3), 522–529.

## Hypercalcaemia and hyperparathyroidism

Cline, J. (2012) Calcium and vitamin D metabolism, deficiency, and excess. *Topics in Companion Animal Medicine* 27(4), 159–156.

Drobatz, K.J. and Casey, K.K. (2000) Eclampsia in dogs: 31 cases (1995–1998). *Journal of the American Veterinary Medical Association* 217(2), 216–219.

Greco, D.S. (2012) Endocrine causes of calcium disorders. *Topics in Companion Animal Medicine* 27(4), 150–155.

Groman, R.P. (2012) Acute management of calcium disorders. *Topics in Companion Animal Medicine* 27(4), 167–171.

Guttin, T., Knox, V.W., and Diroff, J.S. (2015) Outcomes for dogs with primary hyperparathyroidism following treatment with percutaneous ultrasound-guided ethanol ablation of presumed functional parathyroid nodules: 27 cases (2008–2011). *Journal of the American Veterinary Medical Association* 247(7), 771–777.

Holowaychuk, M.K. (2013) Hypocalcemia of critical illness in dogs and cats. *Veterinary Clinics of North America. Small Animal Practice* 43(6), 1299–1317.

Holowaychuk, M.K., Birkenheuer, A.J., Li, J., Marr, H., Boll, A., and Nordone, S.K. (2012) Hypocalcemia and hypovitaminosis D in dogs with induced endotoxemia. *Journal of Veterinary Internal Medicine* 26(2), 244–251.

Kogika, M.M., Lustoza, M.D., Notomi, M.K., Wirthl, V., Mirandola, R., and Hagiwara, M.K. (2006) Serum ionized calcium in dogs with chronic renal failure and metabolic acidosis. *Veterinary Clinical Pathology* 35(4), 441–445.

Luschini, M.A., Fletcher, D.J., and Schoeffler, G.L. (2010) Incidence of ionized hypocalcemia in septic dogs and its association with morbidity and mortality: 58 cases (2006–2007). *Journal of Veterinary Emergency and Critical Care (San Antonio)* 20(4), 406–412.

Milovancev, M. and Schmiedt, C.W. (2013) Preoperative factors associated with postoperative hypocalcemia in dogs with primary hyperparathyroidism that underwent parathyroidectomy: 62 cases (2004–2009). *Journal of the American Veterinary Medical Association* 242(4), 507–515.

Peterson, M.E. and Fluegeman, K. (2013) Cholecalciferol. *Topics in Companion Animal Medicine* 28(1), 24–27.

Pollard, R.E., Bohannon, L.K., and Feldman, E.C. (2015) Prevalence of incidental thyroid nodules in ultrasound studies of dogs with hypercalcemia (2008–2013). *Veterinary Radiology and Ultrasound* 56(1), 63–67.

Schenck, P.A. and Chew, D.J. (2005) Prediction of serum ionized calcium concentration by use of serum total concentration in dogs. *American Journal of Veterinary Research* 66, 1330–1336.

Schenck, P.A. and Chew, D.J. (2010) Prediction of serum ionized calcium concentration by use of serum total concentration in cats. *Canadian Journal of Veterinary Research* 74, 209–213.

Williams, T.L., Elliott, J., Berry, J., and Syme, H.M. (2013) Investigation of the pathophysiological mechanism for altered calcium homeostasis in hyperthyroid cats. *The Journal of Small Animal Practice* 54(7), 367–373.


## Hypocalcaemia and hypoparathyroidism


Drobatz, K.J. and Casey, K.K. (2000) Eclampsia in dogs: 31 cases (1995–1998). *Journal of the American Veterinary Medical Association* 217(2), 216–219.

Holowaychuk, M.K. (2013) Hypocalcemia of critical illness in dogs and cats. *Veterinary Clinics of North America. Small Animal Practice* 43(6), 1299–1317.

Holowaychuk, M.K., Birkenheuer, A.J., Li, J., Marr, H., Boll, A., and Nordone, S.K. (2012) Hypocalcemia and hypovitaminosis D in dogs with induced endotoxemia. *Journal of Veterinary Internal Medicine* 26(2), 244–251.

Kogika, M.M., Lustoza, M.D., Notomi, M.K., Wirthl, V., Mirandola, R., and Hagiwara, M.K. (2006) Serum ionized calcium in dogs with chronic renal failure and metabolic acidosis. *Veterinary Clinical Pathology* 35(4), 441–445.

Luschini, M.A., Fletcher, D.J., and Schoeffler, G.L. (2010) Incidence of ionized hypocalcemia in septic dogs and its association with morbidity and mortality: 58 cases (2006–2007). *Journal of Veterinary Emergency and Critical Care (San Antonio)* 20(4), 406–412.

Milovancev, M. and Schmiedt, C.W. (2013) Preoperative factors associated with postoperative hypocalcemia in dogs with primary hyperparathyroidism that underwent parathyroidectomy: 62 cases (2004–2009). *Journal of the American Veterinary Medical Association* 242(4), 507–515.

Schenck, P.A. and Chew, D.J. (2010) Prediction of serum ionized calcium concentration by use of serum total concentration in cats. *Canadian Journal of Veterinary Research* 74, 209–213.

Williams, T.L., Elliott, J., Berry, J., and Syme, H.M. (2013) Investigation of the pathophysiological mechanism for altered calcium homeostasis in hyperthyroid cats. *The Journal of Small Animal Practice* 54(7), 367–373.


## Diabetes


Aptekmann, K.P., Armstrong, J., Coradini, M., and Rand, J. (2014) Owner experiences in treating dogs and cats diagnosed with diabetes mellitus in the United States. *Journal of the American Animal Hospital Association* 50(4), 247–253.

Davison, L.J. (2015) Diabetes mellitus and pancreatitis – cause or effect? *The Journal of Small Animal Practice* 56(1), 50–59.

Fleeman, L.M. and Rand, J.S. (2003) Evaluation of day-to-day variability of serial blood glucose concentration curves in diabetic dogs. *Journal of the American Veterinary Medical Association* 222(3), 317–321.

Fracassi, F., Corradini, S., Hafner, M., Boretti, F.S., Sieber-Ruckstuhl, N.S., and Reusch, C.E. (2015) Detemir insulin for the treatment of diabetes mellitus in dogs. *Journal of the American Veterinary Medical Association* 247(1), 73–78.

Marshall, R.D., Rand, J.S., and Morton, J.M. (2009) Treatment of newly diagnosed diabetic cats with glargine insulin improves glycaemic control and results in higher probability of remission than protamine zinc and lente insulins. *Journal of Feline Medicine and Surgery* 11(8), 683–691.

Nelson, R.W. and Reusch, C.E. (2014) Animal models of disease: classification and etiology of diabetes in dogs and cats. *The Journal of Endocrinology* 222(3), T1–9.

Rucinsky, R., Cook, A., Haley, S., Nelson, R., Zoran, D.L., and Poundstone, M. (2010) AAHA diabetes management guidelines. *Journal of the American Animal Hospital Association* 46(3), 215–224.

Sako, T., Mori, A., Lee, P., Oda, H., Saeki, K., Miki, Y., Kurishima, M., Mimura, K., Nozawa, S., Mizutani, H., Makino, Y., Ishioka, K., and Arai, T. (2011) Time-action profiles of insulin detemir in normal and diabetic dogs. *Research in Veterinary Science* 90(3), 396–403.

Scott-Moncrieff, J.C.R., Moore, G.E., Coe, J., Lynn, R.C., Gwin, W., and Petzold, R. (2012) Characteristics of commercially manufactured and compounded protamine zinc insulin. *Journal of the American Veterinary Medical Association* 240(5), 600–605.


## Diabetic ketoacidosis


Bresciani, F., Pietra, M., Corradini, S., Giunti, M., and Fracassi, F. (2014) Accuracy of capillary blood 3-β-hydroxybutyrate determination for the detection and treatment of canine diabetic ketoacidosis. *Journal of Veterinary Science* 15(2), 309–316.

Claus, M.A., Silverstein, D.C., Shofer, F.S., and Mellema, M.S. (2010) Comparison of regular insulin infusion doses in critically ill diabetic cats: 29 cases (1999–2007). *Journal of Veterinary Emergency and Critical Care (San Antonio)* 20(5), 509–517.

Gilor, C. and Grave, T.K. (2010) Synthetic insulin analogues and their use in dogs and cats. *Veterinary Clinics of North America. Small Animal Practice* 40(2), 297–307.

Hume, D.Z., Drobatz, K.J., and Hess, R.S. (2006) Outcome of dogs with diabetic ketoacidosis: 127 dogs (1993–2003). *Journal of Veterinary Internal Medicine* 2006; 20(3), 547–555.

O'Brien, M.A. (2010) Diabetic emergencies in small animals. *Veterinary Clinics of North America. Small Animal Practice* 40(2), 317–333.

Reineke, E.L., Fletcher, D.J., King, L.G., and Drobatz, K.J. (2010) Accuracy of a continuous glucose monitoring system in dogs and cats with diabetic ketoacidosis. *Journal of Veterinary Emergency and Critical Care (San Antonio)* 20(3), 303–312.

Sears, K.W., Drobatz, K.J., and Hess, R.S. (2012) Use of lispro insulin for treatment of diabetic ketoacidosis in dogs. *Journal of Veterinary Emergency and Critical Care (San Antonio)* 22(2), 211–218.

Stojanovic, V. and Ihle, S. (2011) Role of beta-hydroxybutyric acid in diabetic ketoacidosis: a review. *The Canadian Veterinary Journal* 52(4), 426–430.

Søren, R.B. (2008) Fluid and electrolyte therapy in endocrine disorders: diabetes mellitus and hypoadrenocorticism. *Veterinary Clinics of North America. Small Animal Practice* 38(3), 699–717.

Weingart, C., Lotz, F., and Kohn, B. (2012) Measurement of β-hydroxybutyrate in cats with nonketotic diabetes mellitus, diabetic ketosis, and diabetic ketoacidosis. *Journal of Veterinary Diagnostic Investigation* 24(2), 295–300.

## Insulinoma

Goutal, C.M., Brugmann, B.L., and Ryan, K.A. (2012) Insulinoma in dogs: a review. *Journal of the American Animal Hospital Association* 48(3), 151–163.

Kraje, A.C. (2003) Hypoglycemia and irreversible neurologic complications in a cat with insulinoma. *Journal of the American Veterinary Medical Association* 223(6), 812–814.

Moore, A.S., Nelson, R.W., Henry, C.J., Rassnick, K.M., Kristal, O., Ogilvie, G.K., and Kintzer, P. (2002) Streptozotocin for treatment of pancreatic islet cell tumors in dogs: 17 cases (1989–1999). *Journal of the American Veterinary Medical Association* 221(6), 811–818.

Northrup, N.C., Rassnick, K.M., Gieger, T.L., Kosarek, C.E., McFadden, C.W., and Rosenberg, M.P. (2013) Prospective evaluation of biweekly streptozotocin in 19 dogs with insulinoma. *Journal of Veterinary Internal Medicine* 27(3), 483–490.

Robben, J.H., Pollak, Y.W., Kirpensteijn, J., Boroffka, S.A., van den Ingh, T.S., Teske, E., and Voorhout, G. (2005) Comparison of ultrasonography, computed tomography, and single-photon emission computed tomography for the detection and localization of canine insulinoma. *Journal of Veterinary Internal Medicine* 19(1), 15–22.

Tobin, R.L., Nelson, R.W., Lucroy, M.D., Wooldridge, J.D., and Feldman, E.C. (1999) Outcome of surgical versus medical treatment of dogs with beta cell neoplasia: 39 cases (1990–1997). *Journal of the American Veterinary Medical Association* 215(2), 226–230.

Trifonidou, M.A., Kirpensteijn, J., and Robben, J.H. (1998) A retrospective evaluation of 51 dogs with insulinoma. *The Veterinary Quarterly* 20, S114–115.

## Acromegaly

Fischetti, A.J., Gisselman, K., and Peterson, M.E. (2012) CT and MRI evaluation of skull bones and soft tissues in six cats with presumed acromegaly versus 12 unaffected cats. *Veterinary Radiology and Ultrasound* 53(5), 535–539.

Lamb, C.R., Ciasca, T.C., Mantis, P., Forcada, Y., Potter, M., Church, D.B., and Niessen, S.J. (2014) Computed tomographic signs of acromegaly in 68 diabetic cats with hypersomatotropism. *Journal of Feline Medicine and Surgery* 16(2), 99–108.

Lourenço, B.N., Randall, E., Seiler, G., and Lunn, K.F. (2015) Abdominal ultrasonographic findings in acromegalic cats. *Journal of Feline Medicine and Surgery* 17(8), 698–703.

Niessen, S.J. (2010) Feline acromegaly: an essential differential diagnosis for the difficult diabetic. *Journal of Feline Medicine and Surgery* 12(1), 15–23.

Niessen, S.J., Church, D.B., and Forcada, Y. (2013) Hypersomatotropism, acromegaly, and hyperadrenocorticism and feline diabetes mellitus. *Veterinary Clinics of North America. Small Animal Practice* 43(2), 319–350.

Niessen, S.J., Forcada, Y., Mantis, P., Lamb, C.R., Harrington, N., Fowkes, R., Korbonits, M., Smith, K., and Church, D.B. (2015) Studying cat (*Felis catus*) diabetes: beware of the acromegalic imposter. PLoS One 10(5), e0127794.

## Pituitary dwarfism

Chastain, C.B. and Panciera, D. (2002) Use of proligestone in the management of three German Shepherd Dogs with pituitary dwarfism. *Small Animal Clinical Endocrinology* 12(3), 3.

Greco, D.S. (2012) Pituitary deficiencies. *Topics in Companion Animal Medicine* 27(1), 2–7.

Kooistra, H.S., Voorhout, G., Selman, P.J., and Rijnberk, A. (1998) Progestin-induced growth hormone (GH) production in the treatment of dogs with congenital GH deficiency. *Domestic Animal Endocrinology* 15, 93–102.

Kooistra, H.S., Voorhout, G., Mol, J.A., and Rijnberk, A. (2000) Combined pituitary hormone deficiency in German Shepherd Dogs with dwarfism. *Domestic Animal Endocrinology* 19, 177–190.

Voorbij, A.M., Meij, B.P., van Bruggen, L.W., Grinwis, G.C., Stassen, Q.E., and Kooistra, H.S. (2015) Atlanto-axial malformation and instability in dogs with pituitary dwarfism due to an LHX3 mutation. *Journal of Veterinary Internal Medicine* 29(1), 207–213.

## Diabetes insipidus

Aroch, I., Mazaki-Tov, M., Shemesh, O., Sarfaty, H., and Segev, G. (2005) Central diabetes insipidus in five cats: clinical presentation, diagnosis and oral desmopressin therapy. *Journal of Feline Medicine and Surgery* 7(6), 333–339.

Blois, S.L., Dickie, E.L., Kruth, S.A., and Allen, D.G. (2010) Multiple endocrine diseases in cats: 15 cases (1997–2008). *Journal of Feline Medicine and Surgery* 12(8), 637–642.

Harb, M.F., Nelson, R.W., Feldman, E.C., Scott-Moncrieff, J.C., and Griffey, S.M. (1996) Central diabetes insipidus in dogs: 20 cases (1986–1995). *Journal of the American Veterinary Medical Association* 209(11), 1884–1888.

Meij, B.P., Voorhout, G., Gerritsen, R.J., Grinwis, G.C., and Ijzer, J. (2012) Lymphocytic hypophysitis in a dog with diabetes insipidus. *Journal of Comparative Pathology* 147(4), 503–507.

Rossi, T.A. and Ross, L.A. (2008) Diabetes insipidus. *Compendium: Continuing Education for Veterinarians* 30(1), 43–52.

Teshima, T., Hara, Y., Taoda, T., Teramoto, A., and Tagawa, M. (2011) Central diabetes insipidus after transsphenoidal surgery in dogs with Cushing's disease. *The Journal of Veterinary Medical Science* 73(1), 33–39.

## Tests

**1. In the diagnosis of thyroid diseases:**

A) TSH is elevated in 90% of hypothyroid dogs.
B) T4T is elevated in 50% of hyperthyroid cats.
C) The measurement of free T4 is the most specific and sensitive test for diagnosis.
D) The measurement of anti-thyroid antibodies is essential to diagnose canine hypothyroidism.

**2. In the diagnosis of adrenal diseases:**

A) The ACTH stimulation test is the most specific test for the diagnosis of Cushing's disease.
B) Stimulation with ACTH is not useful for the diagnosis of Addison's disease.
C) Urinary cortisol/creatinine ratio is the most specific test for the diagnosis of Cushing's.
D) To confirm the type of Cushing's (pituitary or adrenal) in doubtful cases, an MRI or CT scan is essential.

**3. In treatment for Addison's:**

A) Animals with acute symptoms do not need hospitalization, only oral supplementation with gluco- and mineralocorticoids.
B) The acute picture begins to improve simply with the administration of fluid therapy with crystalloids (0.9% NaCl) and a glucocorticoid.
C) With adequate treatment, the recovery of acute cases is usually slow (1 week).
D) In the long term, some animals no longer need medication.

**4. In the treatment of adrenal hyperadrenocorticism (Cushing's):**

A) IV chemotherapy is the treatment of choice.
B) Treatment with mitotane (complete destruction of the adrenal glands) is not a therapeutic alternative.
C) Treatment with trilostane (reduces cortisol levels) is a therapeutic alternative.
D) Tumours are usually benign, so a postoperative follow-up is not necessary.

**5. Hypocalcaemia in dogs and cats:**

A) Is usually caused by parathyroid neoplasms.
B) In severe cases, causes tetany and seizures and requires emergency treatment.
C) Maintenance therapy initially requires the administration of fluid therapy.
D) For long-term treatment, the source of vitamin D of choice is alendronate.

**6. Diabetes mellitus:**

A) In dogs is more common in young to middle-aged neutered females.
B) In cats is more frequent in neutered females.
C) In some hyperglycaemic cats, it is necessary to confirm/rule out stress hyperglycaemia by measuring fructosamine.
D) Can go unnoticed In the dog, and fructosamine should be measured to confirm diagnosis.

**7. In cases of diabetes mellitus:**

A) Animals with ketoacidosis require treatment with regular insulin and fluid therapy.
B) Ketoacidosis is a mild complication that does not require intensive treatment.
C) The insulin of choice for maintenance in the cat is glargine at a high dose.
D) The insulin of choice for maintenance in the dog is Caninsulin at high doses.

**8. Regarding insulinoma:**

A) Diagnostic imaging is not useful, since insulinoma is not usually visualized.
B) The treatment of choice is chemotherapy.
C) Streptozotocin is the drug of choice in all cases, effective against metastasis.
D) The diet in these patients should be rich in carbohydrates and meals should be frequent.

**9. Acromegaly:**

A) In the cat, is caused by a pituitary tumour producing growth hormone.
B) In the cat, is caused by the administration of glucocorticoids.
C) In the dog, is produced by chronic treatment with corticosteroids.
D) Acromegalic cats are usually diabetic and need low doses of insulin.

**10. Regarding central diabetes insipidus:**

A) To confirm the diagnosis, an ACTH test can be performed.
B) To confirm the diagnosis, plasma and urinary osmolality can be measured.
C) It is treated with commercial ADH and has a poor prognosis.
D) It is treated with a renal diet and vasodilators.

**11. Feline hyperthyroidism can be treated with:**

A) Oral or transdermal methimazole.
B) Radiotherapy with cobalt.
C) Diet with a high iodine content.
D) IV chemotherapy.

**12. In relation to canine hypothyroidism:**

A) Lifelong treatment is needed.
B) Some dogs stop needing thyroxine in the medium to long term (months).
C) The initial dose of thyroxine should be reduced by half in periodic reviews.
D) The clinical signs do not resolve with treatment; only the neuromuscular changes improve.

**13. The clinical presentation of hypoadrenocorticism (Addison's):**

A) Progresses rapidly and usually presents as a crisis.
B) Is not usually serious or fatal, regardless of treatment.
C) Is more frequent in geriatric animals.
D) The most frequent symptoms are alopecia, tachycardia, and tachypnoea.

**14. The treatment of hyperadrenocorticism (Cushing's) can be:**

A) Trilostane at a low to moderate initial dose (1–3 mg/kg/d), a treatment that is maintained for life, after adjusting the initial dose.
B) Trilostane at low doses (1 mg/kg/d) and, when symptoms disappear, with a dose of trilostane once a week.
C) Selegiline, which works in 90% of cases.
D) Mitotane for a week to 10 days.

**15. Hypercalcaemia in dogs and cats:**

A) Is always asymptomatic; it is a laboratory finding.
B) To confirm the diagnosis ionized blood calcium should be measured.
C) Does not require urgent treatment under any circumstances.
D) In the long term, only the hypercalcaemia should be treated, not what causes it.

**16. Regarding diabetic ketoacidosis:**

A) It occurs when there is a partial insulin deficiency.
B) Diagnosis should be confirmed by measuring fructosamine levels.
C) It is characterized by metabolic and respiratory acidosis.
D) Mortality is high (30%).

**Answers on page 135**

## Clinical case 1

### Signalment

11-year-old castrated male Common European cat.

### Reason for consultation

He became weak and depressed 2 weeks ago. He has had a bigger appetite for the last 5–6 months; however, over the last 2 weeks he has had little appetite and vomits (once every 2 days); the vomit contains bile and food.

He is also drinking slightly more than before (>500 ml/d) and has polyuria.

There is no other concurrent illness or treatment. He eats everything: canned food and home-cooked food (chicken).

### Physical examination

He is alert and well hydrated, weighs 3.9 kg, and has a body condition score of 4/9. The mucous membranes are pink and CRT is <2 seconds. On cardiac auscultation the heart rate is 200 bpm, with no sign of murmurs. Pulmonary auscultation is normal. Palpable lymph nodes are normal. Temperature is 38.5°C.

On palpation of the neck a slight thickening can be appreciated. The systolic blood pressure (Doppler) is 130 mmHg. Upon palpation, the abdomen is soft; no organomegaly is appreciated.

1. **What are the main problems?**
2. **What are the differential diagnoses?**
3. **What would be your initial diagnostic plan?**
4. **Tests show the following results:**

#### Haemogram

| Parameter | Result | Units | Reference value |
|---|---|---|---|
| Haematocrit | 46 | % | 38–58 |
| Haemoglobin | 15.6 | g/dl | 13–19 |
| Red blood cells | 10.31 | x $10^6$/ µl | 5.5– 8.6 |
| VCM | 50.6 | fl | 62–74 |
| HCM | 15.2 | pg | 21–25 |
| CHCM | 33.9 | g/dl | 31–36 |
| Leucocytes | 5.1 | x $10^3$/µl | 6–17 |
| Basophils | 9 | % | 0–2 |
| Eosinophils | 2 | % | 2–10 |
| Bands | 64 | % | 5–10 |
| Segmented | 19 | % | 46–77 |
| Lymphocytes | | % | 15–43 |
| Monocytes | | % | 1–7 |
| Platelets | 320 | x $10^3$/µl | 150–500 |

*Note*: CHCM, HCM, VCM

#### Blood biochemistry

| Parameter | Result | Units | Reference Value |
|---|---|---|---|
| Glucose | 110 | mg/dl | 70–120 |
| Urea | 64 | mg/dl | 20–40 |
| Creatinine | 1.3 | mg/dl | 0.5–1.4 |
| Total protein | 8 | g/dl | 5.5–7.5 |
| ALT | 313 | IU/l | <80 |
| ALP | 520 | IU/l | <100 |
| Sodium | 148 | mEq/l | 142–152 |
| Potassium | 3.3 | mEq/l | 3.5–5.5 |
| Chlorine | 117 | mEq/l | 110–120 |
| Calcium | 10.0 | mg/dl | 8–11.6 |
| Phosphorus | 5.2 | mg/dl | 3.5–6.5 |
| Total T4 | 11 | µg/dl | 1.5–4.7 |

#### Urinalysis

The urine density is 1.021; the sediment is inactive; pH is 5.5.

The protein/creatinine ratio is 0.4 and the urine culture negative.

#### Abdominal ultrasound

The kidneys are of a size towards the lower normal limit. Urinary bladder is normal. There is slight hepatomegaly and the liver is slightly hyperechogenic. In the small intestine (Figure Clinical case), the muscular layer is thickened and the mucosa is folded and hyperechogenic (compatible with a gastroenteropathy). No lymphadenopathies are observed. The parenchyma is heterogeneous in the pancreas.

#### Ultrasound of the cervical neck region

A 1.5 cm nodule is seen in the right thyroid lobe. The left lobe is normal.

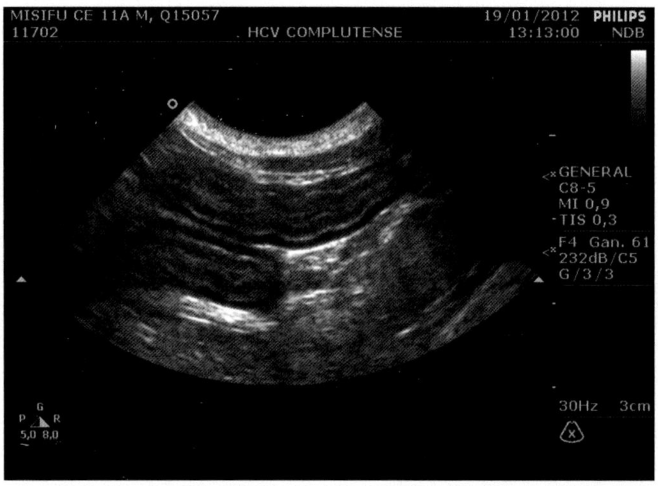


**Figure Clinical case** Courtesy of the HCVC diagnostic imaging service.

**What are the most likely differential diagnoses?**

5. **Would you perform any additional tests?**
   A) PTRrP to evaluate the possible presence of an intestinal neoplasia (lymphoma) that is causing hypercalcaemia.
   B) fPLI to confirm or rule out the presence of chronic pancreatitis.
   C) IGF-1 to assess the possible presence of feline acromegaly.
   D) Echocardiography to evaluate the possible presence of hypertrophic heart disease.
6. **Additional test results:**
   fPLI 25 µg/dl (<5 µg/dl).
   Echocardiography without relevant findings.
   **What treatment would you propose?**

## Clinical case 2

1. **What are the main problems?**
   A) Loss of appetite.
   B) Polydipsia/polyuria.
   C) Vomiting.
2. **What are the differential diagnoses?**
   The differential diagnoses of the three problems can be approached together:
   Renal failure and feline hyperthyroidism are the two most likely diseases, due to age and the presence of these three symptoms. Other diagnoses that may also occur concurrently with the above are diabetes mellitus (initially presented

with polyphagia), pancreatitis, cholangiohepatitis, chronic inflammatory bowel disease, triaditis, pyelonephritis/urinary tract infection, hypercalcaemia, and intestinal neoplasia, among the most probable.

3. **What would be your initial diagnostic plan?**
   Initially a complete blood count, complete biochemistry and levels of T4T, urinalysis and urine culture, and an ultrasound of the neck and abdominal areas.
4. **What is/are the diagnosis/diagnoses?**
   The diagnosis is feline hyperthyroidism, which is what explains the symptoms (PU/PD, vomiting, and the fact that although the patient has now presented with loss of appetite it initially had polyphagia).

   However, it is possible that there is also duodenitis and hepatitis, indicated by ultrasound findings and liver enzymes (although these are also elevated in feline hyperthyroidism). In addition, although there is no abdominal pain on palpation and the ultrasound findings are not significant, the coexistence of pancreatitis should not be ruled out, which would explain the anorexia.
5. **Would you perform any additional tests?**
   fPLI and echocardiography.
6. **What treatment would you recommend?**
   Initially a medical treatment for hyperthyroidism with methimazole at 1.25 mg every 12 h.

   Likewise, a treatment for triaditis with famotidine (long term) and maropitant (1 week), metronidazole (3 weeks), a highly digestible low fat diet (intestinal low fat), and buprenorphine (2–3 weeks).

   Weekly and monthly check-ups to concurrently evaluate levels of T4T, urea/creatinine, UPC, and liver enzyme levels.

   Depending on progression, maintain the adequate dose of methimazole to allow T4T levels to reach 2–4 μg/dl, an intestinal diet, and famotidine. Upon achieving the remission of triaditis, recommend treatment of the thyroid nodule with surgery or radioactive iodine.

## Correct answers

### Test

| | | |
|---|---|---|
| 1. C | 7. A | 13. A |
| 2. A | 8. D | 14. A |
| 3. B | 9. A | 15. B |
| 4. C | 10. B | 16. D |
| 5. B | 11. A | |
| 6. C | 12. A | |

# 4

# Dermatology

Sandra Díaz and Chiara Noli

## Chapter summary



## Introduction

Pruritus, scratching and alopecia are just clinical signs. Therefore, when presented with an itchy dog chewing its paws, it is important not to jump to conclusions; yes, the dog may have allergies, or it may have a *Malassezia* overgrowth secondary to a parasitic problem that glucocorticoid treatment would exacerbate. It´s important to realize that diagnosis based on pattern recognition has its place for simple cases with classical patterns or experienced clinicians, but this approach may lead to omissions.

A problem-based approach to dermatology takes a more global attitude to diagnosis. It seeks to establish a complete problem list and then outline the most likely differentials for those problems. The clinicians have all the information in front of them, and this logical approach makes it easier to identify which are primary and which secondary factors. By identifying the problems and their likely causes, the veterinarian keeps an open mind and is less likely to go down the wrong diagnostic path.

Indeed, it is human nature to look for evidence to back up an assumption, and overlook information that contradicts this conclusion. The problem-based approach to dermatology prevents the clinician from narrowing down their search (in other words, jumping to conclusions) before it is appropriate to do so.

Whilst a problem-based approach may sound lengthy or overly complex, its beauty lies in the logical systematic approach. This makes a misdiagnosis less likely and gives the veterinarian increased confidence to tackle even the most frustrating cases, making for a more satisfying outcome for patient, owner and veterinarian alike.

### Key learning points

- Learn how to take a problem-based approach to dermatology cases.
- Identify primary from secondary skin lesions.

## A problem-based, clinical-reasoning approach to dermatology

When adopting a problem-based, clinical reasoning approach the clinician considers each significant clinical-pathological **problem separately**, before relating them to any other problems presented by the patient.

The alternative approach is to attempt to memorize a long list of diseases that fit the pattern of the animal's clinical signs. This can be relatively simple for common disorders with uniquely recognizable patterns or if the veterinarian has an excellent memory and extensive experience. However, the use of pattern recognition to reach a diagnosis can lead to **errors of omission**.

When a patient displays multiple, non-specific clinical signs (e.g. alopecia, polydipsia and pustules), the use of **pattern recognition is unreliable** as this leads to tunnel vision where the veterinarian pursues their initial diagnostic hunch to the exclusion of other diagnostic possibilities. In turn, subsequent data tend to be interpreted as favourable to this initial impression.

In straightforward cases and with an experienced veterinarian, pattern recognition can lead to a correct diagnosis and successful treatment plan. However, more **complex conditions are not easily identified** using this approach. It is these cases that frustrate veterinarians and pet owners alike.

The problem-based clinical reasoning takes into consideration the pathophysiological basis and the differential diagnosis of the presenting clinical signs before start looking for a pattern. This approach avoids tunnel vision and ensures a more open attitude to all the diagnostic possibilities.

Looking into each clinical problem results in improved identification of any condition(s) which could cause the patterns the patient is presenting with.

The questions that need to be answered are:

- What is/are the problems?
- What body system(s) or area(s) are affected?
- What type of lesions are present?

### *Identify the problem*

For example, the owner reports the dog is losing hair and has 'scab-like' lesions.

**Which problem came first**? Was the hair lost when the scabs loosened and lifted away, or was alopecia present before the crusty lesions developed? The **primary problem must be identified**: crust or alopecia?

**Are there other signs**, such as pruritus? If the animal is itchy, then the alopecia might be self-inflicted. This has the potential to misdirect the clinician's focus of attention – for example, if they fail to identify pruritus as the cause of hair loss, the diagnosis is going to be focused on alopecia and not pruritus, leading to an incorrect diagnosis.

**Identify the affected area of the body** and how it is involved. Decide whether the problem is primary or secondary. For example, are the dog's crusts due to primary disease such as pemphigus foliaceus, or is the crust formation secondary to severe pruritus and self-trauma?

Determine whether this is a **primary dermatologic or systemic problem**. For example, the crusts may have formed secondary to a tick-transmitted disease causing a vasculopathy. The history and the presence or absence of systemic clinical signs like fever and lethargy are very helpful in this step. If there is suspicion of systemic disease, appropriate testing may be needed to confirm or eliminate the clinical suspicion.

### *Identify the location of the lesion*

Observe the patient **at a distance** to determine whether the lesions are:

- localized
- generalized.

Some diseases present with a **classic distribution**, e.g. as sarcoptic mange affecting the margin of the pinnae, elbows, hocks and ventral abdomen. In this case, the distribution of the lesions will help us to quickly develop a list of differential diagnosis.

## *Identify the lesion*

First evaluate the patient from a distance, in order to assess the distribution of the lesions in a **systematic manner**. Then examine the lesions more closely, if necessary using a magnification tool to assess small lesions – indeed, **good lighting** is a prerequisite for this. Be systematic and examine all the skin and mucous membranes, and attempt to determine whether the lesions are **primary or secondary**.

## *Final result*

With this problem-based clinical approach, instead of tunnel vision ('the animal has crusty lesions'), a more enlightening global approach is achieved ('itching is the most likely cause, and the animal is traumatizing the skin and causing alopecia and crusting'). If the alopecia and crusting are secondary lesions, the list of differential diagnoses will be focused on pruritic skin diseases.

## *Examples of differential diagnoses*

### *Pruritic dermatitis:*

Allergic (food allergy, atopic dermatitis, flea allergic dermatitis), parasitic (sarcoptic mange, *Cheyletiella*) and infectious (superficial pyoderma, *Malassezia* dermatitis).

Get into the habit of using a **template for diagnostic examination** (Figure 4.1). This allows you to obtain and organize information to direct the investigation according to the patient's presenting problems.

| Dermatological examination record | |
|---|---|
| Date | Nurse |
| Veterinarian | Type of appointment |
| Date of last examination | |
| Weight | |
| Temperature | |
| Heart rate | |
| Respiration rate | |
| Physical examination (lesions/distribution) | |

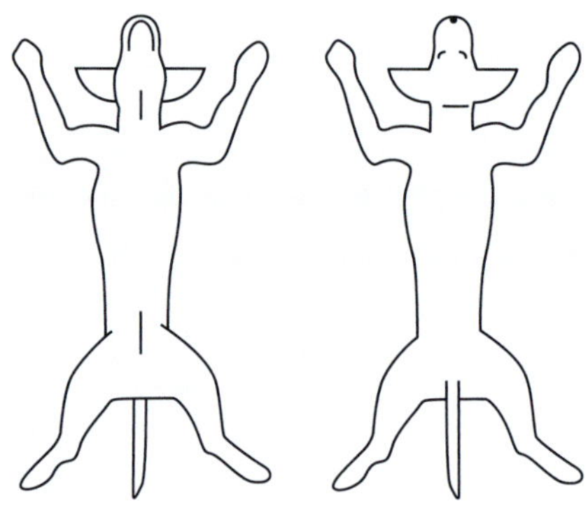

| Problems | Diagnostic plan |
|---|---|
| Different diagnoses | Treatment plan |

**Figure 4.1.** Example of a record chart used for diagnostic examination. Courtesy of the Dermatology Service at the University of Minnesota.

## Dermatological examination

## *Primary reason for consultation*

Team work is vital in dermatology, as the owner's commitment to carrying out treatment is essential to a successful outcome of the case. Part of this means establishing early-on a **relationship of trust** by **identifying why** the client is seeking veterinary help and **the signs** that indicate there is a skin problem (such as pruritus, oily skin or the dog's physical appearance to the general public). Other conditions should be recognised and mentioned, but the focus should remain on the primary reason for consultation.

In summary, the clinician's initial efforts should be directed as follows:

1. definition of **the problem**
2. **definition** of the lesions
3. definition of lesion **distribution**.

This facilitates making a list of differential diagnoses and formulation of an effective diagnostic plan.

## *Signalment*

Keeping the species, age, breed and sex in mind helps to develop a list of differential diagnoses.

### Age

Some dermatological problems only occur at **certain ages** (Table 4.1). When dealing with a chronic problem, it is helpful to ascertain the age at which the symptoms started.

### Breed

The breed can be useful to prioritize the list of differential diagnoses. For example, in a case of crusting dermatitis located in mucocutaneous areas in a Siberian Husky, zinc-responsive dermatitis should be suspected.

### Sex

The sex of the animal helps to identify specific conditions, such as feminization syndrome associated with a testicular tumour, or perianal adenoma, which occur almost exclusively in male animals.

### Coat colour

The coat colour may also indicate predispositions to certain conditions. For example:

White cats are 13 times more likely to develop squamous cell carcinoma.

Animals with diluted coat colours are predisposed to developing colour-dilution alopecia.

## History

A **complete clinical history** is essential and can be time-consuming to obtain. It is important to develop an efficient method of history taking so that no information is overlooked. The history is generally divided into **two sections**.

Table 4.1. Relationship between particular dermatological pathologies and the age of occurrence.

| Patient age | Dermatological pathology |
|---|---|
| < 6 months | Juvenile demodicosis<br>Dermatophytoses<br>Puppy pyoderma<br>Juvenile cellulitis<br>Oral papillomatosis<br>Dietary allergies |
| 6–12 months | Canine acne<br>Colour-dilution alopecia<br>Histiocytoma<br>Oral papillomatosis<br>Zinc-responsive dermatosis |
| 1–5 years | Allergic dermatitis<br>Alopecia X<br>Colour-dilution alopecia<br>Primary idiopathic seborrhoea<br>Autoimmune dermatosis |
| 5 years+ | Endocrinopathies<br>Feminization syndrome (testicular tumour)<br>Neoplasia<br>Bedsores |

### General history

To obtain this the client can be asked to fill in a form before the consultation which can be sent in advance via email or delivered at the time of the visit.

### Dermatological history

This is based on questions aimed at identifying the **main reason** for the visit. For example: Where did the lesions originate? What were the original lesions like and how did they progress? What response was there to previous treatments?

Take care that the questions asked do not lead the owner and suggest an answer. However, sometimes direct questions are appropriate if the client does not mention relevant information, such as linking one problem to another. For example, a dog which presents for excessive licking may have suffered from recurrent otitis but the owner does not think to mention the latter.

Although pruritus is a common cause for consultation, many clients do not specifically know **how severe the itching is**. However, asking appropriate questions can provide a clear idea of the severity involved.

- When did the itching start?
- How many times a day do you see the dog scratching?
- Where is it itchy?
- Does it lick its legs or bite them?
- Does the dog shake its head?
- Does it rub itself on furniture or carpets?
- Does it stop playing to scratch?

Information about the environment in which the animal lives is also important to confirm or rule out certain conditions:

- Does the dog improve if it travels or spends time in kennels?
- Were there any environmental changes before the problem occurred?
- Has there been a change in any cleaning measures?
- Have you used any products in the garden?

It is also very important to determine whether it is **contagious**:

- Are other animals or people affected?

## Physical examination

One advantage of dermatological problems is that they can be seen and felt during the consultation. It is important to have good lighting and a magnifying glass, if necessary, to identify small lesions. The physical examination should be done from two distances:

1. From approximately **1 metre away** to evaluate the general condition and lesion distribution.
2. **Close up**, to identify the type of lesions.

**Skin and mucous membranes** should be examined and palpated systematically, with the animal on its back and side.

Lesions often overlooked include:

- Paronychia (inflammation of the cuticle) (Figure 4.2).
- Interdigital lesions.
- Skin-fold lesions (Figure 4.3).

The coat should be examined:

- Is it soft or hard?
- Dry or oily?
- Does the hair fall out easily?
- If there is alopecia, is it partial or generalized?

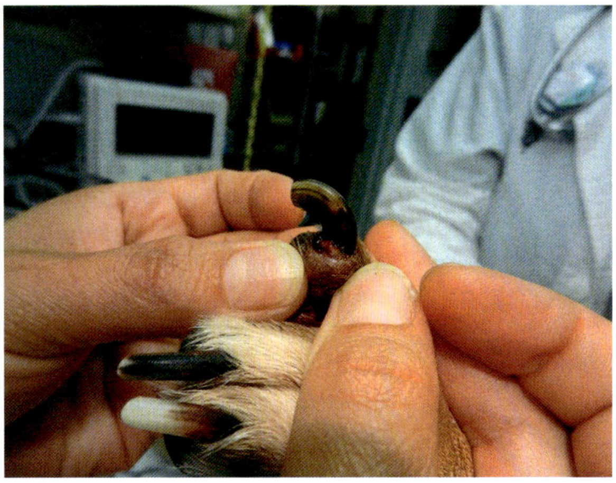

**Figure 4.2.** Paronychia.

## *Identification of lesions*

Skin lesions (Table 4.2) are classified as either:

- **Primary**. Those that **develop early and spontaneously** and reflect the disease; they may be subtle.
- **Secondary**. Those that are **formed from primary lesions** or are produced by trauma, application of medications, inflammation, pruritus or secondary infections.

The appearance of lesions helps determine the origin:

- Linear. May indicate:
  - trauma
  - compromised blood or lymphatic vessels
  - congenital malformation
  - linear granuloma.
- Annular or circular (Figure 4.4). Suggests:
  - superficial pyoderma
  - dermatophytosis
  - demodicosis.

If the lesions are generalized, they suggest a metabolic or systemic problem:

**Table 4.2.** Primary and secondary skin lesions.

| Primary | Secondary | Lesions that may be primary or secondary |
|---|---|---|
| Macule | Epidermal collarette | Alopecia |
| Papule or plaque | Scar | Scaling |
| Pustule | Excoriation | Crust |
| Vesicle or bulla | Erosion or ulcer | Comedone |
| Weal | Fissure | Hyperpigmentation |
| Nodule | Lichenification | Hypopigmentation |
| Cystic tumour | Callus | |

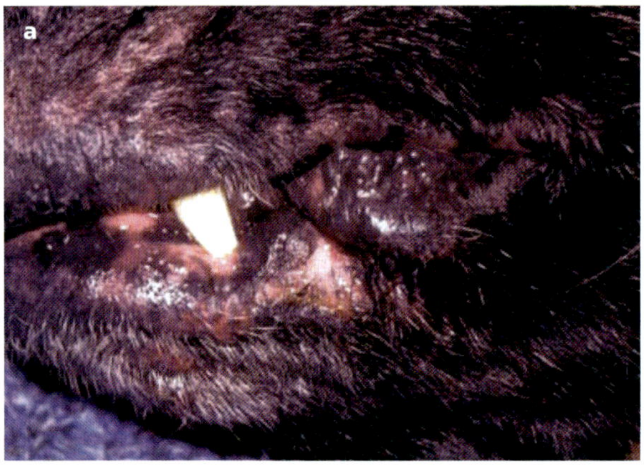



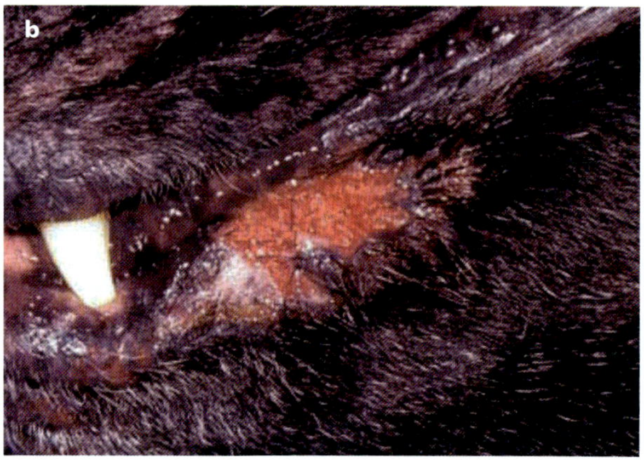



**Figure 4.3.** a, Labial folds; b, mucocutaneous pyoderma.

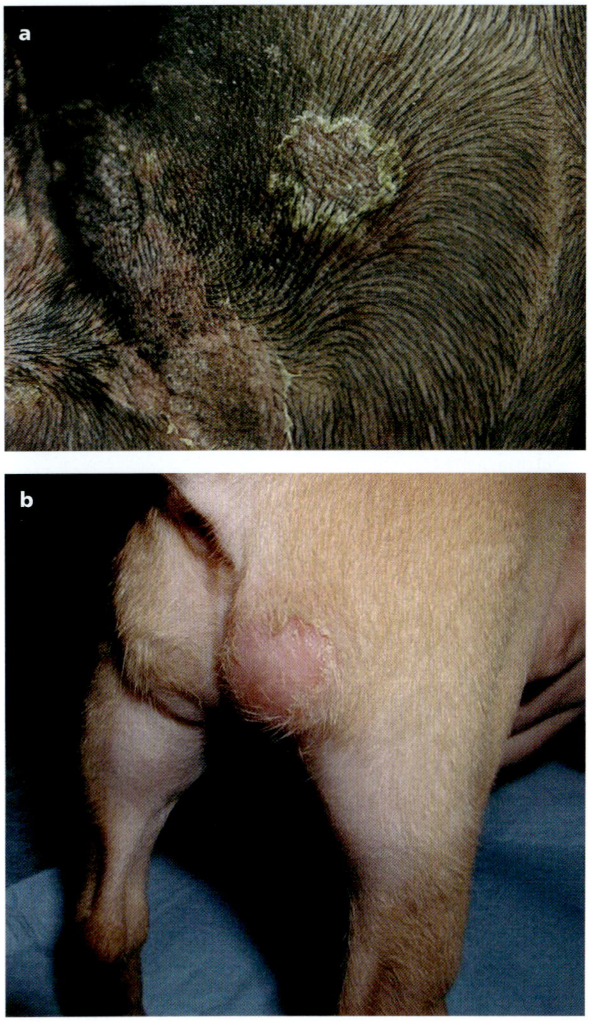


**Figure 4.4.** a, Circular appearance. Epidermal collarette due to a superficial pyoderma; b, area of focal alopecia, dermatophytosis.

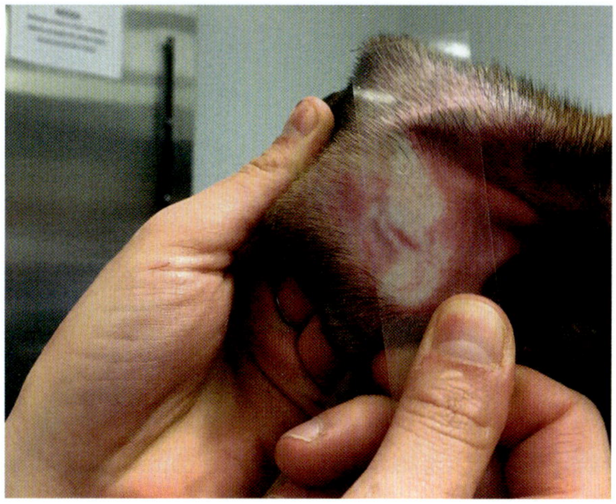

**Figure 4.5.** Diascopy.

- endocrine
- keratinization
- immune-mediated
- allergic dermatitis.

## Skin lesions

### *Primary*

#### *Erythema*

Erythema refers to **redness of the skin** due to congestion of blood vessels in the dermis. It **disappears with diascopy** (Figure 4.5) and may be diffuse or localized.

Dermatoses commonly associated with erythema:

- allergic dermatitis
- ectoparasites
- reactions to medications
- epitheliotropic lymphoma (Figure 4.6).

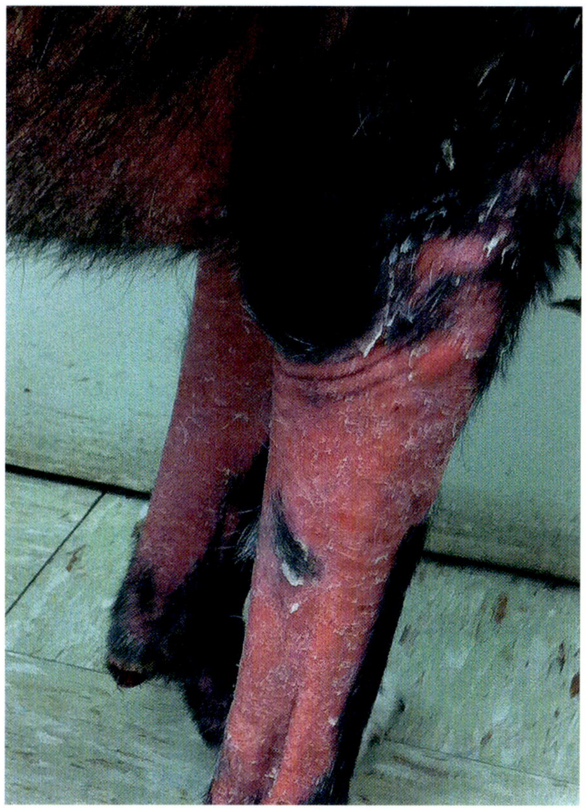

**Figure 4.6.** Severe erythema due to cutaneous epitheliotropic lymphoma.

#### *Purpura*

This refers to **areas of dark red coloration**. Purpura corresponds to extravasation of erythrocytes from the blood vessels and **persists with diascopy**.

Dermatoses that can present purpuric lesions:

- Cushing's syndrome
- vasculopathies
- reactions to medications (Figure 4.7)
- systemic lupus erythematosus.

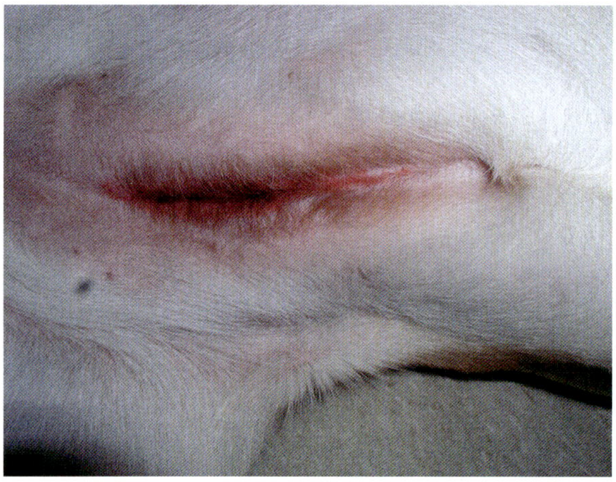

**Figure 4.7.** Purpura on the ventral abdomen due to reaction to gentamicin.

### *Macule*

A macule is a flat area associated with a change in skin colour.

Macules are classified according to the origin and coloration:

#### Hyperchromic

Present in cases of:

- lentigo simplex (Figure 4.8)
- post-inflammatory
- endocrine diseases.

#### Hypochromic

Is associated with:

- vitiligo
- post-inflammatory
- endocrine diseases
- erythema
- haemorrhage.

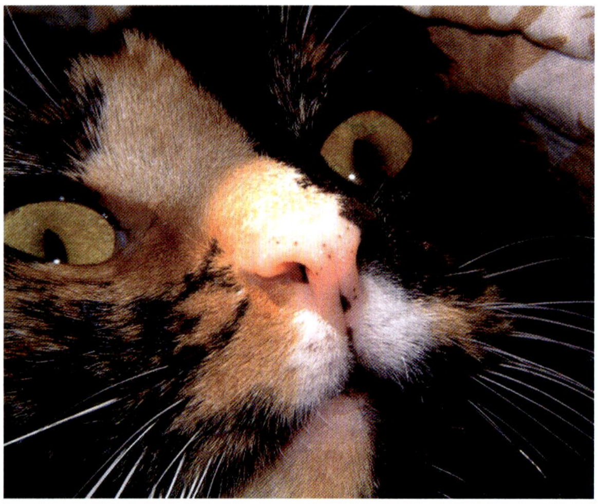

**Figure 4.8.** Macule on the nasal plane due to lentigo simplex.

### *Papule*

Papules are well-circumscribed elevations of the skin with **solid contents and measure less than 1 cm in diameter**.

Papules can appear in different layers of the skin, and are classified as:

- epidermal
- follicular
- dermal.

They can be associated with:

- ectoparasites
- superficial pyoderma
- allergic dermatitis
- calcinosis cutis (Figure 4.9).

### *Wheal*

A wheal is an **elevated oedematous area** with a flattened, rounded or irregular surface.

Hives are wheals that join together forming large lesions.

Wheals are usually associated with a hypersensitivity reaction (Figure 4.10).

### *Plaque*

Plaque is a **prominent area of oedema, measuring more than 1 cm in diameter**. It is formed when papules merge and is seen with chronic inflammatory diseases and neoplasms (Figure 4.11).

### *Pustule*

A pustule is a **small circumscribed elevation** of the epidermis (< 1 cm), **containing purulent exudate**. It may be:

- intra-epidermal
- sub-epidermal

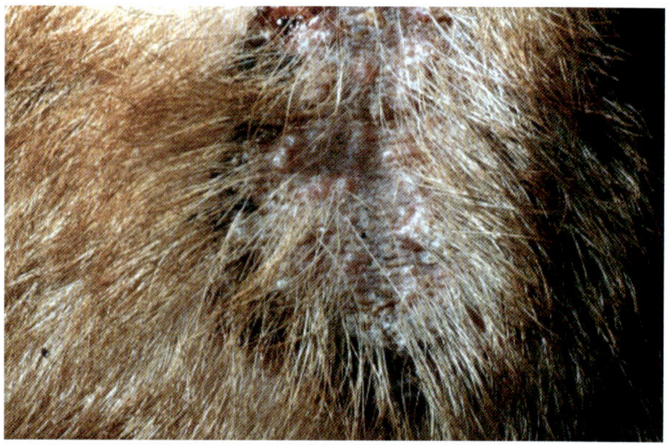

**Figure 4.9.** Calcinosis cutis on the dorsal neck due to iatrogenic Cushing's syndrome.

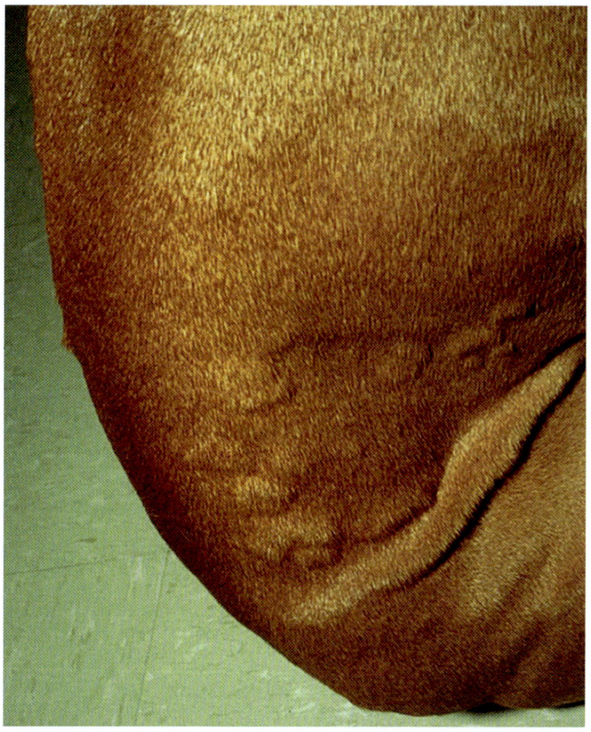

**Figure 4.10.** Wheals on the flank of a Boxer with insect bite hypersensitivity.

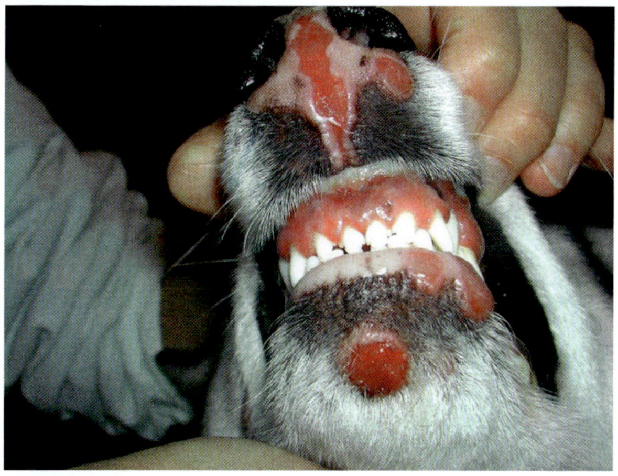

**Figure 4.11.** Plaque on the lower lip due to cutaneous lymphoma.

- follicular
- dermatosis associated with pustular injuries
- superficial pyoderma
- pemphigus foliaceus (Figure 4.12) and erythematosus
- demodicosis
- Leishmaniasis.

### *Vesicle and blister*

Vesicles and blisters are well-circumscribed, **thin-walled, elevated epidermal lesions** (**<1 cm**). They **contain fluid** (serum, lymph or blood) and are fragile and transient.

A blister is a vesicle larger than 1 cm.

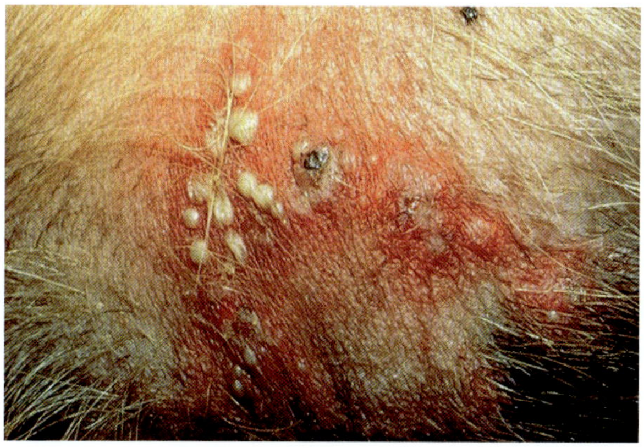

**Figure 4.12.** Pustules on the ventral abdomen due to pemphigus foliaceus.

Vesicles and blisters are uncommon lesions. They can be associated with:

- autoimmune diseases
- contact dermatitis
- viral dermatoses
- severe inflammation
- mucinosis in the Shar Pei (Figure 4.13).

### *Nodule*

A nodule is a **solid, circumscribed elevated lesion** (**>1 cm**). It can originate from different layers of the skin.

Nodular dermatoses include:

- neoplasia
- cutaneous histiocytosis
- hamartoma
- deep pyoderma (Figure 4.14)
- mycobacteriosis
- deep mycosis
- panniculitis.

### *Tumour*

A tumour is described as a **firm elevation with or without defined limits**, which tends to increase in size

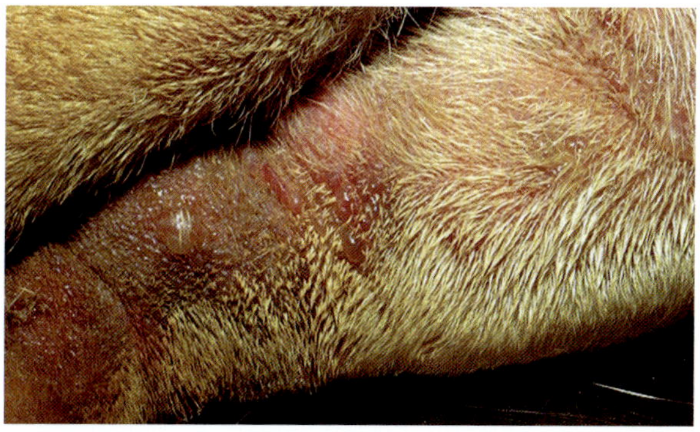

**Figure 4.13.** Mucin vesicle associated with mucinosis on the leg of a Shar Pei.

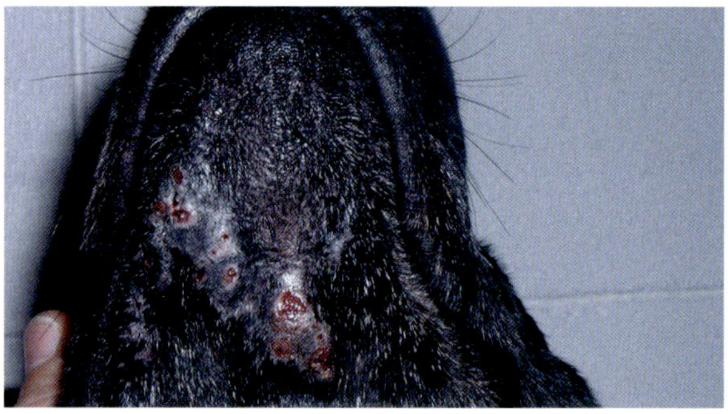

**Figure 4.14.** Ulcerated nodules due to canine acne.

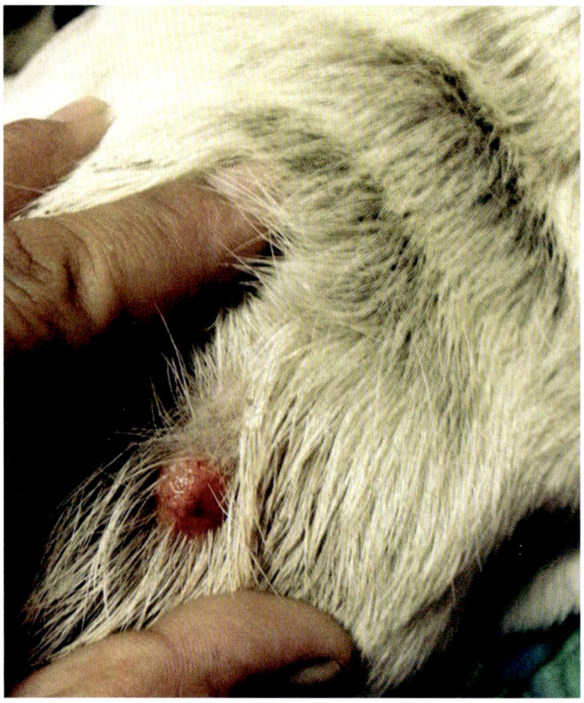

**Figure 4.15.** Histiocytoma.

and be persistent. It can originate from any part of the skin and be **benign or malignant** (Figure 4.15).

### Cyst

A cyst is a raised, sac-like lesion lined by epithelium. It contains liquid or semi-solid material such as keratin or sebum (Figure 4.16).

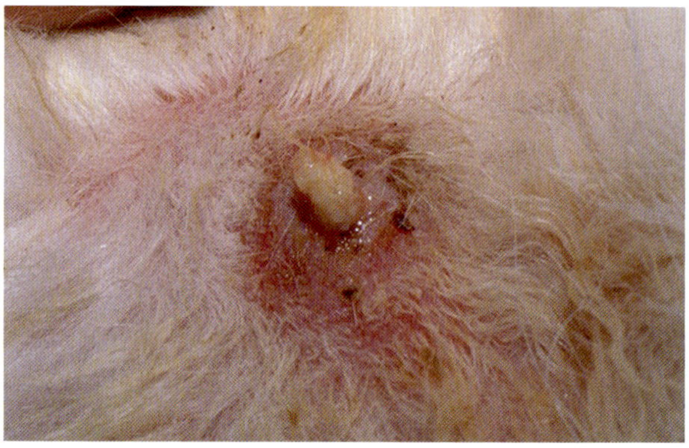

**Figure 4.16.** Infundibular cyst, draining sebum.

## Lesions that can be both primary or secondary

### Alopecia

Alopecia refers to a localized or generalized **lack of hair**. Partial loss of hair is called hypotrichosis. Possible causes are:

- inflammatory
- hormonal (Figure 4.17)
- neoplastic

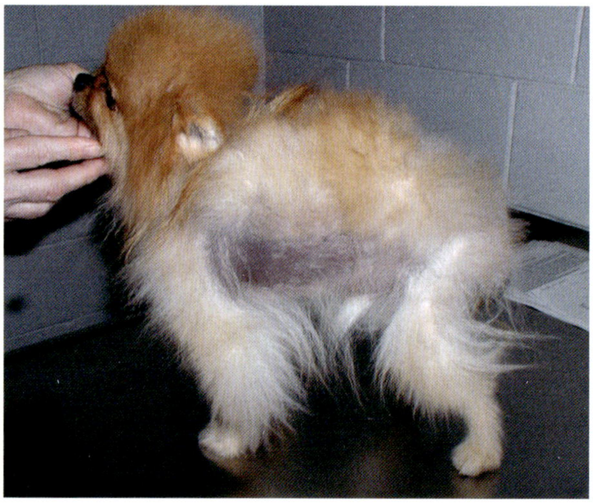

**Figure 4.17.** Alopecia on the flanks. Photograph courtesy of Dr Sheila Torres.

- idiopathic
- congenital.

### Scale

Scales are caused by an **accumulation of loose fragments of the stratum corneum**. Scales that results from a maturation disorder of the epidermis may or may not be associated with a glandular secretion disorder.

Dermatoses that present with scales as a primary lesion include:

- idiopathic seborrhoea in the Cocker Spaniel
- ichthyosis (Figure 4.18)
- sebaceous adenitis
- follicular dysplasia.

### Crust

Crusting is **a form of dry exudate** (serum, blood, pus or microorganisms). It may be the superficial part of another lesion – for example, crusted papules in the case of a flea allergy. If it is secondary, the colour may give an indication of what the original lesion was.

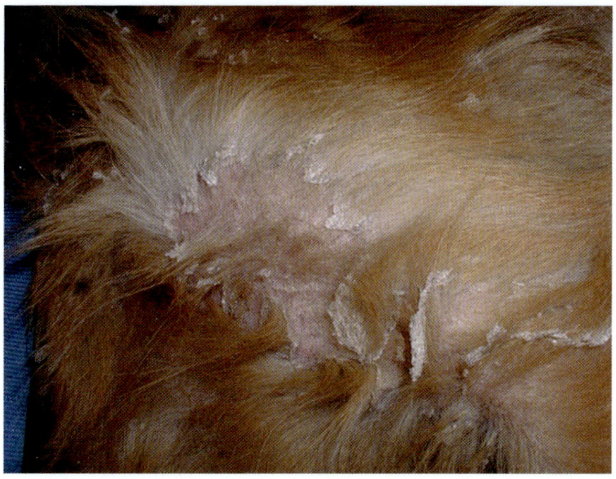

**Figure 4.18.** A Golden Retriever with scales on the body due to ichthyosis.

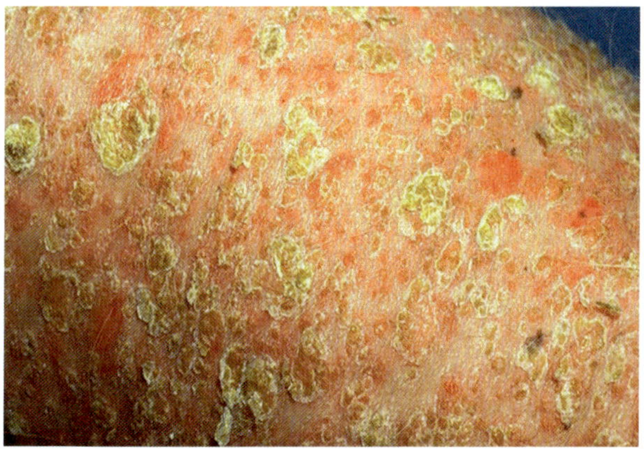

**Figure 4.19.** Generalized crusts due to pemphigus foliaceus.

Crusting sometimes presents as a primary lesion in zinc-responsive dermatitis. It is the most common secondary lesion in cases of pemphigus foliaceus (Figure 4.19).

### Comedone

A comedone is a **dilated hair follicle with black** (Figure 4.20) or **white** (milia) (Figure 4.21) **sebum content**, which may predispose to bacterial folliculitis.

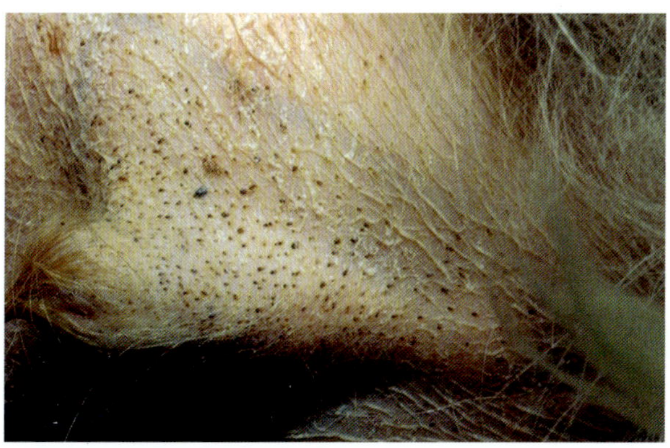

**Figure 4.20.** Comedone on the ventral abdomen due to Cushing's syndrome.

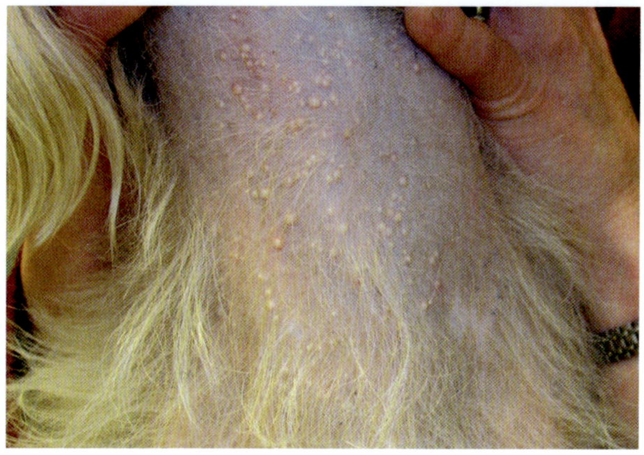

**Figure 4.21.** Milia on the ventral neck due to Cushing's syndrome. Photograph courtesy of Dr Sheila Torres.

The comedone is a *primary lesion* in cases of:

- feline acne
- Schnauzer comedo syndrome
- endocrine dermatoses.

The comedone is a *secondary lesion* in cases of:

- demodicosis
- dermatophytosis.

### Hyper-/hypopigmentation

This refers to **changes to skin colour** and may be macular (lentigo, vitiligo) or diffuse (endocrine problem, albinism, neoplasia) (Figure 4.22).

## Secondary lesions

### Epidermal collarette

An epidermal collarette represents the **remnant of the top of a vesicle, blister or pustule**, and is made up of a circular ring-shaped rim of desquamated keratinocytes. They are common findings in cases of superficial pyoderma (Figure 4.23).

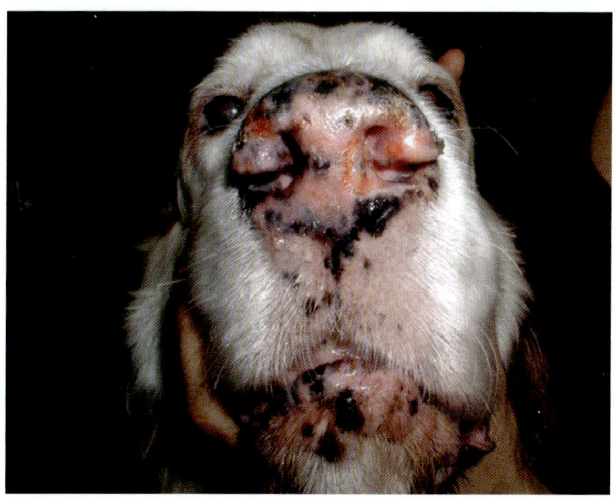

**Figure 4.22.** Depigmentation of the nasal plane and lips due to cutaneous lymphoma.

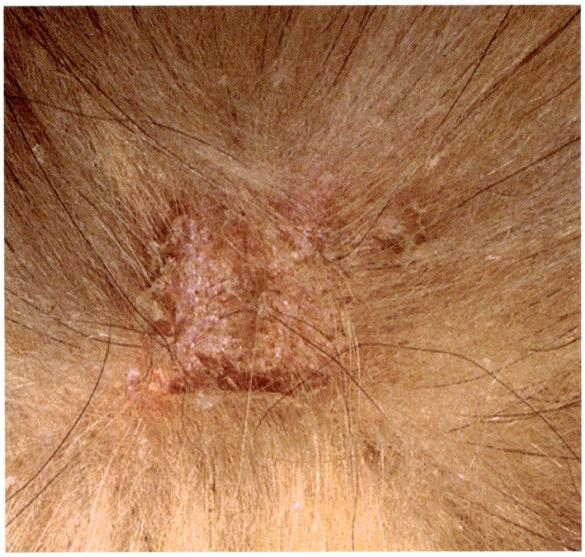

Figure 4.23. Epidermal collarette on the thorax due to superficial pyoderma.

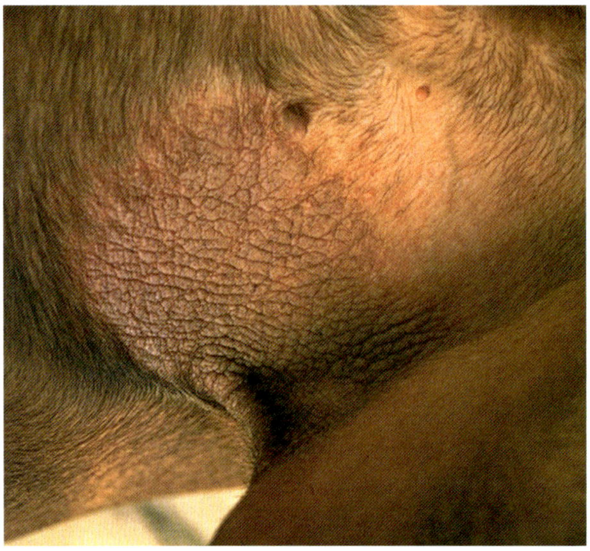

Figure 4.25. Lichenification on the ventral abdomen due to atopic dermatitis. Photograph courtesy of Dr Lynette Cole.

### Erosion/ulceration

Erosions are **partial defects in the epidermis** and, when self-induced, the excoriation is usually linear. An ulcer is a complete defect in the epidermis with exposure of the dermis.

These lesions are seen with:

- pruritic dermatoses
- neoplasms
- deep pyoderma
- Leishmaniasis
- autoimmune diseases
- toxic dermatoses (Figure 4.24).

### Lichenification

Lichenification results from chronic inflammation, as typified by skin thickening, exaggeration of superficial marks and **hyperpigmentation** (Figure 4.25).

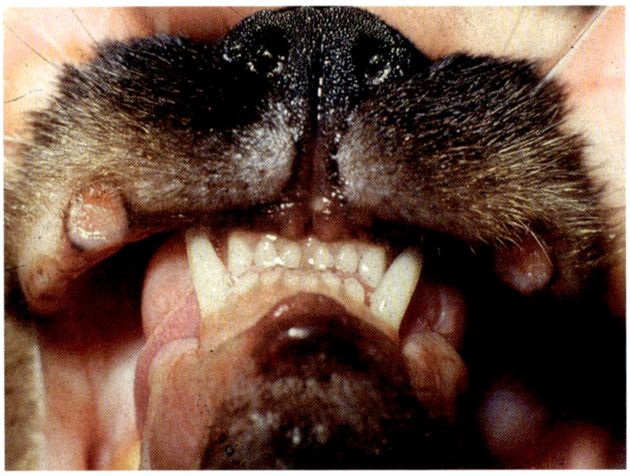

Figure 4.24. Indolent ulcer on the upper lip. Photograph courtesy of Dr Lynette Cole.

### Hyperkeratosis

Hyperkeratosis is defined as an **increase in the thickness of the stratum corneum**. It is common on the pads and nasal surface (Figure 4.26).

### Atrophy

Atrophy refers to a detrimental change in the quality and thickness of the skin. The skin becomes **very thin and loses elasticity**. This is a common response to oral and topical corticosteroids (Figure 4.27).

### Scar

A scar represents an area in which **fibrous tissue** has replaced the dermis and subcutaneous tissue.

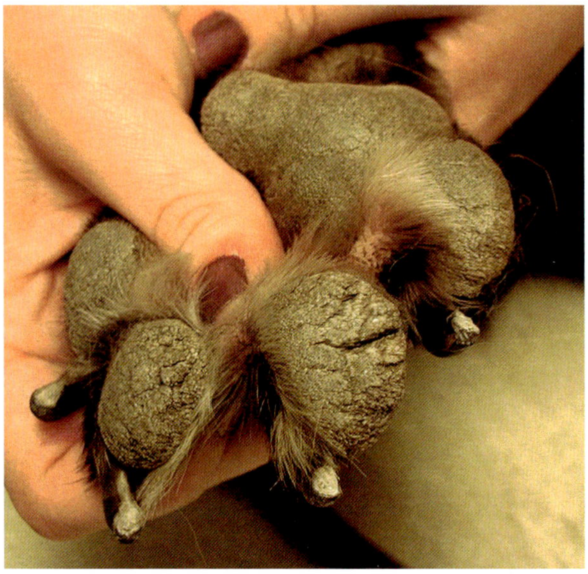

Figure 4.26. Hyperkeratosis on the plantar pads of a Golden Retriever.

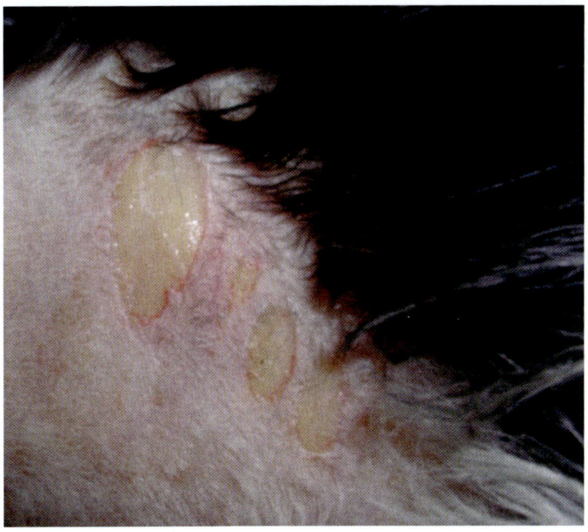

Figure 4.27. Feline cutaneous skin fragility syndrome: atrophy on the ventral abdomen. Photograph courtesy of Dr Sheila Torres.

## Diagnostic tests

In the majority of cases with dermatological lesions, evaluation of skin and ear cytology and skin scrapings are necessary to for a diagnosis to be made. Other frequently used tests include:

- trichogram
- Wood's lamp
- bacterial and fungal cultures
- skin biopsy.

### Skin scrapes

This test is easy to perform and is a simple way to identify parasites. For maximum benefit it is essential to:

1. **Select an affected area** (avoiding highly traumatized areas). To perform the scraping, a spatula or scalpel blade with mineral oil should be used (Figure 4.28).
2. If *Demodex canis*, *injai* or *cati* (follicular) is suspected, the skin should be tightened, released and a deep scraping (until capillary bleeding is observed) should be taken. For other mites (*Sarcoptes*, *Cheyletiella*, *D. gatoi* or *Otodectes*), superficial skin scrapings can be used (Figure 4.29).
3. The material should be transferred to a slide with mineral oil and covered with a coverslip (Figures 4.30 and 4.31).
4. The slide should be examined at 4 or 10x magnification, whilst keeping the condenser low to create contrast (Figure 4.32).

### Flea-remover comb

This tool is useful in the diagnosis of flea allergies and can aid in the identification of other ectoparasites such as *Cheyletiella*, lice and *Demodex gatoi*.

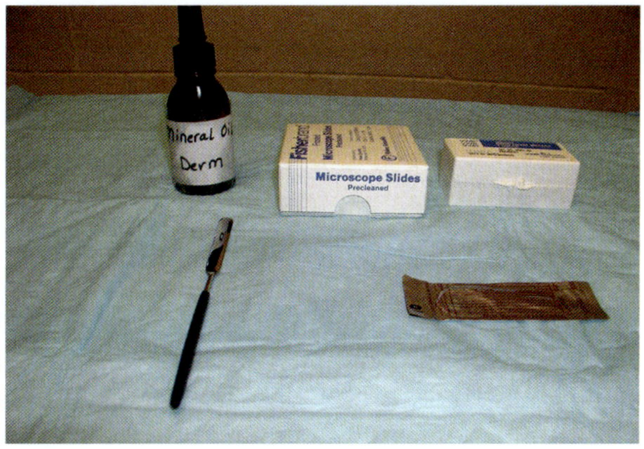


Figure 4.28. Equipment necessary to perform a skin scraping: mineral oil, slide, coverslip, scalpel blade no. 10 and/or spatula.

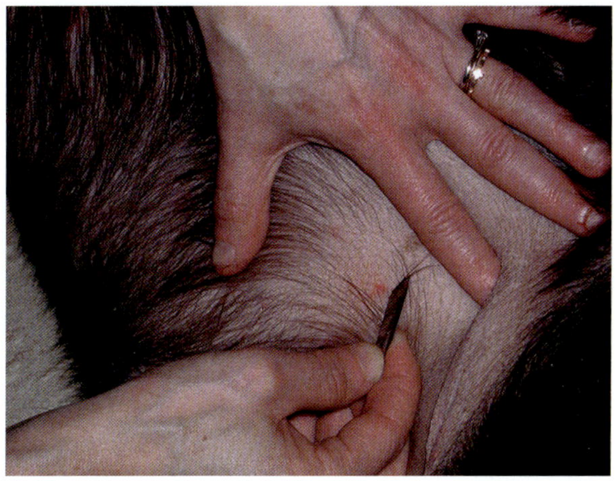

Figure 4.29. Skin scraping. Perform the scraping in the same direction as hair growth, to facilitate collection of material.

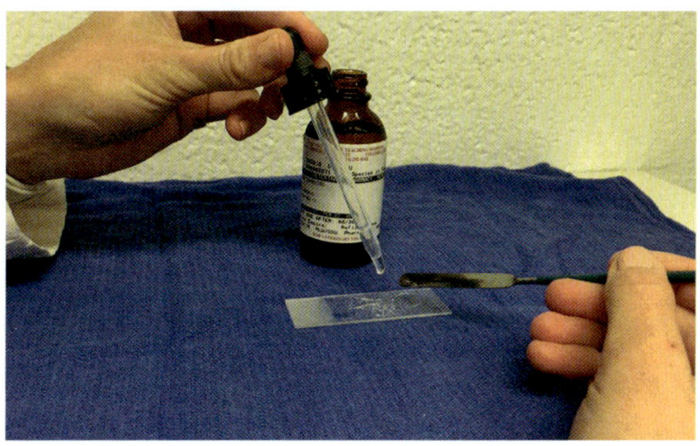

Figure 4.30. Skin scraping. Apply mineral oil to the slide and the spatula or scalpel blade.

It facilitates collection of hairs and scales, which can be transferred to a slide with mineral oil, covered with a coverslip and examined at 4× and 10× magnification, whilst keeping the condenser low.

### Trichogram

A trichogram is useful to **aid the identification of ectoparasites**. It is also helpful in the diagnosis of

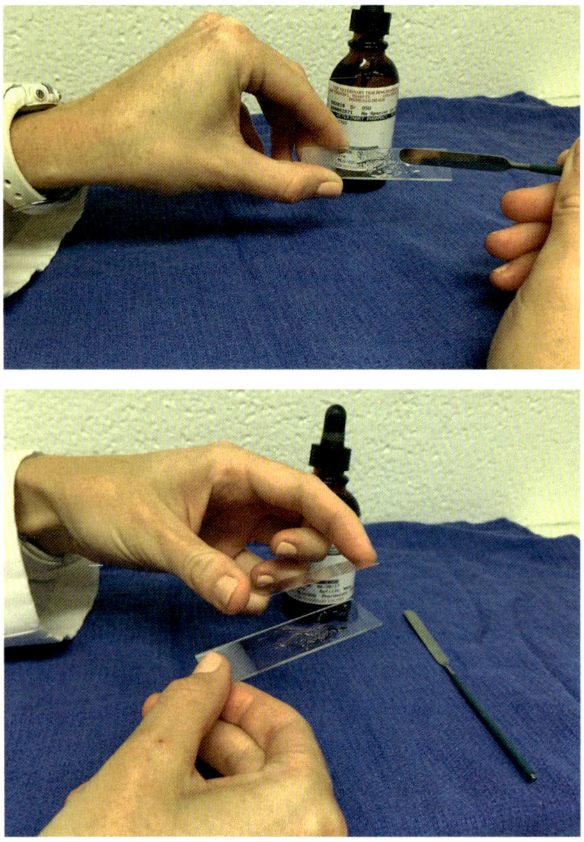

**Figure 4.31.** Deposit the material collected on the slide with mineral oil and cover with a coverslip.

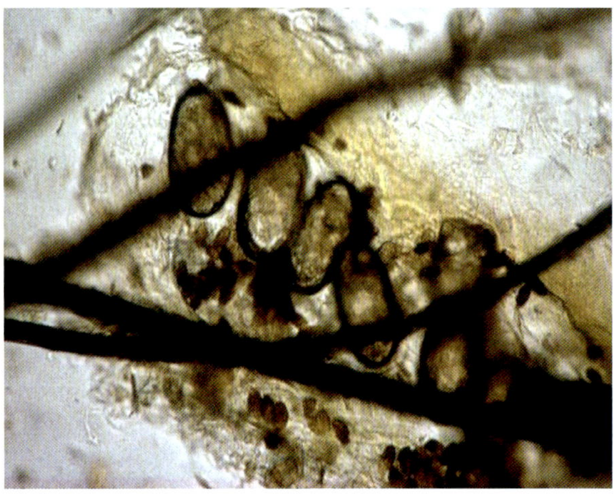

**Figure 4.32.** Superficial skin scraping positive for eggs and faeces in a dog with sarcoptic mange.

dermatophytosis with visualization of hyphae and spores, and allows confirmation of pruritus (damaged hair, identification of roots in anagen and telogen phases) (Figure 4.33) as well as identification of Demodex mites.

### *Cytological examination*

Cytological examination is a **very useful diagnostic tool** that should be used in almost 100% of patients

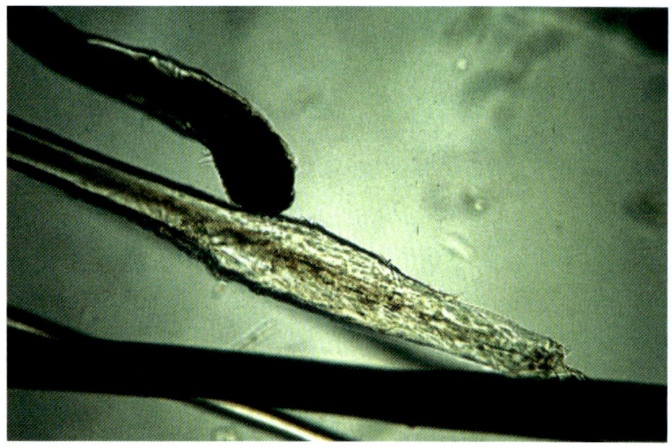

**Figure 4.33.** Roots in anagen phase (pigmented) and telogen phase (end in the form of an arrow).

with dermatological problems. It allows the diagnosis of common infectious diseases (pyoderma, *Malassezia* infections and otitis externa) and uncommon dermatoses (neoplasms and autoimmune diseases). The technique varies depending on the type of lesion and its location.

#### Imprint

This technique is used to study the surface of exudative lesions after opening a pustule or removing a scab (Figure 4.34).

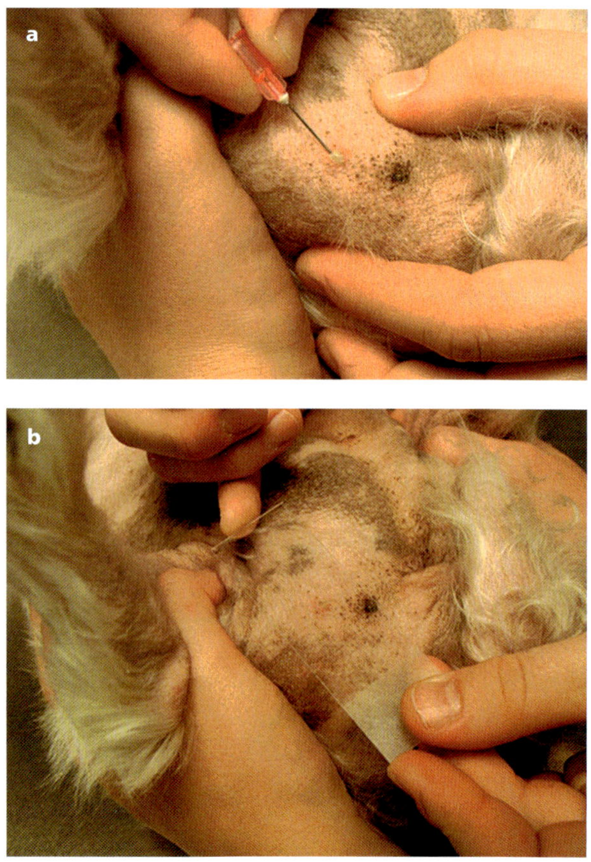


**Figure 4.34.** Imprint of a pustule – superficial pyoderma.

## Sticky tape (transparent)

Used on lesions that are dry, oily or hard to reach with a slide, such as those between the digits. The sample should be stained (omitting the first, Diff-Quik stain), rinsed and allowed to dry. Immersion oil should then be added to the slide with the tape on top, which acts as a coverslip (Figure 4.35). The preparation is examined with a high-objective lens (100x) to identify *Malassezia*. Unstained sticky tape can also be used to identify mites.

## Swab

Useful for taking samples from ears, exudative lesions or under the cuticle in cases of paronychia (Figure 4.36).

## Aspirate

Aspiration is performed with a **20–22 g needle** and 6–12 ml syringe. It allows samples of the following to be obtained:

- nodules
- tumours
- plaques
- abscesses.

An aspirate can be obtained by:

1. Immobilizing the lesion.
2. Inserting the needle with or without the syringe (if only using the needle, it should be reinserted several

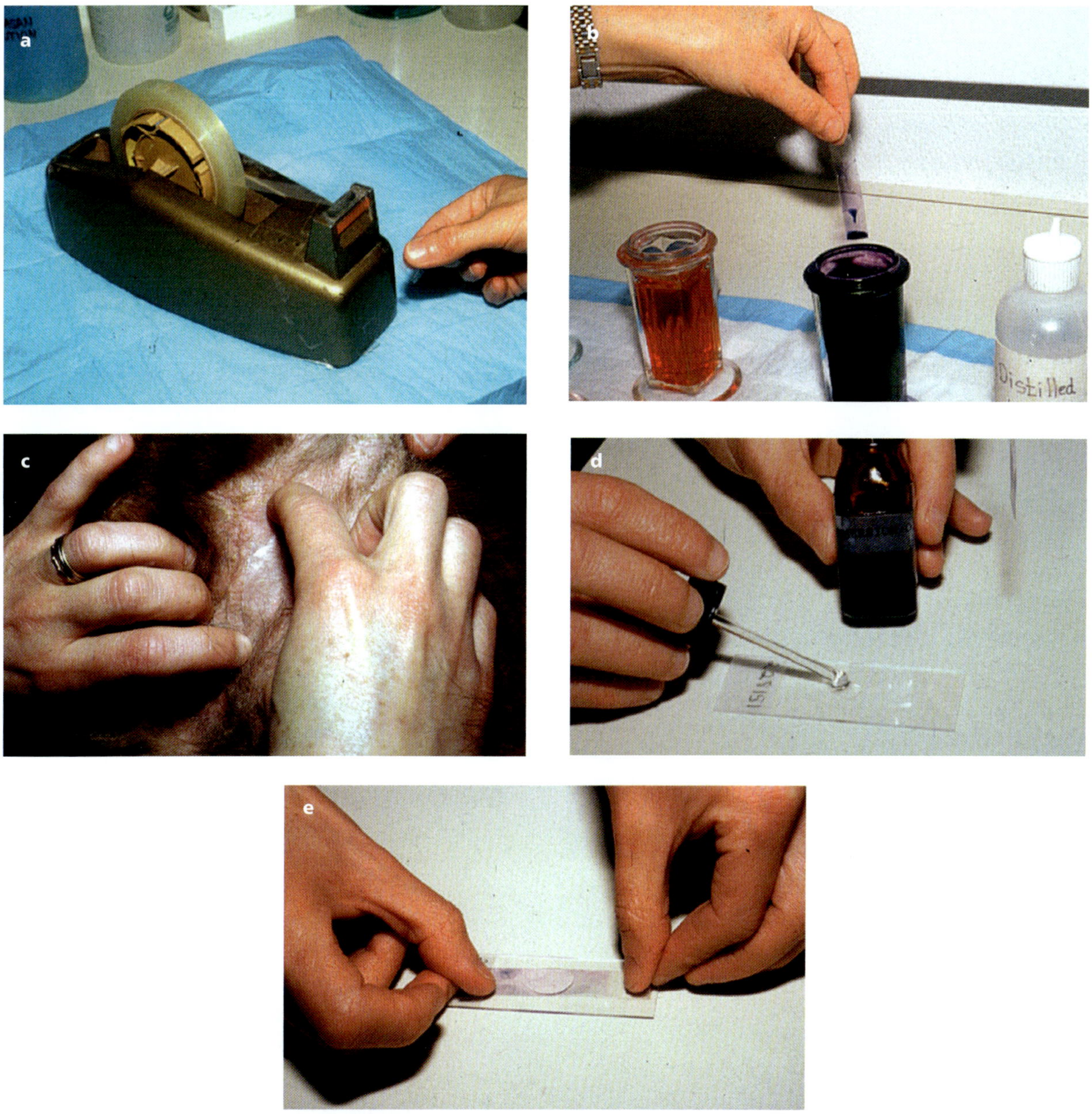


**Figure 4.35.** Sticky tape. Press the tape firmly against the skin, omitting the first Diff-Quik stain, rinse, allow to dry and place the tape on a slide with immersion oil.

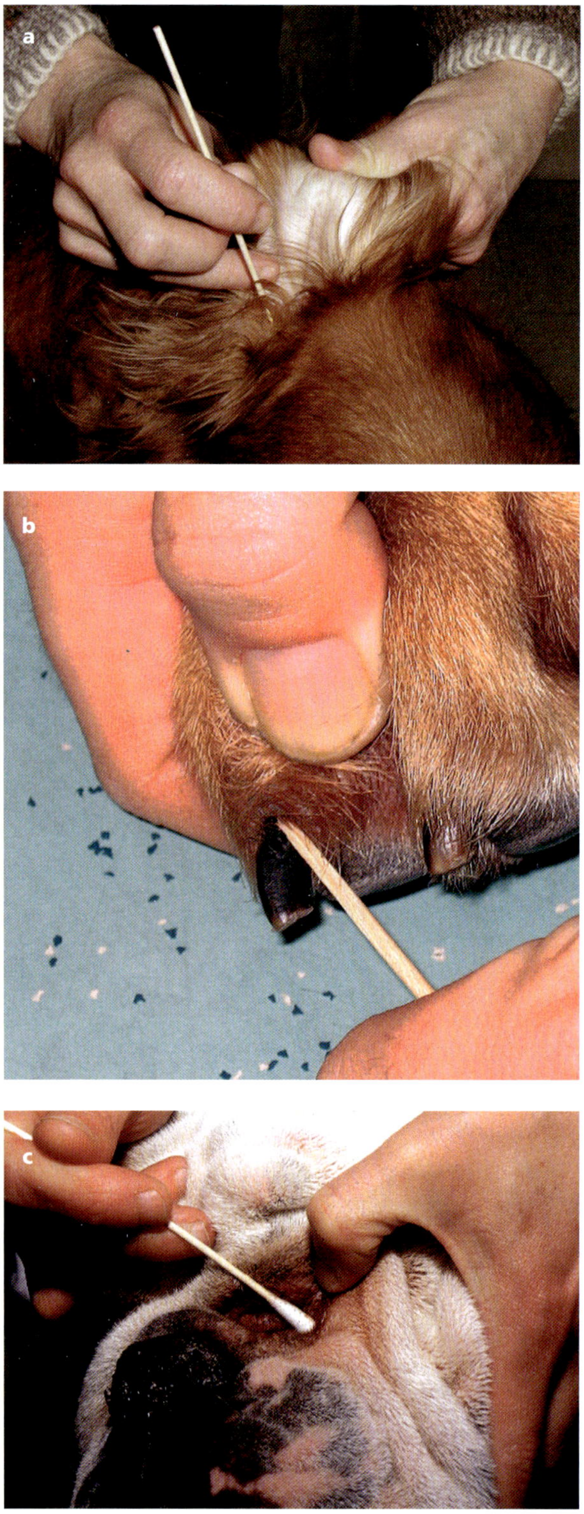


**Figure 4.36.** Swab. a, Ears; b, cuticle; c, exudative lesions.

times and connected the syringe to extract the sample; if the needle is being used with the syringe, the plunger should be pulled to create negative pressure, released and the needle redirected).

3. The syringe should be released before the needle is removed.
4. The sample should be air dried or dried with a lighter.
5. The sample should be stained with Diff-Quik.
6. Examination of the sample:
   a. Examine first with a low objective (4×, 10×) to identify areas of interest (for example, inflammatory cells).
   b. Immersion oil should be used to observe the sample with 50–100× magnification. The condenser should be raised.

### *Wood's lamp*

Used for the **diagnosis of dermatophytosis**. The lamp should be warmed up for 3–5 minutes before the test and placed over the area to be examined for a few minutes. Affected hairs will appear individually with a fluorescent greenish-yellow colour. Scales and scabs do not fluoresce.

The Wood's lamp can give false results:

- **Negative**: only **50% of** Microsporum canis **fluoresces** and not all affected areas show fluorescence. The use of iodine blocks fluorescence.
- **Positive**: due to the **presence of keratin, soaps, Vaseline or certain bacteria** (*Pseudomonas, Corynebacterium*). Fluorescence is not yellowish-green.

### *Bacterial culture and antibiogram*

Used for:

- **Diagnosis of deep lesions** (cellulitis, nodules and tumours) when an infectious cause is suspected.
- Superficial lesions from infections that **do not respond** to empirical treatment.
- Lesions that present **bacilli on cytology**.

The method of sample collection depends on the type of lesion:

- The exudate from a pustule can be taken after opening the pustule carefully with a 25 g needle.
- Samples from epidermal collarette are taken from the edge that is peeling, aiming to choose active lesions.
- In the case of fistulae, the exudate present on the surface of the skin should be cleaned with saline, dried with sterile gauze and a sample of the material obtained after expressing the lesion. Subsequently, the swab should be placed in the transport medium and sent to the laboratory (Figure 4.37).

In the case of deep lesions (papules, nodules or tumours), a tissue sample can be taken for culture. The skin should be prepared surgically and a biopsy taken aseptically, removing the superficial layer of the skin and sending the rest of the sample for analysis. The laboratory should be consulted about the means of transport, but generally swabs in a transport medium are adequate.

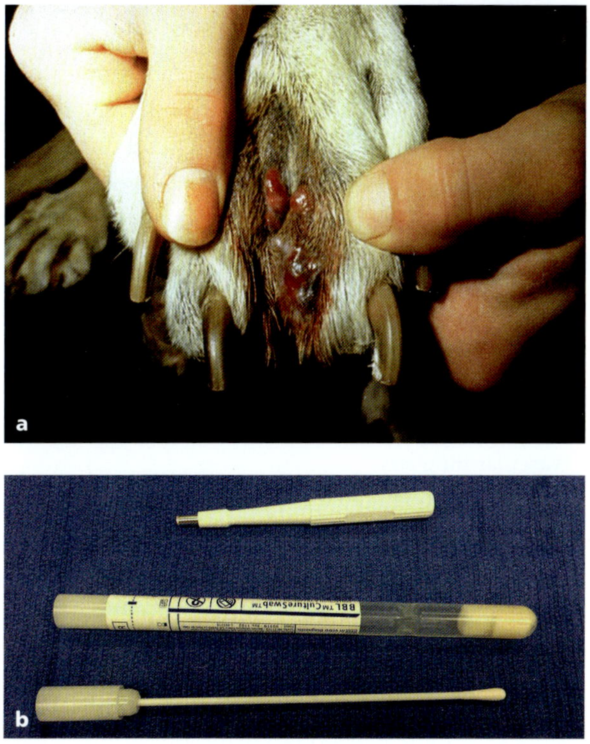

**Figure 4.37.** a, Fistula and haemorrhagic bullae due to deep pyoderma. b, Swab for collection and transport of the sample.

## *Fungal culture*

Fungal culture is the **most sensitive method for diagnosis of dermatophytosis**. Selective dermatophyte agar (DTM) is used, which contains Sabouraud dextrose agar, cycloheximide (antifungal), gentamicin and chlortetracycline (antibacterial) and a pH indicator (phenol red).

Sample collection can be performed with the help of a Wood's lamp (of the hairs that present with fluorescence) and on the periphery of a lesion, including damaged hairs, scales and crusts. If there are no lesions – for example, in an animal suspected of being a healthy carrier – the Mackenzie technique or a sterile toothbrush can be used.

Brush the body for 2–3 minutes, then gently press the brush's teeth into the culture medium. Positive culture is signalled by a colour change followed by colony growth. Dermatophytes change colour at 3–10 days and then, after 10–14 days, so do the pollutants; so, for the first 10 days the culture should be examined every day.

Diagnosis is made by **identifying the macroconidia**. To do this, a piece of adhesive tape should be pressed lightly over the colony and then the adhesive part should be put in lactophenol blue cotton stain, a drop of lactophenol added and then this should be covered with a coverslip. Examine at a magnification of 10–40×. *Microsporum canis* (Figure 4.38), *M. gypseum* and *Trichophyton mentagrophytes* are the most common species in the dog and cat.

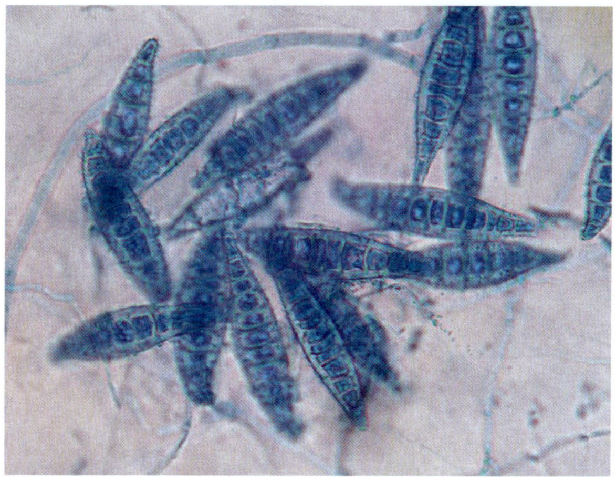

**Figure 4.38.** *Microsporum canis*. The macroconidia are spindle-shaped, 6–15 cells with a spiny protuberance (40x). Courtesy of R. J. Galindo.

## *Skin biopsy*

Necessary for the diagnosis of:

- neoplasms
- autoimmune diseases
- dermatomyositis
- sebaceous adenitis
- zinc-responsive dermatitis
- follicular dysplasia.

Skin biopsy also helps in the diagnosis of certain parasitic, bacterial (mycobacteria), mycotic (deep mycosis), sterile dermatosis and paraneoplastic syndromes.

### When should a biopsy be taken?

When the history and clinical examination suggest a disease that needs to be confirmed by biopsy and the clinical approach has not given a diagnosis, a logical treatment has not worked and when the disease requires prolonged treatment and is associated with serious side effects, nodules, vesicles and ulcers, unusual or severe injuries.

### Where should the biopsy be taken?

If the lesions appear clinically very similar, **1–3 samples** are sufficient (Figure 4.39).

If there are several types of lesion, an attempt should be made to take a sample of each type (see figure 4.19). Different lesions may represent either the evolution of the same pathology or different conditions.

### How should the sample be taken?

Most lesions can be sampled, after infiltrating the skin with a local anaesthetic such as lidocaine, with a **6 mm punch** – or 4 mm for more sensitive places such as the nose and plantar pads. When the punch

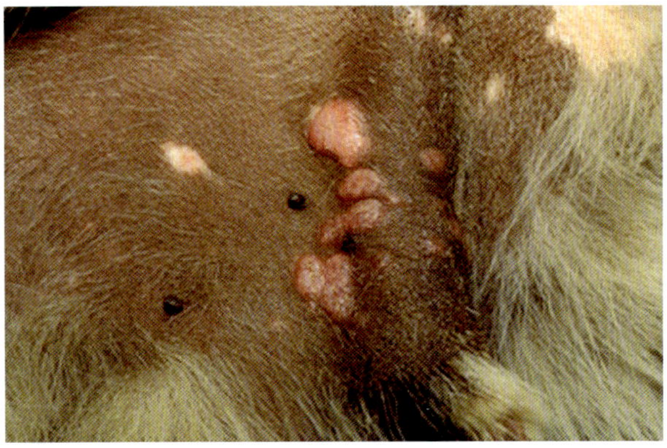

**Figure 4.39.** Inguinal area, papules/alopecic nodules. Although all the nodules are very similar in appearance, one sample is sufficient and is representative of the pathological process.

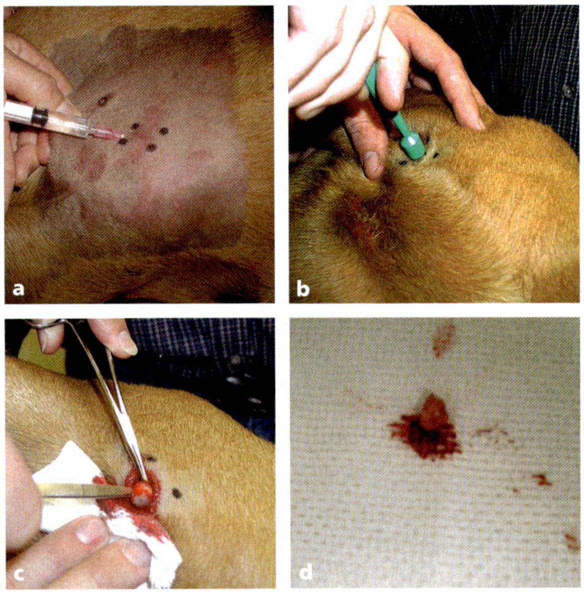


**Figure 4.40.** Infiltration of the skin with 2% lidocaine and sampled with a 6 mm punch.

has penetrated the **full thickness of the skin** it is removed to expose the sample, generally adherent to the subcutaneous tissue, and then the subcutaneous fat must be carefully cut (Figure 4.40). In the process, care should be taken not to damage the sample with the clamp as this can cause artefacts on histopathology. Excess blood should be carefully removed and the sample sent for analysis in 10% formalin. The area can be sutured with suture material or staples.

## Cutaneous manifestations of systemic problems

### *General considerations*

The skin's appearance and integrity are **influenced by systemic factors** such as:

- nutritional state
- hormone levels
- perfusion
- vascular integrity
- overall health.

Since the skin provides innate protection and maintains homeostasis, it is a **sentinel of systemic diseases**. Some cutaneous changes indicate the need to investigate specific systemic diseases. For example:

- **Petechiae or ecchymoses** on the skin or mucous membranes suggest alterations in **haemostasis or vascular integrity**.
- A **yellowish colour** to the mucous membranes indicates jaundice, and possible causes should be evaluated.

Changes in the skin's appearance can be markers of a **pathology occurring in another body system or the presence of a multi-systemic disease**, as occurs with some infectious diseases or systemic lupus erythematosus.

The skin is readily accessible for taking samples that may potentially provide information that helps diagnose systemic disease easily and economically.

### *Skin changes associated with hormonal alterations*

**Endocrine diseases** provide an excellent example of the relationship between systemic disease and the skin. Hypothyroidism, hyperadrenocorticism (HAC) and alterations in sex hormones can alter the appearance and function of the skin.

#### *Hypothyroidism*

#### Pathogenesis

Hypothyroidism causes:

- changes in cornification and melanosis
- increase in the number of hair follicles in **telogen** phase
- accumulation of glycosaminoglycans in the dermis.

#### Clinical signs

Clinically, this translates into:

- Alopecia. Thyroid hormones promote the initiation of the anagen phase of the hair cycle, and therefore many dogs with hypothyroidism have some degree of **alopecia**: Initially it is seen in **areas where there is friction**, on the ventral neck, dorsal part of the tail and pressure points (Figure 4.41).

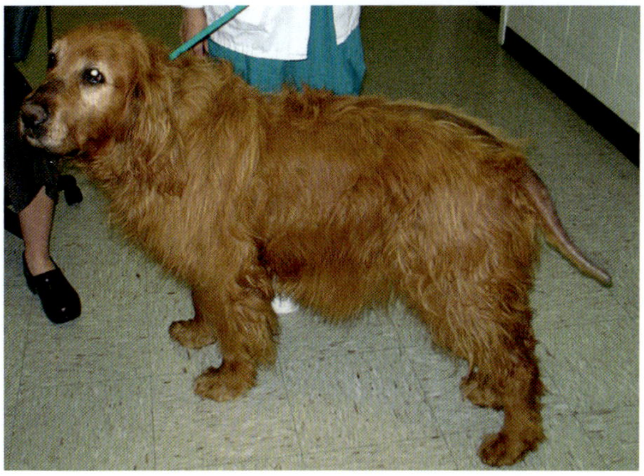

**Figure 4.41.** Alopecia on the dorsal aspect of the tail due to hypothyroidism. Photograph courtesy of Dr David Panciera.

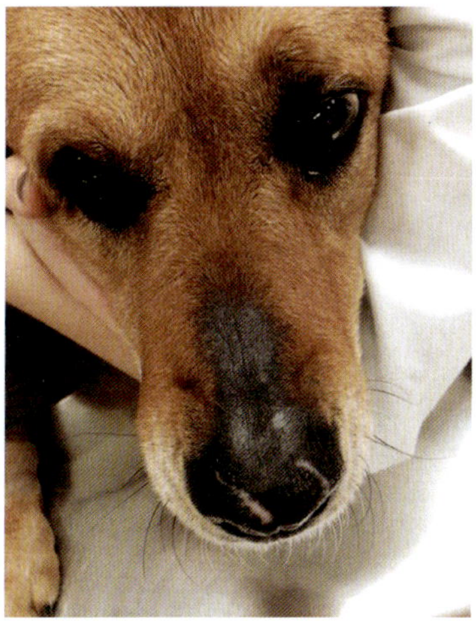

**Figure 4.42.** Focal area of alopecia and hyperpigmentation on the dorsal aspect of the muzzle next to the nasal plane, due to hypothyroidism.

Some animals present with a focal area of alopecia and **hyperpigmentation** on the dorsal part of the snout, next to the nasal plane (Figure 4.42).

**Lack of hair growth after clipping** can be a clinical presentation of hypothyroidism (Figures 4.43 and 4.44).

- hyperpigmentation
- desquamation
- myxoedematous changes
- seborrhoea along the margin of the ear (Figure 4.45).

In some cases of hypothyroidism, the only clinical signs are recurrent pyoderma (Figure 4.46) and otitis externa.

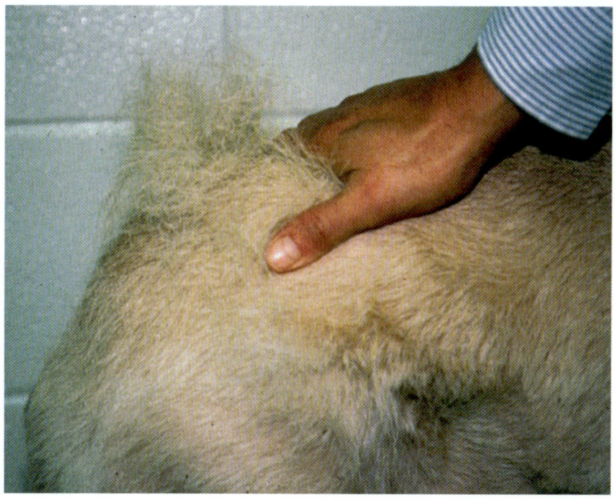

**Figure 4.43.** Dull, brittle hair that falls out easily due to hypothyroidism. Photograph courtesy of Dr David Panciera.

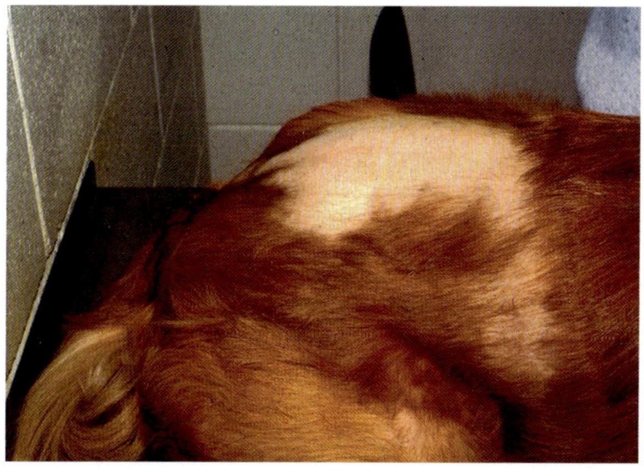

**Figure 4.44.** Lack of hair growth in a dog with hypothyroidism.

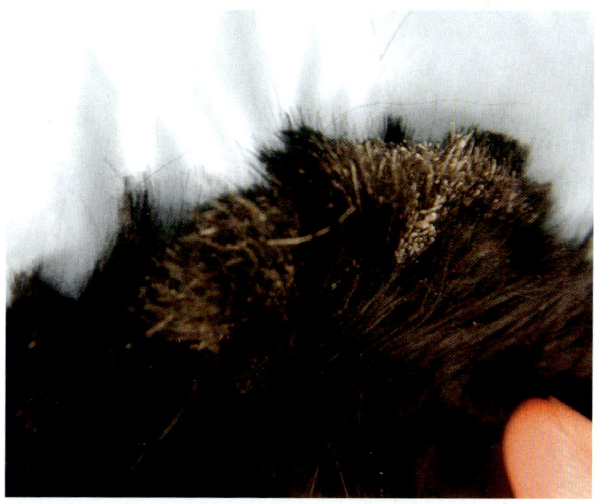

**Figure 4.45.** Seborrhoea of the ear margin due to hypothyroidism.

## *Hyperadrenocorticism*

### Pathogenesis

With hyperadrenocorticism in the dog it is the **excess cortisol that produces dermatological changes**, which include:

- changes in cornification
- inhibition of collagen production
- pilosebaceous and glandular atrophy
- reduced immunity.

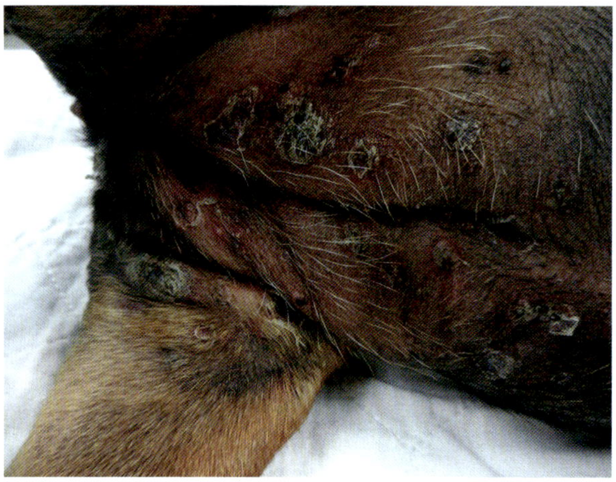

**Figure 4.46.** Epidermal collarettes and crusts due to recurrent superficial pyoderma associated with hypothyroidism.

## Clinical signs

Clinically these changes appear as:

- symmetrical **bilateral alopecia**
- **thin, hypotonic skin** that is prone to bruising (Figure 4.47)
- phlebectasia
- comedones (Figure 4.48)
- calcinosis cutis (Figure 4.49)

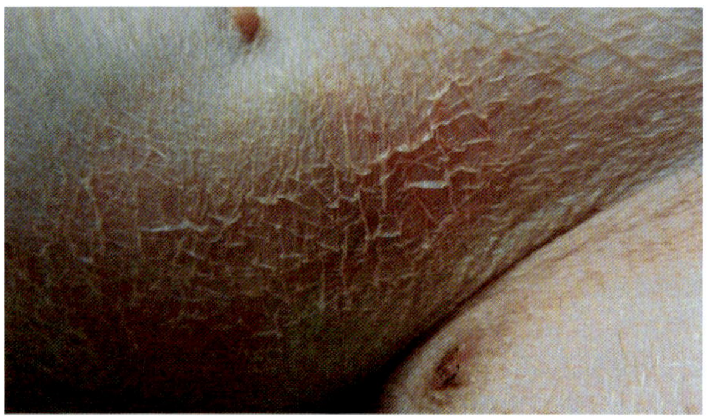

**Figure 4.47.** Thin skin due to hyperadrenocorticism. Photograph courtesy of Dr Sheila Torres.

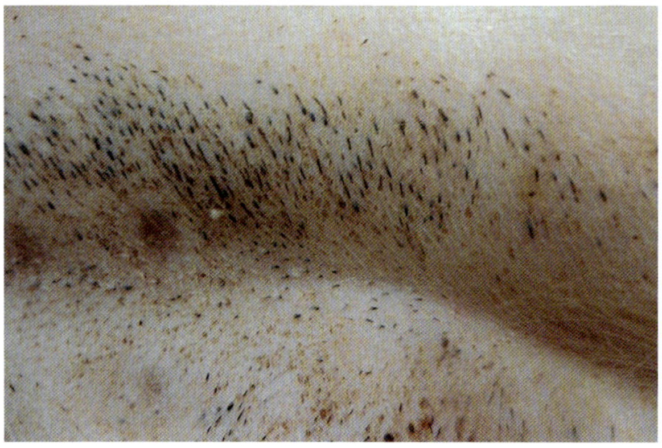

**Figure 4.48.** Comedones in the inguinal region due to hyperadrenocorticism.

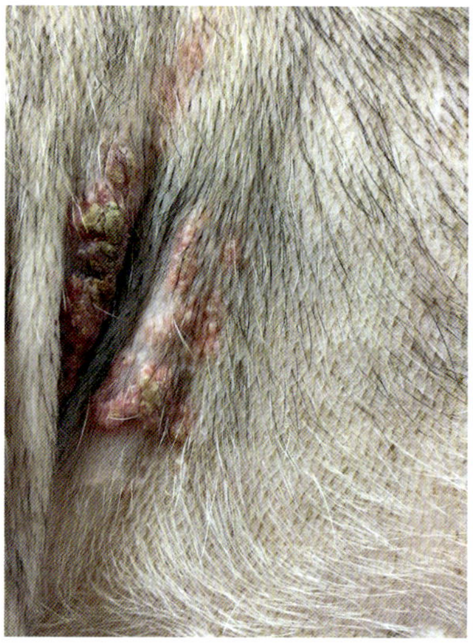

**Figure 4.49.** Calcinosis cutis (papules, whitened plaques and erythema) in the inguinal region due to iatrogenic hyperadrenocorticism. Photograph courtesy of Stephanie Abrams.

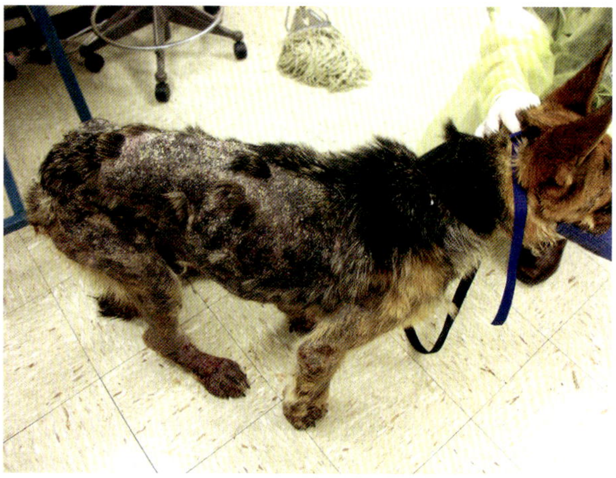

**Figure 4.50.** Generalized Demodicosis due to hyperadrenocorticism.

- recurrent pyoderma
- demodicosis (Figure 4.50).

### *Calcinosis cutis*

#### Definition

This is a broad term and includes all forms of **metastatic dystrophic calcification** of the skin. More specifically, the term is often used for dystrophic calcification secondary to hyperadrenocorticism or iatrogenic hypercortisolaemia.

#### Clinical signs

The lesions include **erythematous papules** that join together to form plaques. Both papules and plaques can ulcerate and develop haemorrhagic scabs.

The lesions develop in **areas that are flexed** (armpit, inguinal area) and on the neck. Dystrophic calcification can also affect the mucous membranes and the tongue.

Metastatic calcification produces **nodular calcium deposits in the skin**, especially in the pads on the feet (documented in dogs and cats with chronic renal failure).

### Prognosis

Cutaneous calcinosis lesions usually resolve over time if the underlying metabolic disorder can be corrected. In some cases, osseous metaplasia can occur, leading to osteoma cutis, which has no cure.

## *Acquired feline skin fragility*

### Aetiopathogenesis

In the cat, acquired skin fragility is associated with the following conditions:

- hyperadrenocorticism
- iatrogenic Cushing's syndrome (Figure 5.27)
- excess levels of progesterone compounds
- hepatic lipidosis (isolated cases)
- hepatic neoplasia (isolated cases).

### Clinical signs

Affected cats have very **thin, fragile skin**, so much so that it is easily traumatized and can be broken with simple handling, and often occurs during the physical examination.

## *Cutaneous paraneoplastic syndromes in the dog and cat*

Tumours are capable of producing **disease at locations distant to them** or their metastases. These diseases are called **paraneoplastic syndromes** and may be more serious than the clinical signs linked to the tumour itself. Removal of tumours is usually accompanied by resolution of paraneoplastic signs.

### Definition

'Para-' is a prefix of Greek origin meaning 'next to' and denotes a proximity in position, a spatial or temporal association. The use of the term '**cutaneous paraneoplastic syndrome**' should be reserved for dermatoses that result **directly from an internal tumour**. Therefore, genodermatoses, skin changes caused by environmental carcinogens and malignant neoplasms of the skin or skin metastases are not included among cutaneous paraneoplastic syndromes.

Because **paraneoplastic syndrome may be the first sign of neoplasia**, it is important to recognize it for early diagnosis and to allow timely treatment of internal neoplasia. It should be taken into account that some of the clinical signs described in paraneoplastic syndromes may present as an isolated finding or occur in association with a benign systemic disease.

### Aetiopathogenesis

The most well-known and **best-characterized paraneoplastic syndrome** is one that results from the **uncontrolled production of cortisol**, a biologically active hormone that is normally secreted by tumoral tissue (Cushing's syndrome).

Although it is suspected that the clinical signs may be the effect of a circulating humoral factor or other by-product of the neoplasm, in most conditions the pathogenesis is unknown. The mechanisms that have been postulated include:

- Production, release or induction of substances such as cytokines or hormones that cause direct or indirect dermatosis.
- A lack of specific substances due to metabolic changes induced by the tumour – for example, lack of amino acids in the case of metabolic epidermal necrosis.
- Aberrant host response to the tumour.

## *Metabolic epidermal necrosis*

### Aetiology

**Metabolic epidermal necrosis** (MEN) is a recognized cutaneous paraneoplastic syndrome in humans. It is associated with pancreatic carcinoma and is known as **glucagonoma syndrome**. In some cases, extra-pancreatic glucagonomas have been reported, and less frequently the syndrome may appear associated with non-neoplastic diseases such as:

- hepatitis
- cirrhosis
- pancreatitis
- coeliac disease
- inflammatory bowel disease
- heroin abuse
- odontogenic abscesses.

In dogs, unlike in humans, glucagonoma is only occasionally identified and the syndrome is most often associated with liver disease, a condition known as hepatocutaneous syndrome.

In cats, this syndrome has been documented in association with pancreatic carcinoma and amyloidosis of the thymus. Few cases have been described, but one of them presented with gingivitis, stomatitis and hepatomegaly. Blood glucose was high and liver enzymes were within normal limits.

### Pathogenesis

Although the exact **pathogenesis of MEN is not known**, it is believed that the skin disease is the result of certain nutrient deficiencies such as:

- amino acids
- biotin
- essential fatty acids
- zinc.

The hyperglucagonaemia resulting from the **secretion of glucagon by the tumour** seems to play a crucial role in the pathogenesis of glucagonoma syndrome. In humans it has been shown that the removal of the tumour, or injection of somatostatin analogues, produces a significant improvement in clinical signs.

The catabolic effect of gluconeogenesis and the subsequent increase in protein and amino acid degradation result in the extremely **low levels of plasma amino acids** observed in affected animals. This could result in depletion of amino acids in the skin and cause necrosis. In addition, **hypoalbuminaemia** could lead to zinc and essential fatty acid deficiency due to a transport defect.

## Clinical signs

In the dog, the clinical signs of glucagonoma cannot be differentiated from those associated with hepatocutaneous syndrome and include:

- erosions
- ulcerations
- alopecia
- exudation.
- **Thick, sticky crusts on the plantar pads** (Figure 4.51) and mucocutaneous junctions (Figure 4.52). Pressure points are also affected.
- depression
- anorexia
- peripheral lymphadenopathy.

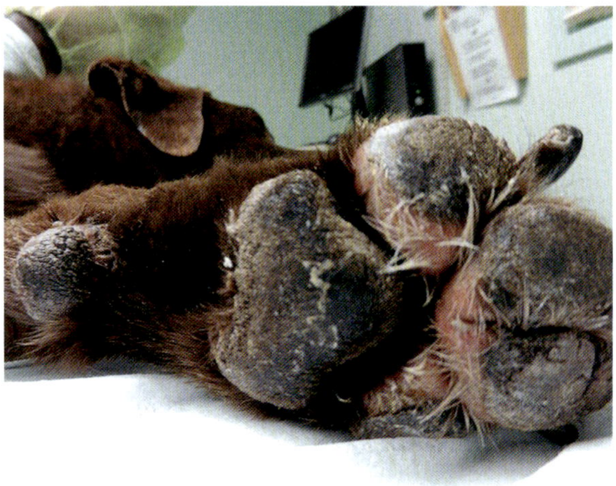

Figure 4.51. Fissures and hyperkeratosis on the pads due to hepatocutaneous syndrome.

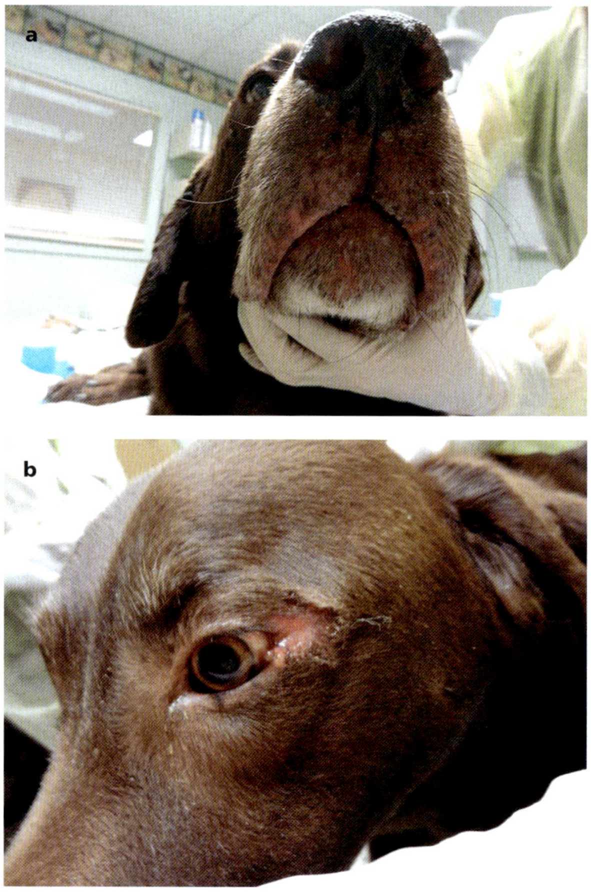

Figure 4.52. Fissures and erosions in mucocutaneous areas due to hepatocutaneous syndrome.

In the cat, the clinical signs described include:

- alopecia
- erythema
- exudate
- desquamation.

## Diagnosis

**Secondary bacterial and yeast infections**, as well as hyperglycaemia, are frequent findings.

**Liver enzymes may be elevated, with low levels of some plasma amino acids.**

In one study, plasma glucagon levels were measured in five dogs and were found to be raised. The levels of amino acids in plasma, glucagon and insulin returned to the normal range in a dog after removal of the pancreatic tumour, showing there was an association.

Abdominal ultrasonography can help identify the tumour and structural changes in the liver in cases of chronic liver disease. A 'Swiss cheese' appearance corresponds to hypoechoic nodules surrounded by hyperechoic parenchyma.

Skin histopathology shows characteristic changes that help with diagnosis, which among others include:

- parakeratoses
- vacuolation
- degeneration of the middle layer of the epidermis
- hyperplasia of the deeper layers.

These changes mean the histopathology has a very characteristic appearance: red (parakeratosis), white (vacuolization) and blue (hyperplasia), like the French flag.

## *Feline paraneoplastic alopecia*

### Epidemiology

This is a **rare condition**. It occurs in animals **over 10 years of age**, without any evidence of sex or breed predisposition.

### Aetiopathogenesis

Associated with:

- pancreatic adenocarcinoma
- bile duct carcinoma.

The association between alopecia and internal cutaneous malignant tumours has been demonstrated in one case with resolution of cutaneous signs after surgical removal of the tumour. However, the pathogenesis of alopecia remains unclear. It is thought that the cutaneous disease (follicular atrophy and loss of the stratum corneum) is mediated by the production of substances (such as cytokines) produced by tumour cells.

### Clinical signs

Clinically paraneoplastic alopecia is characterized by:

- **Symmetric bilateral alopecia** of the ventral area of the body and extremities. Alopecia usually starts in ventral areas but can affect large areas of the trunk.
- **Hair that falls out easily** in non-alopecic areas.
- A Shiny appearance to the skin characteristic of the areas with alopecia (Figure 4.53).
- Affected **plantar pads**: the skin loses the stratum corneum and appears dry and scaly; it can crack and there can be dermo-epidermal separation (Figure 4.54).
- **Pruritus** can be variable but is usually present. Secondary infection with *Malassezia* **pachydermatitis** has been documented, which may exacerbate pruritus.

This skin disease is associated with non-specific systemic signs such as:

- depression
- weight loss
- anorexia
- abdominal pain.

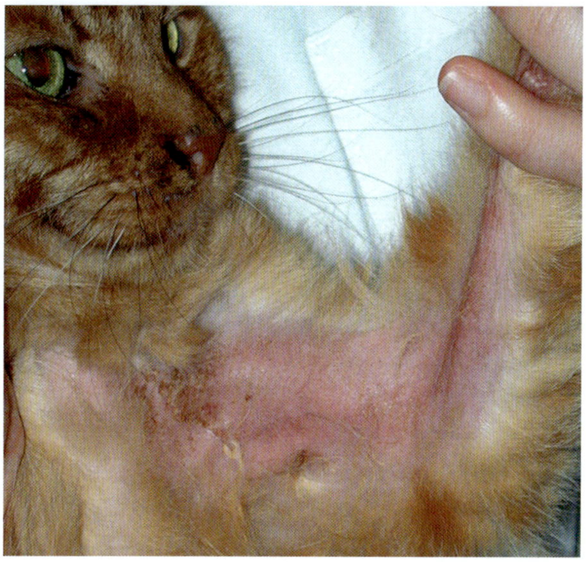

**Figure 4.53.** Alopecia, erythema and skin with a shiny appearance due to feline paraneoplastic alopecia.

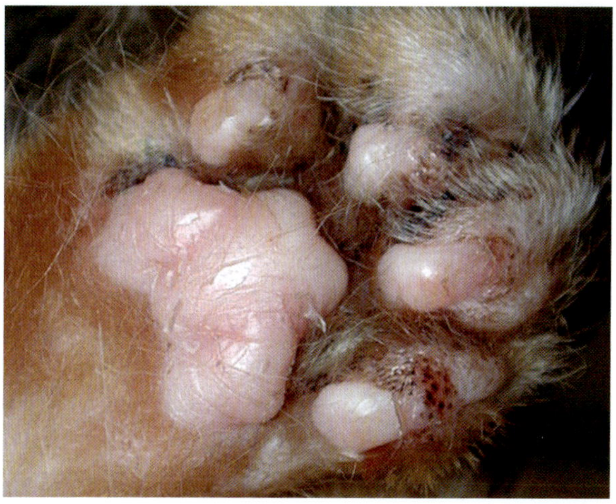

**Figure 4.54.** Loss of stratum corneum and desquamation due to feline paraneoplastic alopecia.

## *Exfoliative dermatitis associated with thymoma*

### Aetiopathogenesis

Exfoliative dermatitis is a **rare disease**, reported in association with **thymoma in cats** and humans.

In humans, paraneoplastic dermatoses (dermatomyositis, scleroderma, pemphigus vulgaris, pemphigus foliaceus and systemic lupus erythematosus) related to thymoma that have been known about for a long time, but exfoliative dermatitis (usually linked to cutaneous lymphoma, leukaemia and neoplasms of the uterus, lung, stomach, prostate, thyroid, liver or larynx) associated with thymoma has also been described recently.

In felines, exfoliative dermatitis can be seen associated with **thymoma, cutaneous lymphoma and drug reactions**. Recently, 18 cases were described in which exfoliative dermatitis was not associated with the presence of thymoma but had histopathological characteristics indistinguishable from those associated with thymoma. In this series, most cases responded to immunosuppressive therapy so it is suspected this was due to an immunopathological reaction to an unknown agent.

Resolution of dermatitis after surgical resection of the thymoma was demonstrated in two cases: the skin returned to normal within 5–6 months. The pathogenesis is not clear. Histopathology shows typical changes of the 'graft-versus-host' reaction and cytotoxic T cells, suggesting a process mediated by autoimmune cells. It is thought that keratinocytes may be attacked by immature autoreactive T cells that have escaped selection, which normally occurs in the thymus.

### Epidemiology

Affected cats are usually **elderly**, but it has also been described in a 4-year-old cat. There does not appear to be any sex or breed predisposition, although a large number of these cats are ginger or ginger/white.

### Clinical signs

Clinically, the condition is characterized by **erythematous, desquamative dermatitis** (Figure 4.55). The signs begin on the **head and the pinna** and then become generalized. In the early stages of the disease the scales are loosely attached to the skin, while in chronic cases they are larger, more tightly adhered and trapped between the hair. Brown, ceruminous deposits can be seen around the lips and eyes, in the auditory canals and the cuticle.

In some ginger cats, the coat lightens or becomes whiter.

### Diagnosis

Blood biochemistry may show **elevated creatinine kinase**, although levels may also be elevated in cats with thymoma without exfoliative dermatitis. Thoracic radiographs usually indicate a mediastinal tumour.

Histopathology of skin lesions shows changes similar to those observed in the 'graft-versus-host' reaction or erythema multiforme. It is characterized by:

- interface dermatitis
- hydropic degeneration of basal cells
- lymphocytic exocytosis
- satellitosis
- apoptotic keratinocytes
- lymphocytic infiltrate in the dermis.

**Thymoma is usually benign.**

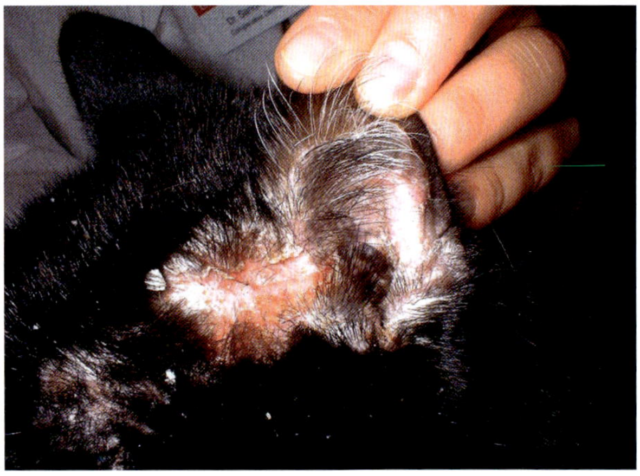

**Figure 4.55.** Erythema and whitened desquamation due to exfoliative dermatitis associated with thymoma.

## Alopecia

### *Focal and multifocal inflammatory alopecia*

#### *Aetiopathogenesis*

Focal or multifocal lack of hair (alopecia, hypotrichosis) is almost always due to an **inflammatory process in the hair follicle**, whether of an infectious, parasitic or immune nature (Table 4.3).

In the case of a bacterial or fungal infection or demodicosis, the hair falls out because the **causal agent results in luminal folliculitis**. However, in immunological diseases the object of the autoimmune attack is the hair follicle structures *per se* (walls, roots, blood vessels, etc.), which makes it impossible for them to produce healthy hair or retain existing hair.

Table 4.3. Causes of focal and multifocal inflammatory alopecia.

| Causes |
|---|
| **Infectious** |
| Bacterial folliculitis |
| Dermatophytoses |
| **Parasitic** |
| Demodicosis |
| **Immune** |
| Vasculitis |
| Alopecia **areata** |
| Dermatomyositis |
| Pemphigus foliaceus |
| **Other possible causes** |
| Epitheliotropic lymphoma |
| Reactions to injections |
| Scars |
| Traction alopecia |

### *Clinical signs*

A focal alopecia can be seen most easily in short-haired animals (Figure 4.56), whilst those with long hair require a more detailed examination of the coat.

The **presence of borders** (Figure 4.57) or scabs at the margins of the areas of alopecia is significant and shows a **bacterial infection or pemphigus foliaceus**.

Hair that can easily be pulled out in strands, with little resistance, indicates a severe follicular problem (for example, infection).

**Inflammatory folliculitis** (i.e. bacterial folliculitis or a reaction to a drug) is suggested by **erythematous skin**, with abrasions or flaking and scabs or scales attached to the hair.

Rounded areas without hair, with scar-like characteristics (lack of growth of new hair, hypopigmentation, smooth and shiny), are seen in cases of:

- healing by secondary intention
- reactions to subcutaneous injections
- traction alopecia (when tight clamps are used)
- vasculitis
- dermatomyositis.

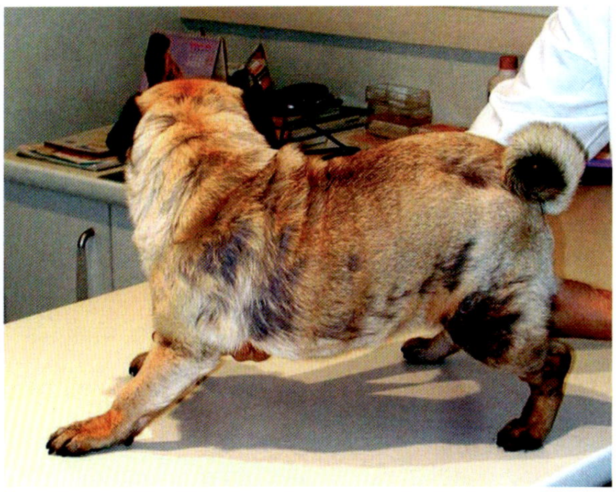

**Figure 4.56.** Multifocal alopecia in a dog with demodicosis.

### *Diagnosis*

#### Skin scrapes

Demodicosis should be searched for in all cases and requires deep skin scrapes and trichoscopic examination of various lesions to check for the presence of *Demodex* spp. mites.

If both deep skin scrapings and trichoscopic examination are negative, it is reasonable to rule out demodicosis. If lesions persist, these tests should be repeated at each subsequent examination.

The presence of *Demodex* spp. mites (Figure 4.58) confirms the diagnosis of **demodicosis**. In addition to specific treatment for demodicosis, the patient should be assessed to see whether there is a **primary underlying immunosuppressive disease** or a secondary bacterial component, especially in cats.

#### Wood's lamp and trichoscopy

Examination with a **Wood's lamp,** along with trichoscopy, is helpful in the search for dermatophytes.

Wood's lamp (Figure 4.59) only gives a **positive result in 50%** of the cases caused by *M. canis* and never in the case of other dermatophytes. A negative result does not rule out a dermatophytosis, but the presence of fluorescence on the hair usually indicates a positive result.

With trichoscopy, spores and hyphae can be seen in the **infected hair shafts** (Figure 4.60). In order to increase the chance of identification, hair samples should be taken from the centre and periphery of the lesion.

#### Fungal culture

If skin scrapings, Wood's lamp examination and trichoscopy are all negative, a mycological culture should be performed with a dermatophyte culture medium,

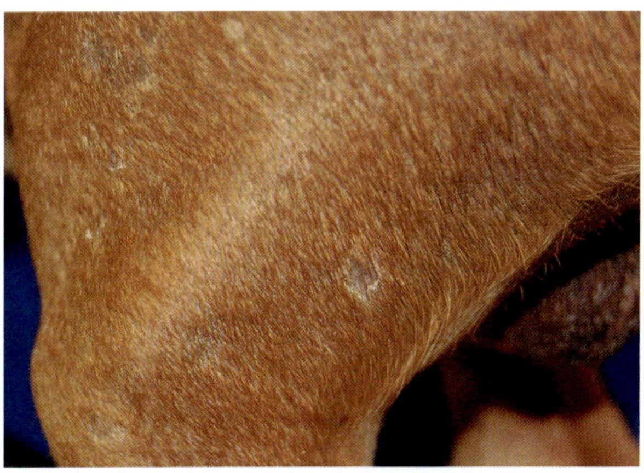

**Figure 4.57.** Areas of multifocal alopecia surrounded by yellow crusts of dry pus in a dog with bacterial folliculitis.

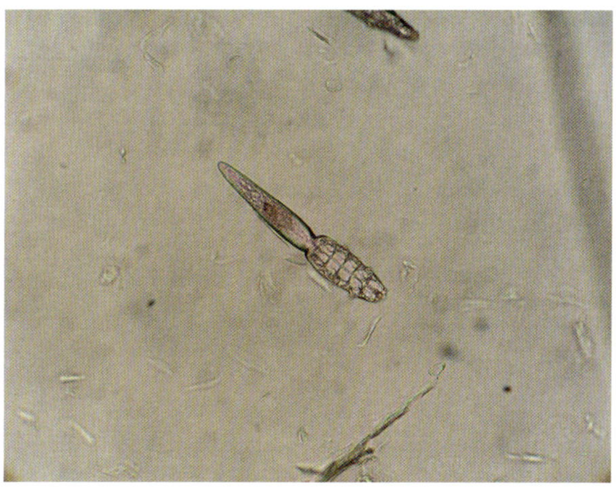

**Figure 4.58.** Adult *Demodex canis.*

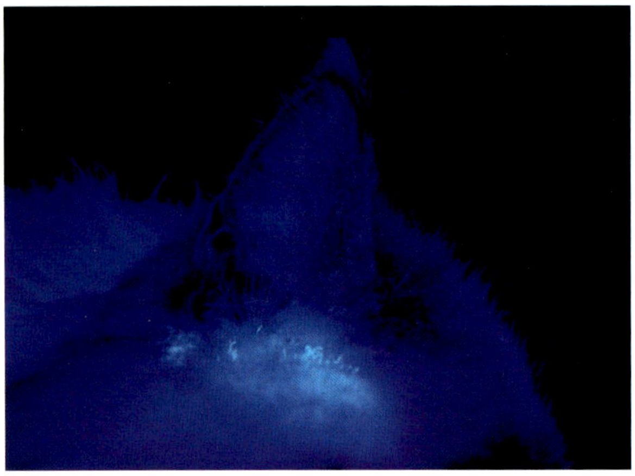

**Figure 4.59.** Image of a positive result for a Wood's lamp examination. Hairs that fluoresce are pulled out and examined under the microscope to confirm the dermatophytosis.

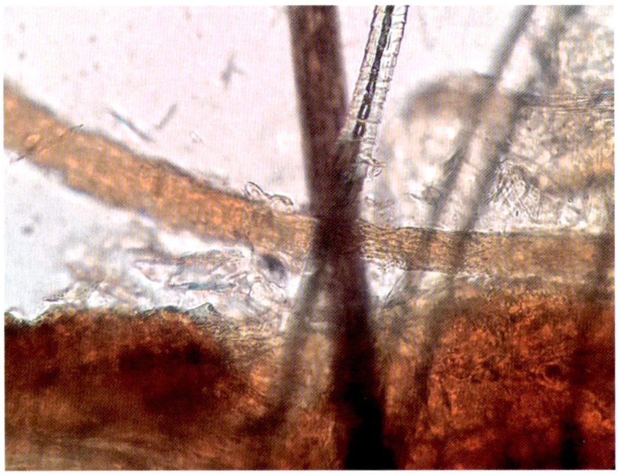

**Figure 4.60.** Hair affected by dermatophytosis. The horizontal hair shaft is invaded by hyphae.

and even Sabouraud's medium can be used if necessary to rule out the possibility of dermatophytosis. Several samples should be taken by cleanly pulling a few hairs from the centre and periphery of the lesions.

### Cytological analysis

If crusts or wheals appear on the margin of the areas with alopecia, the exudate should be collected and examined:

- The presence of degenerate neutrophils with intracellular bacteria suggests a diagnosis of bacterial folliculitis and pyoderma (Figure 4.61).
- Intact neutrophils and acantholytic cells (large, dark blue cells) suggest pemphigus foliaceus. Confirmation requires a skin biopsy.

### Antibiotic tests

If the results of the previous tests do not lead to a diagnosis, an empirical antibiotic treatment can be used to diagnose a bacterial folliculitis by **assessing response to the treatment** (while waiting for the results of fungal culture; generally about 15 days). A **three-week treatment course** should be initiated with one of the following medications, unless these have been prescribed recently:

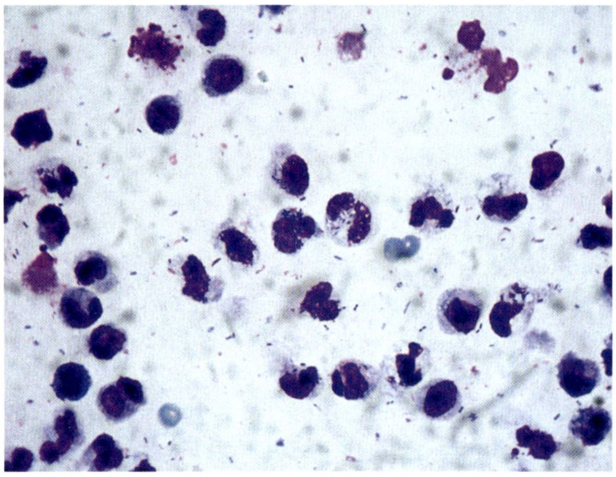

**Figure 4.61.** Neutrophils with intracellular bacteria in a diagnosis of pyoderma.

- *Cefadroxil (20–30 mg/kg/24 h).*
- *Cephalexin (20–30 mg/kg/12 h).*
- *Amoxicillin + clavulanic acid (15–25 mg/kg/12 h).*

The patient should be re-examined after two weeks to assess the results of the treatment, in addition to obtaining the results of the fungal culture.

### Skin biopsy

If fungal culture gives a negative result and the antibiotic test treatment does not produce significant improvement, a **skin biopsy** is recommended to reach a definitive diagnosis. Once any secondary bacterial infection has been eliminated, the possibilities of obtaining histological samples with diagnostic value that allow detection of other rarer manifestations of focal alopecia are optimized, such as:

- pemphigus foliaceus
- alopecia areata
- injection site reactions
- vasculitis
- dermatomyositis
- traction alopecia
- epitheliotropic lymphoma.

## *Canine diffuse alopecia*

### *Aetiopathogenesis*

In the **cat, diffuse alopecia** is almost always due to licking, which is **an indication of pruritus**. Since this should be approached from the perspective of pruritus,

Table 4.4. Causes of non-inflammatory and diffuse alopecia in the dog.

| Causes |
|---|
| **Congenital and hereditary** |
| Bald breeds |
| (Chinese crested, Mexican hairless dog, Sphinx cat) |
| Dysplasia of black hair follicles |
| Colour-dilution alopecia |
| **Hormonal** |
| Cushing's syndrome |
| Hypothyroidism |
| Hormone-producing gonadal tumours |
| **Immune-mediated** |
| Alopecia areata |
| Sebaceous adenitis |
| **Idiopathic** |
| Seasonal flank alopecia |
| Pattern baldness alopecia |
| Alopecia X |
| **Neoplastic** |
| Epitheliotropic T-cell lymphoma |

it will not be discussed in this chapter, and only canine diffuse alopecia will be covered.

Non-inflammatory hair loss is caused by the **telogenization of the hair roots** as a result of (Table 4.4):

- A **systemic metabolic disorder** (for example, hormonal diseases).
- Localized **follicular factors** (for example, alopecia X, pattern baldness alopecia, cyclic or seasonal flank alopecia).
- **Congenital malformations** (bald breeds, colour-dilution alopecia, black hair follicular dysplasia).
- An **inflammatory disease of the hair follicles** (for example, alopecia areata, sebaceous adenitis).

## *Clinical signs*

Non-inflammatory alopecia is manifested by a complete or partial loss of the hair layer (hypotrichosis) with no significant visible alteration of the skin surface. The absence of hair may affect all hair follicles or just some.

If the affected hairs are dark or of a diluted colour, there is a melanization defect (colour-dilution alopecia or black hair dysplasia) (Figure 4.62).

The absence of primary hairs and the presence of undercoat (puppy fur) is common in:

- Nordic breeds
- dogs with a very thick coat
- cases of alopecia X (Figure 4.63)
- cases of testicular tumour.

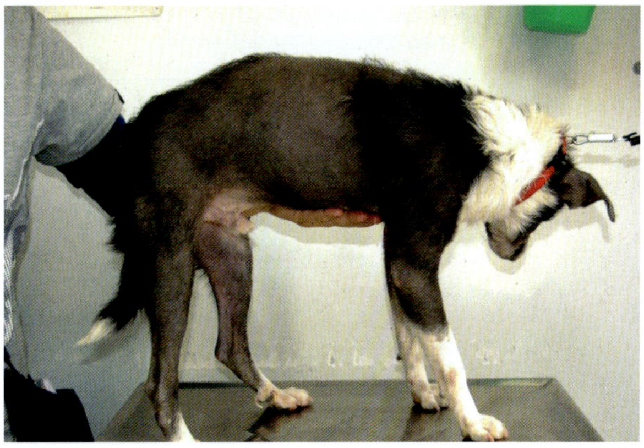

Figure 4.62. Dog affected by black hair dysplasia: the areas with white hair are not affected, while the black hairs display hypotrichosis.

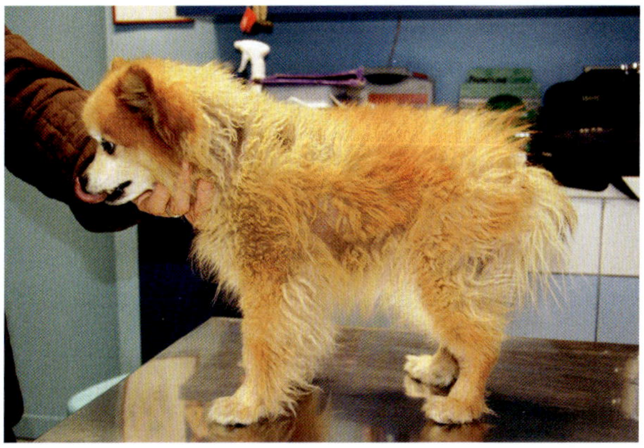

Figure 4.63. Alopecia X in a Pomeranian. The dog has lost its primary hair leaving the finer, drier secondary hair. The coat looks like that of a puppy.

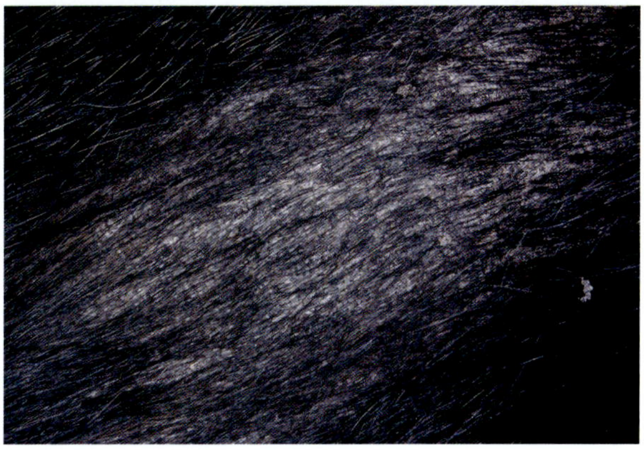

Figure 4.64. Sebaceous adenitis. There is mainly loss of the undercoat, leaving an excess of primary hairs. The coat appears sparse, and scales can be seen on the skin.

The **absence of undercoat** while primary hairs are preserved indicates primary **sebaceous adenitis** (Figure 4.64).

Other important factors to consider are the age of onset of alopecia (Table 4.5), its location (Table 4.6), the breed and the coat type (Table 4.7).

Table 4.5. Most frequent aetiologies of canine diffuse alopecia according to the age of onset.

| Young dogs (<4 years) | Middle-aged dogs (>4 years) |
|---|---|
| Congenital hypotrichosis, bald breeds | Hypothyroidism |
| Diluted coat: colour-dilution alopecia | Hormone-secreting ovarian cysts |
| Black areas: follicular dysplasia of black hairs | Hormone-secreting gonadal tumours |
| Short-haired animals: pattern baldness alopecia | |
| Nordic or thick-haired breeds: alopecia X, alopecia after clipping | |
| Seasonal flank alopecia | |
| Chronic sebaceous adenitis | |
| **Old dogs** | **Dogs** |
| Spontaneous hyperadrenocorticism | Alopecia areata |
| Hormone-secreting gonadal tumours | Iatrogenic hyperadrenocorticism |

Table 4.6. Most frequent aetiologies of diffuse canine alopecia according to the location of alopecia.

| Location of alopecia | Most likely pathology |
|---|---|
| Behind the ears, on the ventral regions of the neck, trunk and abdomen, and on the thighs of short-haired dogs | Pattern baldness alopecia |
| Tail, back of the nose, friction points (ischial tuberosities, neck) | Hypothyroidism |
| Areas of bluish or black hair | Melanization defects (black hair dysplasia, colour-dilution alopecia) |
| Only the trunk | Hyperadrenocorticism<br>Alopecia X |
| Neck | Gonadal tumours<br>Hypothyroidism<br>Alopecia X |
| Flanks | Seasonal cyclical alopecia<br>Hyperadrenocorticism<br>Hypothyroidism |
| Face | Alopecia areata<br>Hypothyroidism (top of the nose) |

In some cases, the appearance of the skin alone is sufficient to suggest a diagnosis:

- **Pattern baldness alopecia** (Figure 4.65) is a perfectly normal part of the coat in terms of colour and consistency.

Table 4.7. Frequency of diffuse canine alopecia according to breed predisposition (without exclusion of other breeds).

| Breed | Most frequent pathology |
|---|---|
| Short-haired breeds | Pattern baldness alopecia<br>Seasonal flank alopecia |
| Nordic or thick-haired breeds | Alopecia X |
| Breeds with a diluted coat colour (black or blue) | Colour-dilution alopecia |
| Small breeds and Boxer | Hyperadrenocorticism |
| Medium or large breeds | Hypothyroidism |
| Akita, Poodle, Viszla, Hovawart, Havanese | Sebaceous adenitis |

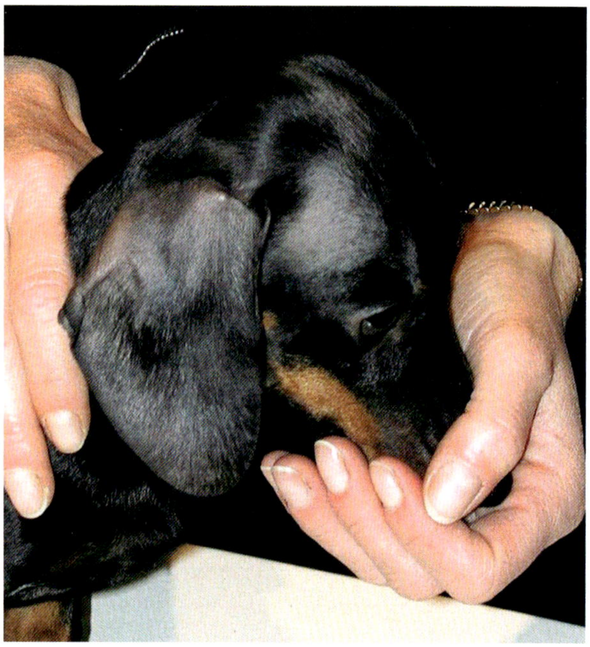

Figure 4.65. Pattern baldness alopecia localized behind the ears and the jaw region.

- With **trunk alopecia** the skin acquires a darker colour (due to sunlight), a change that is not relevant for diagnosis.
- In **congenital alopecia** and **hypoadrenocorticism**, comedones (small keratin plugs that obstruct the follicle opening) may appear.
- With **hypothyroidism and gonadal tumours**, the skin may thicken and become fatty. Secondary colonization and infection with bacteria and *Malassezia* are often seen.

Key indicators that may help diagnosis:

- Follicular plugs (Figure 4.66) indicate sebaceous adenitis.
- Flank alopecia with well-defined margins is characteristic of seasonal cyclic alopecia (Figure 4.67).

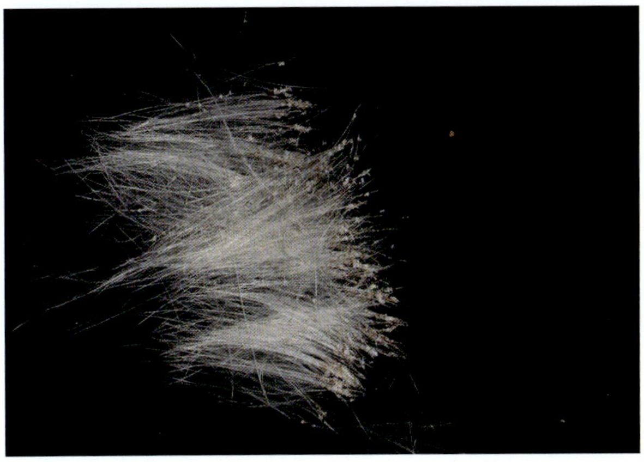

**Figure 4.66.** Follicular plugs stuck to the end of hairs.

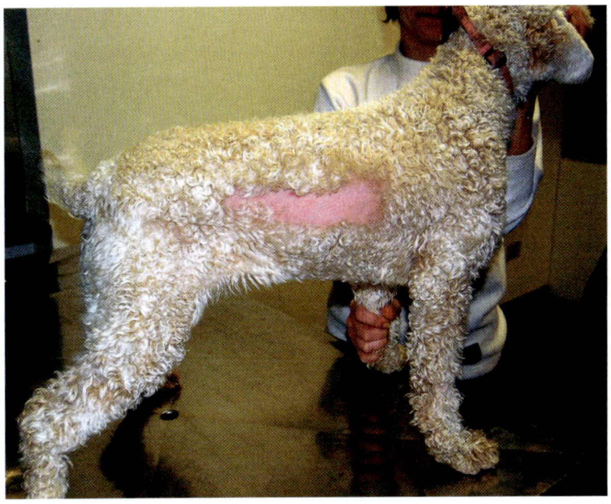

**Figure 4.67.** Cyclic or seasonal flank alopecia in a Lagotto Romagnolo.

- If alopecia only affects black hairs only, not white or light-coloured ones, this indicates a melanization defect.
- The absence of hair on the tail or on the top of the nose indicates hypothyroidism (Figure 4.68).
- The growth of a good tuft of hair in the location of a biopsy indicates alopecia X (Figure 4.69).
- Alopecia behind the ears is characteristic of pattern baldness alopecia (Figure 4.70).

## *Diagnosis*

### Skin scrapes

In all cases of **non-inflammatory alopecia**, it is essential to take one or more deep skin scrapings to **rule out demodicosis** (Figure 4.58).

### Wood's lamp and trichoscopy

If deep skin scrapings are negative, trichoscopy and a Wood's lamp examination, as well as a fungal culture, should be performed to **rule out dermatophytosis** (Figures 4.59 and 4.60).

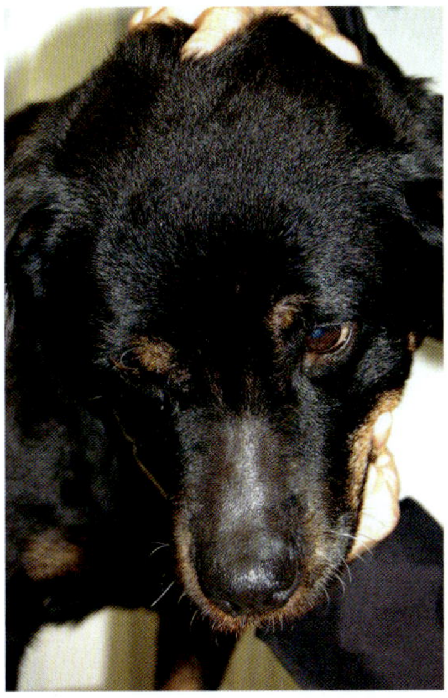

**Figure 4.68.** Alopecia of the nasal plane in a dog with hypothyroidism.

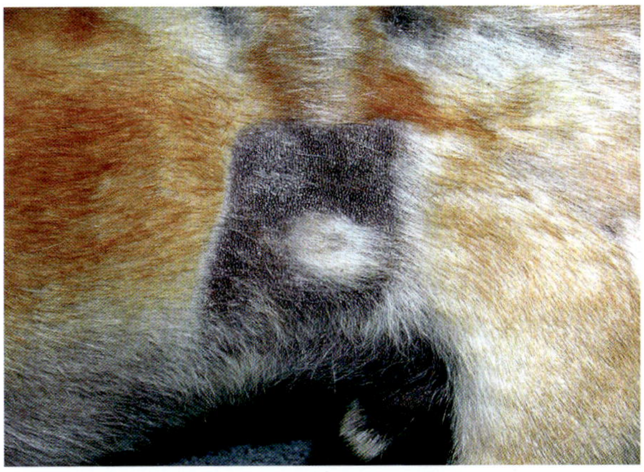

**Figure 4.69.** Alopecia X: hair growth at the site of biopsy.

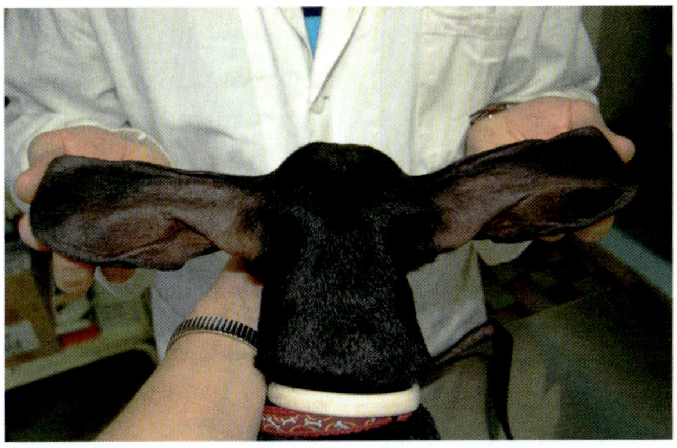

**Figure 4.70.** Alopecia behind the ears with pattern baldness.

### Evaluation of pigmentation

If trichoscopy and fungal culture are negative, it is essential to check for pigmentation defects, observing the distribution of the melanin within the hair whilst performing the trichogram.

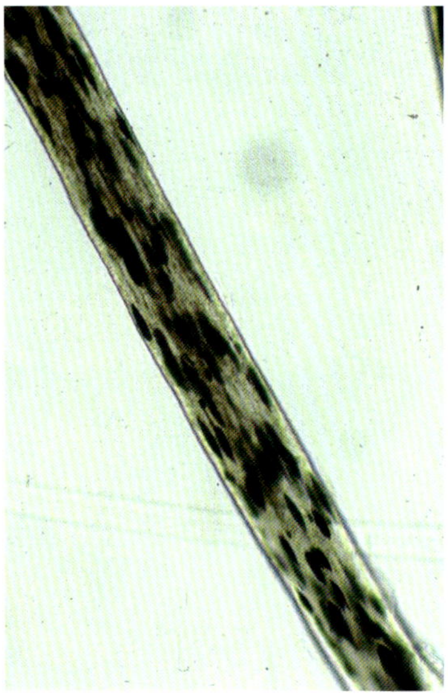

**Figure 4.71.** Microscope image of hair from a dog with colour-dilution alopecia. There are numerous melanosome aggregates in the hair shaft.

If melanin aggregates can be seen, colour-dilution alopecia or black hair dysplasia can be diagnosed (Figure 4.71). In general, in a clinical setting there is a thinning of the coat that does not affect the white or lighter-coloured areas. If the only areas affected are those with black hairs (and undiluted), it is likely to be a black hair dysplasia.

These two diseases are confirmed by skin biopsy. There is no treatment.

The age of the animal, the distribution of alopecia and coat type should be considered:

- If no melanization defects are seen, the age of the animal, distribution of the alopecia and type of coat should be considered.
- In **elderly animals** (>5 years), the possibility of a **hormonal condition** (hyperadrenocorticism, hyperthyroidism or gonadal tumours) should be suspected.
- In **males** it is important to palpate and perform an ultrasound examination of the **testicles**.
- In **small breeds** a test for **hyperadrenocorticism** should be performed.
- In **medium and large breeds**, the first thing that should be ruled out is **hypothyroidism**.
- In **un-neutered females**, especially those with irregular or prolonged seasons, an ultrasound examination to look for **ovarian cysts or tumours** is recommended.

If all of the above tests are negative a skin biopsy should be performed.

In young or middle-aged dogs (0–5 years old), the distribution and type of coat should be considered. In general, the most common key factors are:

- **Short-haired dogs** (6 months – 2 years): pattern baldness alopecia behind the ears, ventral regions of the neck, trunk and abdomen and thighs (Figure 4.65). For this condition, ***melatonin (3–6 mg/dog once a day)*** can be administered until satisfactory results are obtained.
- Dogs with a short, soft or curly coat that present with well-circumscribed, bilateral, circular lesions on the flanks (appear in spring and disappear in summer): **seasonal cyclic flank alopecia**. For this condition, ***melatonin, 3–6 mg/dog once a day*** can be administered until satisfactory results are obtained and then as a preventive measure, for two months after the expected relapse period.
- Dogs 1–5 years old, those with thick fur and Nordic breeds, with persistent undercoats, with a typical puppy coat on the body and alopecia on the neck and perineum (Figure 4.63): **alopecia X**. In uncastrated males use of a **deslorelin implant** every 6 months may be useful, but in castrated males and females it is of no use. Instead **trilostane** can be used, as for Cushing's syndrome, with good results.
- The presence of follicular plugs and alopecia mainly affecting the undercoat: **sebaceous adenitis** (Figure 4.64). In these cases, ***cyclosporine at 5 mg/kg/d***, as well as keratolytic shampoos (*2% sulphur and 2% salicylic acid*) and moisturizing sprays (*75% propylene glycol*) usually contribute towards a significant improvement, although they do not usually provide a complete cure.

### Biopsy

In any of the above cases, a **biopsy** is needed to confirm diagnosis. As these are not systemic diseases and are simply aesthetic, in some cases the owner chooses not to go ahead with biopsy because of its expense and the risk associated with anaesthesia. If alopecia does not fit into any of the above-mentioned groups, alopecia with a hormonal origin and/or skin biopsy can be considered.

## Bacterial diseases

### *Pyoderma*

### Aetiology

In small animals, ***Staphylococci* spp. are the bacteria most frequently isolated** from pyoderma. In the dog *S. pseudintermedius* is the main pathogen, with other coagulase-positive staphylococci and Gram-negative bacteria sometimes isolated. In the cat, the most commonly isolated pathogens are *S. pseudintermedius*, *S. aureus* and *S. simulans*.

### *Classification*

Depending on the depth of infection, pyoderma is classified as:

- surface
- superficial
- deep.

### *Surface pyoderma*

As the name suggests, **surface pyoderma is limited to the most superficial layers** (stratum corneum) and and it is not considered a true pyoderma by some clinicians. This is because **no neutrophils** are observed on cytological examination, **only bacterial growth** which causes erythema and a bad odour is seen.

#### Pyotraumatic dermatitis

Also known as a **hot spot**, pyotraumatic dermatitis is caused by **self-inflicted trauma** due to intense focal itching where the lesion may rapidly enlarge.

Often this disease is secondary to:

- flea bite allergy
- other allergies
- reaction to irritant substances
- ectoparasites.

Dogs with a **long, thick coat** (especially Golden Retrievers, German Shepherds and Newfoundlands) are predisposed. It is more prevalent in the summer months and in humid climates.

A typical lesion has an area of **inflamed alopecia covered with a moist** exudate (Figure 4.72).

On cytology, an abundant bacterial presence is detected, usually without inflammatory cells.

#### Intertrigo, or skin fold dermatitis

Animals with **skin folds** as part of the breed standard (Pug, Bulldog, Pekingese and Persian cat) are predisposed to intertrigo, or skin fold dermatitis. In other breeds it appears in skin folds such as the interdigital spaces and in obese animals (for example, in vulvar folds). **Increases in humidity** (tears in the facial folds or urine in the perivulvar folds, etc.), friction and high temperatures cause **skin maceration**. Macerated skin, together with the accumulation of glandular secretions, is prone to **bacterial and/or yeast colonization** (usually *Malassezia*), microorganisms that cause an inflammatory reaction both by their direct antigen effect and secretion of toxins and metabolites.

When a fold is raised, the skin appears erythematous, moist and covered with a viscous, malodorous secretion (Figure 4.73). In animals with a light-coloured coat, the area stains brown.

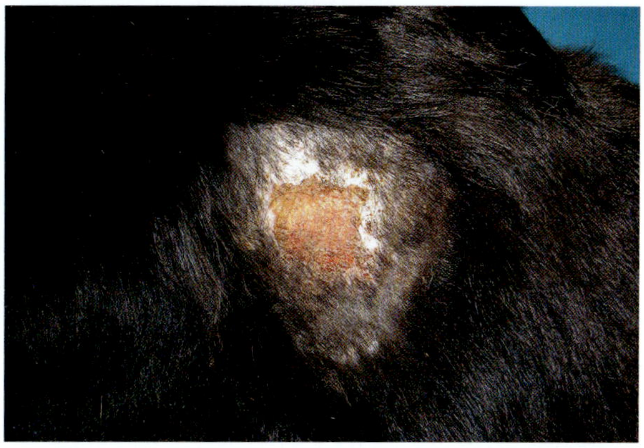

**Figure 4.72.** Hot spot in the lumbar region of a Rottweiler.

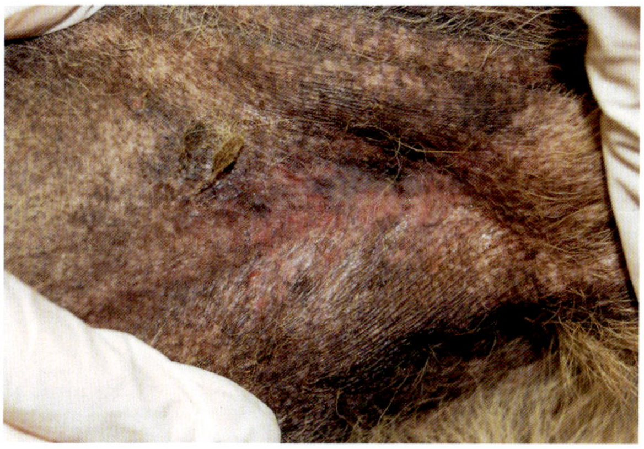

**Figure 4.73.** Skin fold dermatitis in the perivulvar and inguinal regions of an overweight Italian Mastiff.

Cytology shows a large number of bacteria, usually without neutrophils.

#### Secondary bacterial infection

Secondary bacterial infection is characterized by **diffuse erythema** (Figure 4.74). On a simple impression smear of the skin, an **excessive number of bacteria** can be seen. This condition causes itching, desquamation and a foul-smelling odour, and is often associated with

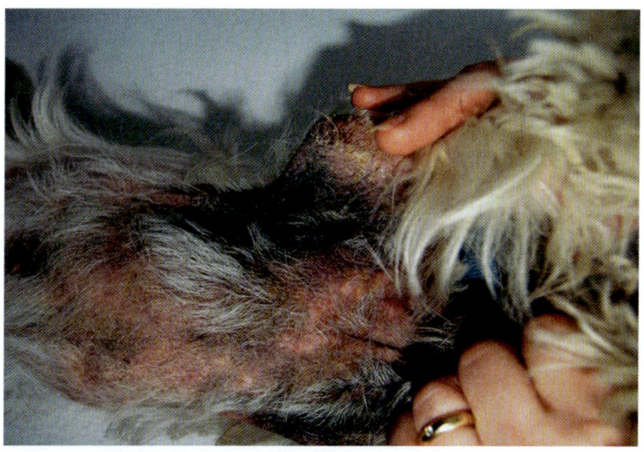

**Figure 4.74.** Lichenification, hyperpigmentation and superficial exudation in a dog with a secondary bacterial infection due to allergy.

an allergic or endocrine disease. Cutaneous signs and pruritus disappear with antibiotic treatment or antibacterial shampoos.

### *Superficial pyoderma*

Superficial pyoderma is described as an infection of the epidermis and hair follicles. It is considered a true pyoderma because on cytological examination bacteria (cocci and/or bacilli) are observed within neutrophils (Figure 4.61).

#### Impetigo

Lesions typical of impetigo are **subcorneal pustules and epidermal wheals** located in hairless areas (abdomen, groin) (Figure 4.75). Normally impetigo is a disease which affects young dogs caused by *S. pseudintermedius*. Cytology of the pustule content reveals neutrophils and bacteria (including intracellular).

#### Superficial bacterial folliculitis

Superficial bacterial folliculitis is defined as an **infection of the hair follicle**. The following cause a predisposition to the disease:

- chronic obstruction of the hair follicle
- inflammation of the hair follicle
- pathologies that alter the immune state (allergy, immune-mediated disease, systemic and metabolic disorders).

The most frequent causes of follicular obstruction are:

- seborrheic keratosis disorders (e.g. sebaceous dermatitis)
- demodicosis
- follicular dysplasia.

The most frequently isolated pathogen is S. pseudintermedius.

The primary lesions of superficial bacterial folliculitis are follicular-based papules and pustules (Figure 4.76) that rupture rapidly to form:

- epidermal wheals (Figure 4.77)
- exfoliation
- focal and multifocal alopecia (Figure 4.78).

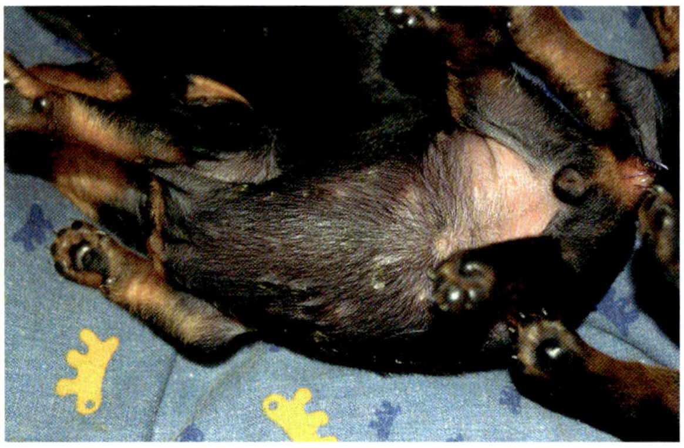

Figure 4.75. Wheals and pustules on the abdomen of a puppy with bacterial impetigo.

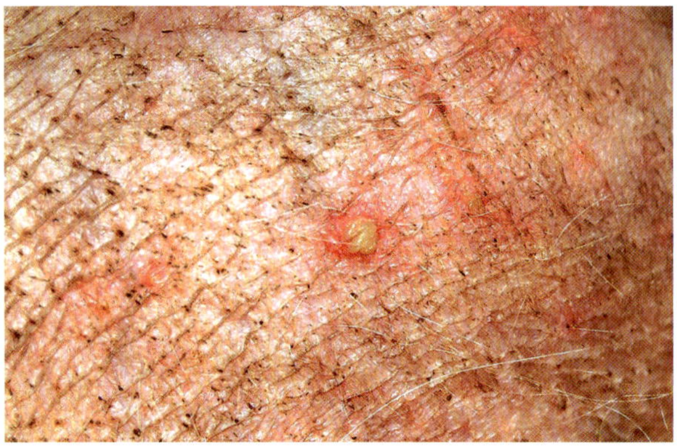

Figure 4.76. Follicular pustule in a dog with bacterial folliculitis.

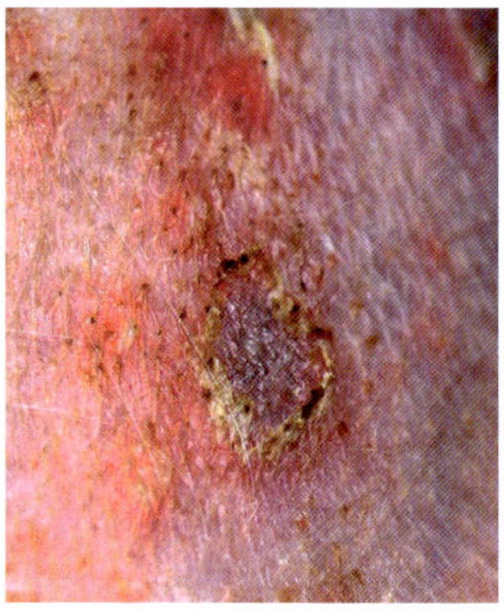

Figure 4.77. Wheal in a dog with bacterial folliculitis.

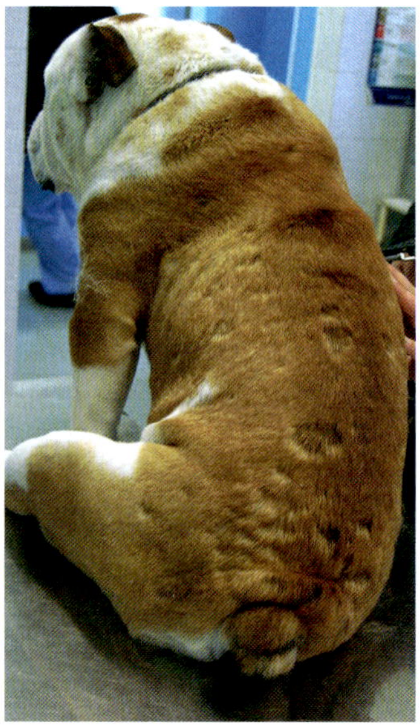

Figure 4.78. Multifocal alopecia in a dog with bacterial folliculitis.

Often bacterial folliculitis is **moderately pruritic**.

Cytological examination of a pustule or a wheal shows the presence of bacteria (cocci or bacilli) in neutrophils.

## *Deep pyoderma*

Deep pyoderma is defined as a **skin infection that reaches the dermis and subcutaneous tissue**. It can be the result of the extension of a deep pyoderma, secondary to either severe folliculitis (furunculosis) or the inoculation of bacteria into deep tissues (abscesses).

The most frequent underlying causes in the dog are:

- demodicosis (Figure 4.79)
- pressure trauma (callus [Figure 4.80], lick granuloma, pododermatitis [Figure 4.81]).

In cats, the most important type of deep pyoderma is chin acne secondary to a keratinization defect.

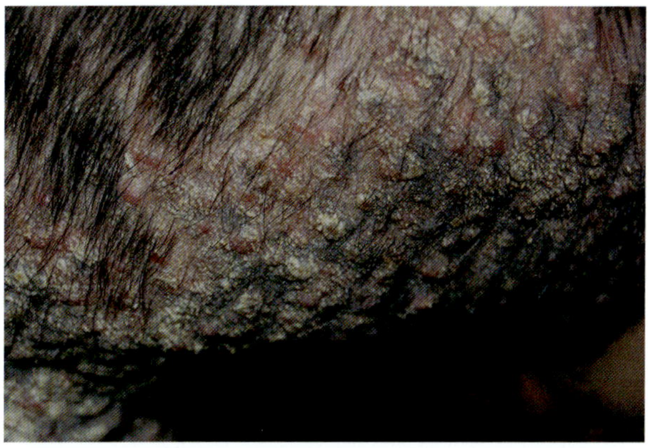

**Figure 4.79.** Papules, pustules and alopecia in a dog with severe pyodemodicosis.

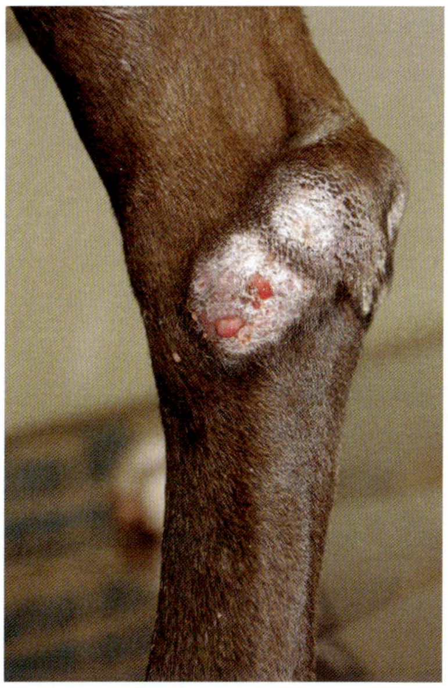

**Figure 4.80.** Infected callus.

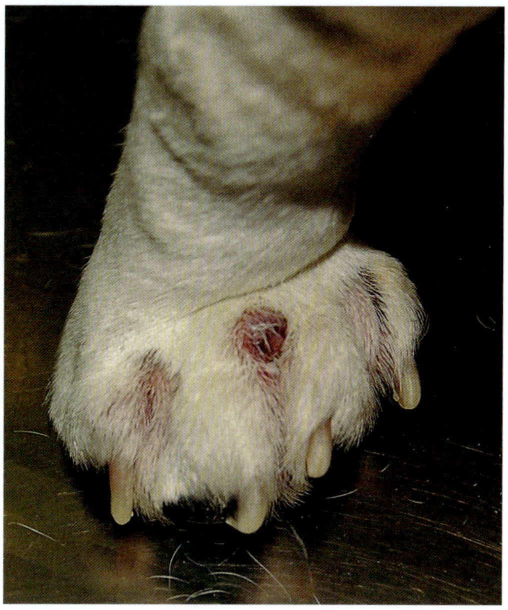

**Figure 4.81.** Furuncle in a case of pododermatitis.

The appearance of deep pyoderma depends on:

- the area affected
- the depth of the disease
- the immune response of the host.

### Appearance

Less severe cases present as **papules** that progress to **haemorrhagic blisters** and then rupture to form **scabby ulcers**. The more severe forms present as an area of painful and often extensive erythema, with numerous fistulae that drain a haemopurulent secretion towards the surface.

Deep pyoderma is diagnosed based on its typical clinical characteristics (haemorrhagic blisters, fistulae and ulcers) and confirmation of the presence of an infection by cytology or bacterial culture. In all cases, culture and sensitivity testing is recommended.

### Treatment

The treatment of bacterial pyoderma is effective if it eliminates symptoms and prevents their reappearance. Since **most of these infections are secondary**, therapeutic success cannot be achieved until the **underlying cause** is identified and treated.

**Surface and superficial pyodermas** (pyotraumatic and intertriginous dermatitis) can be successfully treated with **topical treatments**, applying an antibacterial shampoo (4% chlorhexidine, twice a week) and an antibacterial spray, gel or ointment such as chlorhexidine, mupirocin or fusidic acid. The use of corticosteroids may be justified to control pruritus.

**Deep and superficial pyodermas** that do not respond **to topical treatment require systemic**

**treatment,** possibly in combination with topical therapy. The first signs of superficial pyoderma can be treated empirically with first-line antibiotics. Then, if it does not respond to treatment, **bacterial culture** is indicated. In all cases of deep pyoderma, as well as in those that have already been treated with antibiotics and in which only bacilli are observed on cytology, a bacterial culture to select the correct antibiotic is strongly recommended.

The length of treatment is fundamental:

- Superficial pyoderma should be treated for at **least three weeks**, or for up to a week after its complete disappearance.
- For deep pyoderma, times are doubled.

Before discontinuing treatment it is essential that the veterinarian reassess the patient, bearing in mind that the surface of the skin heals before deeper tissues. Careful palpation is essential to ensure that no source of infection remains.

### First-line antibiotics

First-line antibiotics should be used when empirical antibiotic therapy is administered, although they should also be the first choice if sensitivity tests reveal that bacteria are sensitive to them. These include:

- *cephalexin (15–30 mg/kg/12 h)*
- *cefadroxil (20–30 mg/kg/24 h)*
- *amoxicillin/clavulanic acid (15–25 mg/kg/12 h)*
- *clindamycin (5–10 mg/kg/12 h)*
- *cefovecin (8 mg/kg/15 d SC)* should be used only if oral administration is not possible.

### Second-line antibiotics

Second-line antibiotics should be administered only after corresponding sensitivity tests and only if bacteria are resistant to first-line antibiotics. These are:

- *trimethoprim-sulphonamide (15–30 mg/kg/12 h)*
- *erythromycin (10–15 mg/kg/8 h)*
- *lincomycin (20 mg/kg/12 h)*
- *fluoroquinones (enrofloxacin 5 mg/kg/24 h)*
- *marbofloxacin (2 mg/kg/24 h).*

### Third-line antibiotics (last resort)

These antibiotics should be administered only after corresponding sensitivity tests and only if bacteria are resistant to first- and second-line antibiotics. These drugs are associated with toxicity:

- renal (aminoglycosides)
- hepatic (rifampicin).

These are:

- *rifampicin (5–10 mg/24 h)*. Liver parameters should be checked weekly.
- *chloramphenicol* (empirical dose extrapolated from human medicine: 50 mg/kg/8h).
- *doxycycline* and *aminocycline (5–10 mg/kg/12 h).*
- *fosfomycin, amikacin (in dogs, 15–30 mg/kg/24 h SC).* Renal parameters should be checked before and during treatment.
- *gentamicin (in dogs, 9–14 mg/kg/24 h SC).* Renal parameters should be checked before and during treatment.

### Antibiotics that should never be used

Antibiotics essential for human health should never be administered to dogs, these include:

- vancomycin
- linezolid
- carbapenems (for example, imipenem).

Non-potentiated penicillin (amoxicillin and ampicillin without clavulanic acid) should also not be used, because up to 70% of staphylococcal strains are beta-lactamase-producing.

## Cutaneous mycobacterial infections

### Epidemiology

These are relatively **rare infections** and, in most cases, affect the cat, especially individuals with **FIV or FeLV**.

### Aetiopathogenesis

Atypical mycobacterial infections are chronic in nature and difficult to cure.

The most frequently isolated mycobacteria are:

**Opportunistic mycobacteria** inoculated in the dermis or subcutaneous tissue of the host through a wound or injury inflicted during a fight:

- *M. fortuitum*
- *M. phlei*
- *M. smegmatis*
- *M. thermosensible*
- *M. lepraemurium*, which is transmitted by bites from a rat or infected fleas.

### Clinical signs

Lesions evolve slowly. **Nodules** are formed, with alopecia and erythema, causing ulceration and the formation of sinuous tracts with a haemopurulent exudate (Figure 4.82). They affect subcutaneous tissues and the dermis.

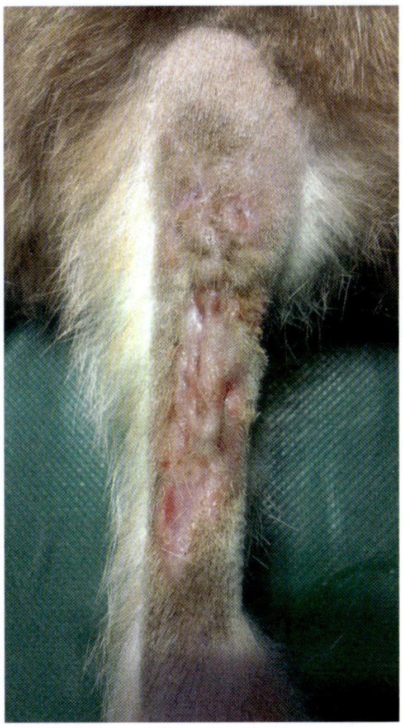

**Figure 4.82.** Fistulation of a mycobacterial infection on the dorsal aspect of a cat's tail.

The most commonly affected regions are:

- the back
- the abdomen
- inguinal areas.

Any surgical intervention in the area heals with difficulty.

### *Diagnosis*

Cytology can reveal **macrophages loaded with acid-fast microorganisms** in the form of bacilli, which do not absorb any stain and, therefore, appear as elongated, empty spaces. Culture is frequently negative because these microorganisms are difficult to culture.

Diagnostic confirmation is by:

- biopsy with special stains for acid-fast bacteria
- polymerase chain reaction of affected tissues.

### *Treatment*

These infections are very difficult to cure. As far as possible, antibiotic therapy should be based on microorganism **culture and sensitivity tests**. Medications used to treat mycobacterial infections include:

- *enrofloxacin 10–20 mg/kg/24 h* (not in cats, because of the risk of retinal degeneration)
- *clarithromycin 15 mg/kg/12 h*
- *doxycycline 5 mg/kg/12 h*
- *rifampicin 10–20 mg/kg/12 h*
- *clofazimine 2–8 mg/kg/24 h*
- *dapsone 1 mg/kg/24 h.*

It may be necessary to combine two or three antibiotics and prolong treatment for 3–6 months.

# Fungal diseases

## *Dermatophytoses*

### *Aetiopathogenesis*

Approximately 98% of feline dermatophytosis are due to *Microsporum canis*. This fungus is well adapted to the **cat as it is its natural reservoir**, and long-haired cats, particularly Persians, are predisposed to it.

**Canine dermatophytosis is less frequent** and is often associated with immunosuppression (transport stress, parasitism in puppies, etc.) or the presence of an infected cat in the environment. *M. canis* is also the main canine pathogen, although there may also be *Trichophyton mentagrophytes* infections caught mainly in rural areas where the soil is infected, affecting areas of the body that are in contact with the ground. The Yorkshire Terrier is predisposed to *M. canis* infection, while in the Jack Russell Terrier the incidence of *Trichophyton* infection is higher.

Infection is by spores or hair fragments, either directly or by means of fomites (bed, brushes, etc.). The **spores are extraordinarily resistant** and can survive up to 18 months in the environment. To cause infection, they must penetrate the epidermis or travel into the hair follicle. Contact does not always cause infection, either because the spores fail to penetrate the epidermis due to the hygiene of the host (especially cats), due to normal epidermal desquamation or through inhibition by the resident cutaneous microflora or the immune system.

Dermatophytes obtain nutrients by decomposing keratin with fungal keratinase. Hairs in the anagen phase are a good medium for fungal growth. The **host's immune response is essential** for elimination of dermatophyte infection.

The following animals are predisposed:

- Those with immunodeficiency.
- Lactating females.
- Gestating females.
- Those with a disease causing weakness or immunosuppression (for example, FIV/FeLV).
- Ectoparasites enable and spread dermatophyte infections. Scratching not only damages the skin and allows penetration of the spores, but also disseminates fragments of contaminated skin into the environment.

### Clinical signs

In general, **cats** are a more tolerant host than dogs to *M. canis*. The former develop **localized or generalized alopecia** (Figure 4.83), often with a minimal degree of inflammation or mild scaling. It is not uncommon for there to be **asymptomatic carriers**, especially among Persian cats.

**Dogs** usually have areas of alopecia with **scaling, inflammation and pruritus**. In young dogs, a form called kerion is most common (Figure 4.84).

### Diagnosis

Dermatophytosis is diagnosed with:

- Wood's lamp (Figure 4.59)
- trichoscopy (Figure 4.60)

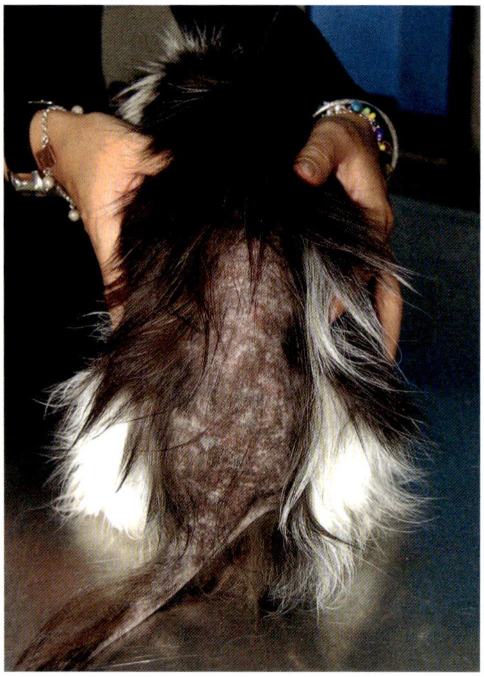

Figure 4.83. Extensive alopecia in a Persian cat due to dermatophytosis.

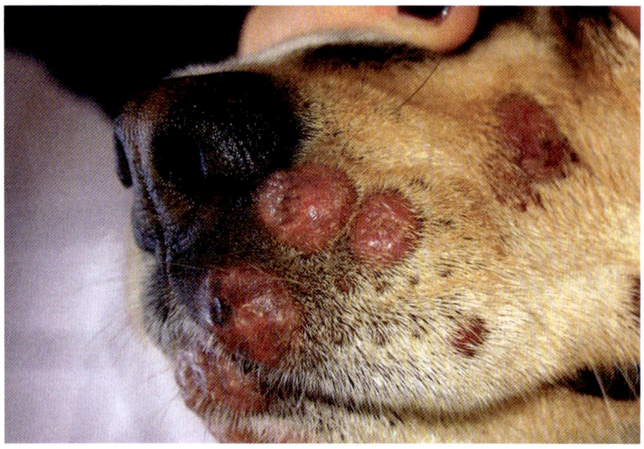

Figure 4.84. Numerous kerions on the snout of a young Husky cross.

- fungal culture
- skin biopsy.

### Treatment

Although dermatophytosis is usually a **self-limiting disease in animals with a normal immune system**, all cases should be treated – especially if it is due to *M. canis*, since transmission to other animals, environmental contamination and the risk of infecting humans are usually significant (more than 50% of people exposed to infected cats will suffer a dermatophytosis, and 15% of human dermatophyte infections are of animal origin).

**Treatment must always be systemic**, even if effects are only localized. The drugs currently used for the systemic treatment of dermatophytosis are:

- **Griseofulvin**. A fungistatic drug that is still widely used in dogs (*50 mg/kg/12 h*), but is better avoided in cats because of its toxicity. Fatty foods help absorption. It is extremely teratogenic, and thus should not be used in breeding animals or before 6 weeks of age.
- **Ketoconazole**. Fungistatic imidazole (*5–10 mg/kg/12–24 h*) that is better absorbed with acidic food. It causes, an elevation in liver enzyme concentrations and, occasionally, hepatotoxicity especially in elderly animals. Liver function must be checked before and during administration to dogs over 6 years of age. It can have gastrointestinal side effects. It should not be administered to pregnant females or to patients less than 6 weeks old.
- **Itraconazole**. Acts in a similar way to ketoconazole, although it is more effective and less toxic. It accumulates in the skin and sebaceous glands and can be administered every other day or every other week (*5–10 mg/kg with food*). In dogs undergoing prolonged treatment at high doses, cases of idiopathic vasculitis with deep, ulcer-like lesions have been described.
- **Terbinafine**. Fungicidal at doses of *30–40 mg/kg/24 h*, on alternate days or weeks. No study has shown that terbinafine is more effective than itraconazole.

Topical treatment reduces the number of spores and hyphae on the skin, as well as environmental pollution, which usually helps reduce the duration of systemic treatment. The usual treatment protocol is a systemic treatment combined with one or two applications per week of a topical antifungal while bathing.

The most effective **topical treatment** consists of azole derivatives (miconazole, ketoconazole, econazole or enilconazole) and calcium polysulfide. **Long-haired animals must be clipped** to make topical treatments more effective. This must, however, be done with care, because trauma to the epidermis provides a gateway to dermatophytes.

Systemic and topical treatment should be administered for a **minimum of 6–8 weeks.** From the end of the fourth week, weekly control fungal cultures should be performed, with samples collected from residual lesions or with the McKenzie brush technique, if there are no lesions. While waiting for results (samples should be cultured for at least 3 weeks), treatment should be continued (topical and systemic), and this can then be suspended once two consecutive negative cultures have been obtained.

**Environmental decontamination** is essential and the area of movement for the animal should also be limited, to minimize its contact with other animals and people. Disinfectants that offer the best results are **common bleach solutions at 1:10–1:100** and enilconazole sprays. Hard surfaces should be cleaned or scrubbed twice per week; curtains and carpets should be vacuumed and even steam-washed; clothes can be washed in a washing machine on cold setting; bowls, toys and brushes should be dipped in diluted chlorine.

## Malassezia *dermatitis*

### *Aetiopathogenesis*

*Malassezia pachydermatis* is considered a **normal inhabitant of the skin**. It is a yeast with 2–7 micrometre-long elliptical cells, appearing as fingerprints on cytological examination (Figure 4.85). Normal desquamation of the skin, the fungistatic properties of the cutaneous hydrolipidic mantle and secretions of the apocrine glands inhibit the excessive growth of *Malassezia*. It can proliferate and **become pathogenic when the skin barrier is broken**, or immunity is weakened. This is what happens, for example, in:

- the skin folds (resulting in skin maceration)
- allergic dermatitis
- hormonal diseases.

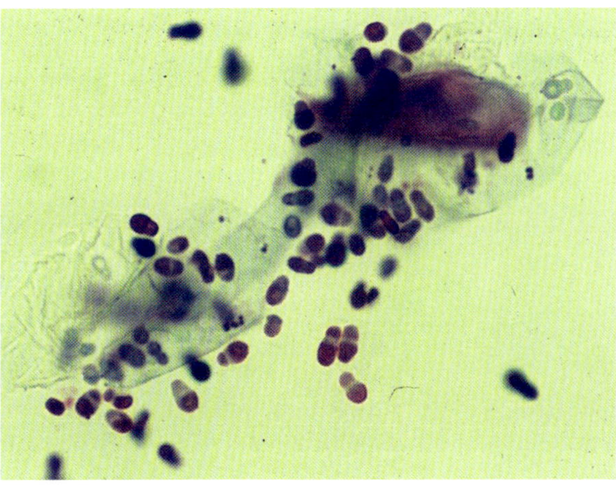

**Figure 4.85.** Cytological image of *Malassezia* yeasts.

In cats, *Malassezia* infection appears with systemic diseases causing immunosuppression, such as:

- feline diabetes
- some tumours
- clinical infections caused by FIV or FeLV.

Excessive *Malassezia* growth may occur simultaneously with *Staphylococcus* spp., suggesting some form of pathogenic synergy.

### *Clinical signs*

Excessive growth of *Malassezia* causes **inflammation, erythema, pruritus** (Figure 4.86) and a **brown discoloration of the nailbed** (Figure 4.87). These yeasts produce lipases that alter the nature of the cutaneous hydrolipidic mantle, creating a layer of wax and fat on the surface. They also express surface antigens against which the host generates an allergic response, increasing itching and inflammation.

### *Diagnosis*

Generally cytological.

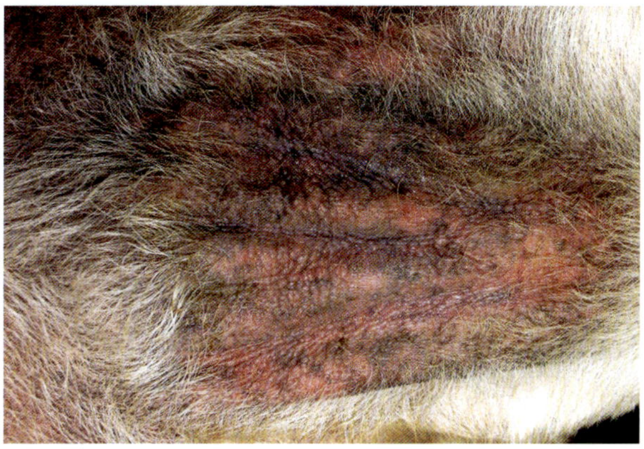

**Figure 4.86.** Inflammation, erythema, alopecia and greasy exudate due to a *Malassezia* dermatitis.

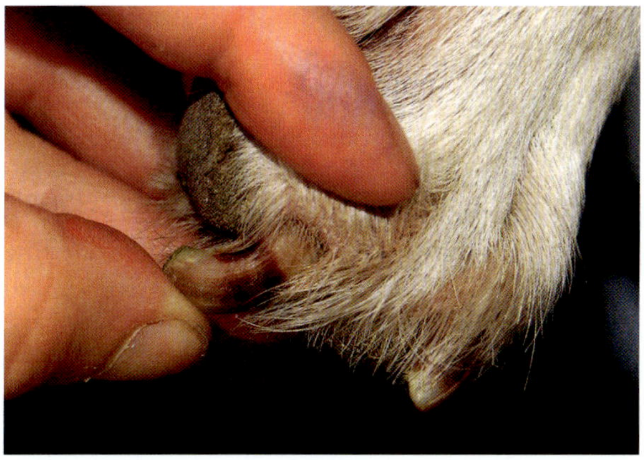

**Figure 4.87.** Brown coloration of the nails caused by a *Malassezia* infection of the nailbed.

### Treatment

The success of treatment depends on the identification and the approach to the underlying cause.

Imidazoles (*ketoconazole 5–10 mg/kg/12 h, itraconazole 5 mg/kg/24 h*) as well as **terbinafine 20–40 mg/kg/24 h**, administered for 2–3 weeks, are effective against *Malassezia*.

Topical treatment alone is also effective, if applied every 2–3 days for 2–3 weeks. Shampoos containing the following are useful:

- 2–4% chlorhexidine
- 2% miconazole + 2% chlorhexidine
- enilconazole.

In cases of resistance or recurrence, periodic treatment with shampoos may be necessary after ceasing systemic therapy.

## Subcutaneous mycoses: mycotic mycetoma and phaeohyphomycosis

### Aetiopathogenesis

Mycetomas and phaeohyphomycosis are deep fungal infections caused by opportunistic soil fungi that penetrate the skin via wounds.

### Clinical signs

They cause a granulomatous reaction with a suppurating fistula which produces a purulent haemorrhagic exudate.

### Diagnosis

Diagnosis is made via cytology with fine-needle aspiration or an impression smear, which reveal a pyogranulomatous reaction with the presence of pigmented fungal hyphae.

Biopsy is recommended in all cases of skin nodules. PAS staining is used to visualize the fungal elements. The fungus causing the infection can be isolated in a fungal culture.

### Treatment

Surgical excision with wide margins is the treatment of choice, although postsurgical recurrence is common. Before the procedure, an antifungal treatment (*itraconazole 5 mg/kg*) should be implemented to reduce the risk of spread, and continued for 3 months after clinical signs appear to have resolved.

### Prognosis

The prognosis depends on the type of fungus and the immune status of the host. In cats, retrovirus infection (FIV, FeLV) should be considered.

## Cryptococcosis

### Aetiopathogenesis

Cryptococcosis is an infection caused by *Cryptococcus neoformans*, a microorganism of the **soil** found commonly, but not exclusively, in the soil, associated with the **faeces of pigeons** and bats. Immunosuppressed individuals (congenital immunosuppression, due to FIV, FeLV or immunosuppressive treatments) are those at highest risk of infection. Cryptococcosis is more common in cats than in dogs.

### Clinical signs

The respiratory system and upper respiratory tract, in particular, are often affected. Infection extends secondarily to other organs, such as the central nervous system, the eyes and the skin. In about 70% of cases where there is upper airway involvement, proliferative lesions appear on the face (Figure 4.88), the nasal plane and the bridge of the nose, which gives rise to a '**Roman nose**' appearance. There may also be ulcerated nodules with fistulae elsewhere on the body, especially on the face and legs.

### Diagnosis

On cytology from an impression smear and fine-needle aspiration, it is common to identify numerous oval or pleomorphic yeast cells, 2–20 µm in length, surrounded by a mucoid capsule (Figure 4.89. Histopathology confirms the diagnosis.

Latex agglutination allows detection of capsule antigens. This test can be used to monitor treatment, although in cats the concentrations drop slowly.

### Treatment

The treatment of choice is based on **imidazole derivatives** (ketoconazole, itraconazole or fluconazole) at doses recommended for treatment of dermatophytes, for at least 4–6 months or until 12 months after apparent clinical resolution.

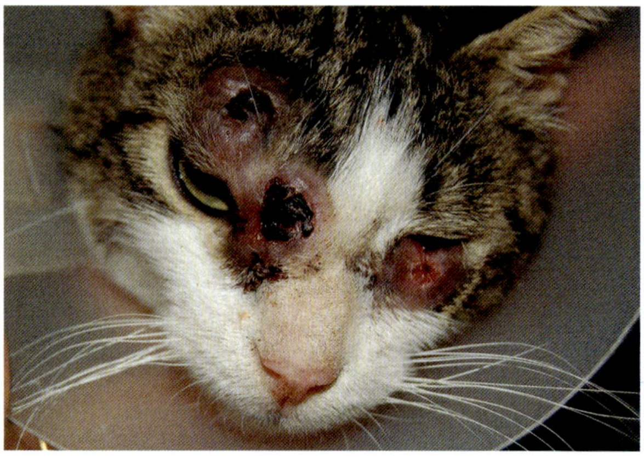

**Figure 4.88.** Ulcerated nodules on the face of a cat with cryptococcosis.

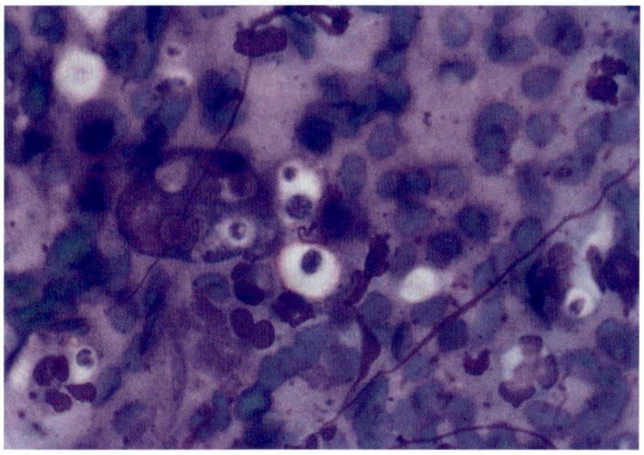

**Figure 4.89.** Cytological image of cryptococcosis: yeast corpuscles surrounded by a transparent capsule together with a macrophage containing other yeasts.

### Prognosis

The prognosis is only favourable in approximately half of cases. Recurrence is common, and cats with central nervous system involvement suffer the worst effects.

## Parasitic diseases

### Ticks

#### Aetiopathogenesis

There is a wide variety of different types of tick, most of which are **visible to the naked eye**. Those of the Ixodidae (hard) family are widespread, encompassing the genera *Ixodes*, *Rhipicephalus*, *Amblyomma* and *Dermacentor* with a life cycle that requires more than one, often wild, host.

Generally, **the tick's life cycle consists of three phases**: larva, nymph and adult, where it feeds on the host, detaches and then returns to the environment. Female ticks produce a large number of eggs.

In the case of *Rhipicephalus sanguineus*, domestic dogs can become infected because **the intermediate stages develop on the same host**. Ticks can survive for prolonged periods in the environment without feeding, even throughout the winter. In temperate zones, transmission occurs mainly in the warmer months.

#### Clinical signs

Although ticks usually cause a simple skin irritation, they may potentially cause paralysis due to the production of toxins as well as being vectors of many diseases, including:

- babesiosis
- *Ehrlichia* or *Rickettsia* infections
- tularaemia
- Lyme's disease.

#### Treatment

To minimize the risk of transmission of infections, **ticks should be removed quickly**, applying a drop of insecticide to them and removing them by gentle traction and rotation. Care should also be taken to also remove the head, otherwise this can cause a foreign body reaction.

Severe infestations can be treated by the administration of an oral isoxazoline.

#### Prevention

Dogs in endemic areas should be given regular **preventative treatment** based on topical liquids containing permethrin or amitraz and/or fipronil, or oral isooxazoline-based products such as fluralaner, afoxalaner or sarolaner. Amitraz, deltamethrin or flumethrin collars are also very effective in preventing ticks from attaching to animals.

### Trombicula

#### Aetiopathogenesis

*Trombicula* mites are **free-living arachnids**, the size of a pinhead (Figure 4.90) and have a characteristic **orange colour**. They live in decomposing organic matter. Their larvae can infect animals but rarely cause infestation, and are generally limited to endemic areas at warmer times of the year.

#### Clinical signs

The lesions they cause almost always appear on **areas of the body in contact with the ground** (legs, abdomen and ears), and consist of pruritic, scabby papules that develop secondarily to the bites of the parasite, causing **alopecia and desquamation**. A **hypersensitivity reaction** to mites is likely to occur, because pruritus may persist after they have been eliminated.

#### Diagnosis

The diagnosis is based on the identification of mites from skin scrapings taken from under the crusts.

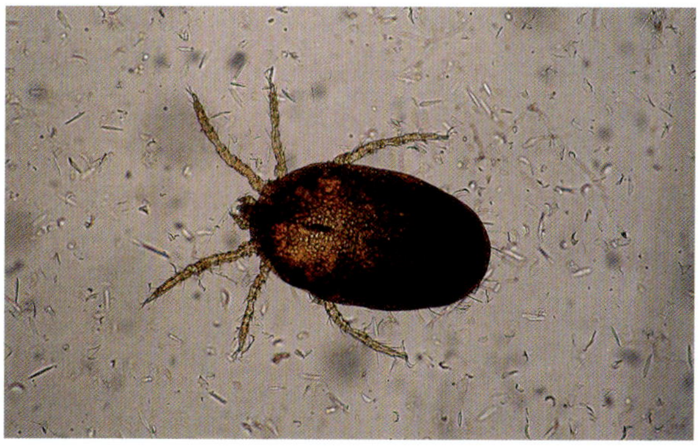

**Figure 4.90.** Microscopic image of a *Trombicula* larva.

#### Treatment

Most **sprays and antiparasitic baths are effective,** although a short course of corticosteroid at anti-inflammatory dosage may be needed to control pruritus.

#### Prevention

The prevention protocol is the same as that for ticks.

### *Ear mites:* Otodectes cynotis

#### Aetiopathogenesis

*Otodectes cynotis* (Figure 4.91) is a psoroptic mite with typically long legs that infests the ears of domestic carnivores. Its **whole life cycle takes place on the epidermis of the host**, almost always **inside the ear**. The eggs take about 3 weeks to evolve into larvae, protonymphs, deutonymphs and then adults. All stages of the life cycle are parasitic, and feed on waste and liquids from the epidermal surface. These mites do not make tunnels. Infection is spread by **direct contact**, especially in younger animals. It is common for infections to be bilateral because the mites move easily from one ear to the other.

When feeding, *Otodectes* mites cause **irritation** in addition to an immune response in the host.

#### Clinical signs

A typical reaction causes a **reddish-brown granular secretion** with a degree of **pruritus** dependent on host sensitivity.

*Otodectes* spp. frequently colonize other parts of the skin and sometimes cause pruritic dermatitis in the periauricular area or on the back, which may look like an allergic dermatopathy (food, fleas or atopic dermatitis).

#### Diagnosis

These mites are identified by **examining secretions from the ears** and skin scrapings from ectopic cases.

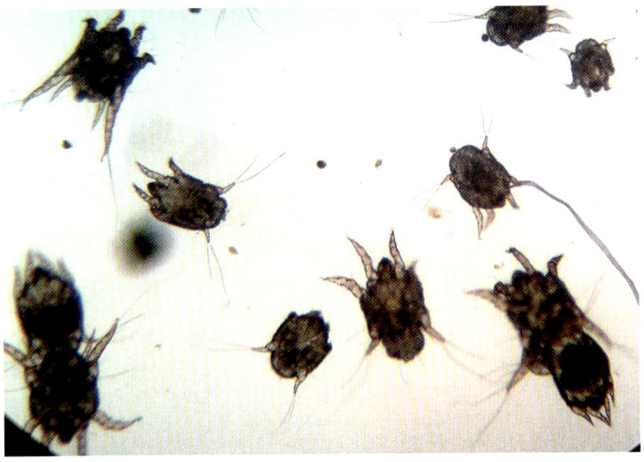

**Figure 4.91.** Microscopic image of *Otodectes cynotis*: numerous mites in the ear wax of an affected cat can be seen.

#### Treatment

*Otodectes* is extremely **contagious**, so all animals in contact with the patient should be considered infected and treated accordingly.

The ears should be cleaned with a suitable ceruminolytic agent. Selamectin, moxidectin and eprinomectin (only for cats) in spot-on form are highly effective, and one to three treatments, 15 days apart, eliminate infection.

### *Cheyletiella*

#### Aetiopathogenesis

*Cheyletiella* spp. (Figure 4.92) are large mites that are easily recognized by their hook-like mouthparts. *Cheyletiella* is a parasite that infects **cats, dogs and rabbits**. The common species are listed below, although the mites are not specific to their host and cross-infestations may occur:

- *C. blakei* is most frequent in cats.
- *C. yasguri* is more typical in dogs.
- *C. parasitivorax* is the most common parasite in the rabbit.

*Cheyletiella* spp. live on the surface of the skin, moving around and perforating the epidermis with their mouthparts and feeding on tissue fluids.

The entire life cycle of the mite takes place on the host's epidermis. Eggs take about 3–5 weeks to evolve into larvae, protonymphs, deutonymphs and adults. Female mites can survive up to 10 days in the environment.

*Cheyletiella* infestations are **highly contagious** by direct contact, environmental contamination and fomites.

#### Epidemiology

Cheyletiellosis is common in animals living in **overcrowded environments**, such as pet shops and breeding kennels.

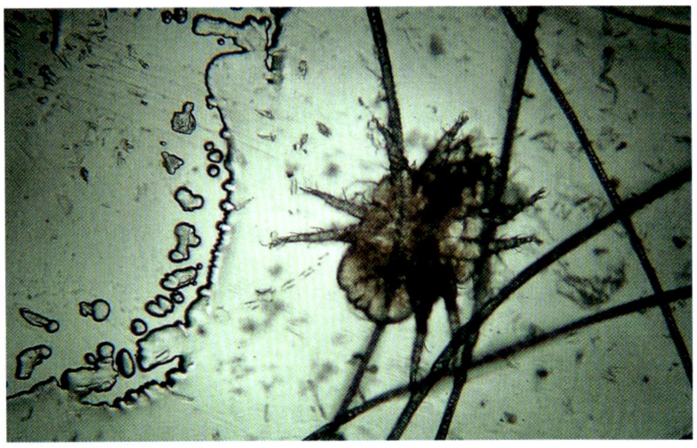

**Figure 4.92.** *Cheyletiella* mite.

### Clinical signs

Affected animals present with typical dry, **small white scales**, located mainly along the back, with a variable degree of pruritus.

*Cheyletiella* spp. can also affect humans, causing pruritic papular dermatitis located on the forearms or abdomen. Owners of an asymptomatic carrier animal may present with symptoms.

### Diagnosis

The diagnosis is confirmed by identifying the mites in:

- A superficial scraping of the scales.
- Collection of scales with transparent adhesive tape.
- Material collected with a flea comb and examined with a faecal flotation solution.

Even if mites are not identified, it does not rule out the diagnosis and, in cases of suspected infestation, a trial treatment is needed.

### Treatment

*Cheyletiella* is sensitive to most topical **antiparasitic products** applied once a week for 3–4 weeks. All animals in contact with the patient, whether symptomatic or not, should be treated.

## Sarcoptic mange

### Aetiopathogenesis

*Sarcoptes scabiei* var. *canis* (Figure 4.93) is the agent responsible for sarcoptic mange. This mite is smaller than *Otodectes* and has shorter legs. *Sarcoptes* is an obligate parasite that **spends the whole of its 3-week life cycle on the host**. The females perforate tunnels in the epidermis, where they deposit faeces and eggs. They feed on tissue waste and tissue. *Sarcoptes scabiei* var. *canis* is a specific canine parasite that rarely affects cats, but can affect foxes and humans, in which it causes pruritic papules. Human infection is self-limiting and resolves when the affected dog is treated. The disease is highly contagious through contact with an infested dog. It is rare that other dogs in contact with the patient do not become infected after a few weeks. After an incubation period of about 15 days, the pruritus, which is intense and of an allergic nature and is not related to the number of mites, progressively increases.

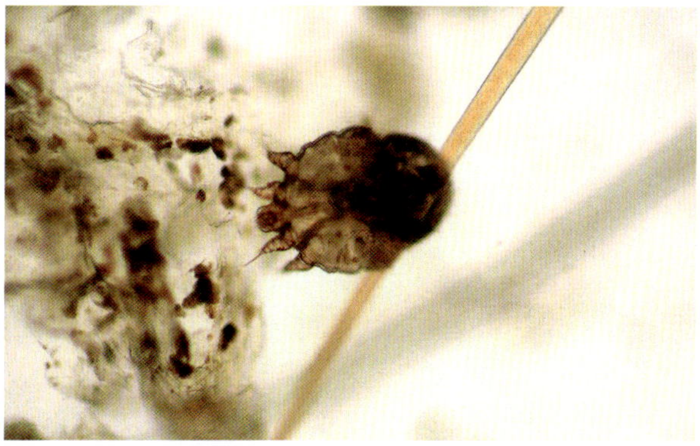

**Figure 4.93.** *Sarcoptes* mite together with a keratin clump containing mite faeces.

### Clinical signs

The first signs are **crusted papules** (Figure 4.94) on the elbows, abdomen and ears. Secondary **alopecia and erythema** appear as a result of self-inflicted trauma. On the lateral aspect of the extremities, alopecia and erythema are observed, indicative of sarcoptic mange (Figure 4.95), as well as desquamation and hyperkeratosis of the edges of the ear and lateral aspects of the elbows.

Dogs scratch incessantly, even in the presence of the veterinarian, and the pruritus is non-responsive to corticosteroids.

### Diagnosis

A **positive pinna-pedal reflex** is an indication of sarcoptic mange.

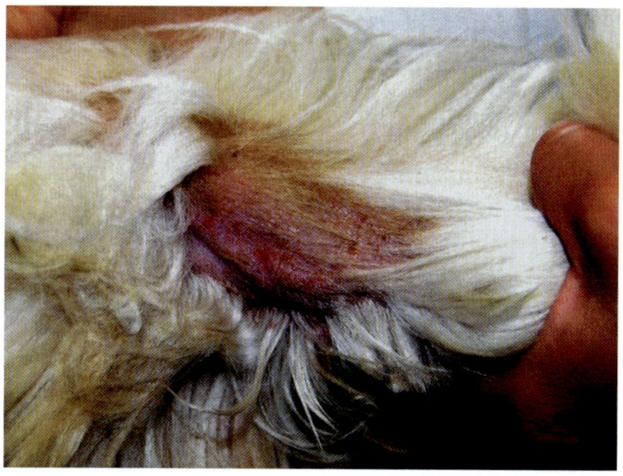

**Figure 4.94.** Papules and crusts on the elbow of a Saluki suffering from sarcoptic mange.

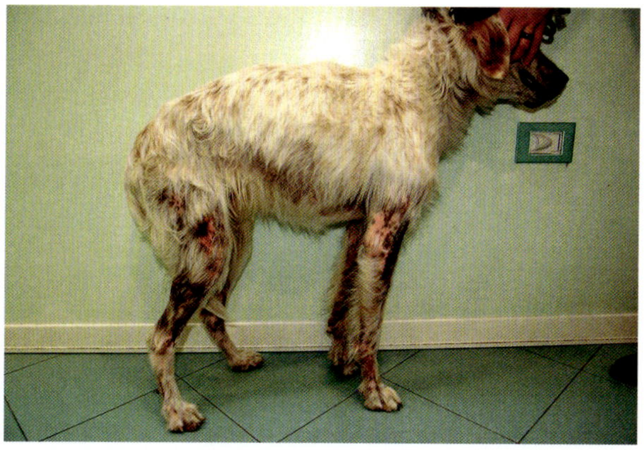

**Figure 4.95.** A dog infected with sarcoptic mange.

The main differential diagnoses are:

- allergic dermatopathy (dietary, allergic dermatitis and flea allergy dermatitis)
- superficial pyoderma.

Diagnosis is confirmed by the presence of mites, eggs or mite faeces (Figure 4.93) on superficial **skin scrapings**. A wide area should be scraped (such as the whole ear) and abundant scales and epidermal residues collected for examination. These mites are very difficult to find, so skin scrapes often give a negative result. In most cases the veterinarian has to resort to a positive response to a trial treatment to confirm the diagnosis.

Another option for diagnosis are serum samples tested for the presence of *Sarcoptes* antibodies. The sample should be taken at least 2–4 weeks after the onset of pruritus, or false negatives may result. When used appropriately, the *Sarcoptes* serology test is 95% reliable in the detection of sarcoptic mange.

### Treatment

Sarcoptic mange is treated by two topical applications of selamectin or moxidectin/imidacloprid every 2 weeks, or by oral sarolaner (*2.5–5 mg/kg*) administration. When mites die, pruritus may increase during the first week of treatment. The pruritus should decrease over the next 3–4 weeks. All dogs in contact with the patient must be treated. Environmental decontamination is not normally necessary because mites can only survive for a short time in the absence of a host.

## Notoedric mange

### Aetiopathogenesis

*Notoedres cati* (Figure 4.96) looks similar to *S. scabiei* but is slightly smaller. The life cycle is similar to that of *Sarcoptes* and the mite is specific to the cat. Notoedric mange is **highly contagious** through contact and appears mostly in feral cats.

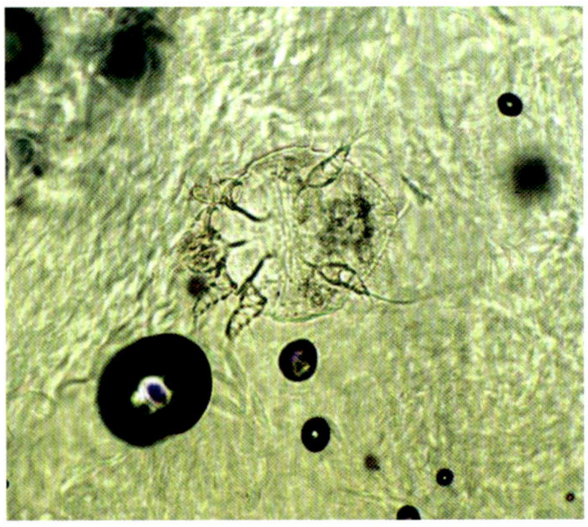

**Figure 4.96.** *Notoedres cati.*

### Clinical signs

The typical lesions are **scales and scabs**, as well as secondary abrasions caused by self-inflicted trauma due to pruritus. It mainly affects the **head and ears** (Figure 4.97), although the infestation extends to the rest of the body when the animal tries to clean itself through licking (for example, forepaws and perineum).

### Diagnosis

The mites are numerous and therefore easy to find on **skin scrapes**.

### Treatment

Cats can be treated with selamectin, moxidectin/imidacloprid or eprinomectin in spot-on form.

Since mites are **extremely contagious**, all cats in contact with the patient should be treated even if they do not present symptoms.

## Canine demodicosis

### Aetiopathogenesis

Three *Demodex* species have been identified in the dog:

- Standard, *D. canis* (Figure 4.58) (250–300 μm), obligate parasite of hair follicles.
- Long-tailed, *D. injai* (Figure 4.98) (334–368 μm), obligate parasite of hair follicles.

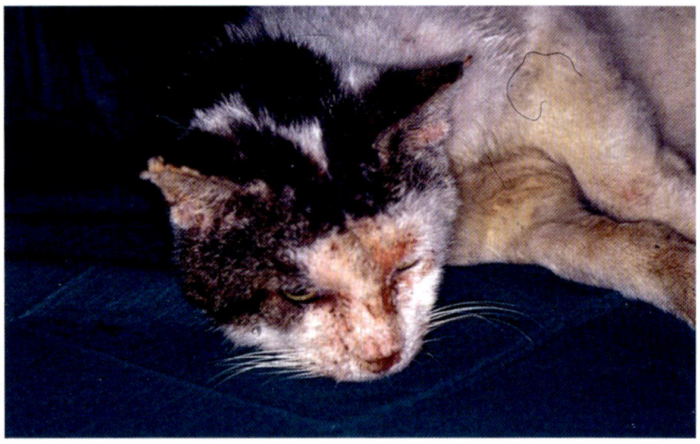

**Figure 4.97.** Cat with notoedric mange: scratches and scabs can be seen on the face due to pruritus.

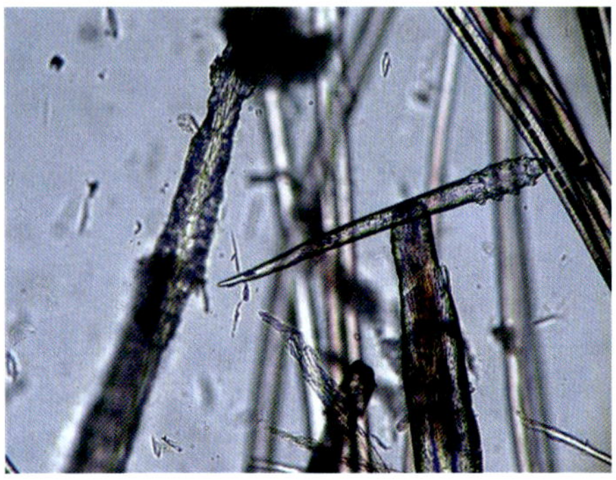

**Figure 4.98.** *Demodex injai.*

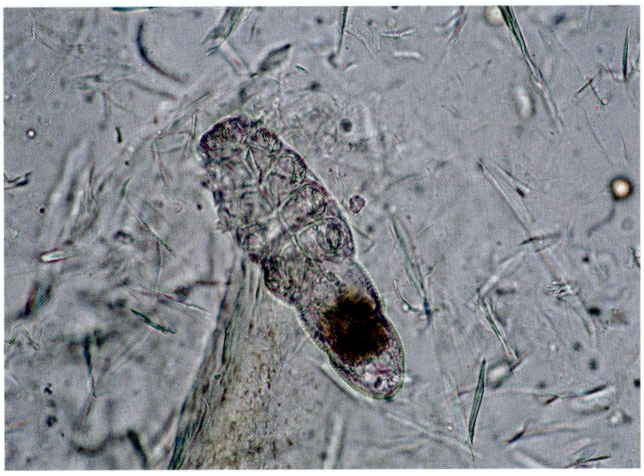

Figure 4.99. *Demodex cornei* (variant of *D. canis*).

- Short, *D. cornei* (Figure 4.99) (90–148 μm), has recently been shown to live in the epidermis and is the same species as *D. canis*.

The **normal cutaneous flora** of mammals contains a small number of *Demodex* individuals. The mite is sensitive to drying and finds survival off the dog difficult. Its life cycle lasts 3–5 weeks, progressing through the different phases of egg, 6-legged larva, 8-legged nymph and adult. It feeds on keratin residues and tissue fluids.

Puppies acquire the infestation during the first days of life, probably when suckling. This explains why the first clinical signs often appear at points of contact with the mother (extremities, face). There is **no intrauterine transmission**: pups born dead or by caesarean section are not infected; they are unlikely to suffer an infestation after 3 days of age.

There is a definite **breed and genetic predisposition** to demodicosis. *D. canis* infestation frequently occurs in the French and English Bulldog breeds, Shar Pei, Great Dane, Dobermann, German Shepherd, Dachshund, Pug and various terriers (especially Bull Terrier and Staffordshire Bull Terrier). Fundamentally in the case of generalized demodicosis, breeding with affected dogs, their siblings or their relatives is strongly contraindicated, (even if they do not present with clinical signs). Cases of isolates of *D. injai* have been published in the Fox and the West Highland White Terrier.

Immunosuppressive drugs (glucocorticoids, progestogens, oclacitinib, etc.) can induce demodicosis, demonstrating the importance of the host immune response in keeping the mite under control.

Systemic diseases associated with outbreaks of demodicosis in adults are:

- spontaneous hyperadrenocorticism
- hypothyroidism
- systemic infections (for example, leishmaniasis)
- neoplasia
- malnutrition
- parasitism
- debilitating systemic diseases.

However, approximately one-quarter of the cases of demodicosis in adults do not present with a detectable underlying disease.

## *Clinical signs*

Two forms of demodicosis are identified:

### Localized

This is usually seen in animals **under 1 year of age**. The lesions consist of **focal alopecia** (between one and five), usually on the **face or limb**. Many cases resolve spontaneously, although some may progress and become generalized.

### Generalized

This may evolve from a localized case, or it can appear suddenly.

Based on the immunological characteristics described above, there are two well differentiated forms:

- **juvenile** onset (in dogs less than 2 years of age)
- **adult** onset.

Generalized demodicosis presents multiple, confluent areas of infestation that affect:

- the **legs** (pododemodicosis).
- the **external auditory canal** (otodemodicosis).

In the absence of a secondary infection and depending on the severity, demodicosis lesions can involve:

- areas of alopecia (Figure 4.56)
- with or without erythema
- hyperpigmentation
- scales
- comedones (Figure 4.100).

With this appearance, the differential diagnoses are:

- bacterial folliculitis
- dermatophytosis
- alopecia areata.

In cases of secondary infection, lesions seen are:

- pustules
- furunculosis
- scabs
- haemorrhagic blisters (Figures 4.79 and 4.101).

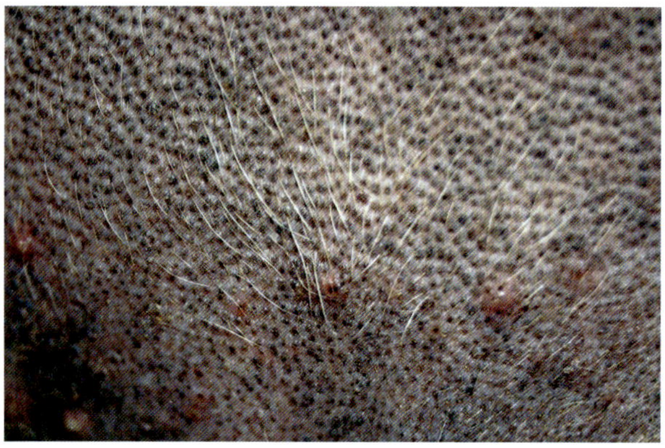

**Figure 4.100.** Numerous comedones and alopecia in a dog with demodicosis.

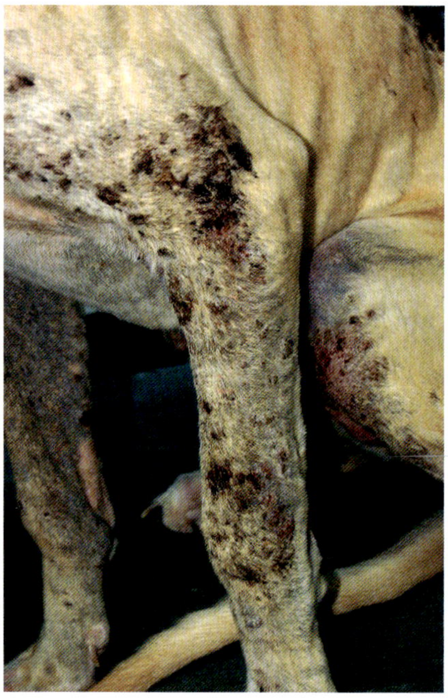

**Figure 4.101.** Alopecia, comedones, pustules, fistula and haemorrhagic crusts in a young Great Dane with generalized demodicosis.

*Staphylococcus pseudintermedius* is the most frequent cause of secondary bacterial infection.

Pruritus is a variable sign. Cases without secondary infection are not usually pruritic, unlike those with severe secondary infections, where pruritus and systemic are usually present, signs such as:

- lymphadenopathy
- fever
- depression.

## Diagnosis

Demodicosis is diagnosed by **deep skin scrapings or trichoscopy**. In most cases the host has a large number of mites, which confirms the diagnosis.

In active infections adults, nymphs, larvae and eggs can be seen.

In cases of otodemodicosis, a large number of mites are seen when examining smears of ceruminous secretion mixed with a drop of mineral oil.

A cytological examination of pustules should be performed in search of bacteria. During staining of the slides, mites may be lost. Unstained mites, with their characteristic shape standing out against a mantle of neutrophils, can be seen.

In chronic fibrotic lesions, such as interdigital granulomas associated with pododemodicosis, in which cutaneous scraping is difficult or impossible, skin biopsy is indicated.

## Treatment

Several authors claim that localized demodectic mange does not require treatment. These claims are based on the fact that **most cases of localized demodicosis resolve spontaneously**. In addition, there is a risk of selecting resistant strains of *Demodex* and masking possible generalized cases that should be **removed from any breeding programme** (together with their siblings and parents). However, if the localized lesions multiply or increase in size, then they should be treated as a generalized demodicosis.

Amitraz, an effective product registered for use in canines in many countries, is a diamine derivative that inhibits monoamine oxidase (MAO). It is an extremely effective acaricide, often providing a rapid reduction in the number of mites that appear on skin scrapings. The commercial product is diluted immediately before application with a sponge over the dog's body.

Dogs with severe infestations or with a long coat should be completely clipped.

Dogs with a secondary infection, excessive desquamation or exudation, or with numerous comedones, are treated with a **2.5% benzoyl peroxide shampoo**, a substance that has disinfectant, astringent and keratolytic properties, as well as the ability to draw waste from hair follicles, facilitating the entry of amitraz. Before applying an amitraz solution, the dog must be dried to avoid dilution of the miticidal agent. Healing rates have been obtained in the range of 80% by applying a 0.125% solution daily, alternating over each half of the body. In cases of moderately intense generalized demodicosis, authors recommend applying 0.05% solution every 2–3 days: medication should be applied with gloves and a sponge all over the skin, including the interdigital spaces, and left to dry on the body without rinsing. The treatment should be administered outdoors or in a well-ventilated room. Side effects are relatively common: up to 40% of patients will experience lethargy, depression or transient pruritus. These signs disappear after a few days, although sometimes they require a reduction in the concentration or an increase in treatment intervals. Occasionally the treatment causes serious side effects such as:

- severe depression
- ataxia
- anorexia
- polydipsia/polyuria.
- Amitraz should not be administered in the following cases:
- In the Chihuahua and miniature breeds, and if at all in very low concentrations.
- In diabetic dogs, because it causes hyperglycaemia (for that same reason, it should not be administered by diabetics).
- Along with certain drugs:
- MAO inhibitors (for example, antihistamines, such as doxepine or hydroxyzine).
- Anaesthetics or sedatives such as α2 adrenergic agonists (xylazine, medetomidine).

Treatment of toxic side effects is by yohimbine administration and supportive treatment.

An alternative to amitraz baths is **spot-on products** based on this active ingredient, which can be applied every 1–2 weeks. Unfortunately, cases of localized or generalized pemphigus foliaceus have been described after the use of these products.

*Milbemycin oxime (0.5–2 mg/kg/24 h PO)* is a good alternative and can be used safely even in dogs that are sensitive to ivermectin, although products which only contain this active ingredient are no longer marketed in Europe.

Moxidectin/imidacloprid applied as a spot-on every 1–2 weeks can be effective in mild cases, and as a preventive treatment once a month for future recurrence of the disease, but is not able to eradicate serious infestations.

It was recently published that **fluralaner,** a new antiparasitic derived from isoxazoline that causes selective inhibition of gamma-aminobutyric acid channels and those controlled by glutamate, characteristic of arthropods, with **insecticidal and acaricidal activity**, is very effective after a **single administration at 50 mg/kg**.

One of the most frequent causes of treatment failure is when treatment is ceased prematurely. Skin scrapings should be examined once a month and treatment should continue until two consecutive negative skin scrapes are obtained at 2-week intervals. It is uncommon for dogs to return after a first check-up with a negative scraping – usually 2–3 months of treatment are needed.

After a period of treatment, if the number of mites is not reduced and especially if they can be seen actively reproducing (eggs, larvae and nymphs are seen), an alternative treatment should be considered.

It is common for there to be a secondary infection, often caused by staphylococci. These cases require antibiotic treatment for 4–6 weeks with:

- *Cephalexin (20–30 mg/kg/12 h)*
- *Cefadroxil (20–30 mg/kg/24 h)*
- *Amoxicillin + clavulanic acid (15–25 mg/kg/12 h).*

If bacilli are observed on cytology, treatment should be based on culture and sensitivity tests.

Any **underlying disease**, especially for adult-onset demodicosis, must be rigorously investigated and treated accordingly. Females should be neutered to avoid the genetic transmission of predisposition to the disease and its recurrence after oestrus and birth.

In all cases of demodicosis, local or systemic administration of drugs that inhibit the host's immune response, preventing healing or inducing recurrence, are **strictly contraindicated**:

- corticosteroids
- progestogens
- other immunosuppressive drugs.

### Prognosis

**Recurrence may occur at times of stress** (oestrus, pregnancy, lactation or with any systemic disease). Cases of onset in adulthood tend to recur if the underlying cause progresses uncontrollably (for example, spontaneous hyperadrenocorticism), if it is not treated or it remains unidentified.

When the underlying causative disease is not identified, prognosis is more reserved, because it could be due to a congenital immunodeficiency.

## Feline demodicosis

### Aetiopathogenesis

Feline demodicosis is associated with three types of *Demodex*:

- *D. cati*. Elongated mite that lives in the hair follicles and sebaceous glands (Figure 4.102).
- *D. gatoi*. Small mite with a short, blunt tail that infests only the superficial epidermis.
- A third species, unnamed.

### Clinical signs

The most common presentation of the disease caused by *D. cati* is a **scaly and erythematous dermatitis** with

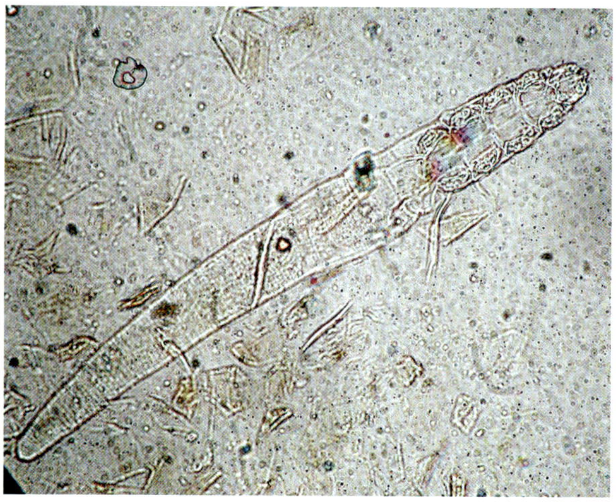

**Figure 4.102.** *Demodex cati.*

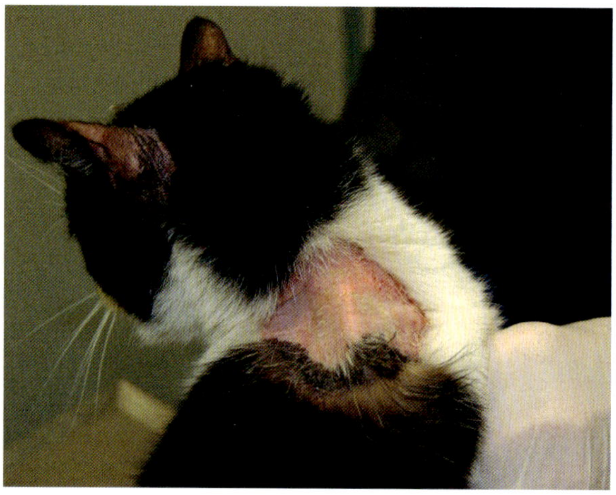

**Figure 4.103.** Demodicosis lesions in a cat treated with various prednisolone acetate depot injections.

a variable degree of pruritus, located on the head and neck, especially on the eyelids and periocular skin; and a ceruminous otitis.

Generalized demodicosis is rare and is associated with an **underlying immunosuppressive disease** such as FIV/FeLV, diabetes mellitus or a tumour (Figure 4.103). These animals have areas of alopecia, scaling and scabs that affect the head and then spread to the rest of the body.

Demodicosis caused by *D. gatoi* is rare and contagious. It can be identified in superficial skin scrapings in cases of pruritus, especially in cats that lick excessively. Some cases present as pruritus, with self-inflicted trauma and scabs, on:

- head
- neck
- shoulders.

It should be differentiated from other, more serious, forms of allergic dermatitis or notoedric mange.

### Diagnosis

Differential diagnoses for feline demodicosis include:

- dermatophytosis
- diseases in which pruritus manifests as excessive licking or self-inflicted trauma:
  - allergies
  - psychogenic alopecia
  - ectoparasites (*Cheyletiella*, *Notoedres*).

### Treatment

These mites are not difficult to eradicate, but it is important to look for an underlying pathological condition, especially in the case of *D. cati*. Generally, amitraz is well tolerated and effective (0.0125–0.0250% every 5 days for 4–6 weeks). Calcium polysulfide-based products are safe and effective. In mild or moderate cases, application of moxidectin/imidacloprid in the form of spot-on once per week is useful.

## Lice

### Aetiopathogenesis

Lice are **species-specific obligate parasites**. The **whole life cycle takes place on the host** and they cannot survive long in the environment. The adult louse has strong legs with appendages that allow it to move and attach firmly to the hairs. Common biting lice of domestic carnivores are:

- The canine louse *Trichodectes canis* (easily recognisable due to its characteristic rounded head).
- The feline louse *Felicola subrostrata*, with a characteristic pointed head.

The female produces eggs called nits, which evolve into adults within 2–3 weeks. Infestation is acquired by contact.

The biting lice **feed on epidermal debris** and irritate the host as they move through the hair.

### Clinical signs

Clinical pediculosis is an infrequent disease, associated mainly with very young or weak animals. Most healthy cats are able to eliminate lice as soon as they are caught. Lice can cause seborrhoea and self-inflicted trauma due to their irritant action.

### Diagnosis

The diagnosis is simple, as lice are visible to the naked eye or with a magnifying glass.

### Treatment

Lice are easy to eliminate with most common insecticides. Two separate treatments are needed approximately 2 weeks apart in order to kill the nymphs that hatch from the nits.

## Fleas

### Aetiopathogenesis

There are more than 2000 species of fleas capable of infesting mammals and birds. In order of prevalence, the fleas that most frequently infest the dog and the cat are:

- cat flea (*Ctenocephalides felis*) (Figure 4.104).
- dog flea, most specific to the canine species (*Ctenocephalides canis*).
- human fleas (*Pulex irritans* and *P. simulans*).
- hen flea (*Echidnophaga gallinacea*).

Fleas spend their whole life on the same host. Since they need an uninterrupted source of blood to feed on, **they rarely move from one animal to another**. After mating, the female flea is capable of producing up to 2000 eggs during its life time, which is about 100 days. Eggs are dry and smooth and fall off the host into the environment, where 2-mm larvae emerge; these are mobile and capable of moving about 1 m per day, presenting positive geotropism and negative phototropism (looking for dark and quiet places underneath carpets, furniture, cracks and recesses, to finish their development). The diet of the larvae consists of organic waste and adult flea faeces (95% blood), and they double their size in just a few days. After two moults, pupae form within a cocoon in which they transform into pre-emergent adults; they can remain in this state for several months until the movement of a potential host stimulates their emergence. Generally, in an environment infested with fleas, pre-emergent adults are much more numerous within cocoons than larval or adult forms.

The larvae require an **ambient temperature higher than 16°C** and a relative humidity above 50%, conditions provided in the microclimate of its secluded environment. Under ideal circumstances, the flea can complete its life cycle in 2 weeks although it can survive in the cocoon phase for up to 1 year. In temperate areas during winter, the cycle cannot be completed outside but they continue indoors, in carpets, furniture, nooks and crannies.

In addition to the irritation they cause the host, fleas have other possible pathogenic effects:

- Saliva is a powerful allergen.
- By feeding on blood, they can cause anaemia.
- They are a vector for pathogens that cause diseases, including:
  - tapeworm (*Dipylidium caninum*)
  - filariasis (*Dipetalonema reconditum*)
  - Lyme's disease
  - plague (*Yersinia pestis*)
  - cat scratch disease (*Bartonella henselae*).

### Clinical signs

In dogs that are allergic to flea bites (Figure 4.105), the **predominant symptom is pruritus** which manifests as:

- scratching
- licking
- biting the skin.

Affected areas are usually:

- base of the tail
- perineum
- lumbar area
- lateral surfaces of the thighs
- inguinal region.

In chronic cases, the entire dorso-lumbar area may be affected and present with:

- alopecia
- hyperpigmentation

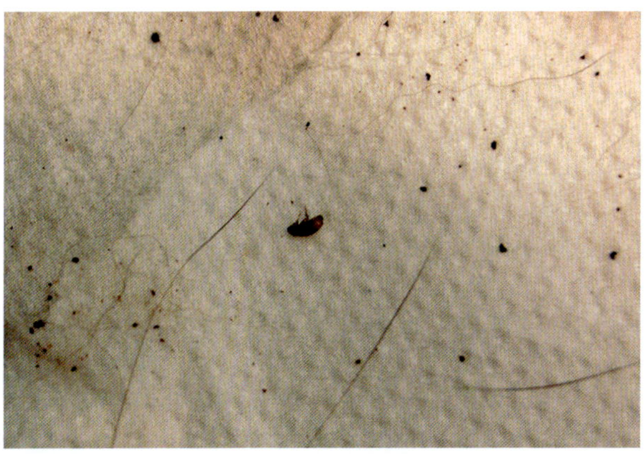

**Figure 4.104.** A flea and its faeces, from the hair of a cat infected with fleas.

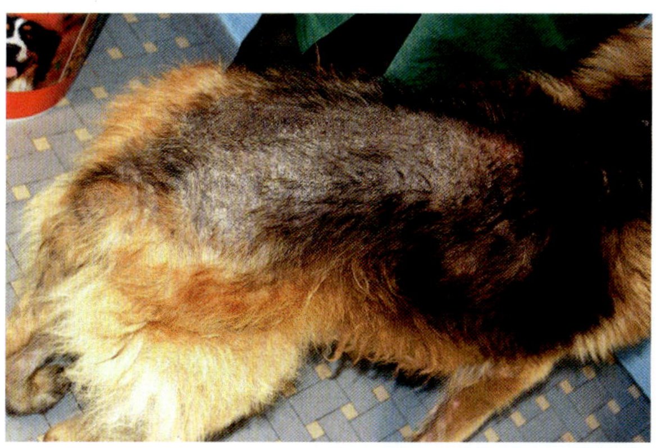

**Figure 4.105.** Serious flea bite allergy in a German Shepherd.

- lichenification
- seborrhoea
- areas of secondary pyoderma (which increases itching).

In cats, the lesions consist of:

- miliary dermatitis
- alopecia caused by licking the abdominal and inguinal regions
- eosinophilic plaques.

Some cats have lumbar signs similar to those in dogs, possibly accompanied by miliary dermatitis on the neck.

## Flea treatment and prevention

Two of the factors most important for successful flea control are efficacy and safety. Efficacy depends on:

- killing adult parasites
- reducing or eliminating environmental reserves
- avoiding new infestations
- residual activity on the pet or objects in its environment.

Substances effective against fleas usually belong to one of these categories:

- those that kill adult fleas (**adulticides**)
- those that inhibit the development of some stage prior to the adult (**insect growth regulators**).

**Adulticides** should be **applied to the animal** before fleas can bite and provoke an allergic reaction. They do not prevent environmental infestation, such as in the home.

**Insect growth regulators** are necessary to **inhibit the development of eggs and larvae**, which constitute the vast majority of the flea population. Used alone for extended periods of time, they can reduce environmental infestation levels but will not prevent the allergic animal from suffering from bites by adult fleas from outside the house. Therefore, to achieve effective flea control, especially in allergic animals, and to break the flea's life cycle at, at least two points, **both types of product are used together**.

### Adulticides

In the cat flea, which is the most frequent species in dogs, cats and ferrets, it has been documented that it has developed resistance to some older insecticides, so new families are constantly being investigated. Molecules with a prolonged residual activity are usually preferred, because they are more convenient for the owner and improve treatment compliance.

#### *Pyrethroids*

Synthetic pyrethroids have anticholinesterase activity, a rapid paralysing effect, relatively low toxicity (some, such as permethrin, should not be applied in cats) and a repellent effect against:

- fleas
- mosquitoes
- *Phlebotumus*.

These compounds do not inhibit larval development, and their main drawback is the relatively short duration of activity. They are usually included in spot-on products and collars.

#### *Nitempyran*

With oral nitempyran, a flea infestation can be eliminated effectively and quickly, the effects being seen 15–30 minutes after administration. Therefore, it is an excellent means of diagnosis if it is administered as soon as the dog enters the clinic, as fleas can be seen falling onto the table during the examination. It should also be administered to any hospitalized animal, to avoid environmental contamination of the clinic. However, the **duration of effect is very short** (elimination of >90% in 24 hours in the dog and in 48 hours in the cat) and therefore it is **not practical as a prevention method** against fleas (it should be administered every 24–48 hours), although it may be a good alternative in animals with very sensitive skin (those that do not tolerate any type of topical application). Nitempyran can be given to cats and dogs >4 weeks of age. In younger animals, fipronil should be applied as a spray.

#### *Fipronil*

Fipronil belongs to the new family of phenylpyrazoles. It is a non-competitive inhibitor of gamma-aminobutyric acid (GABA) that blocks the Cl channels in neurons. It is available in the form of either a 0.25% spray or 10% spot-on formulation, for both dogs and cats. It has a very **low toxicity**, even if swallowed or inhaled, and can be applied to very small puppies (product information from the manufacturer). Its **adulticidal effect can last for 1 month**. However, the paralysing effect of fipronil is minimal, which allows some fleas to feed and reproduce before dying.

Neither the spray nor the spot-on is absorbed through the skin, but is evenly distributed throughout the lipid layer of the entire body's epidermis. To achieve optimal distribution of fipronil, it is important **not to bath the animal during the 3 days before and 3 days following application**. On the third day after administration, the animal can be bathed without the insecticide losing activity.

Fipronil has also been used in association with methoprene to kill flea eggs and larvae, with methoprene and amitraz to improve its anti-tick effect, and recently with permethrin to provide a repellent effect against ticks and flying insects.

Recently a number of generic products have appeared on the market in spot-on format based on fipronil. Since they are different formulations and transporters, there is little information on whether their effectiveness against fleas is comparable to that of the original branded product.

### *Imidacloprid*

Imidacloprid belongs to the chloronicotinyl nitroguanidine family, which binds to the nicotinyl receptors on postsynaptic neurons and blocks neuronal transmission. It is marketed as a spot-on product for dogs and cats, with **efficacy for up to 4 weeks**. It is quickly distributed on the skin after its topical application between the shoulder blades (*10 mg/kg*) and is not affected by heavy rain or sunlight (manufacturer's technical profile on the product).

The paralysing effect of imidacloprid is minimal, which allows some fleas to feed on the animal before dying. Studies show a very low toxicity.

In dogs it has also been associated with permethrin, broadening its effects against fleas, ticks and sandflies; moxidectin as an active endectocide against intestinal nematodes, filarial larvae and skin mites, including *Sarcoptes*, *Notoedres*, *Otodectes* and *Demodex*. Recently, a new collar has been marketed containing imidacloprid and flumethrin, impregnated in an innovative polymer matrix that allows controlled and constant release of the active ingredients for up to 8 months, both for dogs and cats.

### *Selamectin*

Selamectin, an avermectin derived from doramectin, is absorbed systemically and accumulates in sebaceous glands, from which it is released onto the skin. It is registered for administration in both cats and dogs, and is active against:

- fleas
- various mites (not against *Demodex*)
- microfilariae
- some helminths.

In a spot-on format, the product, administered at a dose of 6 mg/kg, is **effective for one month** until its activity declines over time, similar to fipronil and imidacloprid. It takes longer to kill fleas than other products in spot-on formulations (24–36 hours). Selamectin has ovicidal and larvicidal activity, and its spread in flea faeces guarantees a rapid reduction in the number of these parasites in the environment.

### *Pyriprole*

Recently a new phenylpyrazole has been launched, pyriprole (from the same class as fipronil), which is used against fleas and ticks in the form of a **once-monthly spot-on**. It has only been registered for use in dogs and has no larvicidal or ovicidal effect for fleas.

### *Metaflumizone*

Metaflumizone is a parasiticide belonging to a new class of molecules marketed for use in cats and dogs. It is **active against fleas for 6 weeks** (manufacturer's claim).

The product available for dogs also contains amitraz, an excellent acaricidal molecule, which gives it an additional effect against ticks. A recent article reported the appearance of cases of localized or generalized pemphigus foliaceus after the application of the combination of metaflumizone combined with amitraz, which is the reason why it has since been withdrawn from the market in some countries.

### *Spinosad*

Spinosad is a new adulticide for dogs and cats that is administered **orally once per month** and that promises to be at least as effective as topical products, with the advantage that during treatment the animal can be bathed frequently with shampoos. It can be very useful for animals with:

- skin infections
- allergies
- keratinization disorders
- pruritus.

### *Dinotefuran*

Dinotefuran is a fast-acting insecticide that binds to a single point on the nerve synapses of fleas, even without them feeding on blood. The product available for dogs also contains permethrin and pyriproxyfen, to achieve rapid paralysis and an ovicidal and larvicidal effect. The **monthly spot-on preparation** is registered against:

- fleas
- ticks
- lice
- mites
- *Phlebotumus*.

The spot-on product for cats contains dinotefuran and pyriproxyfen.

### *Indoxacarb*

The most recently commercialized compound is indoxacarb, a pro-insecticide with a new concept: it has to be bioactivated by insect enzymes to generate the active *N*-decarboxymethylated metabolite capable of killing fleas and ticks. In mammals, indoxacarb is metabolized into inactive molecules in the liver and is not toxic, so the US EPA has classified it as a reduced risk pesticide. It is sold as a monthly spot-on for cats and dogs.

### *Isoxazolines*

Isoxazolines are a new class of synthetic oral parasiticides that act on insect GABA and glutamate receptors, causing excessive neuronal stimulation and death. Its efficacy has been proven against:

- fleas
- ticks
- mites, including *Sarcoptes* and *Demodex*, although for the latter it is not yet registered.

It is safe in dogs, including those with *MDR1* mutations (breeds such as the Collie and similar), breeding animals, pregnant and lactating bitches, and puppies over 8 weeks of age. Side effects are rare (1–4%) and can cause diarrhoea or anorexia. It seems that there are no interactions with other drugs.

Three isoxazolines have been marketed for domestic carnivores:

- Afoxolaner. Dogs are given a dose of *2.7–6.9 mg/kg PO*, once a month. Eight hours after administration, it is effective for **5 weeks against fleas and for 1 month against ticks**; there is circumstantial evidence of its effectiveness against *Demodex*. The product is absorbed quickly and is highly bioavailable, regardless of the type of food.
- Fluralaner. Administered to dogs at a dose of *25–56 mg/kg PO*. It is **effective against fleas 8 hours after administration**, against Ixodes and Dermacentor **for 12 weeks and** Rhipicephalus **for 8 weeks**. Two recently published articles confirm that it is also effective against *Demodex*. Gastrointestinal absorption is good, although it must be administered with food because of its low bioavailability. Soon a new topical product will be commercialized as a spot-on based on fluralaner, for both dogs and cats.
- Sarolaner. A new oral molecule, this is effective for 5 weeks against fleas, ticks and sarcoptic mange in the dog, and will be marketed shortly.

### Insect growth regulators

Insect growth regulators (IGRs) **interfere with the development of pre-adult stages** that constitute the vast majority of the population (up to 99% of the total flea population. They have a low toxicity in mammals, because they are very specific and act on metabolic pathways in insects. IGRs alone cannot be used to completely eliminate infestations in animals that come and go from the home, because they may bring adult fleas in from outside. For this reason, adulticides should also always be applied periodically to all animals in the household. There are two main classes of IGR:

- chitin synthesis inhibitors
- juvenile hormone analogues.

### *Juvenile hormone analogues*

Juvenile hormone analogues are effective against larval development and egg-hatching stages. Immature larvae need endogenous juvenile hormones for their development but, to reach the pupal stage, concentrations of these hormones have to fall to very low concentrations. Adult fleas need these hormones again to produce eggs, although these eggs must lack them in order to hatch. Therefore, synthetic analogues of these hormones may inhibit the mutation to pupa and egg hatching, thus breaking the reproductive cycle in the environment. Juvenile hormone analogues include:

- Methoprene. Sold in the form of spray or nebulizer for the environment, and as a spot-on (associated with fipronil) for application to the animal. The manufacturer states that, applied to the animal, it can kill newly laid eggs before they fall to the ground. Methoprene has a very low toxicity and a very long residual effect (up to 3–4 months) providing it is protected from direct sunlight, which degrades it rapidly. Therefore, it must be applied by spraying the animal every month.
- Pyriproxyfen. Commercialized as a spray for application in dogs only in association with either micro-encapsulated permethrin or dinotefuran, in a spot-on formulation for dogs and cats. Pyriproxyfen can kill eggs as soon as they are placed on the animal, and is even capable of sterilizing them within the female flea before they are laid (manufacturer's product information). This IGR is effective for approximately 2 months, and the hair of treated animals can prevent the development of fleas in the environment for up to four weeks. A recent study suggests that pyriproxyfen should also be able to kill adult fleas if they are exposed to it for at least 10 days. Both toxicity and effective concentration are very low.

## Formulation

The formulation of an insecticide is an important factor affecting its efficacy and safety.

### Powders

These usually contain pyrethrin, pyrethroids and carbamates. They have a good paralysing effect and are relatively safe, even in puppies and kittens, thanks to their low concentration of active ingredients. The disadvantages of powders are:

- They are usually sticky.
- They dry out the skin and coat.
- They are difficult to distribute evenly over the body.
- They are very short-lasting (up to 1 week).

### Flea collars

Their effects against fleas are usually considered unsatisfactory and are not recommended, but the new imidacloprid/flumethrin-based collar recently marketed is an exception.

### Shampoos

These usually contain pyrethrin, pyrethroids and carbamates. Although very useful for eliminating fleas from the host, unfortunately they do not have even the slightest residual activity after being rinsed off.

### Baths and sprays

These are applied on the coat and left to dry. They usually have a rapid paralysing effect. Depending on the product, this effect can last from 3 days to 2 months. Because some can be toxic to cats or younger animals, it is important to read the instructions carefully; also, toxicity can be increased if applied to damaged skin. Cats do not like sprays, so they can be difficult to treat.

### Spot-on formulations

These can be absorbed (selamectin) or distributed evenly over the surface of the skin without being absorbed (fipronil, imidacloprid, pyriprole, metaflumizone, indoxacarb, dinotefuran). The spot-on formulation is excellent for cats and small dogs, but in large dogs it does not always reach the most distant body regions and has a slow paralysing effect. Some of the products mentioned require that the lipid layer of the epidermis be intact, to allow uniform spread over all body regions – they cannot be applied the same day as a shampoo.

### Oral preparations

Tablets on the market contain adulticides (nitempyran, spinosad, isoxazolides). They flea must bite the animal to be effective.

## Physical control measures

Certain physical measures can help control fleas:

- **Surfaces should be washed** to remove organic matter and the flea faeces on which the larvae feed.
- A **vacuum cleaner** is able to eliminate 20% of larvae and up to 60% of eggs, as well as flea faeces and organic matter. In addition, vacuuming helps sprays penetrate carpets better because it straightens the fibres.
- Bedclothes and other **washable items should be washed at the highest possible temperature**.
- Carpets and upholstered furniture should not be washed, because the humidity favours development of larvae.

### Causes of treatment failure

To achieve the best results, the animal's owner must follow the flea control program exactly. If appropriate active ingredients are chosen, lack of owner compliance is by far the most common reason for treatment failure, more so than resistance. Talking to the owner is almost always sufficient to detect the problem. The veterinarian has to explain to clients how fleas reproduce and the basics of the control programme. If lack of owner compliance is ruled out, treatment failure may be due to:

- Ineffective products being used.
- Insufficient doses being used.
- Not all dogs and cats in the household being treated.
- Products not being used in accordance to the frequency necessary for the levels of infestation and local seasonal factors.
- An adulticide is being applied without an IGR, or vice versa.

## Other parasitic insects

### Aetiopathogenesis

Some species of Hymenoptera (bees and wasps) may sting domestic animals. Mosquitoes and biting flies (for example, *Stomoxys calcitrans*) attack hairless areas, such as the nose, the tips of the ears and the abdomen.

### Clinical signs

Insect bites may be:

- asymptomatic
- symptomatic
- hard papules
- necrosis secondary to vasculitis
- eosinophilic furunculosis.

Reactions to stings can also cause:

- urticaria
- angioedema
- occasionally, anaphylaxis and shock.

### Treatment

In mild cases timely application of a **topical corticosteroid** relieves the symptoms, but prevention is important.

### Prevention

Repellents or insecticides containing microencapsulated permethrin and/or piperonyl butoxide can be applied, especially at times of increased activity of the insects responsible. Repellents alone are sometimes not enough to control hypersensitivity to mosquitoes; therefore, some animals must be confined in a mosquito-proof environment during the afternoon/evening.

## Cutaneous myiasis

### Aetiopathogenesis

Cutaneous myiasis is caused by **fly larvae deposited on the skin**. It is associated mainly with neglected or weak animals, and occurs on **exudative wounds** or those on the perineum, due to maceration caused by urine and faeces. Some isolated cases of tropical forms of aggressive cutaneous myiasis have been seen far from the areas where they usually occur, caused by flies from the genera *Dermatobia*, *Cuterebra*, *Cordylobia* and *Wohlfahrtia* in imported dogs.

### Treatment

The treatment of cutaneous myiasis consists of mechanical elimination (if possible) and the parenteral application of spinosad and/or isoxazolide in cases where there is deep penetration. Antibiotics should be administered to treat possible secondary infections or those transmitted by parasites. Treating the underlying cause is important.

# Approach to pruritus

## Aetiopathogenesis

The **sensation which causes pruritus originates in the unmyelinated nerve endings of the epidermis**, dermis and subcutaneous tissue. The nerve impulses are transmitted by myelin fibres to the grey matter of the dorsal horn of the spinal cord and then to the cerebral cortex. This sensation causes the motor reflex responsible for scratching, and depends on:

- **intensity** of pruritus
- the animal's **tolerance levels**
- degree of **distraction**.

Scratching stimulates pain and mechanical receptors in the skin, which provides a temporary inhibition of the itching sensation through an inter-neuronal block, an effect also achieved by applying heat or cold. The self-mutilation which can be caused as a result of pruritus often generates a vicious circle of itching/scratching, as a result of the trauma inflicted and the subsequent secondary infection. Recently it has been shown that **interleukin 31 is the main mediator of pruritus** in dogs and cats. The main causes of pruritus (Table 4.8) are:

- allergy
- parasites
- infections
- tumours
- immune-mediated pruritus.

The sensation of pruritus is felt only when the stimulus is strong enough to overcome the so-called pruritic threshold. This varies from one individual to another and depends on the **individual's pruritic threshold**. That is why the sensation of pruritus perceived by an individual due to a given stimulus can vary from very

Table 4.8. Causes of pruritus.

| Causes |
|---|
| **Allergies** |
| Flea bite allergy |
| Dietary allergy |
| Atopic dermatitis |
| Contact dermatitis |
| Hypersensitivity to bites or insect bites |
| **Parasites** |
| Sarcoptic mange (**dogs**) |
| Notoedric mange (**cats**) |
| Fleas |
| *Cheyletiella* spp. |
| *Trombicula* spp. |
| **Infections** |
| Bacteria |
| *Malassezia* |
| **Tumours** |
| Epitheliotropic lymphoma |
| **Immune-mediated diseases** |
| Pemphigus foliaceus |

intense and frequent to very slight and occasional. It is also possible that individual factors, each insufficient to overcome the pruritic threshold, combine to overcome it and induce itching. Typical causes of pruritus (allergy, parasites, etc.) combined with factors such as stress, infections, dry skin, heat or contact with water, may exceed the pruritic threshold. Conversely, the elimination of one or more additional factors (for example, the elimination of a bacterial infection in an atopic dog by antibiotic treatment) can provide a significant reduction in pruritus without actually affecting the primary cause.

## Clinical signs

If there are signs of **self-inflicted injuries**, where specific skin lesions cannot be seen, the veterinarian is forced to make deductions based on a detailed history. However, it can be confusing because the owner sometimes underestimates the level of pruritus the animal is suffering from depending on how observant they are, especially in the case of cats, where due to high standards of hygiene these can go unnoticed. On the other hand, exasperated or apprehensive owners often exaggerate the degree of itching. Cutaneous lesions can reveal the location and intensity.

Scratches are the most obvious sign of intense pruritus. They appear in areas of alopecia with broken hairs and dark, often **linear, scabs, formed by dried blood** (Figure 4.106). The skin is reddish in colour and thickened, with hair loss. There may also be pustules, papules and a seropurulent exudate, as well as signs of a secondary bacterial infection (Figure 4.75). Constant licking may indicate mild itching.

In the dog, especially those with light-coloured coats, there is often **brownish staining caused by saliva** (legs, genitals, abdomen, etc.) (Figure 4.107). Another useful sign indicating mild pruritus is the presence of hair in stools, between the teeth or in the gums.

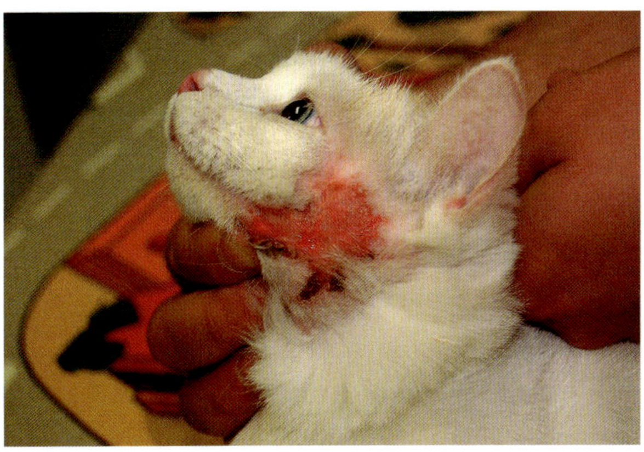

**Figure 4.106.** Alopecia, scratches and crusts due to intense scratching in a cat with a dietary allergy.

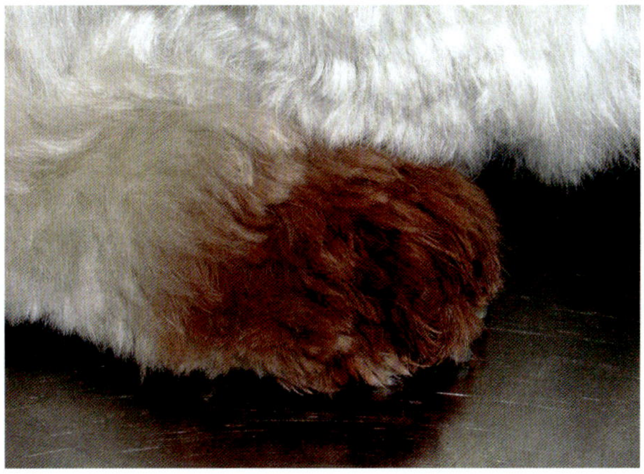

**Figure 4.107.** Brown coloration of hairs due to licking.

## Diagnosis

The **age of onset** of pruritus is of diagnostic value (Table 4.9).

Very young puppies, especially if they come from a suboptimal environment, are predisposed to suffering from:

- fleas
- dermatophytes
- sarcoptic mange
- other ectoparasites.

In **dogs of 3–6 months of age**, the most frequent cause of pruritus is due to **food allergy**.

In those of **1–3 years of age,** it is likely the pruritus is due to **atopic dermatitis**.

In **adulthood**, pruritus is usually due to **flea allergy or immune-mediated diseases**, and less frequently pemphigus foliaceus.

In elderly animals, neoplastic causes should be considered.

The duration of pruritus is also of diagnostic utility: if it is prolonged, it is more likely to be allergic than infectious, parasitic or neoplastic (these diseases tend to cause a rapid deterioration).

**Seasonal pruritus** suggests a flea bite allergy to flea bites or an atopic reaction to a seasonal allergen

**Table 4.9.** Age of onset of pruritus.

| 0–6 months | 1–3 years |
|---|---|
| Cutaneous parasites<br>Dietary allergy | Atopic dermatitis |
| **3–5 years** | **> 8–10 years** |
| Flea bite allergy<br><br>Pemphigus foliaceus | Neoplasia (epitheliotropic lymphoma, mastocytoma)<br>Metabolic (non-cutaneous) |

transported by air (pollen, etc.). However, an atopic reaction to house dust mites or to various plant allergens may manifest as non-seasonal pruritus.

The distribution of pruritus and its lesions is also useful:

- Pruritus located around the caudal area of the back and at the **base of the tail**, which extends to the thighs and abdomen, is likely to be a **flea bite allergy**.
- When located on the **midline of the back** it may indicate a Cheyletiella **infestation**.
- Pruritus located on the **ears and elbows** is suggestive of **sarcoptic mange**.
- Pruritus located on the **abdomen, face and legs** points to **atopic dermatitis or a food allergy.**

A disease that is spread to animals in contact or to people indicates ectoparasites (fleas, *Sarcoptes*, *Cheyletiella*) or dermatophytosis.

## Clinical approach to the pruritic patient

1. Could this be a **contagious parasitic infestation** such as *Sarcoptes* or *Cheyletiella*? Factors to consider include:
   a. Has there been contact with other animals such as foxes, cats, rabbits or other dogs?
   b. Is there free access to the countryside and/or woods?
   c. Has the animal been in kennels recently?
   d. Was the animal purchased recently from a pet shop or a breeder, or has it been in contact with an animal that has been?
   e. Are other animals in the home affected or are any members of the family suffering from itching or red papules?
      - Recent **intense itching**, especially affecting the **ears and elbows** (with desquamation and hyperkeratosis), together with a history of contact with dogs or suspicious environments, or lesions on the owners, suggests **sarcoptic mange**. Normally intense itching due to sarcoptic mange responds poorly to anti-inflammatory doses of corticosteroids. **Superficial skin scrapings**, although important, are often negative. Sarcoptic mange can be eliminated as a diagnosis with a trial treatment of three applications of selamectin or moxidectin in spot-on form at 15–30-day intervals.
      - **Moderate pruritus** on the **dorsal midline** (possibly accompanied by pruritus, papules and dandruff) and a history of contact with other animals (including cats and rabbits) should raise suspicions of **cheyletiellosis.** These mites can be identified in scales collected with a comb or a strip of transparent adhesive tape, although sometimes in too small a number to consider the result positive. Selamectin or moxidectin with imidacloprid, at the doses used to treat sarcoptic mange, are also effective against *Cheyletiella* spp. All in contact animals should be treated, as well as the environment.
      - In endemic areas, seasonal pruritus affecting the **extremities, face and ears** suggests an infestation with ***Trombicula* spp**. The small larvae of these free-living mites can be seen readily with a magnifying glass. They can be treated with any product capable of controlling fleas.

   Is there a bacterial and/or *Malassezia* infection?

   Infection contributes significantly to pruritus. Clinical signs suggestive of an infection (erythematous macules, papules, pustules, focal alopecia and areas of hyperpigmentation and lichenification, covered with exudate) should be checked for. Clinical suspicions are confirmed by a **cytological examination**. Treatment is based on oral antimicrobial agents and disinfectant shampoos for at least 3 weeks. Before the patient is reassessed, a skin parasite control test can be performed at the same time. An acaricide treatment (see point 1) and intensive flea control (see point 3a) can be instituted to assess the response. Broad-spectrum parasiticides (such as isoxazolines) are valid options for this. If the pruritus persists after testing to rule out parasites and infections, the most probable cause is an allergy (without ruling out other possibilities, less common).
2. If there is a **persistent pruritus** but cutaneous parasites and bacterial or *Malassezia* infections have been ruled out, the most likely diagnosis is an allergy. The distribution of pruritus is important.

   A **flea bite allergy** is characterized by an itching that mainly affects the posterior region of the body (especially the base of the tail) and is seasonal. A strict flea control test should be used to start with, even if owners claim never to have seen a flea. All animals in the household should be treated with an adulticide and an ovicide/larvicide for a period of 6–8 weeks. At the end of this period, the patient should be re-screened for residual itching in any area of the body.
3. If pruritus **affects the extremities** (extremities, legs, face and ears), the armpits and the abdominal and inguinal regions, it is **probably due to atopic dermatitis or a food allergy**. In animals **less than 6–8 months of age**, a **food allergy** is more frequent than atopic dermatitis, which may appear similar to sarcoptic mange with intense pruritus and areas with red papules on the abdomen. In any case in which **itching is not seasonal**, performing a rigorous

**dietary elimination test** over an 8-week period is essential, to distinguish atopic dermatitis from a food allergy. The diet should be based on sources of protein and carbohydrates that the animal has never eaten before; it is more accurate if it is done with homemade food than with a prescribed commercial elimination diet. Commercial diets based on low-weight and highly hydrolysed molecules are also a good alternative. In modern commercial dog foods, ingredients such as lamb, veal, corn, soy, fish, chicken, turkey and rice are frequently used, so they do not constitute an elimination diet. In cases of non-seasonal pruritus, there is no need to test for allergens in the environment until a food allergy has been ruled out. Atopic dermatitis is a clinical diagnosis based on the history, the symptoms and ruling out other causes. Allergen tests are not used for diagnosis. A marked positive reaction to suspected antigens, using intradermal tests, suggests an atopic dermatitis, but the absence of a positive reaction does not rule it out. Allergen testing is only necessary if the owner wishes to initiate hyposensitization therapy.

- If the **pruritus is seasonal** and a flea bite allergy has been ruled out, a diagnosis of **atopic dermatitis** is almost certain.
- If the **pruritus occurs for less than 4 months per year**, resorting to **symptomatic treatment** rather than to allergen testing and hyposensitization is often preferable.
- If the pruritus persists after the dietary elimination test and the allergen tests are negative, or if the patient does not respond to hyposensitization treatment, there is little choice but to use a treatment based on corticosteroids or non-steroidal antipruritic drugs, such as cyclosporine or oclatinib (see below).

4. **Pruritus located on contact areas** (legs, lips and sternum) and which is well circumscribed suggests a **contact dermatitis**. The hair has a protective effect, so that sometimes a limiting edge appears between the glabrous areas and those covered by hair. Contact dermatitis is **relatively rare** in dogs and cats, except in areas where certain plants are known to exist. The diagnosis is based on the elimination of suspicious sources, such as known problem plants, plastic bowls, carpets, mats and other possible sources of chemical allergens. In veterinary dermatology the patch test is not usually used.
5. There are other less common causes of pruritus whose clinical signs do not conform to the above descriptions and which require a skin biopsy for diagnosis:
   a. The itchy form of **epitheliotropic lymphoma**, a disease that primarily affects elderly animals, presents in the form of pruritus with erythema and desquamation and does not respond to antibiotics.
   b. A significant proportion of **pemphigus foliaceus** cases may be accompanied by intense pruritus. Cutaneous lesions include papules, pustules, crusts, exfoliation and multifocal alopecia. Scabs and pustules on the medial aspect of the ear, plantar pads and nasal plane, although not always present, indicate pemphigus foliaceus.

## *Treatment of allergic dermatitis*

Allergic dermatopathies are a **chronic condition**. The clinician must ensure the client understands that, unless the causal allergens are identified and eliminated, there is **no possible cure**. Treatment options are **symptomatic treatment or immunotherapy**. Owners need to understand that atopic dermatitis is a multifaceted disease and treatment will probably be lifelong, and it is likely that **relapses will occur** that require treatment adaptation and/or a re-evaluation. The keys to the success when treating allergic dermatitis are:

- owner education
- a combination of therapies adapted to the patient's changing needs.

The simple administration of glucocorticoids, without evaluating the various therapeutic options and constantly reviewing results, usually leads to side effects, treatment failure and loss of the client.

### *Immunotherapy*

**Immunotherapy is the treatment of choice** in cases in which the duration of pruritus **exceeds 4 months per year**. Allergens are administered by subcutaneous injection, and good to very good responses are achieved in 50–80% of dogs and cats which undergo treatment. The mechanism of action of immunotherapy is not fully understood. There are different types of vaccines available:

- Aqueous allergens in phenol-based solutions, which require **subcutaneous injection**.
- **Sublingual hyposensitization**, as a valid alternative recently proposed for dogs that do not tolerate injections.

An improvement in clinical signs can appear at any time between **1 and 8 months after starting treatment**. During the initial phase of immunotherapy, symptomatic treatment is likely to be necessary, even with corticosteroids. Any **secondary infections** or other skin allergies or parasites should also be treated.

Immunotherapy is considered ineffective if no response is achieved within 7–12 months.

If the treatment is effective, a maintenance vaccine is administered for the rest of the patient's life; only a small proportion of cases can be controlled solely with immunotherapy. The vast majority **require concomitant symptomatic treatment**, including corticosteroids, for at least part of the year, and about 75% of cases will require low maintenance doses of cortisone.

## *Symptomatic control*

Symptomatic control consists in the administration of **anti-inflammatory medication** combined with other treatment modalities, to lower the level of the pruritic stimulus to below the threshold.

### Systemic anti-inflammatory medication

**Glucocorticoids** are effective in eliminating the symptoms of atopic dermatitis. Prednisolone is administered at ***1 mg/kg/24 h in the dog*** and ***2 mg/kg/24 h in the cat*** until remission of pruritus (usually 3–5 days); the dose is then reduced to **alternate days** and reduced further to the minimum dose capable of controlling pruritus (generally *0.25–0.5 mg/kg in dogs*). Unfortunately, corticosteroids have diverse and marked side effects:

- polydipsia
- polyurea
- progressive increase in liver enzymes
- muscular atrophy
- predisposition to diabetes mellitus.

Immunosuppression induced by glucocorticoids can in turn cause:

- pyoderma
- *Malassezia* dermatitis
- demodicosis
- other forms of systemic infection (e.g. cystitis).

Cats tolerate corticosteroids better than dogs; however, this does not mean they do not suffer side effects. Those that are overweight are at a higher risk of suffering from type 2 diabetes mellitus. In cases of concurrent infection with FIV, FeLV or Herpesvirus, immunosuppression is a major problem.

Some cases that do not respond to oral prednisone (at anti-inflammatory doses) do so to triamcinolone (*0.3–1 mg/kg/24 h*, followed by a reduction to the lowest effective maintenance dose). As an alternative to oral prednisolone, some authors recommend **methylprednisolone acetate depot injections** (***5 mg/kg/8–12 weeks***).

**Cyclosporine** achieves the same efficacy rate as prednisolone in controlling the symptoms of atopic dermatitis. After starting treatment with cyclosporine, there is a **waiting period of 2–3 weeks** where no response is observed. In cases of severe itching, concomitant administration of other drugs is recommended to control the symptoms (corticosteroids, oclatinib) during the first 2–3 weeks. After one month of treatment, a significant reduction in pruritus can be expected in 75–85% of patients.

In many cases the dose can be halved (or reduced to every other day) after one month, and then **administered twice per week after 2 months**. To maximize absorption, cyclosporine should be **administered 2 hours before a meal**; recent data suggest that administering cyclosporine with food does not alter clinical outcomes. Side effects that have been published include:

- transient vomiting (controlled with metoclopramide, temporarily reducing the dose or administering the drug with food)
- reversible gingival hyperplasia
- hyperkeratosis
- hirsutism.

Cyclosporine is administered at a dose of:

- *Dogs: 5 mg/kg/24 h*
- *Cats: 7 mg/kg/24 h.*

Sporadic **cases of toxoplasmosis** have been reported in **cats treated with cyclosporine**. Therefore, it is recommended that, while under going treatment, they should not be fed raw meat and not be allowed to eat any prey they catch. It should also be confirmed that they are not suffering from infection with FeLV or FIV.

**Antihistamines** inhibit the action of histamine by competitively blocking H1 receptors, but they are not able to block its effects once histamine has bound to the receptor. They are **rarely effective alone** in controlling pruritus, and currently there is not enough evidence to recommend their use. However, they can be useful to reduce the dose of corticosteroids needed to ensure the patient remains asymptomatic. There is evidence of a certain degree of synergy between antihistamines and essential fatty acids. First-generation antihistamines are generally used in dogs and cats (Table 4.10). The only second-generation antihistamines that are of any use in small animal dermatology are oxatomide and cetricin.

In dogs, the most commonly used drugs are:

- chlorpheniramine
- diphenhydramine
- hydroxyzine
- clemastine
- cyproheptadine.

Table 4.10. Most commonly used antihistamines in dogs and cats.

| Drug | Dose |
|---|---|
| Chlorpheniramine | **Dog:** 4–8 mg/kg<br>**Cat:** 2–4 mg/kg/24 h |
| Diphenhydramine | **Dog:** 2 mg/kg/12 h<br>**Cat:** 0.5 mg/kg/12 h |
| Hydroxyzine | **Dog:** 2 mg/kg/8 h<br>**Cat:** 2.2 mg/kg/12 h |
| Clemastine | **Dog:** 0.05–0.1 mg/kg/12 h<br>**Cat:** 0.3–0.6 mg/kg/12 h |
| Cyproheptadine | 0.3–2 mg/kg/12 h |
| Cetirizine | **Dog:** 10 mg/kg/24 h |
| Oxatomide | 1.5 mg/kg/12 h |
| Doxepin | **Dog:** 0.5–2 mg/kg/12 h |
| Amitriptyline | **Dog:** 1 mg/kg/12 h |

In the **cat, chlorpheniramine** seems to be the agent of choice.

Response to antihistamine treatment is variable, and **15-day trial periods of different antihistamines** can be useful to determine which, if any, is the most effective. It is important to observe a period of 5–7 days without treatment between testing different antihistamines, to confirm that any response is due to the one being administered and not to another concomitant treatment.

**Doxepin and amitriptyline** are tricyclic antidepressants with antihistaminic activity. They have been used in atopic dogs whose excitable character could affect the pruritic threshold, with variable success. They have also been administered to **cats** where a psychogenic component is suspected but is known to **cause sedation** and behavioural changes in this species.

In many cases, supplementation with **omega-3 and omega-6 fatty acids** is useful to help control pruritus. However, it usually takes between **6 and 12 weeks of administration until benefits** can be seen. Only a small proportion of patients can be kept under control with fatty acids alone. Between 50 and 75% of dogs treated with essential fatty acids can be controlled with low doses of glucocorticoids, which minimizes the risk of side effects. A certain synergy between treatment with fatty acids and antihistamines or cyclosporine has also been observed to reduce itching. **Linoleic acid (omega-6)** is a polyunsaturated essential fatty acid present in most dog foods. Supplementation with linoleic acid, while improving coat shine, reduces seborrhoea and possibly improves the epidermal barrier, but has little effect on reducing pruritus. Supplementation with **gamma-linolenic acid (GLA)**, an omega-6 metabolite of linolenic acid, or with omega-3 fatty acids, is effective in reducing pruritus in a significant proportion of patients. Sources of GLA include evening primrose, borage and blackcurrant oils. Omega-3 fatty acids are found in linseed oil or in marine fish oils. Omega-6 GLA elongates to form dihomo-GLA. Omega-3 alpha-linolenic acid from linseed oil is converted to eicosapentaenoic acid (EPA) and then to docosahexaenoic acid (DHA). Marine fish oil contains both EPA and DHA.

**Oclacitinib** has recently been registered for the treatment of allergic pruritus in canine atopic dermatitis. It is a Janus kinase (JAK) inhibitor, with a rapid onset of action and is very effective in blocking the pruriginous, pro-inflammatory and pro-allergic effects of cytokines. Testing on laboratory dogs has shown that it improves signs of pruritus induced by IL-31, a pruritic cytokine recently discovered in canine and human species. At **doses of *0.4–0.6 mg/kg/12 h for two weeks*,** followed by once a day, it can rapidly inhibit pruritus safely and effectively, in addition to the clinical signs of canine allergic dermatitis. However, pruritus reappears as soon as the administration of the drug is suspended. Side effects are rare and are not usually serious.

## Topical treatment

In some cases, creams, lotions, topical sprays and shampoos with corticosteroids are useful in reducing the need for systemic medication. **Topical corticosteroids** cause **thinning of the skin** and local immunosuppression and are absorbed systemically (which increases the risk of side effects caused by glucocorticoids). Sprays with a hydrocortisone aceponate base are an exception.

## Shampooing

Shampooing **reduces itching, moisturizes and softens** the skin. In addition, washing eliminates surface allergens, epidermal residues, microorganisms and their toxins. The ingredients of the shampoo must be **hypoallergenic, moisturizing and have good detergent** and antiseptic action. Often dogs with atopic dermatitis have dry skin because of increased water loss through the epidermis, so hydration is very beneficial.

## Hygroscopic agents

Hygroscopic agents (moisturizers) are high molecular weight molecules that are incorporated into the stratum corneum and attract water. These include:

- urea
- glycerine
- lactic acid.

**Propylene glycol**, which has antiseptic properties, is a lipid and keratolytic solvent in addition to helping other drugs to penetrate the skin. Normally propylene glycol is applied at a concentration of 30–40%. When intense keratolytic activity is needed, it is applied at higher concentrations (up to 75%).

Lipids, such as fatty acids and phytosphingosides, are used in shampoos, sprays and spot-on products. They **reduce epidermal water** loss and restore the damaged protective lipid barrier.

### Infection control

Allergic skin is **predisposed to colonization and infection by bacteria and yeasts** (mainly *Staphylococcus* and *Malassezia* spp.), microorganisms that increase pruritus and inflammation, and are part of the pathogenesis of the chronic phase of atopic dermatitis. To detect possible infections, patients should be **checked periodically** (including examination of samples taken with transparent adhesive tape). Any infection that is discovered should be treated with systemic and topical medication.

## Bibliography


Beco, L., Guaguère, E., Lorente Méndez, C., Noli, C., Nuttall, T. and Vroom, M. (2013) Suggested guidelines for using systemic antimicrobials in bacterial skin infections. 1. Diagnosis based on clinical presentation, cytology and culture. *Veterinary Record* 172(3), 72–78.

Beco, L., Guaguère, E., Lorente Méndez, C., Noli, C., Nuttall, T. and Vroom, M. (2013) Suggested guidelines for using systemic antimicrobials in bacterial skin infections. 2. Antimicrobial choice, treatment regimens and compliance. *Veterinary Record* 172(6), 156–160.

Borio, S., Colombo, S., La Rosa, G., De Lucia, M., Damborg, P. and Guardabassi. L. (2015) Effectiveness of a combined (4% chlorhexidine digluconate shampoo and solution) protocol in MRS and non-MRS canine superficial pyoderma: a randomized, blinded, antibiotic-controlled study. *Veterinary Dermatology* 26(5), 339–344.

Fourie, J.J., Liebenberg, J.E., Horak, I.G., Taenzler, J., Heckeroth, A.R. and Frénais, R. (2015) Efficacy of orally administered fluralaner (Bravecto™) or topically applied imidacloprid/moxidectin (Advocate®) against generalized demodicosis in dogs. *Parasites & Vectors* 8, 187.

Frymus, T., Gruffydd-Jones, T., Pennisi, M.G., Addie, D., Belák. S., Boucraut-Baralon, C. et al. (2013) Dermatophytosis in cats: ABCD guidelines on prevention and management. *Journal of Feline Medicine and Surgery* 15(7), 598–604.

Hensel, P., Santoro, D., Favrot, C., Hill, P. and Griffin. C. (2015) Canine atopic dermatitis: detailed guidelines for diagnosis and allergen identification. *BMC Veterinary Research* 11, 196.

Hillier, A., Lloyd, D.H., Weese, J.S., Blondeau, J.M., Boothe, D., Breitschwerdt, E. et al. Guidelines for the diagnosis and antimicrobial therapy of canine superficial bacterial folliculitis (Antimicrobial Guidelines Working Group of the International Society for Companion Animal Infectious Diseases) (2014) *Veterinary Dermatology* 25(3), 163–175.

Miller, W.H., Griffin, C.E. and Campbell, K.L. (2013) *Small Animal Dermatology*, 7 edn. Elsevier, St. Louis, MO, USA.

Moriello, K. (2014) Feline dermatophytosis: Aspects pertinent to disease management in single and multiple cat situations. *Journal of Feline and Medicine and Surgery* 16(5), 419–431.

Mueller, R.S., Bensignor, E., Ferrer, L., Holm, B., Lemarie, S., Paradis, M. et al. (2012) Treatment of demodicosis in dogs: 2011 clinical practice guidelines. *Veterinary Dermatology* 23(2), 86–96.

Noli, C. and Morris, D. (2011) Guidelines on the use of systemic aminoglycosides in veterinary dermatology. *Veterinary Dermatology* 22(4), 379–380.

Olivry, T., DeBoer, D.J., Favrot, C., Jackson, H.A., Mueller, R.S., Nuttall, T. et al. (2015) Treatment of canine atopic dermatitis: 2015 updated guidelines from the International Committee on Allergic Diseases of Animals (ICADA). *BMC Veterinary Research* 11, 210.

Saridomichelakis, M.N. and Olivry, T. (2016) An update on the treatment of canine atopic dermatitis. *Veterinary Journal* 207, 29–37.


## Test

**1. Which of the following lesions can be classified as either primary or secondary?**

A) Alopecia.
B) Weal.
C) Plaque.
D) Lichenification.

**2. Which of the following is an elevated lesion with a flat surface?**

A) Macule.
B) Papule.
C) Plaque.
D) Patch.

3. **What is a comedone?**
   A) The accumulation of keratin stuck to the hair.
   B) The follicular ostium covered and filled with keratin and sebum.
   C) A circular area with a scaly keratin border.
   D) A scab composed of keratin.
4. **Which of the following statements is false with respect to lichenification?**
   A) It is a thickening of the skin.
   B) It results from chronic trauma.
   C) The marks on the skin are more noticeable.
   D) It is usually accompanied by hypopigmentation.
5. **What information is the most useful to make a dermatological diagnosis?**
   A) Location and type of lesions.
   B) Breed.
   C) Sex.
   D) There are other affected animals.
6. **Which of the following is a primary lesion in cases of flea bite allergy?**
   A) Alopecia.
   B) Papule.
   C) Excoriation.
   D) Scales.
7. **What is the name of a solid, well-circumscribed lesion larger than 1 cm in diameter?**
   A) Papule.
   B) Plaque.
   C) Nodule.
   D) Bulla.
8. **Which of the following is not a differential diagnosis in a young dog with a nodule on its snout?**
   A) Foreign body.
   B) Dermatophytosis (kerion).
   C) Bacterial furunculosis.
   D) Cutaneous lymphoma.
9. **What dermatological diseases are common in dogs under 6 months old?**
   A) Dermatophytosis and pemphigus.
   B) Demodicosis and impetigo.
   C) Demodicosis and alopecia X.
   D) Juvenile cellulitis and discoid lupus.
10. **Which of the following should be selected for biopsy?**
    A) Chronic lesions.
    B) Excoriations.
    C) Areas of normal skin adjacent to the lesion.
    D) Primary lesions.
11. **An 11 year-old female Shetland sheep dog presents with hyperkeratosis of the plantar pads, and scabs on the elbows and lips. On the skin biopsy, the pathologist describes a dermatitis with a very particular appearance that shows three bands (red, white and blue). With this pattern on histopathology and clinical lesions, what disease would you suspect?**
    A) Superficial necrolytic dermatitis.
    B) Pemphigus foliaceus.
    C) Zinc-responsive dermatitis.
    D) Sebaceous adenitis.
12. **The pathophysiology of paraneoplastic dermatoses is usually due to:**
    A) Genetic mutations.
    B) Cytokine release.
    C) Unknown causes.
    D) Metastases.

**13. What is the typical location of alopecia in dogs with hypothyroidism?**
- A) Legs and toes.
- B) Abdomen and medial aspect of the thigh.
- C) There is no alopecia.
- D) The tail and top of the nose.

**14. Which breeds are at a higher risk of Cushing's syndrome?**
- A) Giant.
- B) Large.
- C) Medium.
- D) Small and toy.

**15. Which allergy presents most commonly in the cat with pruritus on the head and neck?**
- A) Food allergy.
- B) Flea allergy dermatitis.
- C) Atopic dermatitis.
- D) Contact dermatitis.

**16. Which of these feline parasites is strictly species specific?**
- A) *Cheyletiella*.
- B) Trombicula.
- C) Ctenocephalides.
- D) Felicola.

**17. Which of the following breeds can be an asymptomatic carrier of dermatophytosis?**
- A) Norwegian.
- B) Maine Coon.
- C) Siamese.
- D) Persian.

**18. Where are notoedric mange lesions usually located in the cat?**
- A) Lumbosacral area.
- B) Pinna.
- C) Tail.
- D) Plantar pads.

**Answers on page 195**

## Clinical case 1

The patient in the photograph is a 13-year-old cat with progressive alopecia, which has developed over a 1 month period.

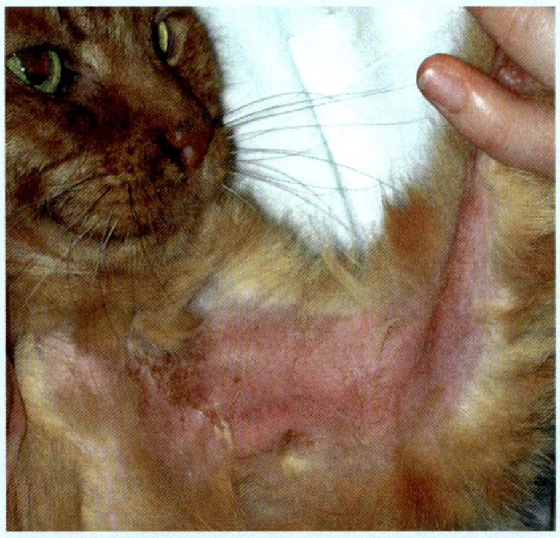

**Figure case 1.1.**

**There is no history of previous dermatological problems. The main differential diagnoses include:**

A) Atopic dermatitis and hyperadrenocorticism.
B) Hyperadrenocorticism and pancreatic carcinoma.
C) Thymoma and hyperthyroidism.
D) Atopic dermatitis and thymoma.

## Clinical case 2

The case in the photograph corresponds to a 14-year-old mixed breed male, who presented with a 2-month history of pododermatitis and severe mucocutaneous pyoderma.

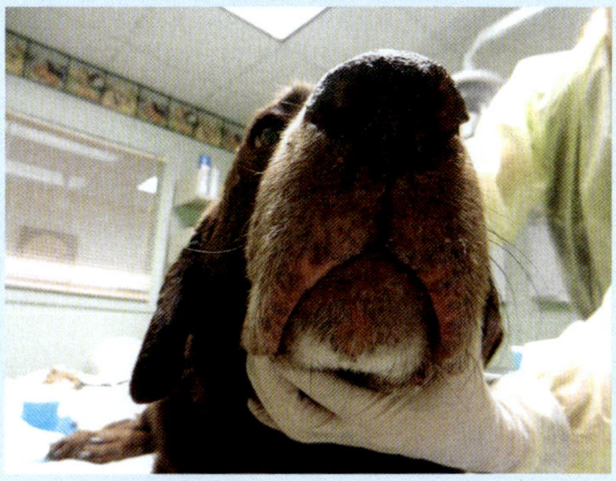

**Figure case 2.1.**

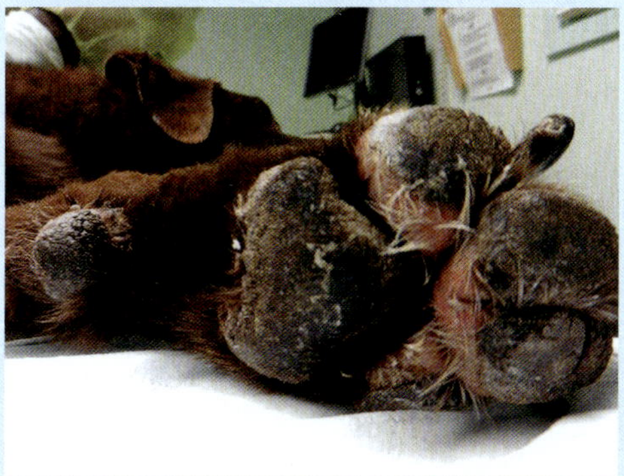

**Figure case 2.2.**

**There was no previous history of dermatological problems. After examining the skin and taking samples for cytology and a skin scraping, what would the next step be?**

A) Thoracic radiography.
B) Abdominal ultrasound.
C) Urinalysis.
D) Complete blood count.

## Correct answers

### Test

| | | |
|---|---|---|
| 1. A | 7. C | 13. D |
| 2. C | 8. D | 14. D |
| 3. B | 9. B | 15. A |
| 4. D | 10. D | 16. D |
| 5. A | 11. A | 17. D |
| 6. B | 12. C | 18. B |

### Clinical case 1

B

### Clinical case 2

B

# 5

# Clinical neurology

Alejandro Luján Feliu-Pascual

## Chapter summary



There's nothing quite like a neurological case for making a clinician feel inadequate. Vague memories of vet school lectures all swill together to form a general impression that this hypermetric dog is a step too far with regards to reaching a definitive diagnosis in first-opinion practice.

Indeed, this may be the case because finding the final answer may depend on an advanced imaging technique, such as MRI or a CT scan. However, this fact alone isn't an escape-clause for the first-opinion practitioner.

A combination of history, physical exam, observation and neurological examination should differentiate what may appear to be primary neurological disease from a systemic problem with neurological signs. Indeed, once the case is confirmed as neurological, even in general practice it is often possible to localize the origin of the problem.

This is because each anatomical part of the nervous system has its own function. Damage or impairment to a particular part results in characteristic deficits. On a clinical examination, recognizing these deficits helps the clinician decide which part of the nervous system is affected, draw up a list of differential diagnosis and decide on the most appropriate tests.

This chapter provides a practical overview of both the signs associated when specific parts of the nervous system are affected and neurological diseases that are actually secondary to systemic disease. This takes the sting out of those tricky neurological cases to enable the clinician to draw up a problem list and decide on the most appropriate course of action for each patient.

## Key learning points

- Understand the link between neurological signs and location of origin.
- Feel confident about performing an reliable neurological examination.
- Differentiate systemic disease with neurological signs from primary neurological disease.

- Recognize the implications of the different reflex tests.
- The pros and cons of various diagnostic tests.

## Neuroanatomy

### *Basic neuroanatomy*

A **sound knowledge of the normal anatomy** of the nervous system (NS) is **fundamental** to the correct localization of neurological lesions and interpretation of diagnostic tests.

The ***Nomina Anatomica Veterinaria 2012*** concisely defines all the structures found in the nervous systems of domestic animals and provides the **correct nomenclature** for the structures covered.

Traditionally, the nervous system is divided into **central (CNS)** and **peripheral (PNS)** areas (Table 5.1). However, from a **functional point of view** the various systems of the nervous system are comprised of components from both these divisions. For example, the **proprioceptive system** is formed from **components of the PNS** (receptors and afferent fibres in the spinal nerves) **and the CNS** (ascending tracts, relay nuclei in the thalamus, connections in the cerebellum, interpretation centres in the cerebral cortex, etc.).

**Each anatomical division of the CNS has its own functions**. If any of these structures are affected, then **characteristic neurological deficits** can be seen. Being knowledgeable of the characteristic neurological functions and signs that appear as a consequence of focal pathologies is fundamental for examination and selection of the most adequate diagnostic tests. Unfortunately, it is not possible to establish the cause of a condition based solely on identifying its location, but identifying the latter greatly helps test selection.

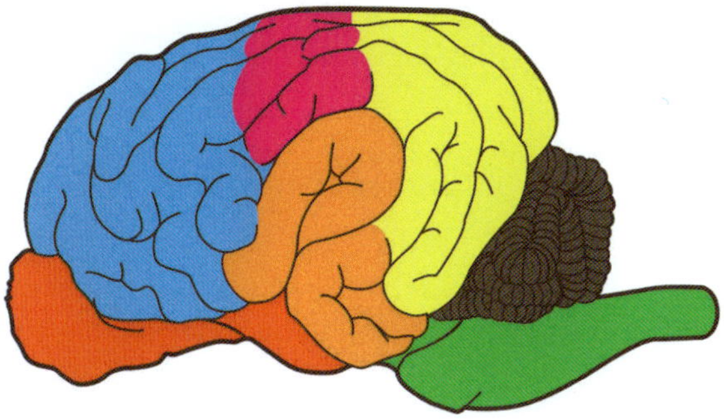

**Figure 5.1.** Encephalon. Frontal lobe (blue), parietal lobe (pink), occipital lobe (yellow), pyriform lobe (red), brainstem (green), cerebellum (brown), temporal lobe (orange).

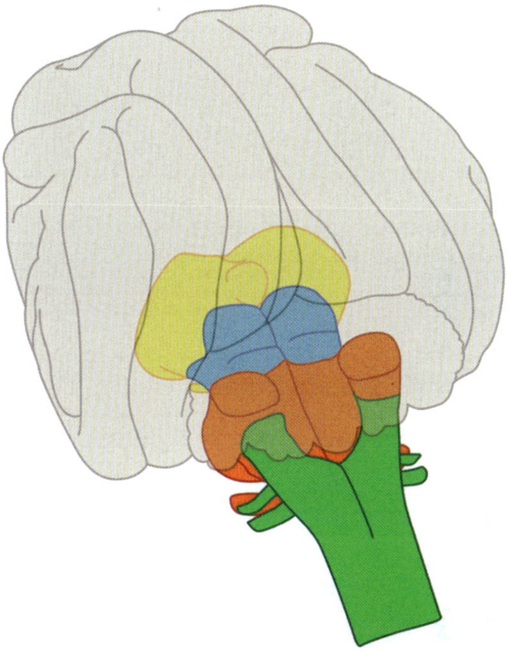

**Figure 5.2.** Brainstem. diencephalon (yellow), mesencephalon (blue), pons (red), myelencephalon (green).

Table 5.1. Key components of the CNS.

| Encephalon | Telencephalon or cerebrum | Frontal lobe | |
|---|---|---|---|
| | (Fig. 5.1) | Parietal lobe | |
| | | Temporal lobe | |
| | | Occipital lobe | |
| | | Piriform lobe | |
| | | Hippocampus | |
| | Brain stem (Fig. 5.2) | Diencephalon | |
| | | Mesencephalon | |
| | | Metencephalon | Dorsal: cerebellum |
| | | | Ventral: pons |
| | | Myelencephalon | |
| Spinal cord | C1–C5 | | |
| | C6–T2 or cervical intumescence | | |
| | T3–L3 | | |
| | L4–S3 or lumbosacral intumescence | | |

The CNS is suspended by a series of ligaments and sheaths and is surrounded by **cerebrospinal fluid (CSF)**, which serves to protect and **nourish the parenchyma**. CSF is **formed mainly in the lateral** and **fourth ventricles** and flows caudally from the first to the third ventricle, the mesencephalic aqueduct, the fourth ventricle and leaves the cranial cavity through lateral openings to surround the brain and spinal cord and flow through the central spinal canal.

In most **dogs**, especially large breeds, as a result of the uneven growth of the spine with respect to nervous structures, the **lumbar, sacral and caudal medullary segments are displaced cranially with respect to their corresponding vertebrae** (Figure 5.3). However, in cats these are located next to the respective vertebrae.

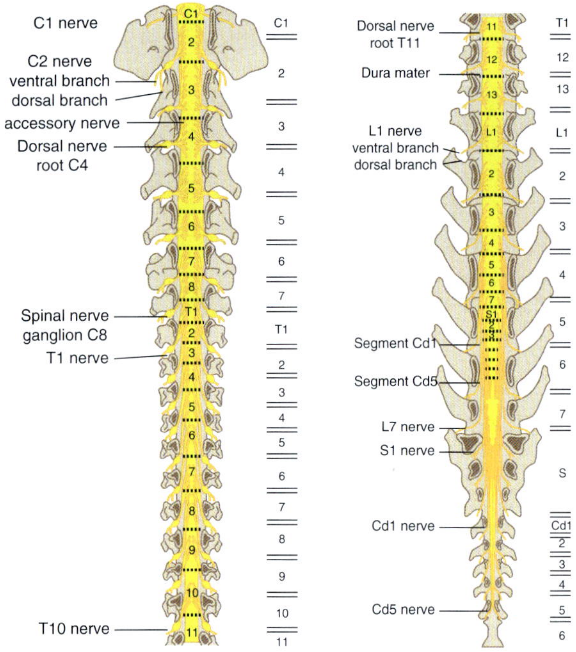


**Figure 5.3.** Image showing the relationship between spinal cord and vertebrae in a large bread of dog.

## Functional neuroanatomy

### The telencephalon or cerebral hemispheres

Table 5.2. Functional neuroanatomy of the different parts of the telencephalon and the cerebral hemispheres.

| Anatomical structure | Function | Consequences of local injuries |
|---|---|---|
| Frontal lobe | Motor cortex and associative reasoning | Behavioural changes, types of aggression<br>Turning<br>Hyperactivity<br>Compulsive pacing |
| Parietal lobe | Sensory cortex | Conscious postural delay<br>Reduction of conscious sensitivity |
| Temporal lobe | Long-term memory and hearing | |
| Occipital lobe | Vision | Contralateral hemianopsia: absence of vision in the contralateral visual field of each eye |
| Piriform lobe | Smell, which is gathered by the olfactory nerve (I), a collection of nerve fibres | Anosmia |

Table 5.2. Continued

| Anatomical structure | Function | Consequences of local injuries |
|---|---|---|
| Hippocampus | Behavioural patterns, personality, short-term memory | |

### Diencephalon

Table 5.3. Functional neuroanatomy of the different parts of the diencephalon.

| Anatomical structure | Function | Consequences of local injuries |
|---|---|---|
| Thalamus | Maintenance of consciousness, centre for ascending and descending connections between the spinal cord and the cerebral cortex. All sensations that are converted into conscious information in the cerebral cortex, or that descend from the cerebral cortex to perform voluntary functions, synapse in the thalamus, with the exception of smell | Obtundation, coma, conscious postural delay, central blindness, etc. |
| Hypothalamus | Control centre of autonomous functions, regulation of body temperature, hunger and satiety, endocrine function through the pituitary gland | Polyuria, polydipsia, anorexia, thermoregulatory changes |
| Optic chiasm | Crossing of optic nerves (II) rostroventral to the diencephalon. In the dog, 75% of the fibres decussate to the contralateral side; in the cat, 65% and in primates approximately 50%, which gives them a different degree of binocular vision | Injuries to the optic nerves or the chiasm produce blindness |

## *Mesencephalon*

Table 5.4. Functional neuroanatomy of the different parts of the mesencephalon.

| Anatomical structure | Function | Consequences of local injuries |
|---|---|---|
| Rostral and caudal colliculi | Ocular and auditory reflexes, respectively. Quick turn of head or body to locate sounds or lights | Absence of ocular and auditory reflexes |
| Motor nuclei of cranial nerves | Oculomotor (III) and troclear (IV). Voluntary extraocular movements and in response to stimulation of the vestibular system | Ipsilateral ophthalmoplegia with ventrolateral eye deviation |
| Parasympathetic nucleus of the oculomotor nerve | Pupillary contraction in response to light stimuli | Ipsilateral mydriasis |
| Mesencephalic nucleus and trigeminal nerve tract | Receives proprioceptive information from the face, masticatory muscles and mouth | Loss of coordination of mandibular movements necessary for normal chewing |

## *Ventral metencephalon (pons)*

Table 5.5. Functional neuroanatomy of the different parts of the ventral metencephalon (pons).

| Anatomical structure | Function | Consequences of local injuries |
|---|---|---|
| Principal sensory nucleus of the trigeminal nerve | Receives sensory information (pressure, pain, etc.) | Lack of sensitivity in face and mouth |
| Trigeminal motor nucleus | Mandibular movements | Atrophy of the masticatory muscles |
| Reticular formation | Diffuse network of interconnected neurons that extend from the diencephalon to the myelencephalon and is responsible for maintaining consciousness, with connections to the respiratory and vasomotor centres | Reduced state of consciousness, alterations in respiratory pattern and blood pressure |
| Abductor nerve nucleus | Extra-ocular movements | Medial deviation of the eyeball |
| Nucleus of the facial nerve | Movement of the facial musculature | Result in facial paralysis/paresis and reduced movement and, in chronic cases, atrophy of the facial musculature |
| Cochlear nuclei | Hearing | Unilateral deafness |

## *Myelencephalon*

Table 5.6. Functional neuroanatomy of the different parts of the myelencephalon.

| Anatomical structure | Function | Consequences of local injuries |
|---|---|---|
| Vestibular nuclei | Integration and coordination of balance and eye movements | Ataxia, head tilting, nystagmus |
| Area postrema | Chemoreceptor trigger zone | Nausea, vomiting |
| Nucleus and solitary tract | Relay of information on the visceral reflexes of the pharynx, larynx, oesophagus, trachea and abdominal and thoracic viscera | |
| Parasympathetic nucleus of the vagus nerve | Motor innervation to the abdominal and thoracic viscera | |
| Parasympathetic nucleus of the glossopharyngeal nerve | Innervation to the salivary glands | |
| Nucleus of the hypoglossal nerve | Motor innervation to most of the lingual muscles | Changes in tongue movement and atrophy |

### *Cerebellum*

The **cerebellum coordinates movement** via inhibition or dampening affects. It receives information from proprioceptive afferent fibres and sends information via efferent fibres to upper motor centres (UMN). There are no direct connections with lower motor nuclei.

Its involvement in a pathological process causes:

- ataxia
- anisocoria
- head and body tremors
- hypermetric movements.

### *Spinal cord*

The organization of the spinal cord is **somatotopic**. **Ascending proprioceptive tracts** are **situated superficially**, have a large diameter and are highly myelinated, and are therefore the first to be affected by a wide range of pathologies, in **particular spinal cord compressions**. (Figure 5.4). **Descending motor tracts** (Figure 5.4 [red]) and ascending somatic tracts are **situated more deeply** (Figure 5.4 [green]). **Ascending deep nociceptive** tracts are **situated around the grey** matter of the spinal cord, which explains why they are the **last to be affected** and their involvement implies severe injury.

## The neurological examination

The neurological examination aims to **identify anomalies** confirming the presence of a lesion in the nervous system. Its second objective is to **locate the lesion** in a particular area of the nervous system (central, peripheral, neuromuscular junction) or musculoskeletal system. In some cases, such as with cranial trauma, identification of the cause and the problem is simple but often a knowledge is required of the basic nervous system because different anatomical areas manifest with different neurological deficits.

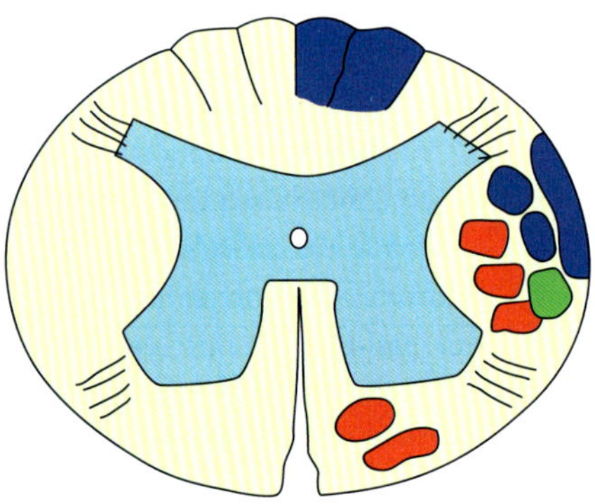

**Figure 5.4.** Organization of the spinal cord.

## *Examination*

### *Clinical history*

An **exhaustive clinical history** can help clarify the underlying cause (such as cranial trauma). However, it must be remembered that it is human nature sometimes for owners to change information. **Other clinical signs** that may appear unrelated to the reason for the consultation (polyuria, polydipsia) should also orientate the neurological examination, and indicate which diagnostic tests should be performed. Special attention should be paid to:

- vaccination history
- de-worming
- exposure to toxins
- diet.

## *Physical examination*

A **thorough physical examination** can identify abnormalities related to the reason for the consultation (for example, heart murmur in cases of collapse; abdominal or laryngeal masses in cases of dysphagia; lack of pulse in aortic thromboembolism). Its importance should never be underestimated.

### *Orthopaedic examination*

Orthopaedic examination is critical, since to the inexperienced eye many **orthopaedic issues can be confused with neurological problems**. Particular attention should be paid to:

- gait evaluation
- palpation and manipulation of joints
- presence of painful points in bones, muscles, tendons and ligaments.

### *Neurological examination*

The neurological examination can be divided into two parts.

- **Observation**. Evaluation of mental state, posture and movement.
- **Handling**. In this following order, evaluation of postural reactions, myotactic spinal reflexes, cranial nerves, nociception and the presence of painful areas in the head and spine.

#### Observation

Whilst taking the history and talking to the owner, **leave the animal loose** in the consulting room. This is useful for observing the patient's mental state, reactions to the environment, evidence of compulsive turning, postural abnormalities, etc.

## Mental state

The owner can indicate whether there has been a change in behaviour with greater reliability than the neurological examination, which may be conditioned by the environment in the consulting room.

There are five mental states.

1. **Normal**. The animal reacts to environmental stimuli in a manner **consistent with the intensity of the stimulus**. It is attentive to what is happening and reacts in an appropriate manner.
2. **obtunded**. Due to neurological causes, **reactions to environmental stimuli are reduced**. The animal does not pay attention to what is going on around it and, although it normally reacts to its name, does so in a slow and inconsistent way.
3. **Delirious**. Reacts inappropriately to the environment, with an **exaggerated response** to the degree of stimulus.
4. **Stupor**. Denotes an **absence of response to visual or auditory stimuli**, although there is a positive response to painful stimuli. Usually occurs in recumbent animals which find it difficult to emerge from this mental state.
5. **Comatose**. The patient **does not respond to any type of stimulus**, even painful ones, and is always in a recumbent position.

An **altered mental state** is indicative that the ascending activating reticular system (AARS) is affected by a **focal lesion of the brainstem** or a **diffuse lesion of the cerebral cortex** (for example, hepatic encephalopathy). Focal lesions in the cerebral cortex do not cause alteration of mental state unless there is increased intracranial pressure and secondary compression of the brainstem.

## Posture

Evaluation of postural reactions can also be made using the clinical history.

In **ambulatory animals**, evidence of limb abduction, head tilt, scoliosis, kyphosis, lordosis, tremors, pleurothotonus, etc. should be sought.

In **non-ambulatory animals**, **decerebrate posture** (opisthotonus with tonic extension of the four limbs) is observed, indicating a **midbrain lesion** with disconnection of cortical inhibitory centres, or decerebellate posture (opisthotonus with tonic hyperextension of the thoracic limbs and pelvic flexion) indicating **disconnection from the cerebellum** (Figure 5.5).

This type of posture should not be confused with the **Schiff–Sherrington posture**, in which there is an increase in the extensor tone of the thoracic limbs as a consequence of an **acute injury to the thoracolumbar** area (Figure 5.6). In this case, postural reaction in the

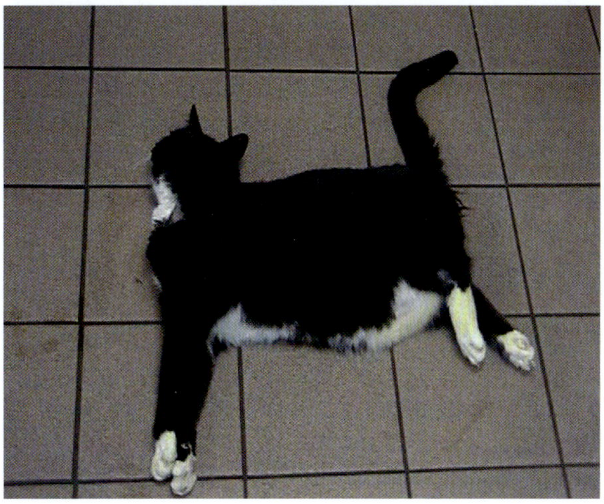

**Figure 5.5.** Decerebrate posture.

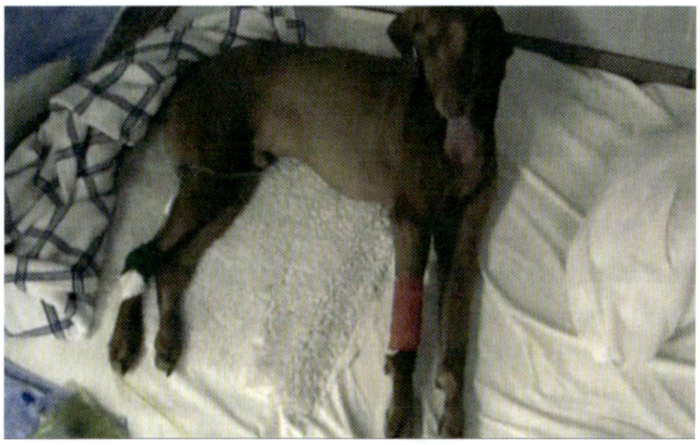

**Figure 5.6.** Schiff–Sherrington posture.

thoracic limbs should be present and mental state will be normal. Identification of this position, although it indicates acute and severe thoracolumbar injury, is of no prognostic value.

## Gait

Gait can be evaluated by walking the animal on **surfaces with different amounts of grip** (grass, cement, carpet) or climbing stairs and observing the presence of lameness, dysmetria, collapse, stumbling, etc. The patient should be examined from all four angles, paying attention to all phases of the gait.

In complicated cases, trot and even canter can be evaluated. In addition, **walking in circles** can reveal alterations in balance and gait, as well as any asymmetry.

## *Performing the neurological examination*

This requires direct, hands-on contact with the patient.

## Postural reactions

**Postural reactions evaluate conscious and non-conscious proprioceptive pathways**. The nervous fibres and tracts carrying this information are **superficial**

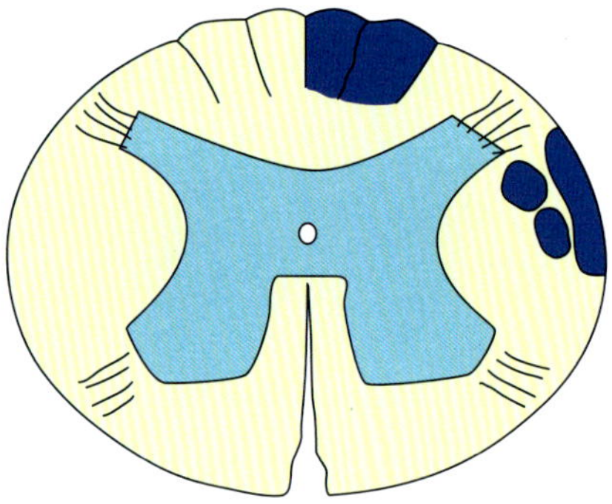

**Figure 5.7.** Conscious and unconscious proprioceptive pathways (shaded dark blue).

in the spinal cord (Figure 5.7) and of a **large diameter**, and therefore they are the **first to be affected** in nervous system or spinal injuries.

Information on the **position of the joints** and muscle tension is collected by **receptors** located in these structures and relayed through ascending medullary pathways, where it is received in the brain. The cerebellum coordinates and initiates the appropriate actions to correct posture, using descending pathways to the effector muscles. Injury to peripheral nerves, the spinal cord or brain can cause a delay in these **postural reactions**, and therefore does **not help much when locating the lesion**.

The tests used most commonly include the following, and preferably use **conscious pathways** up to the cerebral cortex:

- conscious proprioception (knuckling)
- reflex step
- positional visual and tactile reactions (visual and tactile placing).

These tests **do not need voluntary** initiation of a response:

- hemi-walking
- jumping (hopping)
- wheelbarrowing
- extensor postural thrust
- swaying.

All the above reflexes and reactions are **aimed at adjusting body position** and providing the body with a stable position on which to base voluntary movements.

## Spinal reflexes

Evaluation of spinal reflexes provides sufficient information to **locate a neurological lesion** in the **upper motor neuron (UMN) or lower (LMN)** (Table 5.7). Decreased tone, severe muscle atrophy or lack of reflexes indicates injury in the spinal segment or nerve responsible for it.

Table 5.7. Upper (UMN) or lower (LMN) motor neuron signs.

| LMN signs | UMN signs |
|---|---|
| Muscular atrophy >7 days | No muscle atrophy, or minimal disuse |
| Absence or diminution of reflexes | Normal or increased reflexes |
| Reduction in or absence of muscle tone | Normal or increased muscle tone |

## Patellar reflex

The patellar reflex is undoubtedly the **most constant** and reliable of all reflexes to evaluate. The medullary segments involved are **L4–L6**, and it is monosynaptic in nature (direct connection of the sensory neuron with the motor neuron responsible for muscle contraction in the same spinal segment). The reflex may be:

- **absent or reduced** – as a result of a problem:
  - sensory (polyneuropathy)
  - motor (polyneuropathy, alterations in the neuromuscular junction such as with botulism or myopathy)
- **normal**
- **increased** – owing to injury:
  - in the neuromuscular system
  - spinal segments L6–S1 (pseudo-hyperreflexia)
- **clonic** – indicating a chronic injury to the UMN.

## Withdrawal reflex

The flexor, or withdrawal, reflex is **polysynaptic** (with multiple connections between the sensory neuron and the motor neuron through interneurons and with other medullary segments). It may be **reduced but not increased**. If the extension of the contralateral limb occurs when it is being evaluated, the reflex is called a **crossed extensor reflex**, which is pathological in the recumbent adult animal and indicates chronic **damage of the UMN**.

## Cutaneous trunk reflex

With thoracolumbar lesions, evaluation of the **cutaneous trunk reflex** (erroneously called pannicular) is useful. This can be achieved by stimulation of thoracolumbar dermatomes from **L6 to T3** and is mediated by the cutaneous trunk muscle through the lateral thoracic nerve, formed from the ventral roots of the spinal nerves at C8 and T1. Severe **injuries to the spinal cord or spinal nerves** may result in the absence of this reflex bi- or unilaterally.

### Perineal reflex

More caudally, the perineal reflex can be evaluated by stimulating **the skin around the anal sphincter** and observing whether contraction occurs. This way, sensitivity and motor function of pudendal nerves, S1–S3 nerve roots and their connections in the lumbar intumescence can be evaluated.

### Other myotactic reflexes

Other myotactic reflexes, such as the gastronemius, cranial tibial, bicipital and carpo-radial extensor reflexes, are not as reliable and consistent as those mentioned above.

## *Cranial nerves*

Assessment of cranial nerves is based on both observation and functional tests.

The following should be observed:

- symmetry of the face
- muscular atrophy in the masticatory muscles
- deviation of the nose or ears
- narrowing of the palpebral fissures
- deviation of the eyeball and tongue
- enophthalmos or exophthalmos.

### Menace response

The menace response requires the **visual system** (retina, **optic nerve** [**II**], chiasm, optic tract, occipital cortex), cerebellum, mesencephalon and **facial nerve** [**VII**]) to be intact. Conscious processing is necessary, so it is not a reflex but a **learned response** that, in both the dog and the cat, shows for the first time at around **3 months of age**.

### Palpebral reflex

The palpebral reflex does not need processing in the cerebral cortex, and evaluates information on **facial sensitivity** collected by the **trigeminal nerve** (**V**) and the motor response for palpebral contraction by the **facial nerve** (**VII**), as well as its connections in the brainstem.

### Pupillary reflex

The absence of pupillary reflexes may indicate the presence of lesions in the eyeball, **optic nerve** (**II**), optic chiasm, optic tract, mesencephalon and parasympathetic nucleus of the **oculomotor nerve** (**III**) responsible for contraction of the iris.

### Vestibulo-ocular reflex

The vestibulo-ocular reflex allows evaluation of the peripheral vestibular system, **vestibulocochlear nerve** (**VIII**), vestibular nuclei in the myelencephalon, cerebellum, medial longitudinal fasciculus, the motor nuclei and cranial nerves III, IV and VI, which innervate the extra-ocular muscles and are responsible for eye movements.

The presence of **spontaneous nystagmus is always pathological** and suggests a lesion in any of the nuclei or areas mentioned for the vestibulo-ocular reflex.

The majority of **sensory information** from the head is collected through the ophthalmic, maxillary and mandibular branches of the **trigeminal nerve**, although the facial nerve has sensory branches that innervate the inner aspect of the pinna. Pinching the lips with a haemostat should produce facial contraction and withdrawal of the head.

### Swallowing reflex

For evaluation of the swallowing reflex, the mouth should be opened and the tongue or pharynx stimulated, allowing simultaneous detection of weakness or deviation of the tongues muscles. This way, it is possible to evaluate sensory information collected by the facial, glossopharyngeal and vagus nerves, and the motor activity of the glossopharyngeal, vagus and hypoglossal nerves as well as their connections in the brainstem.

## *Nociception*

**Evaluation of pain** should be the last part of a neurological examination. **Palpation of the spine** can be carried out by pressing on vertebral spinous processes in the thoracic and lumbar spine and paraspinal musculature. In the cervical spine, the transverse processes of C1–C6 can be palpated, as well as manipulation and flexion of the neck providing there are no suspicions of possible fracture.

**Superficial pain** is evaluated by **pinching the skin** with forceps. To assess the presence or absence of deep pain, the metacarpal or metatarsal bones can be pressed with mosquito forceps or, better still, the distal portion of the tibia with bone forceps. A concious response consisting of head turning, growling or aggression towards the clinician must be observed. If a superficial pain response is present, evaluation of deep pain is not necessary.

## *Special situations*

Obviously, in some situations, evaluation of all reflexes and reactions is not possible (for example, in comatose patients or those with vertebral fractures). In these cases, the clinician should be able to locate the neurological lesion with **minimal manipulation of the patient**.

- If the animal is in a **coma**, evaluation of **cranial nerves** is important, particularly the pupillary and Vestibulo-ocular reflexes.

- If the animal has suffered **spinal trauma**, evaluation of spinal reflexes and the presence of **superficial and deep pain** is essential.

### *Neurological localization*

Once a complete neurological examination has been performed, the following two questions must be answered.

1. Does the animal have a neurological condition?
2. Where is the neurological lesion located?

To help answer the second question, the most common neurological signs and the location of lesions must be understood. The examples illustrated are from the locations described, but do not necessarily show all the signs listed.

### *Telencephalic lesion*

- seizures
- conscious postural reactions contralateral to the lesion, delayed or absent
- contralateral central blindness with normal pupillary reflexes
- pleurothotonus (Figure 5.8) to the side of the lesion
- compulsive turning towards the side of the lesion
- head pressing on objects or people
- no ataxia
- facial hypoaesthesia
- between obtundation and coma, with a diffuse lesion.

### *Brainstem lesion*

- obtundation, delirium, stupor and coma
- facial paresis/paralysis
- atrophy of the masticatory muscles

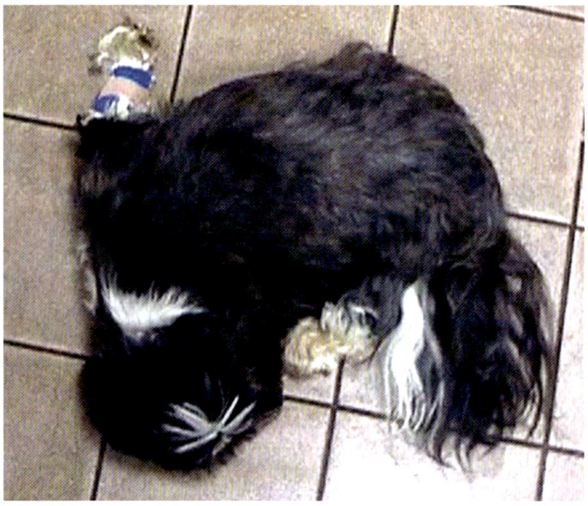

**Figure 5.8.** Pleurothotonus.

- facial hypoaesthesia
- tilting the head towards the lesion
- pathological nystagmus
- decreased pupillary reflexes
- strabismus
- vestibular ataxia.

### *Cerebellar lesion*

- normal mental state
- cerebellar ataxia
- hypermetria
- intention tremor
- head tilting contralateral to the lesion
- wide-based stance
- absent menace response
- strabismus
- pendular nystagmus.

### *C1–C5 lesion*

- normal mental state
- spinal ataxia
- hypermetria
- delay in postural reactions in all limbs
- tetraparesia/tetraplegia
- spinal reflexes present or increased
- normal or increased muscle tone.

### *C6–T2 lesion*

- normal mental state
- delay in postural reactions in all limbs
- tetraparesia/tetraplegia
- decreased spinal reflexes in thoracic limbs
- muscular atrophy of thoracic limbs
- reduced muscle tone in thoracic limbs
- Horner's syndrome.

### *T3–L3 lesion*

- normal mental state
- normal thoracic limbs
- ataxia of the trunk and pelvic limbs
- paraparesia/paraplegia
- spinal reflexes normal or increased in pelvic limbs
- muscle tone of pelvic limbs normal or increased
- changes to or absence of cutaneous trunk reflex
- urinary incontinence (full bladder, difficult to empty).

### *L4–S3 lesion*

- normal mental state
- normal thoracic limbs

- ataxia of pelvic limbs
- paraparesis/paraplegia
- reduced spinal reflexes in pelvic limbs
- muscle tone of pelvic limbs reduced
- decreased or absence of cutaneous trunk reflex
- muscular atrophy of pelvic limbs
- urinary incontinence (full bladder, easy to empty with decreased tone)
- decreased anal tone, sensation and perineal reflex.

### *Neuromuscular injury*

- normal mental state
- decreased spinal and cranial reflexes
- muscular atrophy
- decreased muscle tone
- weakness/collapse
- exercise intolerance
- aphonia.

A good neurological examination shortens the list of differential diagnoses and the time necessary for a diagnosis to be made.

Keep an open mind to the possibility that there may be **two injuries**, which can be confusing when identifying the location of the lesion.

## Diagnostic techniques

Successful diagnosis of a neurological disease starts with a thorough neurological examination for accurate **location of the lesion**. This facilitates preparation of a **list of differential diagnosis** appropriate for the history, progression and lesion location, and in turn selection of the **most appropriate diagnostic tests**.

It is also important to first consider and rule out the possibility of **systemic disease with a secondary effect on the nervous system**, such as hypoglycaemia or Addison's disease, before subjecting the patient to expensive tests that require general anaesthesia such as myelography, electrodiagnosis, MRI or CT scans.

### *Laboratory tests*

A wide range of neurological diseases present with **changes on screening blood tests**. The first step in the investigation should be a thorough evaluation consisting of:

- a complete blood count with blood smears
- electrolytes
- hepatic transaminases
- glucose
- calcium
- creatinine kinase CK
- total proteins and albumin
- urea and creatinine
- **postprandial bile acids** and **ammonium** should also be included, to rule out pathologies with a secondary effect on the nervous system.

### *Serum titres*

The results of serum titres should be **interpreted with caution**. A **positive antibody titre indicates only exposure to the pathogen or vaccination**, not that the neurological sings are caused by the pathogen. This is especially true in the case of endemic diseases such as ehrlichiosis and leishmaniosis.

An increase in serum titre requires a **competent immune system** and a **sufficient response period**, so in early stages of the disease or in cases of infectious diseases that cause immunosuppression (canine distemper virus, FIV) or administration of glucocorticoids, **false negatives can occur**.

Although a serum IgM titre has traditionally been associated with recent exposure to the pathogen, in some infectious diseases **elevated levels** of this immunoglobulin may **persist for months or years**.

Any **positive serum titres** should be accompanied by test results and **clinical signs compatible with the disease** to be considered reliable. Therefore, knowledge of clinical and neurological signs that manifest with different infectious diseases, as well as their method of transmission, is essential. In addition, the possibility of cross-reactivity and contamination of the sample causing a **false positive** should be considered: the presence of a positive serum titre to an infectious disease in an animal with neurological involvement without clinical signs or compatible laboratory results is not reliable.

### *CSF*

Analysis of CSF forms an essential part of the neurological investigation. The analysis must be **performed within 30 minutes** of the sample being obtained to get reliable results.

An increase in the number of **leukocytes in CSF shows inflammation** but does not necessarily prove that the cause is solely inflammatory. **Diagnosis of an infectious disease** affecting the central nervous system should be based on **demonstration of the presence of a pathogen** in CSF or biopsy. Detection of the pathogen by cytology on CSF is possible, providing a definitive diagnosis for the following infections:

- cryptococcosis
- toxoplasmosis
- neosporosis
- angiostrongylosis.

However, the method that has revolutionized the diagnosis of infectious diseases is **polymerase chain reaction (PCR)**, although it also has its limitations. PCR uses short segments of simple-helix nucleotides called primers, whose sequences are complementary to the known DNA of the pathogen. After an amplification process, the target DNA sequences can be detected by gel electrophoresis. In this way, **genetic material of the pathogen** can be identified in different biological samples.

This method is not completely reliable, since false positives can occur when there is contamination (therefore, taking the sample in aseptic conditions and the choice of a reliable laboratory are fundamental), and false negatives can occur due to the presence of PCR inhibitors. It is **not indicated for evaluating response to treatment**, since DNA can persist for a long time after the death of an organism.

The majority of **degenerative and lysosomal diseases** are caused by **genetic mutations** that can be diagnosed by analysis of **DNA from blood or oral mucosa**. Currently, a large number of laboratories offer this type of service and the range of tests will become ever broader in the future. However, it is important to understand both the limitations of these tests and any particularities of the breed, the possibility of false positives and of concurrent diseases.

## Diagnostic imaging

Once the location of the lesion and the list of differential diagnoses have been established, appropriate tests to confirm a diagnosis should be chosen.

- In the case of **focal spinal cord injuries**, spinal radiographs, myelography and CSF analysis may be sufficient.
- In the case of **neuromuscular injuries**, electromyography and nerve conduction studies should be the first choice.
- When **brain injury** is suspected, CT and MRI are the best options.

Both **MRI and CT require deep sedation or general anaesthesia**, options which are contraindicated in some neurological patients until they are stabilized.

Several studies have shown that these two diagnostic methods can reveal abnormalities that are not clinically significant in animals lacking any neurological signs.

It is important to understand the physical principles of how images are obtained, to gauge the advantages and limitations of each of the techniques.

### Plain radiography

Plain radiographs allow detection of **injuries affecting bony structures** or the intervertebral discs. Any **injury that** causes either **lytic or proliferative bone remodelling** can usually be detected on plain radiographs (Figure 5.9).

**Orthogonal projections** under sedation or general anaesthesia are essential for correct interpretation (Figure 5.10).

### Myelography

The injection of iodinated contrast into the **subarachnoid space** at the level of the cerebellomedullary or lumbar cisterns (myelography) is particularly useful for demonstrating the presence of **spinal compressions that justify surgical treatment**, and allows the complete study of the spinal cord without significantly increasing the time or cost of diagnosis (Figure 5.11).

Both myelography and advanced imaging studies (CT, CT with myelography, MRI) can be useful for diagnosis of spinal cord compression. A recent study has shown that, when comparing myelography and MRI for diagnosis of thoracolumbar lesions, there was no difference in treatment outcomes but the cost was higher when MRI was used. Despite this, **MRI** is more sensitive for **detection of vascular spinal cord injuries** that would otherwise go unnoticed.

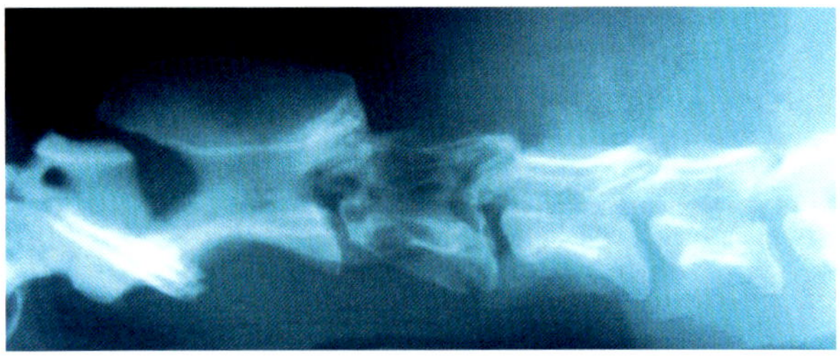

**Figure 5.9.** Lateral radiograph of the cervical spine in a dog with marked osteolysis due to metastasis from a haemangiosarcoma.

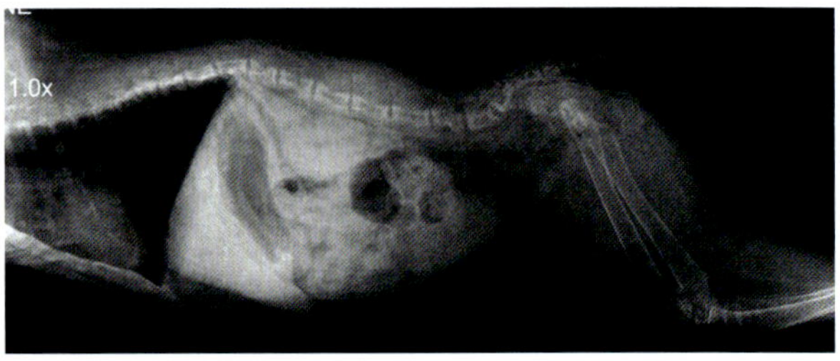


**Figure 5.10.** Lateral radiograph of the spine in a cat with generalized osteopenia due to secondary nutritional hyperparathyroidism.

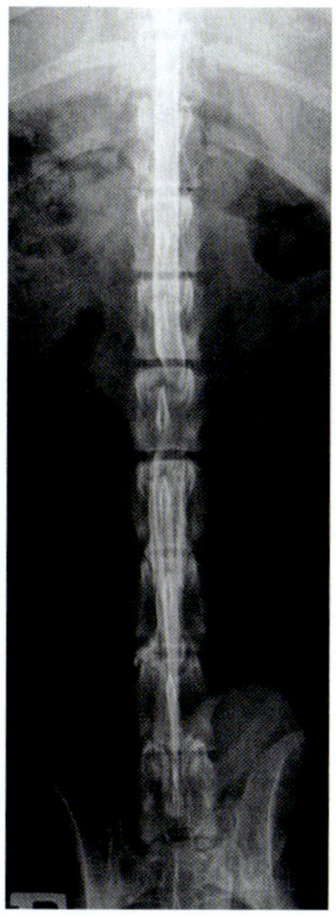

**Figure 5.11.** Lumbar myelography in a 10-year-old Labrador with extradural spinal cord compression due to a vertebral fibrosarcoma.

The imaging techniques mentioned (myelography, CT, myelo-CT and MRI) allow only a definitive diagnosis of fractures and not of other lesions, in particular those which are not compressive.

Advantages of myelography:

- lower cost
- availability
- requires less anaesthesia time than MRI.

Regardless of the technique used, the **experience of the clinician** when interpreting images is fundamental, and a myelography that is well executed and interpreted by an experienced clinician can provide more information than an MRI performed or interpreted by an inexperienced clinician. The most important thing is to reach an accurate diagnosis and implement the appropriate treatment options for that diagnosis.

### *CT*

CT is based on the emission of radio waves that pass through the tissues from a rotating arch which moves around the body, and are then detected by a series of receivers on the opposite side to which they are emitted.

The main advantages of the technique are the:

- good detail available for examining bony structures
- ability to combine with use of intrathecal or intravenous contrast
- ability to perform 3D reconstructions
- speed at which images are obtained, if a helical CT is used.

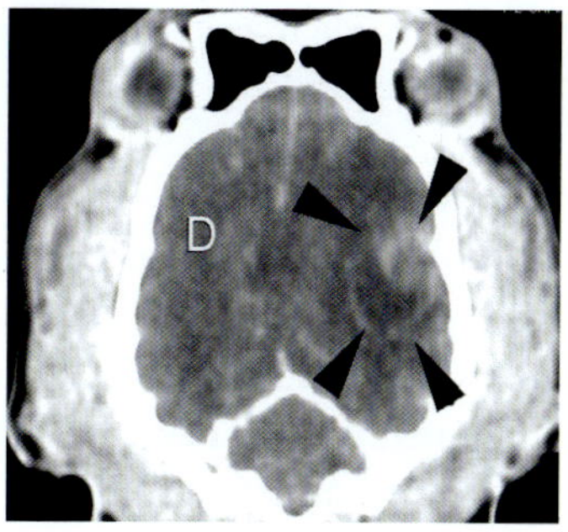


**Figure 5.12.** CT: vascular hamartoma (arrowheads).

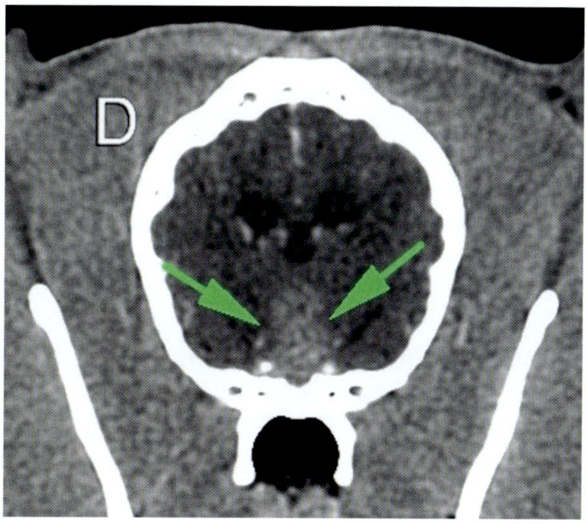


**Figure 5.13.** CT: pituitary macro-adenoma (arrowheads).

However, the **resolution obtained from soft tissues is limited**, and small inflammatory, degenerative lesions – as well as those located next to structures – that cause a high degree of attenuation of radiation (for example, caudo-tentorial structures or metal implants) can go unnoticed (Figures 5.12 and 5.13).

### *MRI*

MRI works by using radio waves to excite protons subjected to an electromagnetic field, hydrogen (present in the body in large quantities) and the detection of the emissions by those protons when they relax.

MRI is particularly useful for visualizing soft tissues such as the brain or spinal cord.

The main drawbacks of MRI are:

- the cost of equipment
- artefacts in the images obtained
- limited resolution of low-field equipment in small animals.

Owing to higher definition of images, detection of some **degenerative diseases** presenting with macroscopic changes is possible, but for a definitive diagnosis other diagnostic tests, such as genetic tests, urinalysis and biopsy, are still necessary.

### Electrodiagnostic tests

When there is **lower motor neuron** (weakness, loss of spinal reflexes, muscle atrophy, etc.) involvement, the most appropriate and least invasive diagnostic method is **electromyography**, which can confirm the presence of spontaneous electrical activity in skeletal muscles suggesting a myopathy or neuropathy. Nerve conduction tests allow **distinction between muscle and nerve involvement**, enabling the type of neuropathy to be characterized before confirmation by muscle and/or nerve biopsy (Figure 5.14). The presence of F-waves can indicate the likely presence of the lesion in the proximal segment of the nerve. In many cases, results from electrodiagnosis, together with clinical history and results of additional diagnostic tests, allow a diagnosis to be reached without having to resort to more invasive or expensive tests, and for treatment to be commenced.

## Neurological manifestations of systemic diseases

The central and peripheral nervous systems (NS) require **large amounts of energy to function**, and any reduction in energy levels or use of energy by systemic conditions can produce varied neurological effects.

Systemic diseases may secondarily affect the nervous system can be classified as follows.

- **Haematological or vascular** anomalies erase may cause a decrease in energy supply to the nervous system, and include:
  - **hypoxaemia** (cardiopulmonary disease, anaesthetic accidents, coagulopathies, cerebral ischaemia).
  - **hypoglycaemia** (sepsis, hyperinsulinism, severe liver disease).
- **Nutritional deficiency** (thiamine, etc.).
- **Electrolyte alterations** disrupting neuronal or muscular functionality ($Na^+$, $Ca^{2+}$, $K^+$).
- **Metabolic changes** producing endogenous neurotoxins, which disrupt the neurochemical balance in the brain:
  - **hepatic encephalopathy** (portosystemic shunt, liver cirrhosis, microvascular dysplasia, hepatitis).
  - **uraemic encephalopathy** (renal failure, urinary obstruction).
- **Endocrine disorders** that result in a myriad of systemic and, secondarily, neurological effects:
  - hypothyroidism, hyperthyroidism.
  - hypoadrenocorticism, hyperadrenocorticism.

## Clinical signs

A **complete history and physical examination** can lead to suspicions of systemic diseases and secondary neurological signs.

- Cyanosis, weak pulse, bradycardia, haemorrhage, abnormal heart or lung sounds are examples of **haematological or cardiovascular alterations** affecting oxygenation and perfusion of the nervous system.
- Symmetrical alopecia, seborrhoea, comedones and hyperpigmentation of the skin raise the suspicion of **endocrinopathy** as the cause of neurological signs.

Neurological signs vary with the location of the lesion, for example: **changes in energy** intake, electrolyte imbalances and endocrine and metabolic diseases often cause **diffuse neurological signs** whereas haematological changes, infectious and immune-mediated

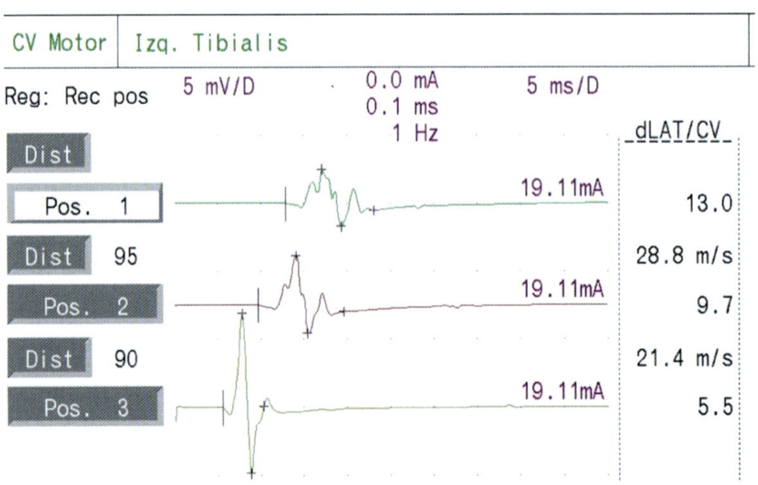


**Figure 5.14.** Motor nerve conduction study in a miniature Schnauzer with demyelinating polyneuropathy showing a delay in nerve conduction.

diseases and paraneoplastic syndromes tend to be **more localized**.

## Diagnosis

The required complementary tests depend on the physical and neurological findings identified during examination.

- A **complete blood count**, including a **blood smear** along with coagulation tests (PT, PTT, ATT, D-dimer and antithrombin III), may show anaemia, polycythaemia, thrombocytopenia and coagulopathies that alter oxygenation or perfusion of the NS.
- Complete **blood biochemistry** including **electrolytes** can show specific changes in other organs that may be responsible for neurological signs (kidney, liver) or electrolyte alterations that interfere with NS or muscle function.
- **Thoracic radiography** and **abdominal ultrasound** can identify pathologies such as pulmonary or aortic thromboembolism, adrenal masses, renal atrophy, neoplasms, etc.

However, these **findings may not be specific** and may **require functional tests** such as the bile acid stimulation test, total T4, free T4/TSH, ammonium, TSH stimulation test or a dexamethasone suppression test to confirm possible diagnoses.

In rare cases, advanced imaging (MRI or CT) is useful for the diagnosis of systemic diseases, but its expense and the need for general anaesthesia mean that its use is not recommended. They can be useful in the following cases:

- pituitary macroadenoma
- cerebrovascular accident
- myelinolysis
- thiamine deficiency (Figure 5.15).

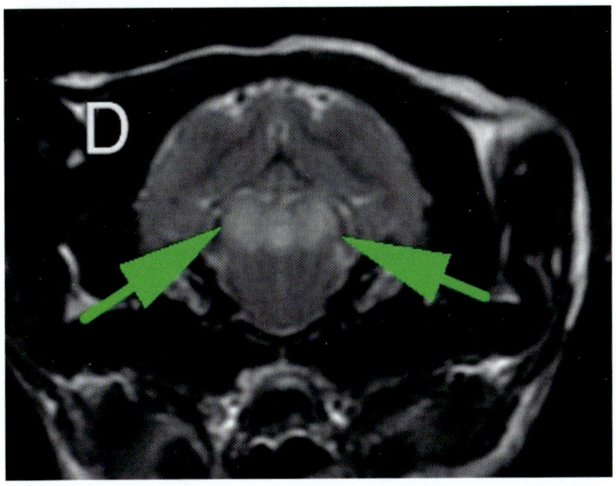


**Figure 5.15.** MRI of a cat with malacia of the caudal colliculi (arrows) as a consequence of vitamin $B_1$ deficiency.

In cases in which neurological examination suggests generalized involvement of **lower motor neurons, electrodiagnostic techniques** are the most appropriate erase tests to be chosen.

## Hypothyroidism

### Aetiology

**Canine hypothyroidism** is most commonly a primary disease with the main cause being **idiopathic atrophy of the gland**, although it can also be due to lymphocytic thyroiditis or hereditary causes.

### Clinical signs

Characteristic systemic signs include:

- weight gain
- seborrhoea
- alopecia
- hyperpigmentation
- anoestrus
- bradycardia.

**Neurological signs** can appear associated with these or independently, among those which have been described are:

- vestibular syndrome
- laryngeal and facial paralysis
- Horner's syndrome
- muscular atrophy
- weakness
- tetraparesis
- ataxia
- megaoesophagus
- focal cerebral signs as a consequence of arteriosclerosis.

Although hypothyroidism has been described in the literature as a cause of seizures in the adult dog, it has not been possible to demonstrate a direct relationship between both. Therefore it is likely that both represent comorbidities. Based on an experimental study, other authors question whether hypothyroidism is responsible for these clinical signs and speculate on the possibility of an immune-mediated pathogenesis.

### Diagnosis

A diagnosis is made by demonstrating a **decrease in free serum T4** measured using equilibrium dialysis with a parallel increase in TSH, or by a TSH stimulation test. Results should be interpreted taking into account that **medications can influence levels of thyroid hormones**, for example glucocorticoids, propanolol, sulfonamides, phenobarbital, potassium bromide and NSAIDs. Electrodiagnostic tests, such as electromyography and nerve conduction studies, show signs compatible with myopathy and neuropathy (fibrillation potentials, positive sharp waves and complex repetitive discharges, decreased conduction velocity).

In animals with peripheral vestibular disease, brainstem auditory evoked response (brainstem potentials) can be used to demonstrate parallel involvement of the auditory system.

### Treatment

Treatment is by **thyroxine supplementation**, which causes an initial improvement in mental state and muscular strength (in a few days, and after this in the remaining neurological deficits), over several months.

Recovery may not be complete in cases of megaoesophagus or laryngeal paralysis, so the latter may require surgical treatment.

## Hyperthyroidism

### Clinical signs

Feline hyperthyroidism has been associated in 12–25% of cases with:

- weakness
- fatigue
- muscular tremors.

Other systemic signs include:

- weight loss
- polyphagia
- hyperactivity
- tachycardia
- PU/PD
- vomiting
- diarrhoea.

### Diagnosis

A diagnosis is reached by demonstrating elevated basal T4 levels together with clinical signs.

### Treatment

Curative treatment consists of surgical removal of the tumour responsible or ablation with radioactive iodine. Medical treatment is not curative.

## Hyperadrenocorticism

### Aetiology

This endocrine disease can be caused by:

- pituitary tumours (70% of spontaneous cases)
- adrenal tumours (30% of spontaneous cases)
- chronic iatrogenic administration of glucocorticoids.

### Clinical signs

Associated clinical signs include:

- PU/PD
- abdominal distention
- hepatomegaly
- thinning of the skin
- symmetrical alopecia
- hypotrichosis.

In parallel, neurological signs can also be seen:

- weakness
- generalized muscular atrophy with proximal muscular hypertrophy
- uneven gait starting in the pelvic limbs.

The diameter of active **pituitary tumours is usually <1 cm**, although occasionally they are larger and cause compression of adjacent structures in the diencephalon.

### Diagnosis

Diagnosis is possible using a **low-dose dexamethasone suppression test** or an ACTH stimulation test. Electromyography allows detection of repetitive complex discharges (pseudomyotonia) that indicate an increase in muscle excitability as a result of histopathological changes in myofibres.

### Treatment

Curative treatment:

- surgical removal of the adrenal mass
- progressive reduction in exogenous glucocorticoids
- trans-sphenoidal hypophysectomy of small pituitary tumours
- radiotherapy.

Despite effective treatment, in some cases muscular signs may persist.

## Hypoadrenocorticism

### Clinical signs

Clinical signs associated with adrenal hormone deficiency are initially non-specific and include:

- lethargy
- vomiting

- diarrhoea
- dehydration
- PU/PD
- hypovolaemic shock
- abdominal pain
- intestinal haemorrhage.

Neurological signs include:

- seizures due to hypoglycaemia
- muscular contractions (spasms).

Hypovolaemic shock and, as a consequence **cerebral hypoperfusion**, can result in severe intracranial sequelae due to cortical necrosis.

Classical clinicopathological abnormalities are:

- hyponatraemia
- hyperkalaemia
- non-regenerative anaemia
- lymphocytosis.

Other alterations such as azotaemia, hypoglycaemia and hyperphosphataemia may also be present.

### Diagnosis

Measurement of **basal cortisol <2 μg/dl has a sensitivity of 100% for hypoadrenocorticism**, although diagnosis should be confirmed using an ACTH stimulation test.

In the presence of hyperkalaemia, an electrocardiogram shows an increase in the amplitude of the T-waves and characteristic changes in the QRS complex.

### Treatment

Treatment of an acute crisis requires the administration of the following until signs improve:

- intensive shock fluid therapy
- intravenous glucose
- insulin
- glucocorticoids.

**Correction of electrolyte abnormalities should be gradual**, in order to avoid pontine myelinolysis.

For maintenance therapy, long-acting mineralocorticoids are sufficient.

### Prognosis

Excellent with mineralocorticoid supplementation.

## Hepatic encephalopathy (HE)

### Aetiology

Causes of HE:

- portosystemic shunt (most common cause)
- hepatic cirrhosis
- acute liver failure
- congenital defects in the urea cycle (very uncommon).

### Clinical signs

Clinical signs are mainly neurological, and the one that manifests earliest is behavioural changes that suggest bilateral cortical involvement. After this, the following can be observed:

- stupor
- blindness
- collapse
- seizures
- deafness
- coma
- growth failure
- anorexia
- fever
- vomiting
- polyurea
- polydipsia
- struvite urolithiasis.

Neurological signs can be episodic and precipitated by the following:

- feeding
- intestinal bleeding
- constipation
- azotaemia
- recent anaesthesia.

### Diagnosis

Diagnosis is possible by demonstrating **high levels of blood ammonia**. In the case of vascular anomaly, there are changes in the enterohepatic cycle so the measurement of **pre- and postprandial bile acids** can also be diagnostic. Given that there are a wide range of causes, the following are necessary for identification of the aetiology:

- complete blood analysis
- radiography and abdominal ultrasound
- urinalysis
- measurement of serum cobalamin.

### Treatment

Treatment may be medical or surgical, depending on the aetiology and the financial situation of the owner.

### Medical
Before surgery, the patient should be stabilized using the following measures:

- low-protein diet
- antibiotic therapy
- lactulose
- *levetirazetam 10–20 mg/kg IV or PO*, if there are epileptic seizures.

### Surgical
Surgical intervention is associated with a longer survival period.

## Hypoglycaemia

### Aetiopathogenesis
**Glucose is the main energy substrate in the nervous system** and is necessary for its effective functioning, so any disease that reduces its availability in the general circulation can cause significant effects.

**Insulinoma** is perhaps the most frequent cause of hypoglycaemia in the dog.

Other diseases that can cause a decrease in serum glucose levels with subsequent neurological signs include:

- liver failure
- insulin overdose
- excessive exercise
- hypoglycaemia in toy dogs
- glycogen storage disease
- xylitol poisoning.

### Clinical signs
**Seizures** are the most frequent neurological sign in cases of hypoglycaemia. There are also other relatively frequent clinical signs, including:

- weakness
- altered mental state
- coma
- trembling
- blindness
- weakness.

In chronic cases, axonal polyneuropathy with progressive weakness and hyporeflexia has been described.

### Diagnosis
The presence of **persistent hypoglycaemia** and **reduced fructosamine levels** indicates a change in blood glucose level. In severe cases malacia may be found on MRI (Figure 5.16) but, in general, advanced imaging is not necessary. Blood glucose should not be measured after a seizure as levels can be reduced by the seizure itself.

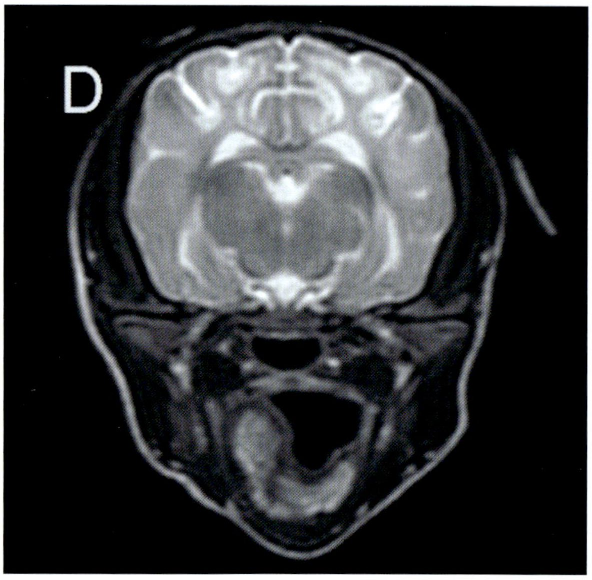


**Figure 5.16.** MRI of a dog after an acute hypoglycaemic crisis causing malacia of the brain.

### Treatment
**Treatment depends on the underlying cause**, and its objective should be to restore normal blood glucose levels because the majority of neurological signs should resolve once blood glucose is restored within normal limits.

## Thiamine deficiency

### Aetiopathogenesis
**Thiamine deficiency** (vitamin $B_1$, a vitamin essential for the metabolism of carbohydrates in the Krebs cycle) is a rare cause of **metabolic encephalopathy**. It has been described in cats and dogs fed diets deficient in the vitamin or due to ingestion of **dietary thiaminase** when fed exclusively on fish.

### Clinical signs
#### Dogs
Clinical and neurological signs in dogs include:

- anorexia
- vomiting
- obtundation
- ataxia
- progressive paraparesis
- ventro-flexion of the neck
- generalized seizures
- opisthotonus
- coma
- death.

### Cats

In cats **vestibular signs** are most common:

- nystagmus
- mydriasis
- absent menace response
- stupor
- death.

#### *Diagnosis*

A definitive diagnosis is made by measurement of blood thiamine levels by a specialized laboratory. Typical findings on MRI may reinforce the suspicion of a deficiency.

#### *Treatment*

Treatment should be aggressive and start as soon as possible. It consists of intramuscular administration of thiamine for several days, which should lead to a complete recovery.

### *Uraemic encephalopathy*

#### *Aetiopathogenesis*

Urinary diseases leading to a decreased excretion of metabolites and electrolyte imbalances can cause clinical and neurological signs.

#### *Clinical signs*

Neurological signs include:

- obtundation or stupor, more frequent in chronic renal failure cases
- generalized seizures, more frequent in cases of acute renal failure
- facial fasciculations
- myoclonus
- weakness.

In the cat, chronic renal failure can cause **hypokalaemia**, which usually manifests as severe neuromuscular weakness with pain and decreased spinal reflexes.

#### *Treatment and prognosis*

The underlying cause should be treated, electrolyte imbalances corrected and associated seizures controlled. Prognosis depends on the cause.

## Epilepsy

The International Veterinary Epilepsy Task Force (IVETF) has recently modified the terminology used when referring to seizures and epilepsy.

- **Epileptic seizure**: clinical manifestation of an excessive synchronous electrical activity of brain cells, which is normally self-limiting.
- **Epilepsy**: disease of the brain characterized by a long-term predisposition for the generation of epileptic seizures.
- **Genetic idiopathic epilepsy**: epilepsy in which a genetic mutation has been shown to cause seizures.
- **Familial idiopathic epilepsy**: epilepsy in which the mutation has not been demonstrated but a genetic cause is assumed since it affects the same breed or family.
- **Idiopathic epilepsy of unknown origin**: the clinical or familial history does not support a diagnosis of familial epilepsy but, after an exhaustive investigation, no biological cause can be found.
- **Structural epilepsy**: the seizures have an intracranial cause.

Seizures can be reactive or epileptic.

- **Reactive**, when they are **due to an extracranial cause**, whether toxic, endocrine or metabolic. This is not considered to be epilepsy, because the seizures resolve after correction of the temporary metabolic state.
- **Epileptic**, which in turn can be divided into two sub-categories.
  - Focal, when they **alter functionality of a part of the brain** and manifest alone or together as rhythmic muscular contractions (motor), episodic behavioural crises (behavioural) or with autonomous signs (autonomic). Focal seizures can evolve into a generalized seizure.
  - Generalized, when they **affect the entire brain**. They usually alter the level of consciousness.

### *Idiopathic epilepsy*

#### *Diagnosis*

The diagnosis of idiopathic epilepsy is **established after excluding all other causes of seizure** and, in most cases, is presumptive.

The most common presentation is in animals **1–5 years old** with a history of repeated seizures that show a complete **return to neurological normality** between episodes.

The most commonly affected breeds are: Golden Retriever, Labrador Retriever, Beagle, Keeshund, Tervueren Belgian Shepherd, Australian Shepherd and Shetland Sheepdog. In some breeds, such as the Hungarian Viszla, Bull Terrier and Labrador Retriever, seizures are focal.

### Treatment

Traditionally, treatment was based on administration of anticonvulsants such as **phenobarbital and potassium bromide**. However, these are effective in only 60–70% of cases. In some cases their **idiosyncratic side effects** mean that substitution is necessary with other, less toxic, anticonvulsants. Regardless of the oral dose, **exhaustive monitoring of serum levels** of both medications is essential since successful treatment is fundamentally related to these levels.

The most widely agreed upon criteria for starting treatment with anticonvulsants are:

- **progressive increase** in the frequency and severity of seizures
- **status epilepticus** or cluster seizures as the first sign of seizures
- presence of **structural epilepsy**
- **severe postictal signs.**

The following should be taken into account when commencing treatment.

- The timing of when treatment is started.
- The most suitable medication and dose for the patient.
- How and when blood levels can be checked, if needed.
- When to add or change an anticonvulsant.
- Ensuring the owner complies with the doses and frequency of administration.

Next, the anticonvulsants used most widely in day-to-day practice are described.

## Phenobarbital

Phenobarbital is the **first-line medication** for the treatment of seizures, regardless of the cause. It acts by potentiating the effect of the inhibitory neurotransmitter GABA-A in the postsynaptic membrane. In the **dog, monitoring of serum levels** of the medication to ensure a minimum therapeutic level due to the induction of hepatic microsomal enzymes is advisable. In the cat the induction of hepatic microsomal enzymes is minimal, so frequent monitoring of serum levels is not required unless other medications that produce this effect (glucocorticoids, chloramphenicol, cimetidine, etc.) are also being administered.

The starting dose is:

- **dogs**: *2–5 mg/kg/12 h*
- **cats**: *7.5–15 mg daily in total,* depending on the size of the animal. It can be administered once or twice daily.

Therapeutic levels have not been established in the cat, although it is thought that they are similar to those in dogs: *14–40 μg/ml.*

Side effects, which are temporary, include:

- sedation
- ataxia
- PU/PD.

Similar to diazepam, phenobarbital is contraindicated for the treatment of hepatic encephalopathy.

## Diazepam

Diazepam exerts its mechanism of action in a similar way to phenobarbital, potentiating the action of GABA-A. In the long term it causes tolerance in the dog, but not in the cat. This means that this anticonvulsant can be used for maintenance therapy in the cat. However, special attention should be paid to **liver enzymes**, since a small proportion of **cats develop fulminant hepatic necrosis** within a few days of administration. Serum levels of ALT and AST should be obtained within a week to identify thsi idiosynchratic reaction early. *Recommended dose: 2–5 mg/8–12 h.*

## Potassium bromide

Potassium bromide is a salt whose mechanism of action occurs on the postsynaptic GABA-A receptors, replacing chloride and hyperpolarizing the membrane. It comes in a master formula or 325 mg capsules, which makes administration in small animals complicated.

The maintenence dose in the **dog** is *30–40 mg/kg/24 h.* **Stable levels are usually reached 3 months** after maintenance therapy is started. In order to accelerate the process, a total loading dose of *450–600 mg/kg* can be administered, divided into as many doses as considered necessary. Hospitalization is advisable during this loading dose period.

**Potassium bromide is not recommended in the cat** because it produces allergic pneumonitis in 50% of cases.

In the dog the possible side effects include:

- sedation
- ataxia
- vomiting
- dermatitis.

Serum levels are reduced by the high amount of salt in the diet, so it is important to **reduce salt intake** as much as possible.

Over the past 15 years, the use of anticonvulsants from human medicine such as levetiracetam, gabapentin, zonisamide and topiramate has made possible a more effective control of seizures in animals afflicted with this condition. However, due to their expense, the use of these medications should be reserved for animals where adequate control of seizures cannot be achieved or for those that suffer from severe side effects.

### Levetiracetam

Levetiracetam is a second-generation anticonvulsant frequently used as additional treatment in the following cases:

- epilepsy refractory to traditional anticonvulsants
- liver or kidney disease.

Its mechanism of action has not been fully elucidated, although it seems to act on the SV2A vesicles in the presynaptic membranes. It is absorbed almost completely orally, and its half-life is 2–4 h, predominantly with renal excretion. An interesting feature of the pharmacokinetics of this drug is that, despite its short half-life, it seems to have a cumulative effect in the brain it can be **administered every 8 h**. Due to the fact there is no hepatic metabolism, it is useful in the **treatment of seizures due to hepatic encephalopathy** or liver damage caused by phenobarbital. In a recent study, its efficacy for the control of seizures has been evaluated as an additional treatment. The author uses an *initial dose of 20 mg/kg/8 h that can be gradually increased*. The only side effects observed have been slight sedation and thrombocytopaenia, but this is rare. Despite its initial efficacy, some animals may develop an aggravation of seizures or even the so-called 'honeymoon effect', with return of seizures in the long term. In the cat, it seems to be as effective as in the dog. Recent introduction of an intravenous presentation makes its use possible in status epilepticus.

### Imepitoin

Imepitoin is the only **anticonvulsant indicated for treatment of idiopathic epilepsy in the dog**. Its mechanism of action is based on partial low-affinity agonism at the point of attachment of benzodiazepines in GABA-A receptors. Its clinical efficacy for reducing the occurrence of seizures is 75%, and it eliminates them completely in 8% of dogs.

Side effects, although less common than with phenobarbital, include:

- hyperactivity
- polyphagia
- sedation (at high doses).

The starting dose is *10–20 mg/kg/12 h*, but this can be *increased to 30 mg/kg/12 h*. There are no studies on interactions with other medications, or for the treatment of structural epilepsy or reactive seizures.

### Gabapentin

Although this medication was introduced into human medicine as a structural analogue of GABA, its anticonvulsant effect is different. This is based on increasing the release and action of GABA and inhibition of neuronal sodium channels, although lately it is believed that it also acts by inhibiting voltage-dependent calcium channels. In the dog, it has good oral absorption and 30–40% hepatic metabolism although it does not induce microsomal enzymes; the half-life is 3–4 h.

The author uses an *initial dose of 10 mg/kg/8 h* that can be gradually increased, except if side effects begin to develop (the most common is sedation). Gabapentin does not seem to be as effective as suggested in recent studies, although it can be reserved for cases in which the cost of other anticonvulsants is prohibitive. In the author's experience, it is more useful for the treatment of neuropathic pain.

### Zonisamide

Zonisamide is an anti-epileptic whose main mechanism of action consists in the inhibition of the presynaptic T-type calcium channels and sodium channels. Its metabolism is mainly hepatic, by microsomal enzymes and, although it does not cause their induction, its **half-life is 15 h**. Due to its hepatic metabolism, higher doses should be used in patients who are being treated with phenobarbital. The author uses a *dose of 5 mg/kg/12 h* in patients who have not been treated with this medication, and *10 mg/kg when animals are already receiving it*. Its efficacy has recently been evaluated in the dog. As with levetirazetam, a 'honeymoon effect' has been observed. Its main disadvantage is the expense.

### Topiramate

Topiramate's mechanism of action is complex, potentiating both the inhibitory action of GABA and the blocking of neuronal calcium and sodium channels and glutamate receptors. Its metabolism does not cause induction of liver enzymes. The recommended dose in human medicine is 2–25 mg/kg/12 h. A gradual increase in dose is recommended. There are **no long-term studies on its efficacy in domestic animals**, but the author has used it in cases refractory to all previously mentioned anticonvulsants with very good results. Again, its disadvantage is the high cost.

### Other anticonvulsants from human medicine

Primidone and phenytoin are no longer used for the treatment of idiopathic epilepsy in domestic animals, since they do not provide any advantage over phenobarbital and there is a higher probability of liver toxicity.

In the dog, **valproate** has a half-life that is considerably shorter in dogs (1.7 h) than in humans (9–16 h), and this means that **dosage is difficult**.

In the dog, **lamotrigine** is metabolized to a **cardiotoxic compound** and is therefore contraindicated.

**Vigabatrin** produces **blood dyscrasias**, which is why it is not recommended.

Oral diazepam has a low absorption (<5%) and is therefore not useful for the control of epilepsy in the dog; **in the cat, diazepam can cause fulminant hepatic necrosis**.

## Vestibular syndrome

Key to **differentiating a vestibular episode from a partial seizure** is recognizing the neurological signs associated with vestibular disease. Both can be episodic, but a complete neurological examination sheds light on the characteristic clinical signs. In addition, since the **vestibular system is able to partially compensate**, performing certain tests during a neurological examination can **reveal hidden vestibular signs**.

The vestibular system is composed of two components.

- A **central component** that includes:
  - vestibular nuclei
  - vestibulocerebellum
  - associated tracts.
- A **peripheral component** that includes:
  - semi-circular canals
  - utricle
  - saccule
  - vestibular nerve.

The vestibular system is responsible for **maintaining the position of the eyes, trunk and limbs** in relation to the position and movement of the head.

### *Unilateral vestibular disease*

The most common neurological sign in **unilateral vestibular disease** is a head tilt. In extreme circumstances the animal may repeatedly **roll**, which is usually **indicative of peripheral disease**. Sight can help to compensate for the lack of balance, and therefore **covering the eyes can exacerbate the signs**.

With **unilateral peripheral disease** the most characteristic neurological sign is **ataxia**, although strength is conserved. However, in **central diseases affecting the vestibular nuclei** there is also **ipsilateral paresis** since lesions usually affect descending vestibular tracts, which are powerful excitators of anti-gravity extensor muscles. In addition, mental state can be affected by lesions that affect the ascending reticular formations in the myelencephalon.

**Nystagmus is an involuntary and rhythmic oscillation of the eyeball**, usually from side to side (horizontal) and almost **always in both eyes**. It typically occurs with a slow phase in one direction and a fast phase in the opposite direction. Physiological nystagmus occurs during examination when the head is moved and is normal. When nystagmus is present in a resting position (horizontal plane) it is called **spontaneous or pathological nystagmus**, whereas the one seen when the head is placed in an unusual or forced position is called **positional nystagmus**. The presence of positional nystagmus is not indicative of central disease. In cases of peripheral disease, nystagmus can be horizontal or rotatory and the **fast phase is always towards the opposite side to the lesion**. In central disease it can be horizontal, rotatory or vertical. Thus, a vertical or changing nystagmus with changes in head position indicates central disease.

**Vestibular strabismus** refers to the ventral or ventrolateral deviation of the eyeball in a forced position, which is usually corrected when the head is moved to a different position. Eyeball deviation is ipsilateral to the vestibular lesion (Figure 5.17).

### *Central unilateral vestibular disease*

- **Head tilting** is ipsilateral to the lesion.
- The quick phase of **nystagmus** is to the opposite side of the lesion.
- **Strabismus is ipsilateral**, as with most central diseases.

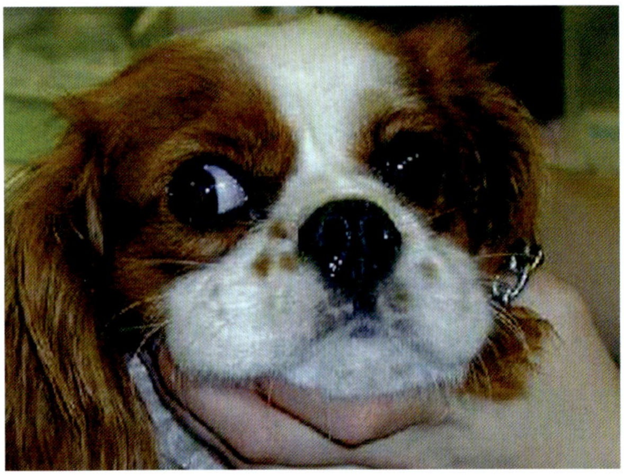

**Figure 5.17.** Right vestibular strabismus.

- With **central vestibular disease** there is a **delay in postural reactions** and **altered mental state**.

## *Paradoxical central vestibular disease*

Occurs with injuries in:

- caudal cerebellar peduncle
- rostral and medial vestibular nuclei
- flocculonodular cerebellar lobe
- fastigial nucleus in the cerebellum.

In these cases, the following can be seen:

- contralateral head tilting
- quick phase of nystagmus towards the side of the lesion
- only postural reaction deficits are ipsilateral to the lesion, which makes them the most reliable sign for localization.

## *Clinical signs of bilateral vestibular disease*

Bilateral vestibular disease is characterized by **symmetrical ataxia** where strength is maintained. Animals display a characteristic **head movement from side to side** (head sway) without pathological or physiological nystagmus. In severe cases, they remain crouched with a broad-based stance.

### *Diagnosis*

Obtaining a complete clinical history with the help of the owner is essential, including information relating to:

- course of the disease
- associated clinical signs
- history of previous trauma
- administration of ototoxic medications
- vaccination history
- diet
- previous ear disease.

The presence of **obtundation**, **paresis, postural deficits** or other neurological signs not associated with the vestibular system is indicative of **central nervous system disease**.

Diagnostic tests should include:

- comprehensive complete blood count and biochemistry
- total T4/TSH.

If peripheral disease is suspected, the following are recommended.

- **Otoscopic examination under general anaesthesia**. Lack of findings does not rule out otitis media.
- **Radiographs of the tympanic bullae**. Lack of findings does not rule out otitis media.
- **CT or MRI**. These are the most sensitive methods to demonstrate accumulation of fluid or neoplasia in this location. They can also show enhanced contrast uptake of the vestibulocochlear and facial nerves.
- Obtaining **fluid samples for culture after myringotomy**, in order to confirm the diagnosis and suggest the most appropriate antibiotic.

If central nervous system disease is suspected, the following are essential.

- Advanced imaging tests (CT or MRI).
- Obtaining a **CSF sample**, unless contraindicated because of increased intracranial pressure. The following help with diagnosis.
  - Routine tests (differential blood count and proteins).
  - Titrations or PCR on CSF for **infectious diseases**. The pathogens commonly involved in vestibular diseases are distemper virus, FIP, toxoplasma, neospora, cryptococcus or different bacteria due to expansion of otitis media.

If results of tests on CSF suggest inflammation in the **absence of infectious agents**, the most likely cause is **immune-mediated meningoencephalitis**.

## *Idiopathic vestibular disease*

### *Diagnosis*

**Idiopathic vestibular disease is common** in the dog and cat, with a higher likelihood in **old animals**.

The key to its diagnosis is the **absence of structural, metabolic or inflammatory diseases**, as in peripheral vestibular syndrome.

### *Treatment*

Treatment is supportive. Recurrence is possible.

## *Vascular diseases*

In recent years, vascular diseases such as **cerebellar infarctions** have been diagnosed more frequently. The characteristic images on MRI make them easily recognizable by the expert eye (always along with the clinical history), although other pathologies such as tumours or inflammation can show similar image characteristics. **Underlying diseases should be ruled out**, such as endocrine or coagulation disorders; in more than 50% of cases, the primary cause is not found.

### Others

The presence of **lysosomal diseases** or **congenital vestibular syndrome** in young animals without findings on diagnostic tests, including MRI, is less common. In some lysosomal diseases, a screeninng of abnormal organic acids, amino acids or oligosaccharides in urine may be positive.

## Discospondylitis

Discospondylitis is one of the most **common** diseases to **affect the intervertebral discs and, by proximity, the surrounding structures**. It is caused by infection of the intervertebral discs and osteomyelitis of the adjacent vertebrae.

### Aetiology

Infection may be due to:

- migration of foreign bodies
- bacterial and fungal infections that migrate to the intervertebral discs from the urogenital tract, skin, heart or mouth
- iatrogenic contamination during epidural anaesthesia
- abscess due to foreign bodies.

The most frequently isolated pathogen is *Staphylococcus intermedius*. *Streptococcus* spp., *B. canis* or *E. coli* bacteria may also be isolated, and *Aspergillus* spp. among the different types of fungi.

### Clinical signs

The most common clinical sign is the presence of **local pain** that can be improved with NSAID administration. There may also be:

- peaks of fever and obtundation
- lameness
- apparent abdominal pain
- fistulous tracts.

In order to cause neurological signs, infection must extend into the epidural space (epidural empyema) and there must be involvement of the nerve roots or fractures/pathological dislocations with displacement.

### Diagnosis

From a radiological point of view, different pathologies that can affect the intervertebral discs cannot be distinguished 100% reliably, even with MRI. It is the combination of clinical signs, laboratory findings and imaging results that allows a diagnosis to be reached with a maximum degree of reliability. Therefore, the following tests are essential:

- thoracic radiography
- abdominal ultrasound
- urinalysis.

**Fungal discospondylitis** usually affects multiple intervertebral spaces, but does not cause much bone destruction and is usually **chronic**.

#### *Diagnostic imaging*

#### Plain radiography

Plain radiographs of the painful area are usually sufficient. Bone remodelling, osteolysis, collapse of the intervertebral space and, in chronic cases, sclerosis and osteophyte production, can be observed (Figure 5.18).

#### Myelography

Myelography can be used to document the compression caused by epidural empyema adjacent to the discospondylitis.

#### CT

CT can show bone destruction on the few occasions when plain radiographs are normal or inconclusive.

#### MRI

With MRI, detection of foci of discospondylitis not apparent on radiography is possible, or with a CT scan in 12% of spaces that are affected. Despite its apparent sensitivity, it does not differentiate between fungal and bacterial infections, so culture of samples is still necessary for confirmation.

#### Bone scintigraphy

This technique can be used to detect foci of infection in other parts of the body.

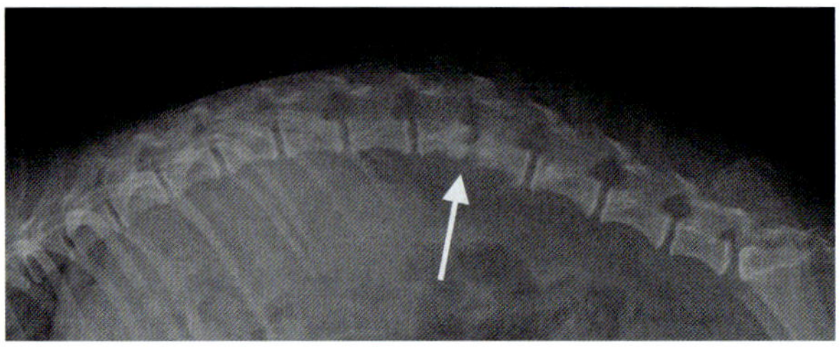

**Figure 5.18.** Lateral radiograph of the lumbar spine in a dog with discospondylitis.

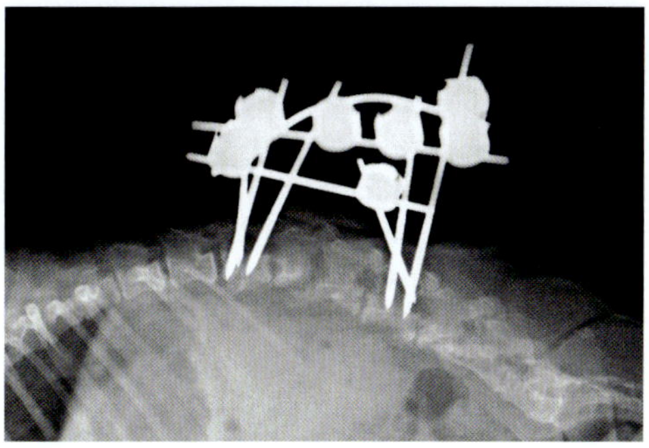

Figure 5.19. Surgical treatment of a dog with fungal discospondylitis using external fixation.

### *Laboratory tests*

**Leukocytosis** is usually found only in the **case of endocarditis**. Blood cultures may be positive in 45–75% of cases, urine cultures in 25–50% of cases and fine needle aspiration of the intervertebral disc by fluoroscopy, in 75% of cases.

## *Treatment*

**Medical treatment is sufficient** in the vast majority of cases, and should be based on the results of the culture and **antibiotic sensitivity tests**. Biopsy is necessary only in cases where there is no response to initial treatment, or to treat compression caused by subluxation and in cases refractory to medical treatment, where surgical stabilization may be necessary (Figure 5.19).

Clinical check-ups are performed using plain radiography. It is important to warn the owner of the radiological deterioration that precedes improvement.

# Bibliography


Aghighi, S.A., Tipold, A., Piechotta, M., Lewczuk, P. and Kastner, S.B. (2012) Assessment of the effects of adjunctive gabapentin on postoperative pain after intervertebral disc surgery in dogs. *Veterinary Anaesthesia and Analgesia* 39(6), 636–646.

Auger, J., Dupuis, J., Quesnel, A. and Beauregard, G. (2000) Surgical treatment of lumbosacral instability caused by discospondylitis in four dogs. *Veterinary Surgery* 29(1), 70–80.

Babu, C.S., Satishchandra, P., Sinha, S. and Subbakrishna, D.K. (2009) Co-morbidities in people living with epilepsy: Hospital based case-control study from a resource-poor setting. *Epilepsy Research* 86(2–3), 146–152.

Bailey, K.S., Dewey, C.W., Boothe, D.M., Barone, G. and Kortz, G.D. (2008) Levetiracetam as an adjunct to phenobarbital treatment in cats with suspected idiopathic epilepsy. *Journal of the American Veterinary Medical Association* 232(6), 867–872.

Battersby, I.A., Giger, U. and Hall, E.J. (2005) Hyperammonaemic encephalopathy secondary to selective cobalamin deficiency in a juvenile border collie. *Journal of Small Animal Practice* 46(7), 339–344.

Bauer, J., Ben Menachem, E., Kramer, G., Fryze, W., Da Silva, S. and Kasteleijn-Nolst Trenite, D.G.A. (2006) Levetiracetam: A long-term follow-up study of efficacy and safety. *Acta Neurologica Scandinavica* 114(3), 169–176.

Berent, A.C. and Tobias, K.M. (2009) Portosystemic vascular anomalies. *Veterinary Clinics of North America: Small Animal Practice* 39(3), 513–541.

Berry, W.L. and Leisewitz, A.L. (1996) Multifocal *Aspergillus terreus* discospondylitis in two German Shepherd dogs. *Journal of the South African Veterinary Association* 67(4), 222–228.

Blevins, L.B., Fenn, J., Segal, H., Newcomb-Gayman, P. and Carroll, K.C. (1995) False-positive cryptococcal antigen latex agglutination caused by disinfectants and soaps. *Journal of Clinical Microbiology* 33(6), 1674–1675.

Boothe, D.M. and Perkins, J. (2008) Disposition and safety of zonisamide after intravenous and oral single dose and oral multiple dosing in normal hound dogs. *Journal of Veterinary Pharmacology and Therapy* 31(6), 544–553.

Brady, C.A., Vite, C.H. and Drobatz, K.J. (1999) Severe neurologic sequelae in a dog after treatment of hypoadrenal crisis. *Journal of the American Veterinary Medical Association* 215(2), 222–225, 210.

Braund, K.G., McGuire, J.A., Amling, K.A. and Henderson, R.A. (1987) Peripheral neuropathy associated with malignant neoplasms in dogs. *Veterinary Pathology* 24(1), 16–21.

Braund, K.G., Steiss, J.E., Amling, K.A., Toivio-Kinnucan, M., Case, L.C., Kemppainen, R.J. et al. (1987) Insulinoma and subclinical peripheral neuropathy in two dogs. *Journal of Veterinary Internal Medicine* 1(2), 86–90.

Butterworth, S.J., Barr, F.J., Pearson, G.R. and Day, M.J. (1995) Multiple discospondylitis associated with Aspergillus species infection in a dog. *Veterinary Record* 136(2), 38–41.

Cabassu, J. and Moissonnier, P. (2007) Surgical treatment of a vertebral fracture associated with a haematogenous osteomyelitis in a dog. *Veterinary and Comparative Orthopaedics and Traumatology* 20(3), 227–230.

Caldwell, G.W., Wu, W.N., Masucci, J.A. et al. (2005) Metabolism and excretion of the antiepileptic/antimigraine drug, topiramate in animals and humans. *European Journal of Drug Metabolism and Pharmacokinetics* 30(3), 151–164.

Carrera, I., Sullivan, M., McConnell, F. and Goncalves, R. (2011) Magnetic resonance imaging features of discospondylitis in dogs. *Veterinary Radiology and Ultrasound* 52(2), 125–131.

Chandler, K. (2006) Canine epilepsy: What can we learn from human seizure disorders? *Veterinary Journal* 172(2), 207–217.

Churcher, R.K., Watson, A.D. and Eaton, A. (1999) Suspected myelinolysis following rapid correction of hyponatremia in a dog. *Journal of the American Animal Hospital Association* 35(6), 493–497.

Daminet, S. and Ferguson, D.C. (2003) Influence of drugs on thyroid function in dogs. *Journal of Veterinary Internal Medicine* 17(4), 463–472.

Davidson, M.G. (1992) Thiamine deficiency in a colony of cats. *Veterinary Record* 130(5), 94–97.

Davis, M.J., Dewey, C.W., Walker, M.A., Kerwin, S.C., Moon, M.L., Kortz, G.D. et al. (2000) Contrast radiographic findings in canine bacterial discospondylitis: A multicenter, retrospective study of 27 cases. *Journal of the American Animal Hospital Association* 36(1), 81–85.

De Decker, S., Gielen, I.M., Duchateau, L., Van Soens, I., Bavegems, V., Bosmans, T. et al. (2010) Low-field magnetic resonance imaging findings of the caudal portion of the cervical region in clinically normal Doberman pinschers and foxhounds. *American Journal of Veterinary Research* 71(4), 428–434.

De Lahunta, A. (2004) Neurological examination. In: Braund, K.G. (ed.) *Clinical Neurology in Small Animals: Localisation, Diagnosis and Treatment*. IVIS.

Dewey, C.W. (2003) Encephalopathies: disorders of the brain. In: Dewey, C.W. (ed.) *A Practical Guide to Canine and Feline Neurology*. Iowa State Press, Iowa, USA, pp. 99–178.

Dewey, C.W., Guiliano, R., Boothe, D.M., Berg, J.M., Kortz, G.D., Joseph, R.J. et al. (2004) Zonisamide therapy for refractory idiopathic epilepsy in dogs. *Journal of the American Animal Hospital Association* 40(4), 285–291.

Di Terlizzi, R. and Platt, S.R. (2009) The function, composition and analysis of cerebrospinal fluid in companion animals: Part ii – analysis. *Veterinary Journal* 180(1), 15–32.

Duesberg, C.A., Feldman, E.C., Nelson, R.W., Bertoy, E.H., Dublin, A.B. and Reid, M.H. (1995) Magnetic resonance imaging for diagnosis of pituitary macrotumors in dogs. *Journal of the American Veterinary Medical Association* 206(5), 657–662.

Fischer, A., Mahaffey, M.B. and Oliver, J.E. (1997) Fluoroscopically guided percutaneous disk aspiration in 10 dogs with diskospondylitis. *Journal of Veterinary Internal Medicine* 11(5), 284–287.

Fukunaga, K., Saito, M., Muto, M., Yoshioka, R., Mishima, K., Fujiwara, M. et al. (2010) Steady-state pharmacokinetics of zonisamide in plasma, whole blood, and erythrocytes in dogs. *Journal of Veterinary Pharmacology and Therapy* 33(1), 103–106.

Garosi, L. (2009) Neurological examination of the cat. How to get started. *Journal of Feline Medicine and Surgery* 11(5), 340–348.

Garosi, L.S., Dennis, R., Platt, S.R., Corletto, F., de Lahunta, A. and Jakobs, C. (2003) Thiamine deficiency in a dog: Clinical, clinicopathologic, and magnetic resonance imaging findings. *Journal of Veterinary Internal Medicine* 17(5), 719–723.

Gaskill, C.L., Burton, S.A., Gelens, H.C., Ihle, S.L., Miller, J.B., Shaw, D.H. et al. (1999) Effects of phenobarbital treatment on serum thyroxine and thyroid-stimulating hormone concentrations in epileptic dogs. *Journal of the American Veterinary Medical Association* 215(4), 489–496.

Gaskill, C.L., Miller, L.M., Mattoon, J.S., Hoffmann, W.E., Burton, S.A., Gelens, H.C. et al. (2005) Liver histopathology and liver and serum alanine aminotransferase and alkaline phosphatase activities in epileptic dogs receiving phenobarbital. *Veterinary Pathology* 42(2), 147–160.

Gendron, K., Doherr, M.G., Gavin, P. and Lang, J. (2011) Magnetic resonance imaging characterization of vertebral endplate changes in the dog. *Veterinary Radiology and Ultrasound*, https://doi.org/10.1111/j.1740-8261.2011.01861.x

Gerritzen-Bruning, M.J., van den Ingh, T.S. and Rothuizen, J. (2006) Diagnostic value of fasting plasma ammonia and bile acid concentrations in the identification of portosystemic shunting in dogs. *Journal of Veterinary Internal Medicine* 20(1), 13–19.

Gilmore, D.R. (1987) Lumbosacral diskospondylitis in 21 dogs. *Journal of the American Animal Hospital Association* 23, 57–61.

Goossens, M.M., Feldman, E.C., Theon, A.P. and Koblik, P.D. (1998) Efficacy of cobalt 60 radiotherapy in dogs with pituitary-dependent hyperadrenocorticism. *Journal of the American Veterinary Medical Association* 212(3), 374–376.

Greene, C.E., Lorenz, M.D., Munnell, J.F., Prasse, K.W., White, N.A., Bowen, J.M. (1979) Myopathy associated with hyperadrenocorticism in the dog. *Journal of the American Veterinary Medical Association* 174(12), 1310–1315.

Greenhalgh, S.N., Dunning, M.D., McKinley, T.J., Goodfellow, M.R., Kelman, K.R., Freitag, T. et al. (2010) Comparison of survival after surgical or medical treatment in dogs with a congenital portosystemic shunt. *Journal of the American Veterinary Medical Association* 236(11), 1215–1220.

Hardy, B.T., Patterson, E.E., Cloyd, J.M., Hardy, R.M. and Leppik, I.E. (2012) Double-masked, placebo-controlled study of intravenous levetiracetam for the treatment of status epilepticus and acute repetitive seizures in dogs. *Journal of Veterinary Internal Medicine*, https://doi.org/10.1111/j.1939-1676.2011.00868.x

Hasegawa, D., Kobayashi, M., Kuwabara, T., Ohmura, T., Fujita, M. and Orima, H. (2008) Pharmacokinetics and toxicity of zonisamide in cats. *Journal of Feline Medicine and Surgery* 10(4), 418–421.

Hay, R.J. and Mackenzie, D.W. (1982) False positive latex tests for cryptococcal antigen in cerebrospinal fluid. *Journal of Clinical Pathology* 35(2), 244–245.

Isoherranen, N., Yagen, B., Soback, S., Roeder, M., Schurig, V. and Bialer, M. (2001) Pharmacokinetics of levetiracetam and its enantiomer (r)-alpha-ethyl-2-oxo-pyrrolidine acetamide in dogs. *Epilepsia* 42(7), 825–830.

Jaderlund, K.H., Egenvall, A., Bergstrom, K. and Hedhammar, A. (2007) Seroprevalence of *Borrelia burgdorferi* sensu lato and *Anaplasma phagocytophilum* in dogs with neurological signs. *Veterinary Record* 160(24), 825–831.

Jaggy, A. (1990) Seizures in hypothyrotic dogs. *Proceedings of* [ ] Bern, Switzerland, pp. 51–52.

Jaggy, A. (2000) Neurologic manifestations of canine hypothyroidism. In: Bonagura, J.D. (ed.) *Current Veterinary Therapy xiii*. W.B. Saunders, Philadelphia, PA, USA, pp. 974–975.

Jaggy, A., Oliver, J.E., Ferguson, D.C., Mahaffey, E.A. and Jun, T.G. (1994) Neurological manifestations of hypothyroidism: A retrospective study of 29 dogs. *Journal of Veterinary Internal Medicine* 8(5), 328–336.

Jeffery, N.D. (2001a) Neurological examination of dogs 1. Techniques. *In Practice* 118–130.

Jeffery, N.D. (2001b) Neurological examination of dogs 2. Interpretation of findings. *In Practice* 187–196.

Jones, J.C. and Inzana, K.D. (2004) Subclinical CT abnormalities in the lumbosacral spine of older large-breed dogs. *Veterinary Radiology and Ultrasound* 41(1), 19–26.

Kantrowitz, L.B., Peterson, M.E., Trepanier, L.A., Melian, C. and Nichols, R. (1999) Serum total thyroxine, total triiodothyronine, free thyroxine, and thyrotropin concentrations in epileptic dogs treated with anticonvulsants. *Journal of the American Veterinary Medical Association* 214(12), 1804–1808.

Kraje, A.C. (2003) Hypoglycemia and irreversible neurologic complications in a cat with insulinoma. *Journal of the American Veterinary Medical Association* 223(6), 812–814, 810.

Lamb, C.R. (1998) Ultrasonography of portosystemic shunts in dogs and cats. *Veterinary Clinics of North America: Small Animal Practice* 28(4), 725–753.

Lappin, M.R. (2010) Update on the diagnosis and management of *Toxoplasma gondii* infection in cats. *Topics in Companion Animal Medicine* 25(3), 136–141.

Luján Feliu-Pascual, A. (2006) Cual es tu diagnóstico: Aspergilosis generalizada en un pastor alemán. *Clínica Veterinaria de Pequeños Animales* 26(3), 276–278.

Lynch, B.A., Lambeng, N., Nocka, K., Kensel-Hammes, P., Bajjalieh, S.M., Matagne, A. et al. (2004) The synaptic vesicle protein sv2a is the binding site for the antiepileptic drug levetiracetam. *Proceedings of the National Academy of Science USA* 101(26), 9861–9866.

Marks, S.L., Lipsitz, D., Vernau, K.M., Dickinson, P.J., Draper, W., Larsen, J.A. et al. (2011) Reversible encephalopathy secondary to thiamine deficiency in 3 cats ingesting commercial diets. *Journal of Veterinary Internal Medicine* 25(4), 949–953.

Meierkord, H., Boon, P., Engelsen, B., Göcke, K., Shorvon, S., Tinuper, P. et al. (2010 EFNS guideline on the management of status epilepticus in adults. *European Journal of Neurology* 17(3), 348–355.

Meij, B., Voorhout, G. and Rijnberk, A. (2002) Progress in transsphenoidal hypophysectomy for treatment of pituitary-dependent hyperadrenocorticism in dogs and cats. *Molecular and Cellular Endocrinology* 197(1–2), 89–96.

Meij, B.P., Voorhout, G., van den Ingh, T.S., Hazewinkel, H.A., Teske, E. and Rijnberk, A. (1998) Results of transsphenoidal hypophysectomy in 52 dogs with pituitary-dependent hyperadrenocorticism. *Veterinary Surgery* 27(3), 246–261.

Meij, B.P., Voorhout, G., van den Ingh, T.S. and Rijnberk, A. (2001) Transsphenoidal hypophysectomy for treatment of pituitary-dependent hyperadrenocorticism in 7 cats. *Veterinary Surgery* 30(1), 72–86.

Mooney, C.T. (2005) Hyperthyroidism. In: Ettinger, S.J. and Feldman, E.C. (eds) *Textbook of Veterinary Internal Medicine*. Elsevier Saunders, St Louis, MN, USA, pp. 1544–1563.

Moore, S.A., Munana, K.R., Papich, M.G. and Nettifee-Osborne, J. (2010) Levetiracetam pharmacokinetics in healthy dogs following oral administration of single and multiple doses. *American Journal of Veterinary Research* 71(3), 337–341.

Moore, S.A., Munana, K.R., Papich, M.G. and Nettifee-Osborne, J.A. (2011) The pharmacokinetics of levetiracetam in healthy dogs concurrently receiving phenobarbital. *Journal of Veterinary Pharmacology and Therapy* 34(1), 31–34.

Morales, C. and Montoliu, P. (2012) *Neurología Canina y Felina*. Multimédica Ediciones Veterinarias, Barcelona, Spain.

Muñana, K.R. (2013) Management of refractory epilepsy. *Topics in Companion Animal Medicine* 28(2), 67–71.

Nghiem, P.P. and Schatzberg, S.J. (2010) Conventional and molecular diagnostic testing for the acute neurologic patient. *Journal of Veterinary Emergency and Critical Care (San Antonio)* 20(1), 46–61.

Niederhauser, U.B. and Holliday, T.A. (1989) Electrodiagnostic studies in diseases of muscles and neuromuscular junctions. *Seminars in Veterinary Medicine and Surgery (Small Animals)* 4(2), 116–125.

Palus, V., Penderis, J., Jakovljevic, S. and Cherubini, G.B. (2010) Thiamine deficiency in a cat: Resolution of MRI abnormalities following thiamine supplementation. *Journal of Feline Medicine and Surgery* 12(10), 807–810.

Parry, A.T., Harris, A., Upjohn, M.M., Chandler, K. and Lamb, C.R. (2010) Does choice of imaging modality affect outcome in dogs with thoracolumbar spinal conditions? *Journal of Small Animal Practice* 51(6), 312–317.

Patterson, E.E., Goel, V., Cloyd, J.C., O'Brien, T.D., Fisher, J.E., Dunn, A.W. et al. (2008) Intramuscular, intravenous and oral levetiracetam in dogs: Safety and pharmacokinetics. *Journal of Veterinary Pharmacology and Therapy* 31(3), 253–258.

Patterson, J.S., Rusley, M.S. and Zachary, J.F. (1985) Neurologic manifestations of cerebrovascular atherosclerosis associated with primary hypothyroidism in a dog. *Journal of the American Veterinary Medical Association* 186(5), 499–503.

Paull, L.C., Scott-Moncrieff, J.C., DeNicola, D.B., Glickman, N., Refsal, K.R. and Glickman, L.T. (2003) Effect of anticonvulsant dosages of potassium bromide on thyroid function and morphology in dogs. *Journal of the American Animal Hospital Association* 39(2), 193–202.

Penderis, J., McConnell, J.F. and Calvin, J. (2007) Magnetic resonance imaging features of thiamine deficiency in a cat. *Veterinary Record* 160(8), 270–272.

Perucca, E. (2001) Clinical pharmacology and therapeutic use of the new antiepileptic drugs. *Fundamental Clinical Pharmacology* 15(6), 405–417.

Pettigrew, R., Fyfe, J.C., Gregory, B.L., Lipsitz, D., Delahunta, A., Summers, B.A. et al. (2007) CNS hypomyelination in rat terrier dogs with congenital goiter and a mutation in the thyroid peroxidase gene. *Veterinary Pathology* 44(1), 50–56.

Platt, S.R., Adams, V., Garosi, L.S., Abramson, C.J., Penderis, J., De Stefani, A. et al. (2006) Treatment with gabapentin of 11 dogs with refractory idiopathic epilepsy. *Veterinary Record* 159(26), 881–884.

Renwick, A.I., Dennis, R. and Gemmill, T.J. (2010) Treatment of lumbosacral discospondylitis by surgical stabilisation and application of a gentamicin-impregnated collagen sponge. *Veterinary and Comparative Orthopaedics and Traumatology* 23(4), 266–272.

Rossmeisl, J.H. (2010) Resistance of the peripheral nervous system to the effects of chronic canine hypothyroidism. *Journal of Veterinary Internal Medicine* 24(4), 875–881.

Rothuizen, J. (2009) Important clinical syndromes associated with liver disease. *Veterinary Clinics of North America: Small Animal Practice* 39(3), 419–437.

Ruland, K., Fischer, A. and Hartmann, K. (2009) Sensitivity and specificity of fasting ammonia and serum bile acids in the diagnosis of portosystemic shunts in dogs and cats. *Veterinary Clinical Pathology*, https://doi.org/10.1111/j.1939-165X.2009.00178.x

Rundfeldt, C., Gasparic, A. and Wlaź, P. (2014) Imepitoin as novel treatment option for canine idiopathic epilepsy: Pharmacokinetics, distribution, and metabolism in dogs. *Journal of Veterinary Pharmacology and Therapeutics* 37(5), 421–434.

Sahaya, K., Goyal, M.K., Sarwal, A. and Singh, N.N. (2010) Levetiracetam-induced thrombocytopenia among inpatients: A retrospective study. *Epilepsia* 51(12), 2492–2495.

Saito, M., Olby, N.J., Obledo, L. and Gookin, J.L. (2002) Muscle cramps in two standard poodles with hypoadrenocorticism. *Journal of the American Animal Hospital Association* 38(5), 437–443.

Saito, Y., Ogawa, T., Nagaishi, J., Inoue, T., Maegaki, Y. and Ohno, K. (2008) Laminar cortical necrosis in adrenal crisis: Sequential changes on MRI. *Brain and Development* 30(1), 77–81.

Schrauwen, E. (1991) Clinical peripheral polyneuropathy associated with canine insulinoma. *Veterinary Record* 128(9), 211–212.

Schultz, R.M., Johnson, E.G., Wisner, E.R., Brown, N.A., Byrne, B.A. and Sykes, J.E. (2008) Clinicopathologic and diagnostic imaging characteristics of systemic aspergillosis in 30 dogs. *Journal of Veterinary Internal Medicine* 22(4), 851–859.

Shahar, R., Rousseaux, C. and Steiss, J. (1985) Peripheral polyneuropathy in a dog with functional Islet B-cell tumor and widespread metastasis. *Journal of the American Veterinary Medical Association* 187(2), 175–177.

Shamir, M.H., Tavor, N. and Aizenberg, T. (2001) Radiographic findings during recovery from discospondylitis. *Veterinary Radiology and Ultrasound* 42(6), 496–503.

Siao, K.T., Pypendop, B.H. and Ilkiw, J.E. (2010) Pharmacokinetics of gabapentin in cats. *American Journal of Veterinary Research* 71(7), 817–821.

Streeter, A.J., Stahle, P.L., Holland, M.L., Pritchard, J.F. and Takacs, A.R. (1995) Pharmacokinetics and bioavailability of topiramate in the Beagle dog. *Drug Metabolism and Disposition* 23(1), 90–93.

Swinney, G.R., Foster, S.F., Church, D.B. and Malik, R. (1998) Myotonia associated with hyperadrenocorticism in two dogs. *Australian Veterinary Journal* 76(11), 722–724.

Theon, A.P. and Feldman, E.C. (1998) Megavoltage irradiation of pituitary macrotumors in dogs with neurologic signs. *Journal of the American Veterinary Medical Association* 213(2), 225–231.

Van Ham, L., Braund, K.G., Roels, S. and Putcuyps, I. (1997) Treatment of a dog with an insulinoma-related peripheral polyneuropathy with corticosteroids. *Veterinary Record* 141(4), 98–100.

Volk, H.A., Matiasek, L.A., Lujan Feliu-Pascual, A., Platt, S.R. and Chandler, K.E. (2008) The efficacy and tolerability of levetiracetam in pharmacoresistant epileptic dogs. *Veterinary Journal* 176(3), 310–319.

Von Klopmann, T., Boettcher, I.C., Rotermund, A., Rohn, K. and Tipold, A. (2006). Euthyroid sick syndrome in dogs with idiopathic epilepsy before treatment with anticonvulsant drugs. *Journal of Veterinary Internal Medicine* 20(3), 516–522.

Von Klopmann, T., Rambeck, B. and Tipold, A. (2007) Prospective study of zonisamide therapy for refractory idiopathic epilepsy in dogs. *Journal of Small Animal Practice* 48(3), 134–138.

Watt, P.R., Robins, G.M., Galloway, A.M. and O'Boyle, D.A. (1995) Disseminated opportunistic fungal disease in dogs: 10 cases (1982–1990). *Journal of the American Veterinary Medical Association* 207(1), 67–70.

## Test

1. **The frontal lobe of the encephalon is involved in:**
   A) The conscious visual interpretation of images from the retina.
   B) Memory and hearing.
   C) Initiation of conscious movements and associative reasoning.
   D) Smell.
2. **With regard to neuroanatomy, indicate which statement is true:**
   A) From a functional perspective, the nervous system is divided into central and peripheral areas.
   B) For the correct interpretation of findings during a neurological examination, knowledge of neuroanatomy is necessary.
   C) From an anatomical perspective, the spinal ganglia are part of the central nervous system.
   D) Lower motor neurons always have their origin in the spinal cord.
3. **Indicate which of the following statements is true:**
   A) CSF is predominantly produced in the subarachnoid space.
   B) Production of CSF is dependent on intracranial pressure.
   C) Medullary proprioceptive tracts are adjacent to the grey matter.
   D) The ventral midbrain is responsible for coordination of movements throughout the body.
4. **After a neurological examination you should be able to:**
   A) Establish whether the animal presents a neurological problem, and its location.
   B) Estimate the severity of the neurological lesion.
   C) Prepare a list of differential diagnoses based on the location and clinical history.
   D) All of the above are true.
5. **With regard to the neurological examination, which of the following statements is true?**
   A) Postural reactions are reduced only in cases where there is spinal cord involvement.
   B) Mental state is usually affected by chronic focal lesions in the telencephalon.
   C) The patellar reflex is the most reliable for evaluation of lower motor lesions in the pelvic limbs.
   D) All of the above are true.
6. **Regarding imaging tests for neurological diseases, indicate which statement is false:**
   A) Myelography can be used to show spinal compressions that require surgical decompression.
   B) CT is especially useful in diseases that affect bony structures.
   C) MRI allows a definitive diagnosis to be reached for a large number of neurological diseases.
   D) In spinal diseases, success of treatment is not influenced by the diagnostic method used (MRI versus myelography).
7. **Indicate which statement is true in relation to polymerase chain reaction (PCR):**
   A) Allows the presence of genetic material from different pathogens in biological samples to be demonstrated.
   B) Is useful for monitoring the response to treatment.
   C) Is an unspecific technique.
   D) When detecting infectious diseases, it does not matter whether the sample is contaminated.

**8. Indicate which answer is true with regard to the clinical signs of hypothyroidism:**

A) They have been associated with the acute development of thyroid neoplasia.

B) A direct relationship with the presence of seizures has been demonstrated.

C) The results of thyroid hormone tests are not influenced by glucocorticoid administration.

D) The total absence of thyroid hormone is not the cause of polyneuropathy in hypothyroid patients.

**9. With regard to hyperadrenocorticism, indicate which is the correct answer:**

A) It is an acute disease which develops rapidly and generally results in death.

B) Surgical treatment of adrenal masses can be curative.

C) Neurological signs include generalized weakness, postural delays and decreased spinal reflexes.

D) In a nerve conduction study, a delay in conduction is detected.

**10. With regard to hepatic encephalopathy, indicate which of the following is true:**

A) Neurological signs that are seen suggest focal involvement of the cerebral cortex and include head tilting, nystagmus and seizures.

B) If the animal has seizures, the most appropriate anticonvulsant is bromide because it does not rely on hepatic metabolism and has a rapid mechanism of action.

C) Surgical treatment is associated with a longer survival period.

D) Measurement of ammonium in blood can be done using an external laboratory because it does not degrade with transport.

**11. Idiopathic epilepsy of unknown origin:**

A) Is caused by pathogens that live in humid environments.

B) Probably has a structural cause even though it has not been found during an extensive investigation.

C) Is one in which no neurological abnormalities are found during a neurological examination.

D) Has a dark origin related to lunar phases.

**12. In uraemic encephalopathy:**

A) In the case of acute renal failure, the occurrence of seizures is frequent.

B) Hypokalaemia associated with chronic renal failure in the cat produces muscle spasticity and tremors.

C) The most suitable anticonvulsant for renal failure is potassium bromide.

D) The vomiting observed is due to an increase in intracranial pressure which, as a consequence, compresses the vomiting centre in the myelencephalon.

**13. With regard to seizures in domestic animals, indicate which statement is true:**

A) The most effective antiepileptic is phenobarbital.

B) Partial seizures cannot be of genetic origin.

C) Idiopathic epilepsy can be diagnosed only on post-mortem.

D) The most appropriate antiepileptic to control seizures in kidney patients is potassium bromide.

**14. With regard to seizures in domestic animals, indicate which statement is true:**

A) They do not need treatment since they resolve on their own.

B) Cluster seizures are neurological emergencies that must be treated quickly.

C) Serum phenobarbital levels should be measured at most every 6 months.

D) The administration of phenobarbital does not influence metabolism of levetiracetam.

**15. Discospondylitis:**

A) Affects the lumbosacral space most frequently.

B) It is treated empirically by testing different antibiotics.

C) The treatment period is restricted to 7–10 days.

D) Has a large hereditary component.

**16. With respect to discospondylitis, which is the correct answer?**

A) Must be treated surgically to achieve a faster and longer-lasting recovery.

B) Urine and blood cultures always successfully identify the organism.

C) Fungal infections are restricted to the intervertebral discs.

D) The pathogen involved most commonly are Staphylococcus spp.

**Answers on page 224**

## Clinical case 1

**Signalment**: Two-year-old male Podenco cross-breed with an acute history of lethargy and ataxia over the last 7 days. The dog was found on the edge of the road 8 months ago, and its vaccination history is unknown. A month before examination he presented with an episode of recurrent coughing and, a week before, he had hyperthermia. He was treated with doxycycline and clindamycin for a week, but no clinical improvement was obtained.

**Physical examination**: Capillary refill time, cardiac auscultation and abdominal palpation were considered normal. Rectal temperature, 39.5°C.

**Neurological exam**: Mental state: mild obtundation. Ataxic gait. Delayed postural reactions in all limbs. Presented constant myoclonus of the left pelvic limb and the left eye that did not cease whilst sleeping. Examination of the cranial nerves showed bilateral mydriasis with diminished pupillary reflexes and vertical nystagmus. The remainder of the spinal and cranial reflexes and responses were normal.

1. **Where is the neurological location of the lesion?**
2. **Make a list of differential diagnoses for the clinical history and location.**
3. **What plan would you propose to reach a diagnosis?**

## Clinical case 2

In the answers section for the first part of the case (page 224), review the results of the diagnostic tests and, using what you see, answer the following questions.

1. **Interpret the results.**
2. **Which diagnostic test would you perform next?**
3. **Justify why distemper can be the cause of the neurological signs in this animal.**

## Correct answers

### Test

| | | |
|---|---|---|
| 1. C | 7. A | 13. A |
| 2. B | 8. D | 14. B |
| 3. A | 9. B | 15. A |
| 4. D | 10. C | 16. D |
| 5. C | 11. B | |
| 6. C | 12. A | |

### Clinical case 1

1. **Where is the neurological location of the lesion?**

Obtundation may indicate diffuse involvement of the cerebral cortex or a focal brainstem lesion affecting the function of the ascending reticular system.

Ataxia may be due to a focal lesion in the cerebellum or spinal cord affecting ascending proprioceptive pathways or their connections in the cerebellum.

Similarly, alteration of postural reactions may represent a spinal cord injury to the ascending proprioceptive pathways.

Myoclonus may be due to lesions in the upper motor nuclei in the brainstem, to an independent pacemaker in the lower motor neurons of the ventral horn of the spinal cord and the motor nucleus of the facial nerve, or to instability of muscle fibres.

Bilateral mydriasis with decreased pupillary reflexes suggests involvement of the mesencephalon, where the parasympathetic nucleus of the oculomotor nerve responsible for pupillary contraction is located.

Vertical nystagmus implies changes in the central vestibular system.

Because there is not a single location that can explain all neurological signs, it is most likely that it is a multifocal problem that affects the brainstem, the cervical spinal cord and, possibly, the cerebellum.

2. **Make a list of differential diagnoses for the clinical history and location.**

The multifocal localizations of the neurological signs, together with hyperthermia and the history of recurrent coughing a few weeks before the onset of neurological signs following the mnemonic role of VITAMIN-D, suggest the following differential diagnoses:

- **Vascular:** Immune-mediated vasculitis with intra-axial haemorrhages.
- **Inflammatory/infectious:** Toxoplasmosis, neosporosis, distemper, meningo-encephalitis of unknown origin, pyogranulomatous meningoencephalitis.
- **Neoplasia:** Intravascular lymphoma, multicentric lymphoma, choroid plexus carcinoma, multifocal metastasis.

3. **What plan would you propose to reach a diagnosis?**

In the first place, a complete blood analysis that includes blood count and biochemistry, chest radiography and abdominal ultrasound is essential, as well as ruling out infectious diseases by means of adequate tests for the clinical picture and possible differentials. In order to demonstrate whether there is inflammation of the central nervous system, a cerebrospinal fluid sample should be taken and tested. To obtain reliable results, this must be processed within 30 minutes after collection.

The results from the complete blood count show slight anaemia and lymphopenia with monocytosis suggestive of an immunosuppressive process (Table case 1.1).

Table case 1.1. Blood test results.

| Parameter | Results | Normal range |
|---|---|---|
| RBC | 5.05 | 5.5–8.5 × $10^{12}$/l |
| Haematocrit | 0.347 | 0.37–0.55 l/l |
| Haemoglobin | 120 | 120–180 g/l |
| MCV | 68.7 | 60.0–77.0 fl |
| MCH | 23.8 | 18.5–30.0 pg |
| MCHC | 347 | 300–375 g/l |
| RDW | 15.3 | 14.7–17.9 % |
| Reticulocytes (%) | 0.3 | |
| Reticulocytes | 13.5 | 10–110 K/µl |
| WBC | *15.82 | 5.5–16.9 × $10^9$/l |
| Neutrophils (%) | *64.0 | |
| Lymphocytes (%) | *1.7 | |
| Monocytes (%) | *31.5 | |
| Eosinophils (%) | *2.2 | |
| Basophils (%) | *0.6 | |
| Neutrophils | *10.11 | 2–12 × $10^9$/l |
| Lymphocytes | *0.28 | 0.5–4.9 × $10^9$/l |
| Monocytes | *4.98 | 0.3–2 × $10^9$/l |
| Eosinophils | *0.34 | 0.1–1.49 × $10^9$/l |
| Basophils | *0.1 | 0–0.1 × $10^9$/l |
| Platelets | 216 | 175–500 × $10^9$/l |
| MPV | 16.5 | fl |
| PDW | 25.7 | |
| Platelets | 0.36 | |

There are no significant alterations in the biochemistry profile that explain the clinical picture (Table case 1.2).

Table case 1.2. Biochemistry profile.

| Parameter | Results | Normal range |
|---|---|---|
| Glucose | 5.55 | 4.11–7.94 mmol/l |
| Urea | 10.71 | 2.5–9.64 mmol/l |
| Creatinine | 114.92 | 44.2–159.12 µmmol/l |
| Total protein | 74 | 52–82 g/l |
| Albumin | 34 | 23–40 g/l |
| Globulin | 39 | 25–45 g/l |
| ALT | 118 | 10–100 U/l |
| ALP | 147 | 23–212 U/l |

Table case 1.3. Results for serology infectious disease tests.

| Results | Interpretation |
|---|---|
| Anti-*Neospora caninum* antibodies <1/80 | Negative |
| Canine anti-Toxoplasma IgG antibodies 1/40 | Acquired or evolving immunity |
| Canine anti-Toxoplasma IgM antibodies negative | Negative |
| Anti-distemper virus IgG antibodies 1/160 | Unvaccinated: positive >1/20 |
| Anti-distemper virus IgM antibodies negative | Unvaccinated: negative <1/20 |
| *Cryptococcus neoformans* Negative | Negative except recent vaccination |
| *Anti-Ehrlichia platys* antibodies <1/80 | Negative |

The results of the serology tests for infectious diseases (Table case 1.3) suggest exposure to canine distemper virus but, as the dog's vaccination status is unknown, it is difficult to know whether to attribute it to infection or previous vaccination. The slight positive toxoplasma titre also indicates previous exposure, but does not establish whether it was recent or if it is clinically significant.

No notable alterations were found in thoracic and abdominal radiographs.

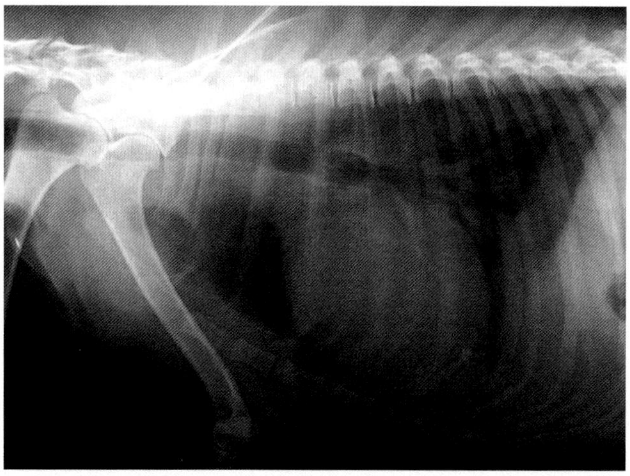

Figure case 1.1. Thoracic radiograph.

A CSF sample was obtained from the cerebello-medullary cistern under general anaesthesia and analysed within 30 minutes of collection. These were the results:

- Total count: 13 cells/µl (reference value <6).
- Pandy test: positive moderate (negative reference).
- Differential count: 95% mature lymphocytes, 3% monocytes and 2% non-degenerate neutrophils.

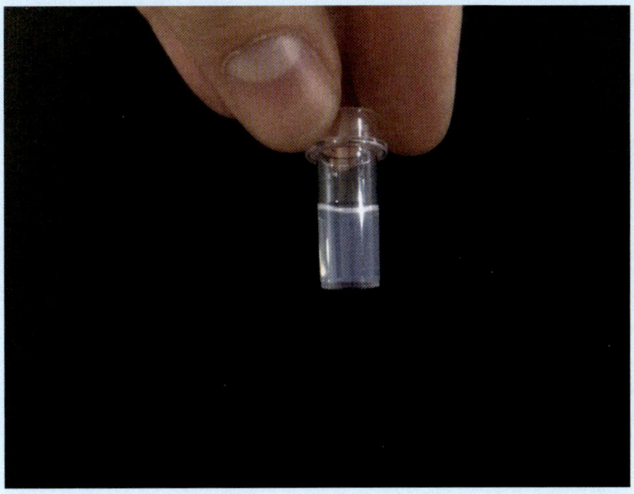

**Figure case 1.2.** Pandy test.

## Clinical case 2

1. **Interpretation of results**
   The presence of a high number of white cells (pleocytosis) indicates inflammation of the CNS and/or meninges. In this case it is slight, which may be a reflection of emerging inflammation, although it can also be seen in immune-mediated, neoplastic, traumatic, viral and necrotizing inflammatory processes.
   A positive reaction to the Pandy test occurs when there are high levels of globulins in CSF, due either to intrathecal production or a permeable blood–brain barrier. The predominant cell type in this case is lymphocytes, which indicates chronic inflammation, although this can also be due to viral infections.
2. **Which diagnostic test would you perform next?**
   Given the results from CSF analysis, infectious processes should be ruled out. For this, the most specific test for detection of genetic material from infectious agents is PCR, since it detects the microorganism itself rather than the immunological reaction it produces, which can be influenced or hidden by other factors unrelated to the infection.
   PCR was performed for *Toxoplasma gondii*, *Neospora caninum*, *Cryptococcus* spp., *Leishmania* spp., *Ehrlichia* spp. and canine distemper virus, and was found to be positive to the wild strain of the distemper virus.
3. **Justify why distemper can be the cause of the neurological signs in this animal.**
   Canine distemper virus is a neurotropic Morbillivirus that can infect the brain and cause encephalomyelitis, despite a correct vaccination programme. When exposure to the wild virus occurs, immunocompetent animals are able to organize an adequate immune response and eliminate the virus. However, despite this effective systemic response, the virus can cross the blood–brain barrier and infect neural tissue. There it can locate within the glial cells and replicate, avoiding contact with the immune system and subsequently altering brain function. In this case, the presence of a multifocal syndrome in the brain and spinal cord with fever suggests an infectious cause. The results of serum titres should be interpreted with caution, since these indicate only exposure to the infectious agent. As the dog's vaccination status is unknown, it is difficult to be sure that this positive result has been caused by infection, and not because of exposure. Typical findings in CSF show mild pleocytosis with an increase in globulins due to intrathecal production. The predominant cell type is mature lymphocytes. The presence of genetic material from the wild virus, determined by PCR analysis of bodily fluids (CSF, urine, serum), shows infection if clinical signs are compatible. An advantage of this test is that it can be determined whether genetic material is derived from a vaccine or wild strain in recently vaccinated animals.

# 6

# Urinary tract diseases

María Dolores Tabar Rodríguez

## Chapter summary

## Introduction

Good management of renal disease makes a profound impact on the patient's prognosis and life expectancy. Whilst a 'happy ending' is not always possible, approaching each case in a logical manner increases the probability of identifying underlying factors, which when corrected may greatly improve that individual's outlook. Conversely, when no trigger for renal disease is identified, optimal medical management goes a long way to improving patient quality of life and longevity.

Of course, the urinary tract is so much more than just the kidneys (important as they are). Conditions affecting the bladder are common and a cause of much distress for both the animal and owner. From the blocked cat to the dog with a recurrent UTI, these cases need not be a headache when use is made of a logical diagnostic pathway. The answer can often be found in simple tests (such as SG and a urine dipstick) available in-house (such as a urine sediment exam.), along with imaging such as ultrasound.

For those more complex cases, this chapter guides the reader through selecting the most appropriate tests and imaging options. And, for the most complex cases – such as the clinician faced with an oliguric patient – there is guidance on how to manage the case and to correct electrolyte imbalances and acid–base disturbances. All in all, the aim is to provide a helpful and logical overview of the best approach to urological cases as they are likely to present in practice.

### Key learning points

- Differentiating pre-renal, renal and post-renal azotaemia, and the importance of identifying acute vs chronic renal disease.
- Management of patients with renal disease, including treatment of underlying causes and managing complications.
- Indications and contraindications for renal biopsy.
- Interpretation of urine sediment exams and management of urolithiasis cases.
- Optimal treatment of complex and/or recurring UTIs.

## Upper urinary tract pathologies

### *General considerations*

Over their lifetime, animals have a **limited number of nephrons**, which are the **functional unit of the kidney**. The loss of between **2/3 and 3/4 of the functional capacity** of the two kidneys implies the presence of **renal insufficiency**. This may present as chronic renal failure, better known as **chronic kidney disease** (**CKD**), or as acute renal failure, more accurately referred to **as acute kidney disease** (**AKD**).

It is important to **determine whether renal disease is acute or chronic**, since this affects the focus of the case with differing causes, treatment and, ultimately, prognosis. To differentiate between acute and chronic disease requires information obtained from the clinical history, physical examination and laboratory tests.

An **understanding of the following concepts is crucial: renal failure is** a clinical syndrome that **occurs when 75% of nephrons are not functioning**, and therefore the kidney **is not able to maintain its regulatory, excretory and endocrine functions**. The term **uraemia refers to the set of clinical signs** appearing as a consequence of this critical loss of nephron function. The term renal disease infers the presence of morphological and/or functional changes in one or both kidneys, independent of extent.

**Azotaemia is defined as an increase in non-protein nitrogen compounds in blood,** mainly **urea and creatinine**. The presence of azotaemia does not expressly indicate an intrinsic renal alteration, since **the origin may be pre-renal** (as a result of reduced renal perfusion), **renal or postrenal** (due to interference with urine excretion). Differentiating between these origins is established via the medical history, physical examination, laboratory tests and imaging techniques.

## Diagnostic techniques and urinary tract pathologies

In patients with clinical signs suggestive of kidney disease, a systematic approach is required to establish the following:

- **Confirm** the presence of kidney disease.
- **Characterize** the renal disease (glomerular, interstitial, tubular or mixed).
- Determine its **extent**.
- Determine whether it is **acute or chronic** in character.
- Identify the **primary cause**, plus the complications thereof or concomitant diseases that perpetuate kidney injury.
- Apply a symptomatic and/or aetiological **treatment**.
- Define the **prognosis**.

Before performing diagnostic tests, it is essential to start with a thorough evaluation of the **patient's signalment** (age, breed, sex), **clinical history** (duration and evolution of clinical signs, access to nephrotoxic substances, vaccinations, area of residence and travel history, other previous illnesses, etc.) and complete

**physical examination**. Based on the changes detected, the diagnostic protocol is defined that may include blood and urine tests, blood pressure measurement, imaging techniques and cyto-/histopathological study.

## *Laboratory tests*

As a minimum, a **complete blood count**, **biochemistry** profile and **urinalysis** should be performed. In addition, there are new **biochemical markers** that help evaluate renal functionality, as well as tests to more accurately assess **glomerular filtration rate** (renal clearance tests).

### *Complete blood count*

Although non-specific for kidney disease, changes may include:

- **non-regenerative anaemia** in animals with CKD
- **leucocytosis** in some animals with pyelonephritis, infectious diseases, etc.

### *Blood biochemistry*

In patients with kidney disease, several biochemical changes can be detected.

#### Azotaemia

Azotaemia is represented by an **increase in serum urea and creatinine**. These are **not very sensitive** markers, as they remain normal until functionality of 75% of the renal mass is lost. **Azotaemia can be pre-renal, renal or postrenal** (Table 6.1).

Table 6.1. Differentiation of renal, pre-renal and post-renal azotaemia.

| Azotaemia | Mechanism | Differentiation |
|---|---|---|
| Pre-renal | Decreased renal perfusion (dehydration, hypovolaemia, etc.) | Concentrated USG except in conditions that alter urine concentration mechanisms (for example, hypoadrenocorticism, pyometra, hypercalcaemia, medications [diuretics, glucocorticoids], etc.)<br>Normalization after fluid therapy |
| Post-renal | Interference with urine excretion from the body (urinary tract rupture, urinary obstruction, etc.) | Clinical history (trauma, presence of stranguria/dysuria/oliguria)<br>Physical examination (balloon bladder, uro-abdomen, etc.) |
| Renal | Changes to renal parenchyma | Low USG<br>Other changes on tests and diagnostic imaging |

USG, urine specific gravity.

**Urea** is derived from endogenous and exogenous **protein catabolism** and, in the kidney, it undergoes filtration, reabsorption and diffusion events. Its production is not constant, and may be increased by variables of non-renal origin (gastrointestinal bleeding, high-protein diet, fasting, fever, administration of glucocorticoids or diuretics, etc.). Therefore, it is **not very specific and is not used to monitor kidney disease**.

**Creatinine** arises from the **metabolism of muscle creatine**, which is filtered and excreted by the kidney. Its **excretion is constant** and therefore reflects glomerular filtration rate (GFR) better than other parameters, and its **values increase** in situations where there is a **decrease in GFR**. Creatinine values are higher in breeds with a larger muscle mass. Ideally, creatinine levels should be compared to levels from prior tests and any trends and variations observed. The **relationship between serum creatinine and GFR is curvilinear**. This means that, at the start, significant decreases in GFR can lead to small changes in serum creatinine. However, over time, creatinine can increase dramatically with relatively small changes in GFR. **Creatinine levels are used to monitor kidney disease** and, in the International Renal Interest Society (IRIS) classification of chronic kidney disease.

#### Hyperphosphataemia

**Phosphate levels increase with a decrease in GFR**, and are used in the monitoring and treatment of CKD. Hyperphosphataemia is also related to secondary renal hyperparathyroidism.

#### Hypokalaemia and hyperkalaemia

**Potassium levels are dependent on urine production**, since potassium is eliminated by passive mechanisms (urine flow). Potassium may be increased in cases of oliguria, or reduced in some cases of chronic renal failure. If it is **high, the presence of urinary obstruction** (post-renal azotaemia) or anuria should be ruled out. Hypokalaemia is more frequent and clinically relevant in cats with CKD, as it results in decreased appetite and muscle weakness (it should be supplemented PO and/or IV).

#### Calcium

Calcium may be high, normal or low.

#### Metabolic acidosis

Metabolic acidosis occurs as a result of lower proton excretion, lower phosphate and sulphate filtration and lower tubular proton secretion.

### *Urinalysis*

The way a urine sample is obtained and its handling are critical for an accurate interpretation of the analysis.

Ideally, the urine should be **collected by cystocentesis** early in the day, after the patient has been fasted, and the test performed shortly thereafter (within 1 hour):

- Measure urine specific gravity (USG).
- Test with a urine test strip.
- Urine sediment examination.

Part of the sample should be **stored aseptically**, in case other tests such as **urinary culture** and/or **protein/creatinine ratio** measurement are necessary at a later date. It is assumed that samples obtained by spontaneous urination will be contaminated with bacteria, cells and debris from the urogenital tract, and also skin and hair, but may be useful for initial tests, especially when collected and stored correctly.

### *USG*

USG is measured using a **refractometer**. This measures the total concentration of solutes in the urine and allows evaluation of the **functionality of the renal tubules** and their ability to conserve or excrete water. If the urine is very cloudy, the sample should be centrifuged and SG measured using the supernatant. USG can help confirm the presence of polyuria and, in some cases, establish the patient's hydration status. A healthy animal can have a USG between 1.001 and >1.050 (Table 6.2). Any USG value can be considered normal, depending on certain factors such as the patient's hydration status and the presence or absence of azotaemia. Urine is considered to be **'normally concentrated' if the USG is >1.030 (dog) or >1.030 (cat).** It is important that USG is interpreted together with diagnostic tests and the animal's clinical history (prior to administration of fluids, diuretics, glucocorticoids, etc.).

In order for the urine to concentrate, the presence of antidiuretic hormone (ADH), a good response to ADH (interaction with ADH receptors) and adequate maintenance of the hyperosmolarity of the interstitial fluid in the renal medulla are necessary. **Water consumption** and urine production (water balance) are regulated by the hypothalamus, pituitary gland and kidney, through complex interactions between **plasma osmolarity, intravascular fluid volume and the thirst centre** (Figure 6.1).

Urine specific gravity values help confirm or rule out the presence of kidney disease:

- **1.035**. Indicates that the kidneys have retained their ability to concentrate urine, and therefore **rules out the possibility of renal failure**. If the patient presents with azotaemia, **pre-renal causes** (dehydration, hypovolaemia, etc.) should be investigated. It is important to remember that at least 1/3 of functional nephrons are required to concentrate urine, and consequently USG >1030 does not rule out the possibility of renal pathology.
- **1.013–1.029 (dog) or 1.013–1.034 (cat)**. If the animal presents with azotaemia or dehydration, these values indicate an **inadequate capacity to concentrate urine**. The patient may suffer from kidney failure or other pathologies that prevent it from concentrating urine (for example, pyelonephritis, diabetes). In hydrated animals and without further evidence of kidney injury or other diseases, it may be useful to repeat the USG measurement before continuing further with the diagnostic protocol.
- **1.008–1.012**. Specific plasma density (**isosthenuric urine**). The production of urine with this specific gravity implies a **total lack of water conservation** in the renal tubules. In combination with azotaemia, an animal with this USG will suffer from renal failure. As an exception, certain diseases or drugs that may interfere with the capacity for renal concentration (for example, diabetes, glucocorticoids, diuretics, hypercalcaemia) should be taken into account. Therefore, it is possible that a patient suffering from one of these diseases is dehydrated (and with pre-renal azotaemia) and is not able to concentrate urine.
- **<1.008**. Implies that the the **renal tubules are functional** (since they are actively diluting glomerular filtration) and, therefore, the possibility of renal failure can be ruled out. It occurs in situations such as **primary polydipsia**, in the absence of ADH (central **diabetes insipidus**) or if there is interference with the action of ADH in the collecting tubules (nephrogenic diabetes insipidus, hypercalcaemia, hyperadrenocorticism, pyelonephritis, pyometra, hypokalaemia, hyponatraemia, hepatic insufficiency or erythrocytosis). Also, if there is spinal lavage or changes in the reabsorption of solutes with the consequent loss of hypertonicity of the medullary interstitium (use of diuretics, hypo-adrenocorticism, tubular lesions with glycosuria, diabetes mellitus, use of fluids with glucose).

Table 6.2. Urinary specific gravity values and terms used to define it.

| Term | Urine specific gravity | |
|---|---|---|
| | Dog | Cat |
| Hyposthenuria | <1.008 | <1.008 |
| Isosthenuria | 1.008–1.012 | 1.008–1.012 |
| Minimally concentrated urine | 1.013–1.030 | 1.013–1.040 |
| Hypersthenuria | >1.035 | >1.045 |

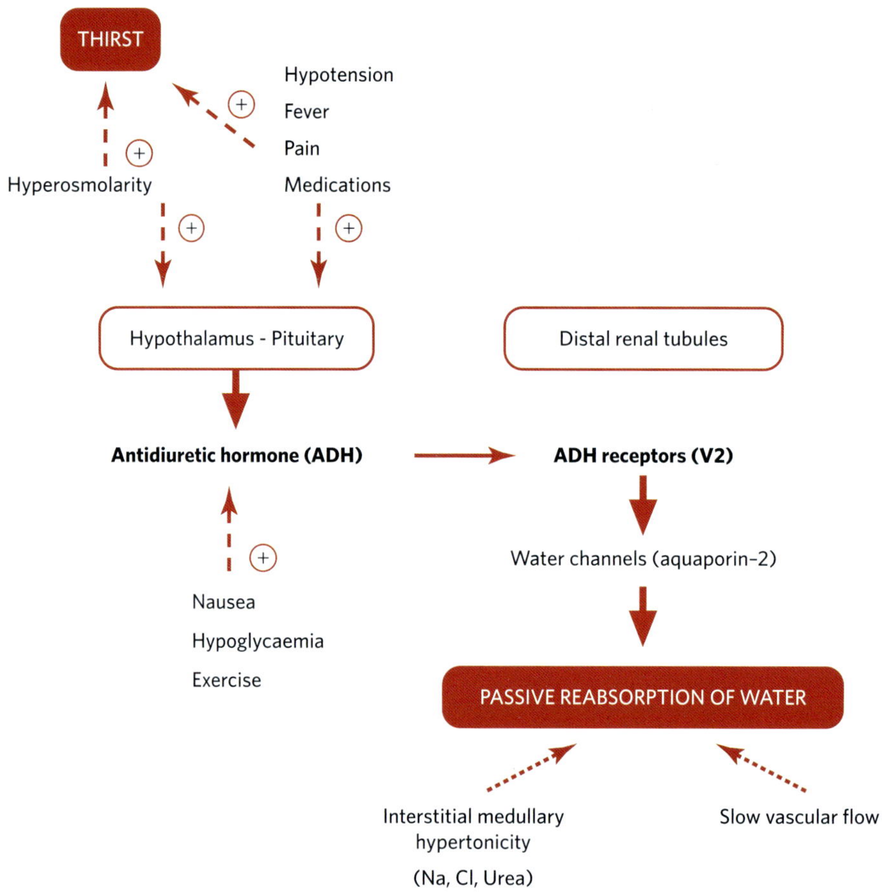


**Figure 6.1.** Regulation of water balance.

## Urine biochemistry

Fundamental to urinary analysis is the interpretation of a test strip, together with urinary specific gravity and a sediment exam (cells, cylinders, bacteria, crystals, etc.).

The following parameters must be evaluated on test strips:

- **pH**. Varies depending on diet and blood pH. There are tubular diseases that lead to significant changes in urine pH (tubular acidosis). Urine pH can contribute to the formation of crystals and uroliths, and is one of the factors that should be monitored in patients with urolithiasis.
- **Proteins**. Evaluation of proteinuria is important (addressed later in more detail). A urinary test strip gives a semi-quantitative assessment, and then quantitative techniques such as the **protein/creatinine ratio** (**UPC**) can be used.
- **Glucose**. When blood glucose levels exceed the reabsorption capacity of the renal tubules (300 mg/dl), glucose appears in the urine. This is typical of patients with **diabetes mellitus**, but it can also be a consequence of **stress** (especially in cats), the administration of fluids with glucose or tubular diseases (Fanconi syndrome). Certain medications (especially some antibiotics) can give false positives.
- **Occult blood.** A positive urine strip test involves the presence of red blood cells, haemoglobin or myoglobin. In urine samples with an abnormal colour suggestive of haematuria, it is important to differentiate between haematuria (red blood cells in the urine) and pigmenturia (presence of haemoglobin or myoglobin in the urine) by centrifuging the urine sample (Figure 6.2).

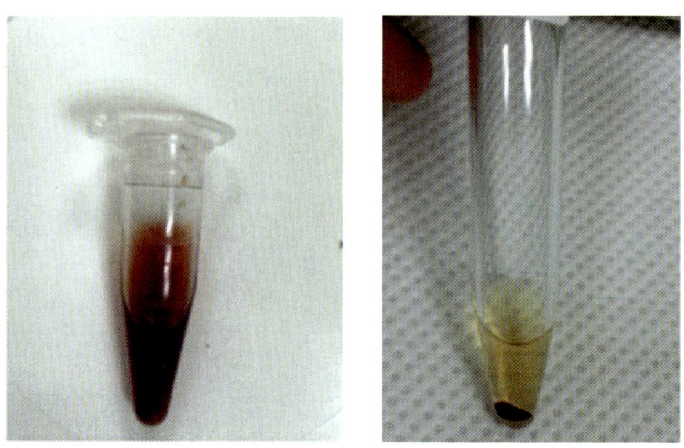

**Figure 6.2.** Difference in appearance between haemoglobinuria (left) and haematuria (right).

- **Bilirubin**. In the **dog, small amounts of bilirubin are normal** but in the cat the presence of bilirubinuria is always pathological. Urobilinogen has no diagnostic utility.
- **Ketone bodies**. Can be detected in patients with diabetic ketoacidosis (urine test strips detect acetoacetate but not β-hydroxybutyrate), but also in other circumstances such as prolonged fasting, low-carbohydrate diets, persistent fever and hypoglycaemia.
- **Leukocytes**. The chemical reaction that detects the presence of leukocytes in urine is **not very sensitive or specific** (especially in the cat), and must always be interpreted together with sediment evaluation.

## Urine sediment

- **Red blood cells**. When red blood cells are present in urine it is important to **determine their origin** (coagulopathies or upper or lower urogenital tract disease, whether due to inflammatory causes, urolithiasis, neoplasia, trauma or kidney disease [renal infarction, vascular malformation, glomerular disease, haematoma in the renal pelvis, etc.]). Renal haematuria usually presents with cylinders of red blood cells.
- **Leukocytes**. Their presence in urine normally implies inflammation of the urinary or genital tract.
- **Epithelial cells**. It is **normal to find some transitional epithelial cells** in urine. However, if they are found in large quantities or show dysplastic changes, the possibility of neoplasia or inflammation of the urinary tract should be considered.
- **Cylinders**. Structures that **form in the lumen of the renal tubules**. It is normal to find small amounts of hyaline or granular cylinders. When hyaline cylinders are present in greater quantities, this suggests the presence of a nephropathy with proteinuria. Granular cylinders are usually seen in toxic nephropathies; cells can be either red blood cells (renal haematuria), leukocytes (pyelonephritis) or renal epithelial cells (tubular necrosis or pyelonephritis).
- **Bacteria** or other infectious agents (parasites, fungi, etc.) (Figure 6.3).
- **Crystalluria**. Detection of crystals of no clinical significance (struvite, amorphous phosphate, oxalate) is common in dog and cat urine. Solubility of the crystals depends on urinary pH, temperature and USG. In cases of urolithiasis, the detection of crystals and their identification can help predict the type of urolith present.

## UPC

Allows **quantification of protein loss** in urine and determines the presence of **glomerular disease.** A value **>0.5 in the dog or 0.4 in the cat indicates**

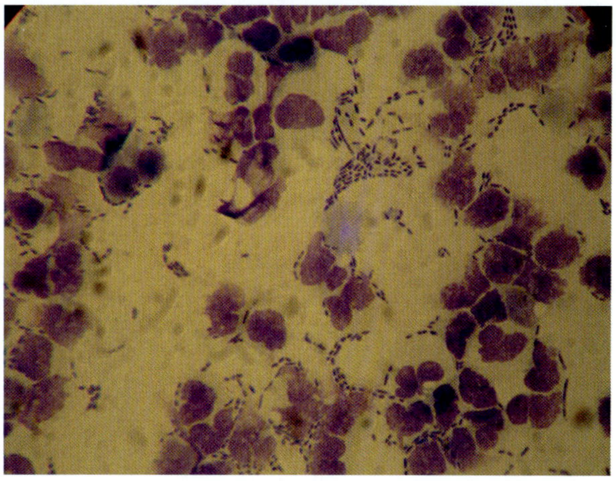

**Figure 6.3.** Urinary sediment from a dog with pyelonephritis. A large number of neutrophils and phagocytosed bacteria can be seen.

**proteinuria**, although it does not define the origin. The degree to which this is increased can help differentiate tubular proteinuria (0.5–2.5), glomerulonephritis (0.5–15) and glomerular amyloidosis (0.5–40). UPC should be performed in the dog with evidence of significant proteinuria on a urine test strip, and in all cats to assess proteinuria.

## Urine culture

In cases of suspected urinary infection and when monitoring patients with kidney disease, **culture and an antibiogram** are important. Urine culture samples should be obtained by **cystocentesis**.

## *Other biochemical markers*

### Cystatin C

**Cystatin C is a protease inhibitor** constantly produced by all tissues. It is freely filtered at the glomerular level, without undergoing tubular secretion, and is almost completely reabsorbed by tubular cells at the proximal tubules. Therefore, serum cystatin C concentration could be a **marker of GFR**. However, it is not widely used mainly because there is **controversy** over whether serum values could be altered in the presence of inflammation and/or neoplasia.

### Symmetric dimethylarginine (SDMA)

This is a new renal biomarker derived from the metabolism of certain amino acids.

**SDMA** is a derivative of the intranuclear methylation of L-arginine residues, released into the cytoplasm after proteolysis and **excreted by the kidneys**. The measurement of SDMA, **together with creatinine, urea and urinalysis**, can help in the **early diagnosis of CKD. SDMA is raised before creatinine**, and this is specific for kidney disease. Recent studies indicate that SDMA increases by an average of 17 months before creatinine in cats with CKD (which happens with **losses of 40% of GFR**), or about 9.5 months before creatinine in dogs with CKD. Muscle mass does not interfere with SDMA levels (unlike creatinine, which may be interesting when monitoring patients with CKD and loss of muscle mass). The reference range established for the dog and cat is the same: 0–14 μg/dl.

### Genetic tests

Genetic tests are available for certain hereditary kidney diseases in breeds in which the molecular defect responsible for the lesion is known, for example:

- certain glomerulopathies in the Cocker Spaniel, Samoyed and Soft-coated Wheaten Terrier
- polycystic kidney disease in the Persian cat.

### Renal clearance tests

**Measurement of GFR is the most accurate way to assess renal function** and is especially useful in early stages of renal failure without azotaemia. Currently, there are several validated methods in both the dog and cat for measuring GFR – for example, plasma clearance tests with non-radioactive markers such as iohexol, which are easier to perform than urinary clearance tests: the test is performed by the administration of an IV marker and blood samples taken repeatedly over a certain period of time, with GFR calculated by an established formula.

## *Diagnostic imaging*

### *Radiology*

Radiology (Figures 6.4 and 6.5) is useful for:

- assessing the size and shape of the kidneys
- detecting renal mineralization
- visualizing radiodense uroliths.

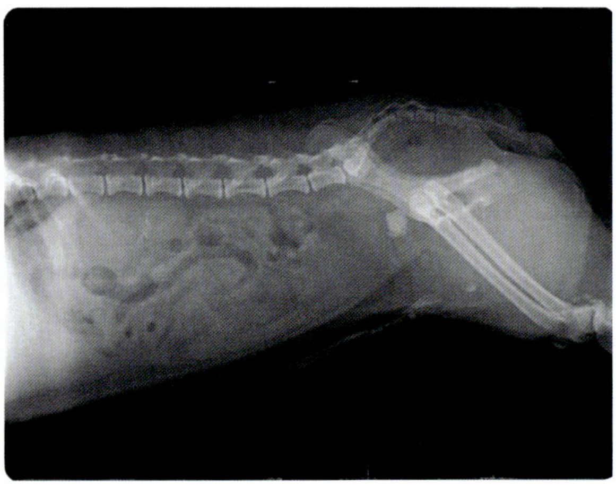

**Figure 6.4.** Urolith in the bladder and penile urethra.

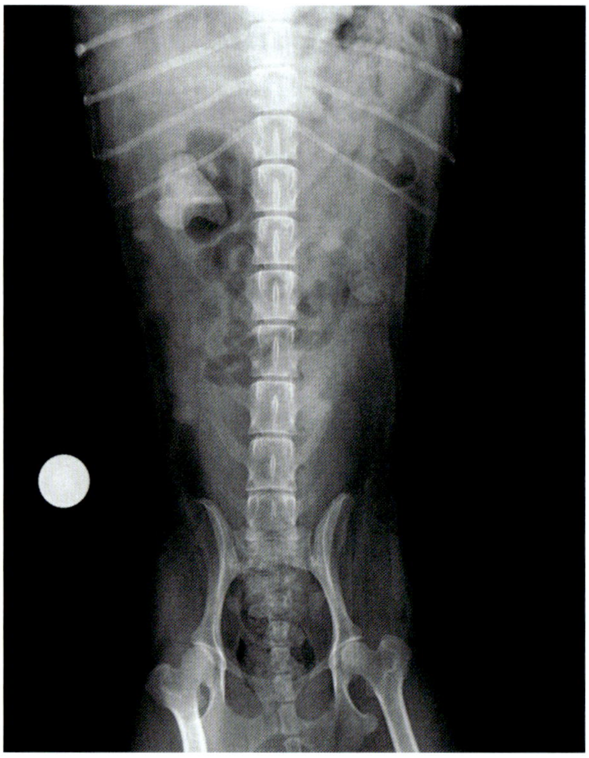

**Figure 6.5.** Nephrolithiasis.

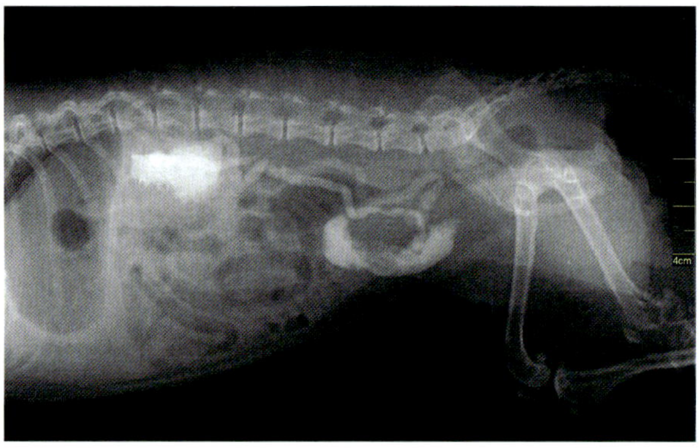

**Figure 6.6.** IV urography in a patient with transitional cell carcinoma of the bladder. A defect in bladder filling can be seen, and dilatation of the renal pelvis.

The use of contrast media by retrograde urethrography or IV pyelography (Figure 6.6) allows the diagnosis of:

- congenital conditions (ectopic ureter).
- diseases of the renal pelvis and ureters
- rupture of urinary tracts.

The use of IV contrast agents should be avoided if renal function is not good (i.e. dehydrated or uraemic animals).

### *Ultrasound*

A normal appearance on renal ultrasound does not rule out kidney disease, but this is a useful complementary

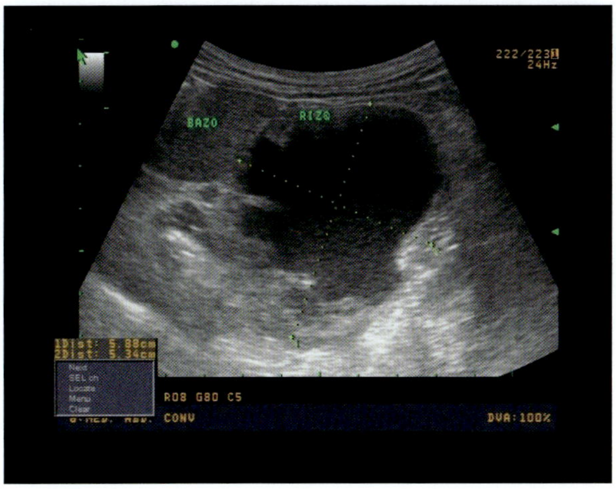


**Figure 6.7.** Severe dilatation of the renal pelvis in a dog with pyelonephrosis.

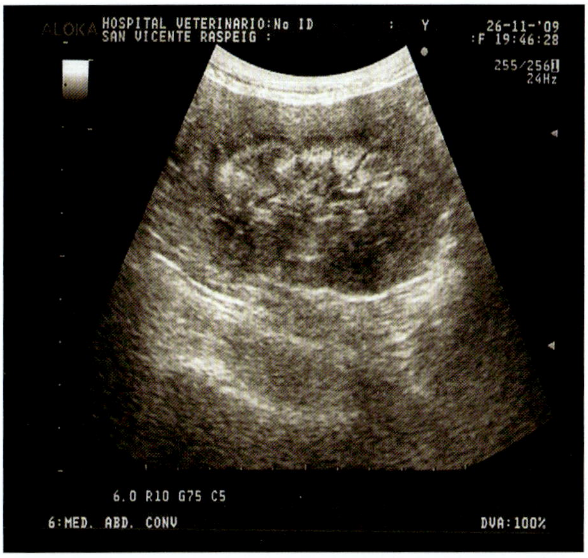


**Figure 6.8.** Nephrocalcinosis in a dog with lymphoma and hypercalcaemia.

test since the presence of different patterns of hypo- or hyper-echogenicity and their distribution can narrow down the differential diagnoses. Ultrasound is especially valuable for the **detection of structural abnormalities** in the upper and lower urinary tract (dilation of the renal pelvis, tumours and other diseases of the renal parenchyma, dilation of the ureters and presence of uroliths, and diseases of the urinary bladder, etc.). It also allows the **evaluation of the rest of the abdomen** and, therefore, the diagnosis of underlying diseases (Figures 6.7 and 6.8).

### *Advanced imaging tests: computerized axial tomography and magnetic resonance imaging*

These techniques can provide valuable information in complicated cases, complementing the information obtained via other more conventional imaging tests (radiology and ultrasound) (Figure 6.9).

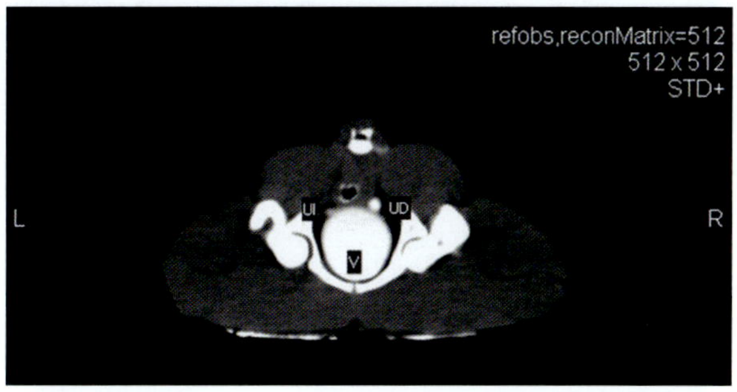


**Figure 6.9.** Ectopic ureter in a bitch.

### *Scintigraphy*

At present available only at certain **university hospitals**, the test assesses the flow of **radioisotopes**.

### *Cystoscopy*

This is a useful technique in the diagnostic approach to patients with **lower urinary tract pathologies**.

### *Arterial pressure*

The importance of **arterial blood pressure** in the diagnosis and treatment of renal failure will be discussed later.

**Direct arterial pressure** is measured using **invasive** methods (arterial puncture with a needle connected to a transducer) that are generally used only in intensive care units or anaesthetized animals.

There are two **indirect methods** for measurement of arterial blood pressure:

- **Doppler**. Detects blood flow in arteries by means of an **ultrasound transducer** (Figure 6.10). With this technique, **only systolic** pressure can be measured.
- **Oscillometry**. Detects **vibrations in the arterial wall** (Figure 6.11). Enables measurement of **systolic and diastolic** pressure.

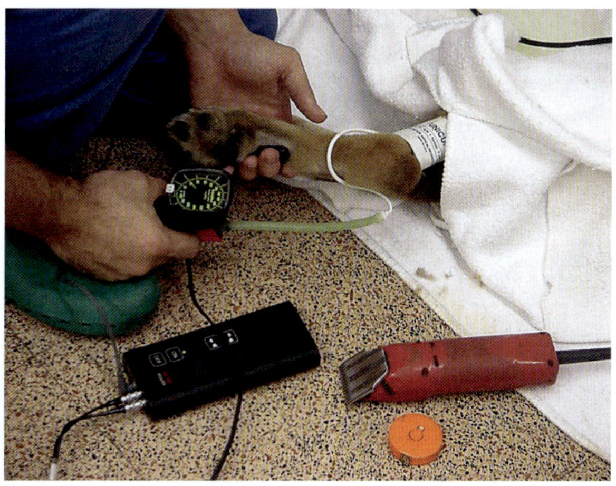

**Figure 6.10.** Measurement of arterial pressure using the Doppler method.

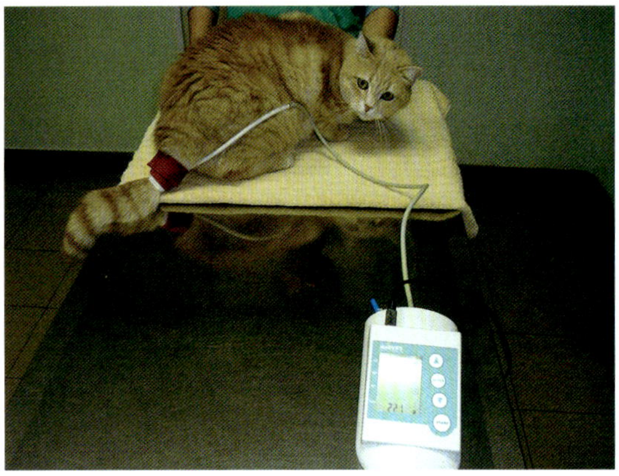


**Figure 6.11.** Measurement of arterial pressure using high-definition oscillometry.

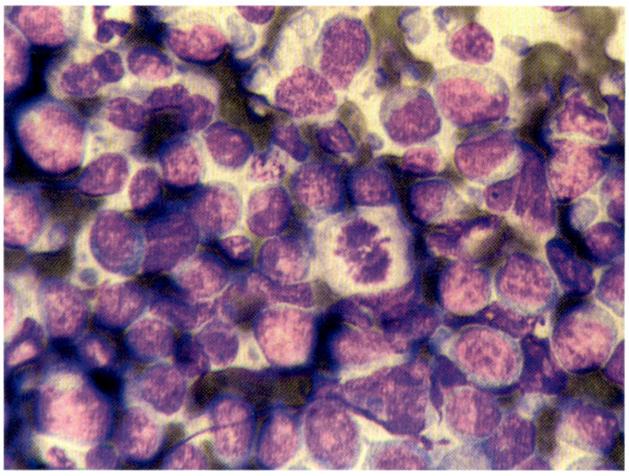

**Figure 6.12.** Renal lymphoma diagnosed using renal cytology.

## Recommendations for the measurement of arterial blood pressure

- Choose a **quiet room** away from other animals, if possible in the presence of the owner. Let the patient acclimatise for 5–10 minutes (should not be sedated).
- Place the animal in a **comfortable position**, preferably lying down, with the heart at the same height as the cuff.
- The **width of the cuff should be 30–40% the width of the limb or tail** where it is placed (record the cuff used and the measurement site in the notes to make future measurements under the same conditions).
- Ignore the first result and then take **5–7 consecutive measures**. If values that differ by more than 20 mmHg are observed, measurements must be repeated. The highest and lowest values should be discarded and the average of the remainder of the annotated values calculated.
- If possible, in the case of hypertension **repeat after 30 minutes**, before administering antihypertensive treatment.

Each technique has advantages and disadvantages (for example, movement of the animal can interfere with oscillometry) but, in general, the two techniques give reliable values and are useful if they are executed following a correct protocol. It is important to standardize the technique if you want to compare values recorded on different visits.

## *Renal biopsy*

Renal biopsy should be considered when the information derived from it would influence treatment. In some cases, **renal cytology** allows an initial, less aggressive, approach that can provide valuable information (for example, in the case of suspected renal lymphoma [Figure 6.12]).

Before performing a biopsy, consider:

- If indicated (that is, if the results will be of clinical use).
- The procedure (obtaining adequate samples safely).
- The samples should be evaluated by a pathologist with experience in nephropathology and with access to the appropriate equipment (optical microscopy, electron microscopy and immunofluorescence).
- Renal biopsy is indicated in the following cases (Figure 6.13):
- **proteinuric** renal disease

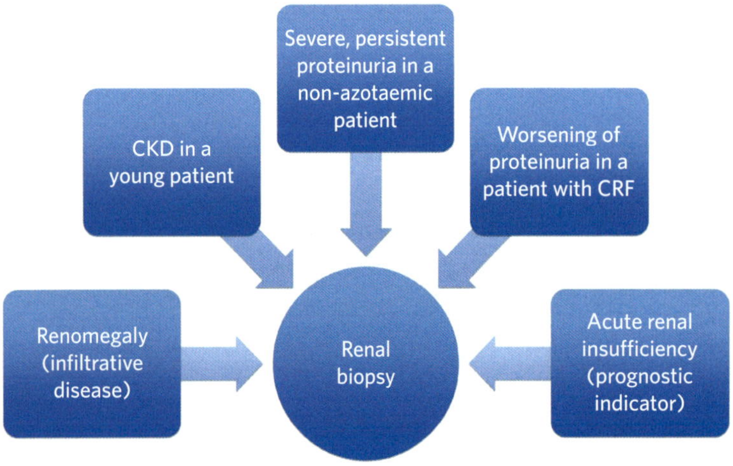


**Figure 6.13.** Situations where renal biopsy is indicated.

- **nfiltrative disease** of the renal parenchyma
- **young animals** with CKD.

It is contraindicated in:

- severe **coagulopathies** (test coagulation beforehand)
- presence of **cavitated lesions** (hydronephrosis, renal cysts, abscesses, vascular abnormalities)
- patients with **advanced renal disease**.

**Haemorrhage** is the most frequent complication, so it is important to keep the patient on fluids after the biopsy to eliminate possible blood clots from the ureters that could cause an obstruction.

It is essential that the biopsy (sampling and interpretation of it) is carried out by experienced personnel and analysed using various techniques, not limited to optical microscopy but also including electron microscopy and immunofluorescence, which are essential to obtain the necessary information.

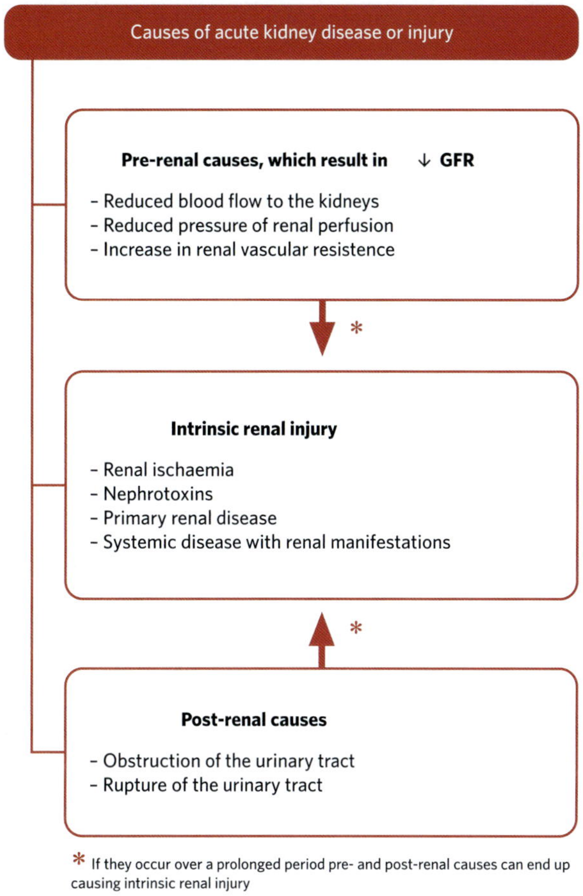


**Figure 6.14.** Causes of acute renal injury.

## AKD

### *Definition*

The terms '**acute renal injury**' or '**acute renal disease' (AKD)** now replace the term 'acute renal failure' (ARF).

This is because '**acute renal failure**' refers to a **subpopulation** of patients with acute renal injury associated with a **high risk of mortality** . The new concept of '**acute kidney disease**' encompasses a **wider spectrum** of patients with varying degrees of functional injury, from milder to more severe manifestations (with ARF).

**AKD** is defined as a **rapid loss** (within hours to days) of **nephron function**, which causes **azotaemia, water, electrolyte and acid–base balance disturbances and uraemia**.

### *Pathophysiology*

The symptoms of AKD include **pre- and post-renal** conditions that can be either **independent or combined** with an intrinsic renal lesion depending on the origin, extent and duration of the conditions responsible for the AKD. **Patients with acute uraemia** are recognized in which pre-renal, intrinsic renal and/or post-renal components are identified with a thorough diagnostic and therapeutic approach (Figure 6.14).

In AKD, **four pathophysiological stages** can be identified which **occur consecutively**. (Figure 6.15):

1. **Initial phase**. This refers to the immediate **insult** (nephrotoxic, ischaemic) responsible for the renal damage.
2. **Expansion phase**. Continuous **hypoxia and the inflammatory response** spread renal damage.

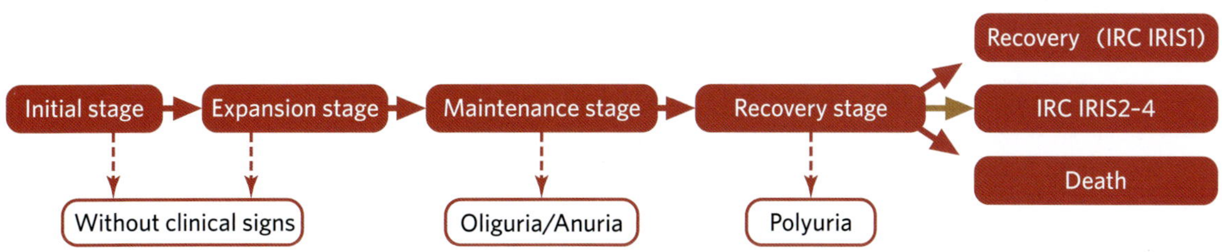


**Figure 6.15.** Stages of AKD.

These first two phases can last **less than 48 hours**, and clinical or laboratory changes are not always seen while they are occurring.

1. **Maintenance phase**. Characterized by **azotaemia and uraemia** and can last from **days to weeks**. In this phase, urine production is very variable and may be increased or decreased, and there has already been a critical level of irreversible kidney damage.
2. **Recovery phase**. Lasts from **weeks to months**. Azotaemia improves and there is repair of the renal tubules, this entails a **polyuria** marked by the partial recovery of tubular function and osmotic diuresis by the accumulated solutes. This may involve a volume depletion that can interrupt recovery.

A patient with AKD can progress and worsen until death, or may partially (remaining in different stages of CRI 1–4) or totally recover.

## IRIS classification

In human medicine, a system was defined to **grade renal injury** in patients with **acute renal injury**, taking into account variations in creatinine, glomerular filtration rate and urine production. This was based on studies that demonstrated a **relationship between the stage and mortality.** The acronym RIFLE (from the words 'Risk', 'Injury', 'Failure', 'Loss' and 'End-Stage Kidney Disease') was used.

In 2013 the **IRIS** company established a classification system to **grade the severity of AKD** in dogs and cats. Unlike the IRIS classification for chronic kidney disease, the IRIS grade for AKD ('IRIS AKI Grade') represents a specific moment in the course of the disease that will change as the condition worsens, improves or evolves into chronic kidney disease.

The **objective is to facilitate classification, functional stratification and treatment decisions**. The classification is based on serum creatinine levels, urine production and the need for renal replacement therapy (dialysis, transplantation, etc.) (Table 6.3).

## Aetiology

The main **causes of AKD** in **dogs** are:

- infectious diseases
- nephrotoxicity
- haemodynamic instability
- immune-mediated diseases
- miscellaneous and idiopathic.

In **cats**:

- Nephrotoxins (lilies, non-steroidal anti-inflammatory drugs [NSAIDs], ethylene glycol, aminoglycosides, doxorubicin, vitamin D and food contaminants such as melamine and cyanuric acid). These account for 50% of cases.
- Ischaemic injuries.
- Pyelonephritis.
- Neoplasia.
- Sepsis.
- Prolonged ureteral or urethral obstruction.

Table 6.3. AKD classification according to IRIS.

| AKD grade | Serum creatinine | Clinical description | Sub-class |
|---|---|---|---|
| **Grade I** | <1.6 mg/dl | Non-azotaemic AKD:<br>Documented ERA (evidence of acute renal injury from clinical history findings, examination, laboratory tests and imaging techniques) and/or<br>Progressive increase (without azotaemia) of creatinine: ≥0.3 mg/dl in 48 hours<br>Oliguria (<1 ml/kg/h) or anuria in a 6-h period | Each grade or class is further classified into:<br>1. Non-oliguric or oligoanuric<br>2. In need of renal replacement therapy |
| **Grade II** | 1.7–2.5 mg/dl | Mild AKD:<br>Documented AKD and static or progressive azotaemia<br>Progressive increase (with azotaemia) of creatinine: ≥0.3 mg/dl in 48 hours, or response to volume expansion (increase in urine production to >1 ml/kg/h in 6 hours and/or decrease in creatinine to baseline values in 48 h)<br>Oliguria (<1 ml/kg/h) or anuria in a 6-h period | |
| **Grade III** | 2.6–5.0 mg/dl | Moderate–severe AKD: | |
| **Grade IV** | 5.1–10.0 mg/dl | Documented and variable AKD, increased severity of azotaemia and functional renal failure | |
| **Grade V** | >10 mg/dl | | |

### *Pre-renal causes*

Any condition that **decreases renal blood flow** can produce **pre-renal azotaemia** which, if prolonged, can lead to intrinsic renal injury due to ischaemia and which, in turn, is an important cause of azotaemia in hospitalized patients or those undergoing treatment (Figure 6.16).

Situations that **decrease renal blood flow** include: **dehydration, hypovolaemia, hypotension**, decrease in effective circulating volume (heart failure, liver cirrhosis, nephrotic syndrome), anaesthesia, hypo-adrenocorticism, trauma, surgery, shock, heat stroke, hypoalbuminaemia and reduced renal perfusion (NSAIDs, angiotensin-converting enzyme inhibitors [ACEI]).

The kidney has a **self-regulatory mechanism** that allows it to maintain glomerular filtration rate in cases of hypotension/hypovolaemia. This is achieved by **vasodilation of the afferent glomerular arterioles** by prostaglandin and the **constriction of efferent arterioles** by the renin–angiotensin system. However, when mean blood pressure drops below 80 mmHg, these compensatory mechanisms begin to fail and glomerular filtration rate decreases. At first this is reversible through the administration of fluids and the correction of hypovolaemia but, if left untreated, in many cases irreversible kidney damage occurs.

**Angiotensin-converting enzyme inhibitor drugs (ACEI)** alter glomerular haemodynamics and may produce pre-renal azotaemia which results in intrinsic renal injury. **NSAIDs** inhibit prostaglandin-mediated vasodilation, so it is essential to monitor patients undergoing treatment with NSAIDs as well as avoid administration in situations where there is reduced renal perfusion (dehydrated, hypovolaemic patients, etc.) NSAIDs inhibit COX-1 and COX-2 enzymes. COX-1 is expressed in the healthy kidney and is responsible for the synthesis of prostaglandins, necessary for maintaining the glomerular filtration rate in situations of hypotension/hypovolaemia. COX-2 can be induced by toxins, cytokines and others, but it is also constitutively expressed in the kidney, especially in situations where there is hypovolaemia, contributing to the synthesis of vasodilatory prostaglandins. Therefore, **even the use of selective COX-2 inhibitors can lead to kidney damage** in dehydrated, hypotensive animals, etc. The International Society of Feline Medicine and the American Association of Feline Practitioners have published a consensus with guidelines on the use of NSAIDs in cats. In summary, based on current studies, the authors state that the proper use of NSAIDs (adequate doses in clinically stable cats) is associated with a very low risk of kidney damage.

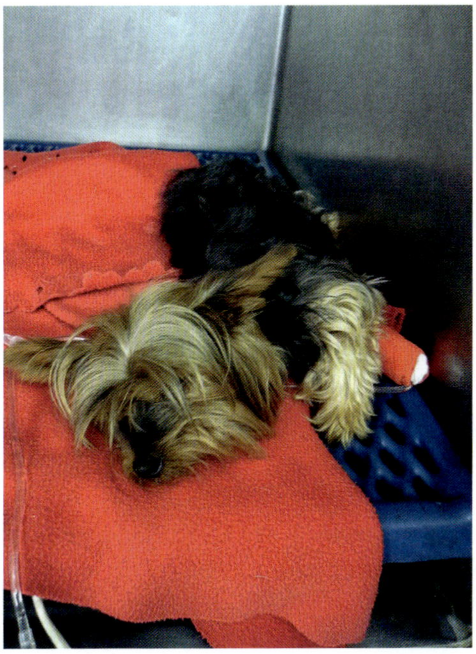

**Figure 6.16.** A Yorkshire Terrier with pre-renal azotaemia due to hypovolaemia as a result of hypo-adrenocorticism.

### *Intrinsic renal injury*

Prolonged **pre-renal hypoperfusion** leads to intrinsic renal injury, with ischaemia implicated in the occurrence of acute kidney disease.

Various **infectious diseases** may also be involved in the onset of AKD:

**Bacterial pyelonephritis** is usually caused by bacteria **ascending from the lower urinary tract**, although their arrival can also be haematogenous, and certain conditions (bacterial endocarditis, pyometra, discospondylitis, etc.) may favour its development. **Gram-negative bacteria**, including *Escherichia coli*, are those most frequently implicated in urinary tract infections.

**Leptospirosis** is a bacterial zoonosis with a worldwide distribution, caused by *Leptospira* spp., of which more than 250 serovars have been identified, grouped into antigenically related serogroups. Among other problems, leptospirosis can cause **acute interstitial nephritis**. Leptospirosis should be suspected in dogs suffering from fever, acute renal failure, liver failure, uveitis, pulmonary haemorrhage or abortion. With new serovars, clinical cases of polyuria/polydipsia, glomerulopathy or chronic pyelonephritis, among others, are sometimes seen. Azotaemia is not continuous and may be present in only 50–60% of cases.

There are many potentially **nephrotoxic substances**, the most frequent being:

- In the dog: ethylene glycol, NSAIDs, cholecalciferol and aminoglycosides.
- In the cat: ethylene glycol, cholecalciferol and lilies.

Table 6.4. Causes of intrinsic kidney damage responsible for acute kidney disease.

| | |
|---|---|
| **Ischaemic conditions** | Shock symptoms (hypovolaemic, haemorrhagic, hypotensive, septic)<br>Decreased cardiac output (CHF, arrhythmias, pericardial effusion, etc.)<br>Anaesthesia, trauma, hyper-/hypothermia, skin burns<br>Transfusion reactions, DIC, renal vessel thrombosis<br>Hyperviscosity, polycythaemia<br>NSAIDs |
| **Nephrotoxins** | Endogenous toxins (haemoglobin, myoglobin)<br>Exogenous toxins (heavy metals, organic compounds, lily plants in cats, grapes in dogs, cholecalciferol, etc.)<br>Medications (antibiotics, antifungals, antivirals, chemotherapeutic agents, immunosuppressants, NSAIDs, ACEI, diuretics, radiocontrast agents, etc.)<br>Hypercalcaemia, melanin, cyanuric acid |
| **Primary renal disease** | Infections (pyelonephritis, leptospirosis, borreliosis, etc.)<br>Immune-mediated diseases (acute GN, SLE, vasculitis, etc.)<br>Neoplasms (lymphoma, adenocarcinoma, sarcoma, nephroblastoma, etc.) |
| **Systemic diseases with renal manifestations** | Infectious (FIP, leishmaniosis, babesiosis, bacterial endocarditis, etc.)<br>Sepsis, SIRS, DIC, multiorgan failure, haemolytic anaemia, etc.<br>Pancreatitis, hepatorenal syndrome, etc. |

ACEI, angiotensin-converting enzyme inhibitors; CHF, cardiac heart failure; DIC, disseminated intravascular coagulation; DIC, disseminated intravascular coagulation; FIP, feline infectious peritonitis; GN, glomerulonephritis; NSAIDs, nonsteroidal anti-inflammatory drugs; SIRS, systemic inflammatory response syndrome; SLE, systemic lupus erythematosus.

Other primary renal diseases of **immune-mediated** or **neoplastic** origin can also cause AKD, as well as systemic diseases that alter renal haemodynamics or cause a systemic inflammatory response (Table 6.4).

## Post-renal causes

**Obstruction of the ureters**, urethra or renal pelvis by calculi, mucous plugs, blood clots or masses can cause acute kidney damage if it **lasts more than 1 week** (Figure 6.17). Conditions such as **ureterolithiasis** are detected more frequently in the **cat** as being responsible for acute azotaemia.

**Rupture of the urinary tract** can produce acute uraemia. The presence of **uro-abdomen** causes an inflammatory tissue reaction which leads to sterile or septic peritonitis (if there was urinary infection), requiring an emergency surgical approach.

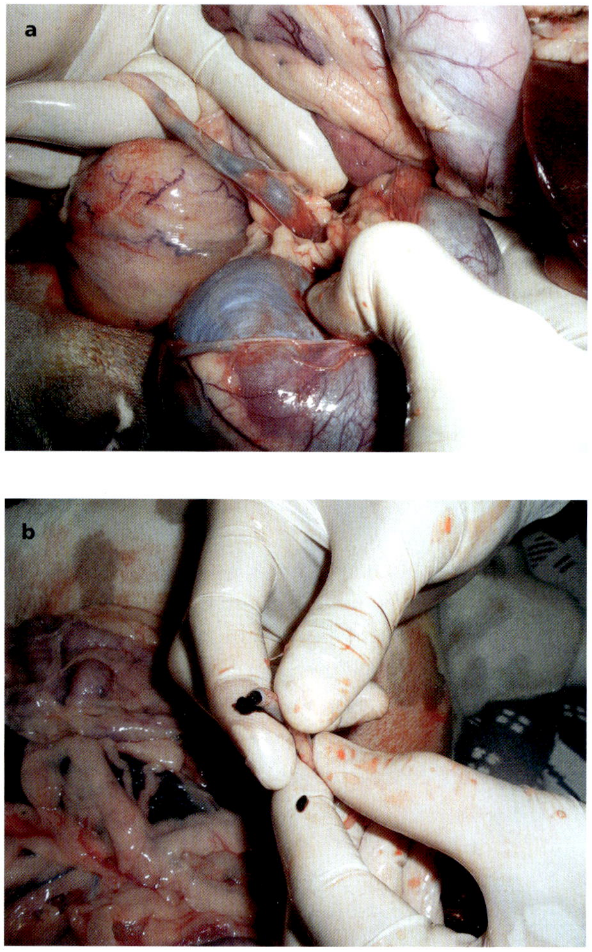


Figure 6.17. Images from a post-mortem on a patient with ureteral obstruction due to a blood clot.

## Clinical signs

In addition to a **systematic physical examination,** it is essential to take a **thorough history**, including the **risk factors** (Table 6.5) for acute renal injury (especially in hospitalized animals), in order not to miss information that is key to diagnosis and treatment.

### History

In animals presenting with symptoms compatible with renal insufficiency, a good clinical history gives an idea about the type (acute or chronic), possible aetiology and evolution of the disease.

The **signalment** (age, sex, breed) can give important clues. For example, **young animals** are prone to **food indiscretion** (access to objects with zinc, lilies, grapes, nephrotoxic medications) and, in **geriatric animals**, **neoplasms** are more frequent (although lymphoma and nephroblastoma are also seen in young patients).

The **previous and current** clinical history (concurrent diseases, episodes of urolithiasis, urinary infections, recent sedation, treatments administered), vaccinations,

Table 6.5. Risk factors for acute uraemia.

| In hospitalized or animals undergoing treatment |
|---|
| **Renal hypoperfusion** |
| Anaesthesia |
| Sepsis |
| Gastric dilatation volvulus |
| Signs of shock |
| **Electrolyte and acid–base changes** |
| Increased nephrotoxicity of radiological contrast media if there is hyponatraemia |
| Increased gentamicin nephrotoxicity if there is hypokalaemia, metabolic acidosis, hypocalcaemia or hypomagnesaemia |
| **Nephrotoxic medications** (especially if combined) |
| Aminoglycosides; avoid using these for more than 7–10 days, administer less frequently (every 24 hours), in hydrated and normovolaemic patients, review other medications administered simultaneously, and monitor |
| Out-of-date tetracyclines (cause tubular damage) |
| Penicillins (cause hypersensitivity symptoms) |
| Sulphonamides (lead to the formation of crystals in renal tubules) |
| NSAIDs |
| Diuretics |
| **Previous conditions** |
| Renal or hepatic insufficiency |
| Pancreatitis |
| Diabetes mellitus |
| Cardiovascular disease |
| Neoplasia |
| Trauma |
| Extensive burns |
| Old age |
| Fever |
| Vasculitis |

the pet's usual environment, **travel history**, access to **nephrotoxins** (especially lilies), grapes, zinc, ointments with calcipotriol, antifreeze, rodenticides (with cholecalciferol), contact with other animals, exposure to vectors of infectious disease, the possibility of trauma (suggesting uro-abdomen), etc.

A thorough summary of clinical signs should also be compiled, including their duration and nature (urinary and non-urinary). Some animals with **chronic renal failure may suffer from decompensation** and present with typical symptoms of acute uraemia:

- weight loss
- poor body condition
- previous presence of polyuria–polydipsia (PUPD, suggests a chronic course).

The following signs are suggestive of **lower urinary tract disease**:

- dysuria
- stranguria
- polyuria.

### *Physical examination*

A thorough physical examination includes assessment of **hydration** status, **body condition**, a **rectal** examination and an **eye** examination.

Typical changes can lead to suspicions of certain conditions such as:

- **Icteric mucous membranes** (leptospirosis in icteric dogs with azotaemia [Figure 6.18]).
- **Uveitis** (leptospirosis, lymphoma).
- Pale mucous membranes and **haemoglobinuria** (haemolytic anaemia due to zinc poisoning, babesiosis, etc.).
- **Bradycardia** (hypo-adrenocorticism).
- **Abdominal pain** (pancreatitis, pyelonephritis, etc.).
- **Neurological** disorders (ethylene glycol poisoning).
- Lymphadenomegaly (infectious diseases, lymphoma [Figure 6.19]).

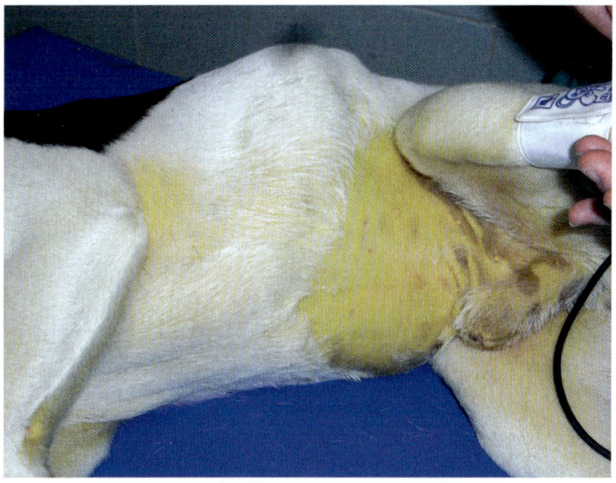

Figure 6.18. Icteric dog with AKD due to leptospirosis.

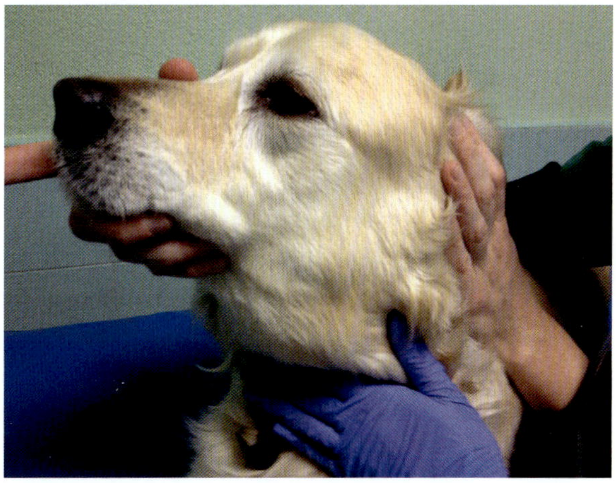

Figure 6.19. Lymphadenomegaly in a bitch with AKD due to hypercalcaemia and lymphoma.

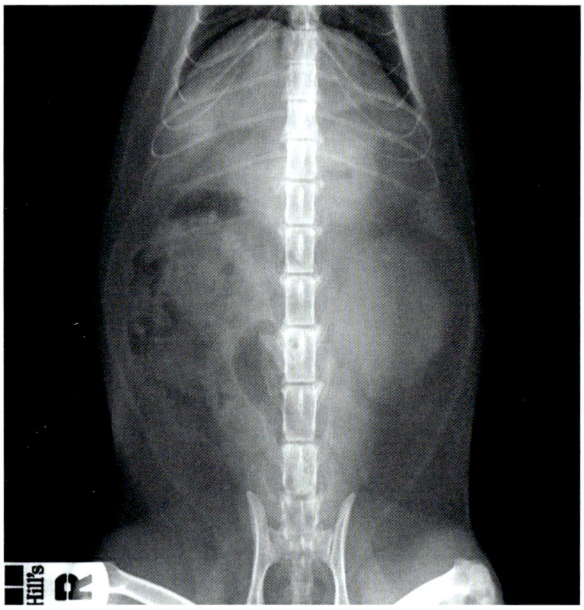

Figure 6.20. Radiograph of a cat with renal asymmetry due to ureteral obstruction.

- Urethral thickening and/or urolithiasis.
- **Anal gland masses** (neoplasia especially adenocarcinoma of anal glands with hypercalcaemia).

When palpating the kidneys, their size, symmetry and the presence of pain should be evaluated. Small kidneys suggest a chronic condition with acute deterioration, while bilateral renomegaly suggests nephrotoxicity, infectious or neoplastic causes (lymphoma). In cats with renal asymmetry (one large and one small), ureteral obstruction should be suspected (Figure 6.20).

## Diagnosis

Evaluate each patient as an individual to formulate a diagnostic plan based on clinical suspicions. Investigation should focus on the **origin of the azotaemia** (pre-renal, renal or post-renal) and **the cause**, along with identifying **clinical consequences** that require specific treatment.

### Blood tests

The results of the **blood count are usually not specific**, although a **stress or inflammatory leukogram** may be observed (indeed, its absence in a patient with a suggestive clinic picture should lead to a suspicion of hypoadrenocorticism). Although anaemia is more common in patients with CKD, it is also seen in those with AKD in cases of haemolysis due to infections caused by pyroplasmids, zinc poisoning or gastric ulcers, etc.

The following can be detected on blood biochemistry:

- Different degrees of **azotaemia and hyperphosphataemia**.
- **Hyperkalaemia**, common in animals with oliguria or anuria (also due to post-renal causes).
- **Hypercalcaemia**. The most common causes of hypercalcaemia in dogs are neoplasia, kidney disease, hypo-adrenocorticism, hyperparathyroidism and intoxication due to vitamin D derivatives; and, in the cat, idiopathic feline hypercalcaemia. Draw up a list of differential diagnosis in order to undertake appropriate investigation (Figure 6.21).
- **Hypocalcaemia and/or hyperglycaemia** and, in some cases, hyperphosphataemia in patients with ethylene glycol poisoning.
- **Elevation of liver enzymes and bilirubin** in some dogs with leptospirosis.

If there is suspicion of pancreatitis, measurement of specific canine or feline pancreatic lipase is recommended.

### Urinalysis

Urinalysis can detect **isothenuria** and, depending on the aetiology, other changes such as proteinuria, glycosuria, haematuria, pyuria, bacteriuria, crystalluria (calcium oxalate crystals in ethylene glycol poisoning) and cylindruria.

**Urine culture** is indicated in all patients with acute azotaemia of unknown cause (a negative result does not completely exclude the possibility of pyelonephritis).

### Diagnostic imaging

These techniques are fundamental to assess the **structure of the urinary tract** and adjacent tissues, and to detect urolithiasis, masses and abdominal free fluid.

Specific cases may require radiological studies (with contrast to detect rupture of the urinary tract or uroliths), abdominal ultrasound or more advanced techniques.

**Ultrasound** is useful in the diagnosis of **renal tumours**, such as renal lymphoma, and to **facilitate cytological sampling** and biopsies. With ethylene glycol poisoning there are specific ultrasound changes such as an increase in renal cortical echogenicity and the presence of a hypo-echogenic band at the corticomedullary junction (Figure 6.22). Dogs with leptospirosis may show renomegaly, pyelectasia, a hyperechoic renal cortex, perirenal fluid and a hyperechoic medullary band.

### Other tests

In patients with acute renal injury, **blood pressure** should be monitored. In addition, depending on clinical suspicions, **infectious diseases** should be tested for (serologies and/or PCR for leptospirosis, babesiosis, borreliosis, etc.), **abdominal free fluid** should be

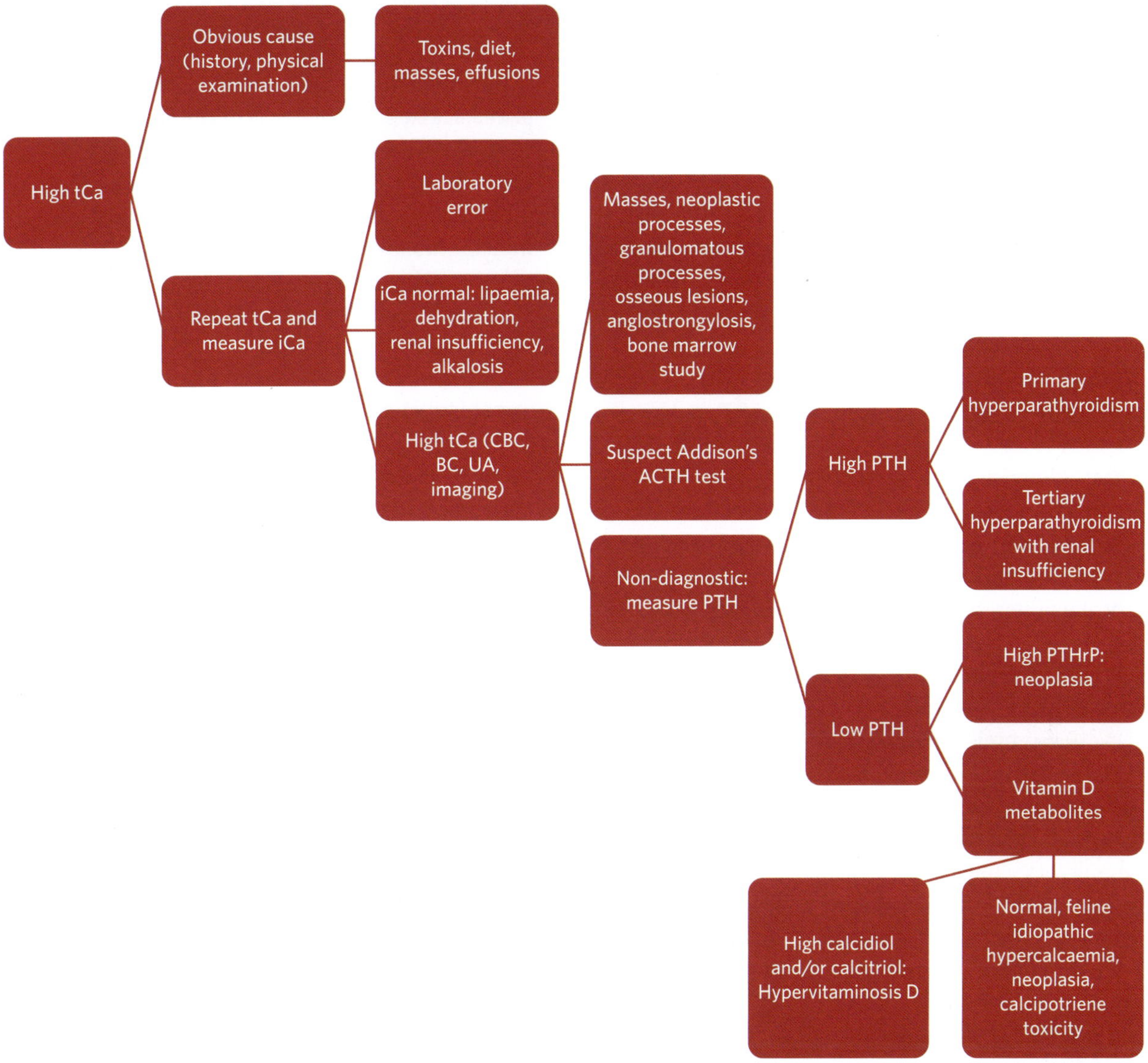


**Figure 6.21.** Diagnostic approach in the hypercalcaemic patient.

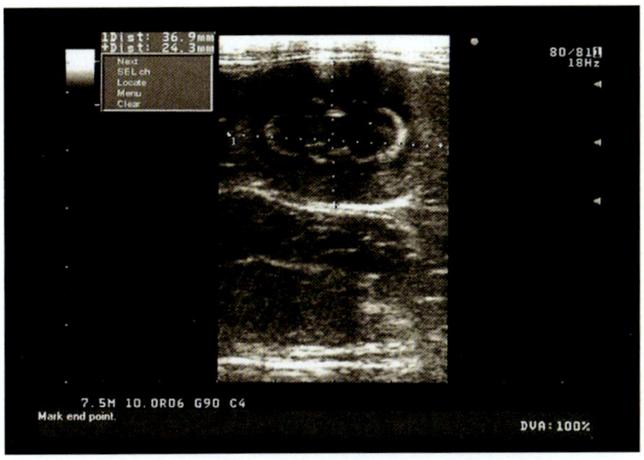

**Figure 6.22.** The presence of a hypo-echogenic band at the corticomedullary band in a patient with ethylene glycol poisoning.

analysed and tests to detect ethylene glycol and zinc, etc. can be performed.

Although more veterinary studies are needed and the techniques are not widely available, there is currently considerable interest in the study of **biomarkers** that serve to detect early kidney injury. Some of these include **serum cystatin C** or urinary markers for tubular lesions such as **GGT** (gamma-glutamyl transpeptidase), **NAG** (*N*-acetyl-beta-D-glycosaminidase) and 'retinol-binding protein'. The **GGT/creatinine urine ratio** has sometimes been used to monitor the occurrence of acute tubular injury in patients receiving nephrotoxic treatments.

### *Renal biopsy*

In specific cases renal biopsy may be indicated, when less invasive means have failed to yield information about the definitive cause, the extent of the lesion, chronicity and the prognosis. It is also indicated for the **diagnosis of neoplasia** (although lymphoma can be diagnosed by cytology in most cases). Biopsy is particularly recommended when considering options such as peritoneal dialysis or haemodialysis.

## Treatment

The therapeutic approach to acute kidney disease is based on **supportive treatment, eliminating the underlying cause** and **correction of the haemodynamic and biochemical** consequences of uraemic syndrome. When it is not possible to control the clinical signs or the clinical pathological changes with medical management, more advanced therapies such as haemodialysis can be applied, provided they are available.

### Specific treatment

**Correct or eliminate** the cause of the AKD:

- **Stop administration** of drugs with nephrotoxic potential.
- With ethylene glycol poisoning, vomiting can be induced (if ingestion was within the previous 3 hours) or administer substances such as 4-methylpyrazole or ethanol to prevent metabolism of ethylene glycol.
- Where leptospirosis is suspected, administer antibiotics (doxycycline or penicillins).
- In cases of **pyelonephritis, fluoroquinolones** may be a good first option, with positive action against Gram-negative bacteria and good penetration of renal tissue. However, treatment should be guided based on the results of culture and an antibiogram.
- With **NSAID poisoning**, improve renal perfusion with **fluid therapy** and consider administration of **prostaglandin analogues such as misoprostol**.

### Supportive treatment

#### Fluid therapy

The mainstay of treatment is **intravenous fluid therapy**, with **strict monitoring** of hydration status, renal function, acid–base status and electrolyte levels. The aim is to determine the type and amount of fluids required to maintain an adequate blood pressure, blood volume and cardiac output.

##### *Monitoring patients with AKD receiving fluid therapy*

Physical examination:

- heart and respiratory rate, pulse, capillary refill time, mucous membrane colour, mental state, temperature
- presence of oedema in the conjunctiva, peripheral oedema.

Body weight:

- Weight should be monitored at least three times per day.

Approximate calculation of fluid loss or gain:

1 kg of weight = 1 l of fluid

##### *Urine production*

- **Urine production** is measured via a urinary catheter, placed in a sterile manner with a **closed collection system** or using **absorbent pads** (weigh before and after urination to estimate the volume of urine produced). In cats, urine can also be measured directly from the litter tray.

Thus, fluid therapy can be adjusted to the amount of urine produced.

##### *Haematocrit and total protein*

- Performed using **centrifuge analysis** (microhaematocrit) (Figure 6.23).

These are useful for assessing changes in water balance, but it should also be taken into account that they may vary due to other factors (haemorrhage, proteinuria, effusion etc.).

##### *Central venous pressure (CVP)*

- Evaluate changes or trends but, in general, CVP <0 cm $H_2O$ indicates hypovolaemia while CVP >10 cm $H_2O$ reveals volume overload.

**Patients with AKD are at risk of volume overload**, which is associated with increased mortality. Very high fluid therapy rates were traditionally recommended; however, a more **careful approach** is now favoured, observing the response to the **monitored** administration of fluid therapy boluses, sometimes in combination with **vasoactive drugs**.

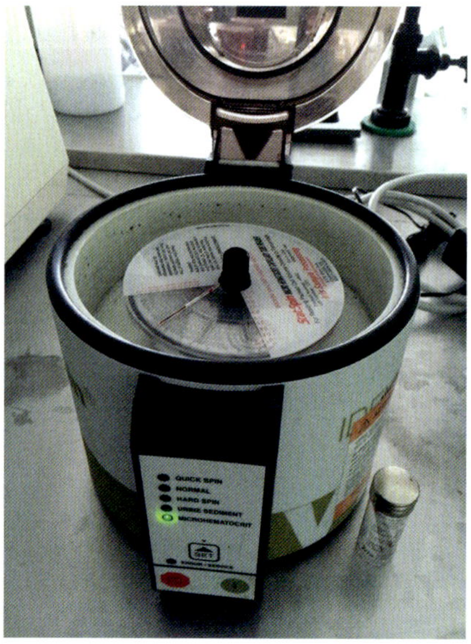

**Figure 6.23.** Measurement of haematocrit by centrifugation.

It is unclear which is the best vasopressor drug to maintain good renal perfusion. Dopamine has been used for this purpose for a long time, but its use is not currently recommended since no beneficial effect has been demonstrated at the renal level, and also due to the risk of its possible adverse effects. Current evidence points towards a greater beneficial vasopressor effect with **norepinephrine or vasopressin**.

Calculate the initial volume of fluid according to the animal's weight and the level of dehydration. This **water deficit should be replenished within the first 4–6 hours** to normalize renal blood flow as soon as possible. Maintenance fluid requirements (44–66 ml/kg/day) are administered plus the **estimated fluid loss due to vomiting and diarrhoea**. **Monitoring of urine production** is essential; if necessary, a urinary catheter can be placed, whilst always considering the possible inconvenience of this due to the risk of urinary infections. The latter is minimized by a catheter placed under sterile conditions, a closed urine collection system used and the catheter is changed every 2–3 days (maximum).

In human patients with AKD, the use of **isotonic crystalloid solutions** (rather than colloids) is recommended for **intravascular volume expansion**. This recommendation is based on studies demonstrating that 4% albumin solutions did not show any benefits when compared to saline. Other studies relate the use of hydroxyethyl starch (Hemohes) with significant renal dysfunction in addition to coagulation abnormalities. Therefore, isotonic solutions such as **Lactated Ringer's or 0.9% saline without potassium** are initially administered in cases of hyperkalaemia (demonstrated or suspected by the presence of oliguria or anuria). After rehydration, the type of fluid is adjusted according to the state of hydration and electrolyte levels of the patient.

The **duration of fluid therapy** depends on the patient's response. Ideally, the renal parameters should be normalized before therapy is withdrawn. However, it can take several days of treatment until **azotaemia values plateau and no longer decrease**. This point is achieved when the **renal values in a well-hydrated patient do not change in a 24-hour period.** From that moment, although renal recovery can continue for months, the administration of additional fluids will probably not provide additional benefits and a decision to begin the gradual withdrawal of fluid therapy can be made whilst observing whether this is tolerated by the patient.

### *Management of the oliguric and anuric patient*

When the patient is adequately hydrated, **urine flow should increase rapidly to 2–5 ml/kg/h**. However, if insufficient urine output is observed, circulating blood volume should be assessed to see if it is adequate. For this, the state of hydration should be assessed visually during the physical examination by means of jugular vein pressure, haematocrit and total protein, and the size of the cardiac chambers and the pulmonary vessels should be assessed using thoracic radiography and echocardiography, etc. If the circulating volume is estimated to be adequate, fluid therapy should be adjusted to avoid volume overload. For this, maintenance fluid requirements should be managed according to **insensitive losses (22 ml/kg/day)** plus urine production in the previous interval, while reassessing fluid therapy at short intervals of time.

Table 6.6. Medications promoting urine production in the oliguric or anuric patient.

| Medication | Administration |
|---|---|
| Furosemide | 1–2 mg/kg IV bolus, followed by constant infusion at 0.25–1 mg/kg/h |
| 20% mannitol | 0.5–1 g/kg IV bolus<br>In continuous infusion, 1–2 mg/kg/min<br>Contraindicated if there is volume overload, pulmonary oedema or congestive heart failure |
| Fenoldopam | Continuous infusion At 0.8 μg/kg/min (0.1–1) |

**Medications can be used to increase urine production**, such as diuretics and vasopressors (Table 6.6):

- **Furosemide**. Its use has been highly debated and is **not recommended** for this purpose. However, it can be useful in helping to avoid volume overload (its use as a continuous infusion is more effective than administration as an isolated bolus).
- **Mannitol**. Osmotic diuretic with other beneficial effects, such as the inhibition of renin release and its antioxidant effect as a result of its action on free radicals.
- **Dopamine**. Widely used in oliguric patients, its use is **currently discouraged** based on studies in patients who did not show a clinical benefit and on possible harmful effects in the evidential absence of efficacy in animals.
- **Fenoldopam**. Selective dopamine D1 receptor agonist. It has been shown to be renoprotective in studies in humans, and in small initial studies in the dog and cat, but recent studies (2015) show no significant differences.

### *Correction of electrolyte disturbances and acid–base balance*

**Animals that recover from an oliguric phase**, and those with milder kidney lesions that do not develop azotaemia, often have **profuse polyuria** and may suffer electrolyte abnormalities such as **hyponatraemia and**

**hypokalaemia**, which must be adequately corrected (supplemented with fluid therapy and/or orally).

Many patients with AKD suffer from **metabolic acidosis** due to:

- reduced ability to reabsorb and recycle bicarbonate
- reduced excretion of hydrogen ions through the renal tubules
- production of lactic acid due to poor renal perfusion
- decrease in phosphate elimination leading to reduced excretion of acid in urine.

In most cases **administration of bicarbonate is not necessary**, since diuresis often corrects this acidosis. Indeed, bicarbonate supplementation can lead to significant complications and is recommended only if blood pH is <7.2 or serum bicarbonate levels are <14 mEq/l despite improved perfusion with fluid therapy.

**Hyperkalaemia** may develop as a result of metabolic acidosis and reduced elimination of potassium in patients with oliguria or anuria. When this is detected, the first action is to attempt **restoration of urine production**.

In animals with **severe hyperkalaemia** or persistent oliguria, other treatments are needed that are **cardioprotective and to reduce potassium levels**; these include calcium gluconate, sodium bicarbonate and the joint administration of glucose and insulin or terbutaline.

### *Nutrition*

**Nutritional support** is very important in the recovery of animals with AKD, since they need an adequate supply of protein and energy for the regeneration of damaged renal tissue. **Enteral nutrition** is preferred (with **oesophagostomy or gastrostomy tubes** if necessary), although parenteral nutrition may be indicated in some cases.

### *Management of uraemic signs*

In uraemic patients, **vomiting and anorexia** are frequent gastrointestinal sequelae. **Uraemic toxins** stimulate the central and peripheral receptors that **trigger nausea**, and hypergastrinaemia caused by **reduced renal excretion of gastrin** can result in **gastric inflammation and ulceration**. Therefore, the use of **anti-emetic drugs** (metoclopramide, maropitant, dolansetron, ondansetron, etc.) and substances that **inhibit the production of gastric acid** (famotidine, ranitidine, omeprazole, pantoprazole) should be considered.

Arterial pressure should be monitored in patients with AKD, as **systemic hypertension is common** (some studies indicate that it affects 37–87% of affected dogs). In the presence of hypertension, fluid therapy should be reduced and, ideally, dialysis should be carried out to remove excess fluid. **Diuretics or antihypertensives** can be administered, taking care not to induce hypotension and compromise renal perfusion. Oral hypotensive drugs such as **amlodipine or ACEIs** may be used, but the use of ACEIs is controversial due to their negative effects on glomerular filtration rate.

The administration of oral medications can be problematic in animals with persistent vomiting. There are intravenous antihypertensive drugs (e.g. nitroprusside, hydralazine), but their use must be strictly monitored. The efficacy of rectal administration of amlodipine dissolved in saline solution has been described anecdotally.

### *Renal replacement therapy*

In AKD patients with persistent oliguria or anuria despite medical management and that have refractory hyperkalaemia, with volume overload or to extract certain toxins that can be dialysable (such as ethylene glycol), if available, various renal replacement therapies such as peritoneal dialysis, intermittent haemodialysis and continuous therapy can be an option.

## *Prognosis*

The **prognosis of cases of ARF is reserved to poor**, although this depends on many factors such as the cause, any delay in treatment and the patient's response to treatment. A lack of access to renal replacement therapies should also be included as a negative prognostic factor, although even with these survival is not guaranteed (studies of cats with AKD that received these treatments showed survival rates of 44–60%).

In some studies, the following have been **identified in the dog**:

### *Negative prognostic factors*

- presence of severe azotaemia (creatinine >10 mg/dl)
- worsening of azotaemia despite treatment
- presence of concurrent systemic diseases such as pancreatitis or sepsis.

### *Markers of renal recovery*

- increase in GFR
- urine production
- sodium clearance fraction.

Various studies indicate that **in the cat**:

### *Negative prognostic factors*

- hyperkalaemia
- hypo-albuminaemia

- low levels of bicarbonate
- low urine output.

The initial severity of azotaemia not prognostic, but its reduction in the first 3 days is related to longer survival times.

## Chronic kidney disease

### *Epidemiology*

**Chronic kidney disease (CKD) is the more common type of kidney disease in dogs and cats.**

The prevalence of CKD is 0.5–7% in dogs and 1.6–20% in cats. This prevalence increases among older patients so that, in geriatric patients, routine check-ups are recommended for its detection.

### *Definition and aetiology*

**CKD is defined as the presence of structural or functional changes of one or both kidneys for at least 3 months.**

Although the terms chronic kidney disease (CKD) and chronic kidney insufficiency (CKI) are often used interchangeably, it should be remembered there is a difference. This is that an animal in CKI has a more advanced form of CKD, having lost approximately 2/3 of its functional renal capacity.

To avoid confusion between terms such as kidney disease, kidney failure and renal insufficiency, it is preferable to use the staging system proposed by IRIS. The latter is based on creatinine levels and the presence of proteinuria and systemic hypertension (Figures 6.24 and 6.25) thus giving a more consistent picture of the patient's stage.

However, the patient's stage can be dynamic and change, for example, after the administration of antihypertensive or antiproteinuric treatments, and therefore the IRIS stage and the sub-stage should be re-evaluated periodically.

Once a renal injury has occurred in a specific area of the nephron (glomerulus, tubules, peritubular capillaries or interstitial tissue), the lesion may progress and affect the remainder of the kidney.

The **initial injury** can be triggered by a **congenital or acquired problem**. Congenital origins should be suspected according to the patient's age, breed and specific findings from imaging tests.

**Congenital changes** have been described in:

**Cats:**

- Abyssinian (medullary amyloidosis)
- Persians (polycystic kidneys).

| IRIS study | DOG Creatinine (mg/dl) | CAT Creatinine (mg/dl) | * Incorporation of SDMA (preliminary recommendations by IRIS in December 2015) |
|---|---|---|---|
| 1 | <1.4 | <1.6 | **Persistent increase >14 µg/dl** |
| 2 | 1.4–2 | 1.6–2.8 | With poor body condition, **SDMA ≥25 µg/dl** may indicate that the level of renal dysfunction has been underestimated. Consider treatment recommendations for IRIS **Stage 3** CKD in this type of patient. |
| 3 | 2.1–5 | 2.9–5 | With poor body condition, **SDMA ≥45 µg/dl** may indicate that the level of renal dysfunction has been underestimated. Consider treatment recommendations for IRIS **Stage 4 CKD** in this patient. |
| 4 | >5 | >5 | |

* The classification is based on creatinine levels, after at least two measurements in the stable patient (well hydrated, eating and drinking), preferably after 12 hours of fasting with free access to water. For sub-staging, persistent renal proteinuria and a correct blood pressure measurement (measured 2–3 times over a period of several weeks) are considered.

| | DOG UPC value | CAT UPC value |
|---|---|---|
| Not proteinuric | <0.2 | <0.2 |
| "Borderline" proteinuria | 0.2–0.5 | 0.2–0.4 |
| Proteinuric | >0.5 | >0.4 |

| | DOG/CAT Systolic AP (mmHg) | DOG/CAT Diastolic AP (mmHg) | Risk of future injury to target organ |
|---|---|---|---|
| Normal blood pressure | <150 | <95 | Minimum |
| "Borderline" hypertension | 150–159 | 95–99 | Low |
| Hypertension | 160–179 | 100–119 | Moderate |
| Hypertension severe | >180 | >120 | High |

**Figures 6.24 and 6.25.** CKD staging according to IRIS guidelines.

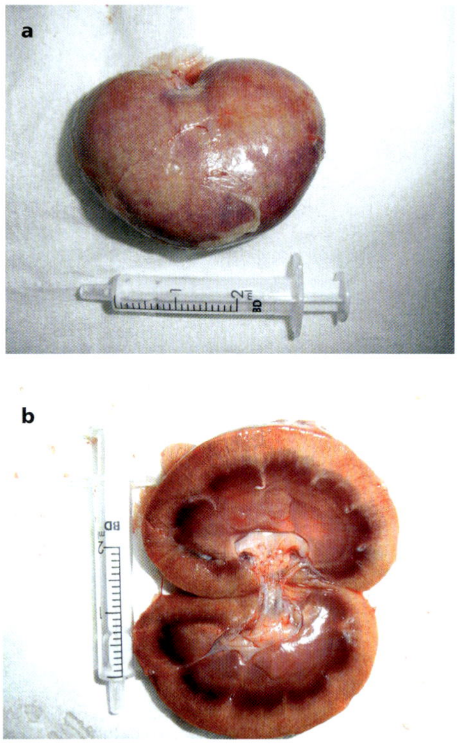

**Figure 6.26.** Kidney on post-mortem from a Shar-Pei with CKD caused by renal amyloidosis.

**Dogs**:

- Basenji (alteration in proximal tubular reabsorption)
- Shar-Pei (amyloidosis; Figure 6.26)
- Chow Chow (renal dysplasia)
- Cocker Spaniel (defect in type IV collagen similar to Alport syndrome in humans)
- Doberman Pinscher (familial glomerulopathy)
- Lhasa Apso (renal dysplasia)
- Samoyed (type IV collagen defect)
- Shih-Tzu (renal dysplasia)
- Soft-coated Wheaten Terrier (renal dysplasia with proteinuria)
- Standard Poodle (glomerular atrophy).

**Acquired causes** that can trigger chronic renal failure include:

- pyelonephritis
- neoplasia
- glomerulopathies of infectious, immune-mediated or neoplastic origins
- hypercalcaemia
- nephrolithiasis
- primary systemic hypertension.

When the primary cause is not identified, this is termed **idiopathic chronic renal failure** (Table 6.7).

Table 6.7. Causes of CKD.

| **Infectious** |
|---|
| Parasitic (leishmaniosis) |
| Bacterial (pyelonephritis, leptospirosis) |
| Viral (FIP, FeLV) |
| Fungal (*Candida*, blastomycosis) |
| **Metabolic** |
| Hypokalaemia |
| Hypercalcaemia |
| **Obstructive nephropathy** |
| Bilateral hydronephrosis (castration granuloma, transitional cell carcinoma in the bladder trigone) |
| Ureteroliths |
| Nephroliths |
| **Neoplasia** |
| Lymphoma |
| Carcinoma |
| Nephroblastoma |
| **AKD sequelae** |
| Renal ischaemia |
| **Tubulo-interstitial disorders** |
| Chronic exposure to nephrotoxins |
| Medications (NSAIDs, antibiotics, etc.) |
| **Proteinuric renal disease** |
| Amyloidosis (Figure 6.26) |
| Primary and secondary glomerulopathies |
| **Idiopathic** |
| **Familial or congenital kidney disease** |
| Amyloidosis (**dogs:** Shar-Pei, English Foxhound, Beagle; **cats:** Abyssinian, Siamese, Oriental Shorthair) |
| Renal dysplasia (several breeds) |
| Fanconi syndrome (Basenji) |
| Glomerulopathy (several breeds) |
| Multifocal renal cystadenocarcinoma (German Shepherd) |
| Polycystic kidney disease (**dogs:** Cairn Terrier, Bull terrier, West Highland White Terrier; **cats:** Persians, Himalayan) |
| Telangiectasia (Pembroke Welsh Corgi) |
| Reflux nephropathy with segmental hypoplasia (Boxer) |

## *Clinical signs*

Animals with chronic renal failure often **show clinical signs for a period of weeks to months** prior to diagnosis (Table 6.8). Thus, they present with a persistent chronic history of loss of appetite and weight, vomiting and diarrhoea, among other signs (Figure 6.27). **Urine production is usually increased** by polyuria and compensatory polydipsia, but there may also be an **oliguric or anuric presentation** in the case of an exacerbation of chronic renal failure or in terminal phases.

**Uraemia or uraemic syndrome** is the set of clinical signs that appear as a result of the loss of renal functionality, due to alteration of glomerular, tubular and endocrine functions that leads to the **retention of toxic metabolites**, changes in the volume and composition

Table 6.8. Differentiation between AKD and CKD.

| | AKD (potentially reversible) | CKD (irreversible and ± progressive) |
|---|---|---|
| **Appearance of clinical signs** | Acute | Present for at least 3 months |
| **Body condition** | Good | Weight loss, poor nutritional status and poor coat quality |
| **Anaemia** | No (may be present due to other causes) | Yes |
| **Other** | | Progressive increase in creatinine and/or persistent proteinuria for >3 months<br>Decreased renal size, renal asymmetry<br>Skeletal disorders (renal osteodystrophy due to secondary renal hyperparathyroidism) |

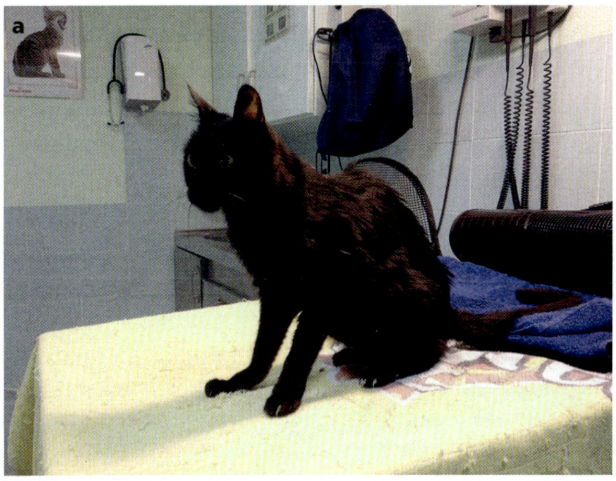

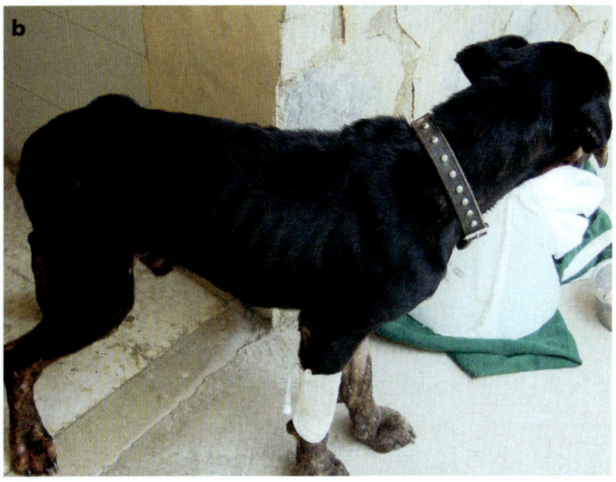

**Figure 6.27a.** Poor bodily condition in a cat with CKD; b, dog with CKD due to leishmaniosis.

of body fluids and deficiencies or excesses of certain hormones.

Clinical signs can be classified into several groups:

- **Urinary**: Polyuria, oliguria, anuria, dysuria, polyuria and haematuria.
- **Gastrointestinal**: Diarrhoea, vomiting, halitosis and ulcers.
- Caused by **systemic hypertension:**
  - ocular (acute blindness due to retinal detachment, haemorrhages)
  - **neurological** (seizures, mental depression, etc.)
  - **cardiac** (cardiac hypertrophy)
- Others: weight loss, apathy, muscle weakness, ventroflexion of the neck (in cats with hypokalaemia), oedema, ascites, signs of renal osteodystrophy and lumbar back pain (in some cases of pyelonephritis).

## Diagnosis

When presented with a patient with suspected CKD, information from the **history and physical examination** should be thoroughly reviewed. The aim is to prioritize the search for specific problems that need investigation in greater depth, to **determine the type of kidney disease present** and the **underlying cause** and to identify concomitant diseases or **complications** of CKD (such as hypertension, anaemia, secondary renal hyperparathyroidism, etc.; Table 6.9). Minimum laboratory investigations include **blood tests** (blood count and biochemistry) and **complete urine tests**.

## Treatment

Therapeutic management consists of:

- **Treatment of the primary cause**. Treatment for leishmaniosis, surgery to correct congenital disorders, extraction of uroliths, antibiotic treatment in pyelonephritis, etc.
- **Symptomatic treatment**. Treatment to control clinical signs of uraemia, restore electrolyte, vitamin and mineral changes, maintain a balanced nutrition and slow the progression of kidney injury and treat secondary complications.

In general, the following should be done:

- **Discontinue the use of potentially nephrotoxic drugs**. Those that are eliminated exclusively through the renal route should be used with caution, especially in animals at stages 3 and 4, adjusting doses and/or frequency as necessary.
- Identify and **treat any pre- or post-renal** changes.
- Rule out or treat urinary or non-urinary tract diseases that can perpetuate the kidney injury (such as

Table 6.9. Data to be collected in patients with CKD.

| In all patients |
|---|
| **Clinical history**<br>Review medications administered |
| **Thorough physical examination**<br>Including examination of eye fundus |
| **Blood test**<br>Complete blood count<br>Blood biochemistry: creatinine, urea, electrolytes (K, Cl, Na), blood gases and serum bicarbonate, calcium, phosphorus and albumin. (Others: SDMA, ALT, T4 in cat, etc.) |
| **Urinalysis**<br>USG, urine strip, urinary sediment<br>Urine culture<br>Protein/creatinine ratio |
| **Measurement of arterial blood pressure**<br>**Diagnostic imaging of the urinary tract**<br>Kidneys: determine size, shape, location and number, evaluation of renal parenchyma<br>Urinary bladder: size, shape, location<br>Presence of masses or urolithiasis in kidney, ureter, bladder or urethra |
| **In certain cases** |
| **Measurement of glomerular filtration rate**<br>**Ionised calcium and PTH**<br>**Skeletal radiography**<br>Evidence of renal osteodystrophy<br>**Carbamylated haemoglobin**<br>**Ultrasound of parathyroid glands**<br>**Testing for infectious diseases**<br>Serology, PCR, bone marrow biopsy, etc.<br>**Echocardiography (suspected bacterial endocarditis, etc.)**<br>**Renal biopsy** |

pyelonephritis, urolithiasis, systemic infectious diseases, pyometra or endocrine diseases).

- Monitor **blood pressure and proteinuria**.
- At certain times (from IRIS CKD stage 2, or earlier in patients with UPC >2), a **renal diet** can be fed, which helps control hyperparathyroidism and hyperphosphataemia, hypertension, proteinuria, hypokalaemia and azotaemia. The palatability of renal diets, although currently greatly improved, may be a problem in some inappetent patients, especially cats.

Other problems that can be resolved include the following.

### *Dehydration*

**Fluid therapy** should be administered in cases where signs of **dehydration or hypovolaemia** are detected, and there should be continuous access to water (fresh water, several water locations, fountains, etc.).

### *Systemic hypertension*

If **arterial pressure >160 mmHg** is seen persistently, or if there is evidence of **injury to target organs** (central nervous system, retina or heart), measures should be put in place in order to keep it below 160 mmHg (Tables 6.10 and 6.11).

### *Proteinuria*

Treatment of all patients with persistently **elevated UPC ratios** (dog: >0.5, cat: >0.4) with anti-proteinuric drugs is currently recommended, whilst at the same time investigating the causes of proteinuria. Animals with a borderline UPC should be strictly monitored.

### Considerations in patients with proteinuria

- Look for diseases or **concurrent conditions** that can be treated.
- Consider whether performing a **renal biopsy** is necessary to identify the underlying disease.
- **ACEIs** and renal diet. ACEIs are contraindicated in dehydrated or hypovolaemic patients, and dehydration must be corrected before these are administered.
- In dogs, **low-dose acetylsalicylic acid (1–5 mg/kg/day)** if albumin <2 g/dl (in the cat it is controversial, but can be used at doses of 1 mg/kg every 72 h).
- **Treatment monitoring** and disease progression. Creatinine and UPC ratio:
  - Stable creatinine levels and a decrease in UPC are signs of a positive response.

Table 6.10. Management of systemic hypertension.

| | Dog | Cat |
|---|---|---|
| **1.** | Reduce sodium intake: low-salt renal diet (there is no evidence of its effectiveness as a sole measure; it should be introduced progressively and together with the administration of anti-hypertensives) | Reduce sodium intake: low-salt renal diet (there is no evidence of its effectiveness as a sole measure; it should be introduced progressively and together with the administration of anti-hypertensives) |
| **2.** | Start ACEI at standard doses (or angiotensin receptor blockers [ARB]) | Start CCB (amlodipine) treatment |
| **3.** | Double the dose of ACEI | Increase the dose of amlodipine up to 0.5 mg/kg/day |
| **4.** | Combine ACEI with calcium channel blockers (CCB) | Combine CCB with ACEI, or BRA |
| **5.** | Combine ACEI, CCB and hydralazine | |

Table 6.11. Anti-hypertensive drugs available and recommended oral doses.

| Anti-hypertensive drugs | | Oral doses used |
|---|---|---|
| **Angiotensin-converting enzyme inhibitors (ACE inhibitors)** | Benazepril | D: 0.5–2.0 mg/kg/12 h C: 0.5–2.0 mg/kg/24 h |
| | Enalapril | D: 0.5–2.0 mg/kg/12 h C: 0.5–2.0 mg/kg/24 h |
| | Ramipril/Imidapril | D/C: 0.25–1.0 mg/kg/24 h |
| **Angiotensin receptor blockers** | Losartan | D/C: 0.25–1.0 mg/kg/24 h D: 0.5–1.0 mg/kg/24 h |
| | Irbesartan | D: 1–5 mg/kg/12–24 h |
| **Calcium channel blockers** | Amlodipine | D/C: 0.1–0.75 mg/kg/24 h |
| **β-blockers** | Atenolol | D: 0.25–1.0 mg/kg/12 h or 6.25–12.5 mg/12 h |
| **Aldosterone antagonists** | Spironolactone | D/C: 1.0–2.0 mg/kg/12–24 h |
| **α-Blockers** | Prazosin | D: 0.5–2.0 mg/kg/8–12 h C: 0.25–0.5 mg/cat/24 h |
| | Phenoxybenzamine | D: 0.25 mg/kg/8–12 h or 0.5 mg/kg/24 h |
| **Direct vasodilators** | Hydralazine | C: 2.5 mg/8–12 h or 5 mg/24 h |
| | Acepromazine | D: 0.5–2.0 mg/kg/12 h (start with a dose at the lower end of the range) C: 2.5 mg/12–24 h |
| **Diuretics: thiazides** | Hydrochlorothiazide | D/C: 0.5–2.0 mg/kg/8 h |
| **Loop diuretics** | Furosemide | D/C: 2–4 mg/kg/12–24 h D/C: 1–4 mg/kg/8–24 h |

- Progressive increases in creatinine or UPC ratio indicate that the disease is progressing.

### *Phosphorus intake*

There is evidence that a **reduction in phosphorus intake is beneficial** for CKD patients. The aim is to maintain **serum levels at 2.7–4.6 mg/dl**, although in more advanced stages values below 5–6 mg/dl are acceptable since it is difficult to obtain values in the previous ideal range.

Factors for the reduction of serum phosphorus levels:

1. Dietary **restriction of phosphorus**: Feed a renal diet.
2. If hyperphosphataemia persists, **enteric phosphorus chelates** (e.g. aluminium hydroxide, aluminium carbonate, calcium carbonate or calcium acetate) can be added at progressive doses **until the desired effect** is achieved. The dose limits are marked by toxicity according to the chosen drug. **Calcium and phosphorus levels should be monitored** every 4–6 weeks until they stabilize, and then at least every 12 weeks.
3. **Careful use of calcitriol** (1.5–3.5 ng/kg) in dogs with stage 3 or 4 CKD may prolong survival if phosphorus is controlled and ionic calcium and PTH levels are monitored. There is currently no evidence of its effectiveness in the cat.

### *Metabolic acidosis*

Once the condition has been stabilized with a renal diet, if **serum bicarbonate or total carbon dioxide levels remain <16 mmol/l in the cat or <18 mmol/l in the dog**, then the use or oral sodium bicarbonate or potassium citrate can be considered. The aim is to maintain the former value at 16–24 mmol/l (cat) or 18–24 mmol/l (dog).

### *Anaemia*

If anaemia is affecting the patient's quality of life (generally **haematocrit <20%**), treatment with erythropoietin (EPO) should be considered. Human recombinant EPO can be used, although it is not approved for veterinary use, or, preferably, **darbepoetin, which is less antigenic**.

### *Vomiting, nausea, inappetence*

In patients with these signs, the use of **antacids** (ranitidine, famotidine, omeprazole) or **anti-emetics** (metoclopramide, maropitant, ondansetron, etc.) should be considered. It should be noted that in cats the presence of uraemic gastropathy has not been proven, and it is probable that digestive signs are more likely to be the consequence of circulating uraemic toxins with a central effect, so the use of antacids is controversial.

### *Hypokalaemia*

**Hypokalaemia is more frequent in cats** (Figure 6.28) and is identified in 20–30% of cats with CKD, especially those that are hypertensive. Potassium is supplemented through **dietary intake** (commercial renal diets for cats are higher in potassium) or with **oral supplements** (potassium gluconate 2–6 mEq/cat/day, divided into 2–3 doses; potassium citrate 40–60 mg/kg/day, divided into 2–3 doses).

## *Prognosis*

Before giving a prognosis, factors such as severity of clinical signs, uraemic complications, the patient's age and the cause of primary disease (amongst other

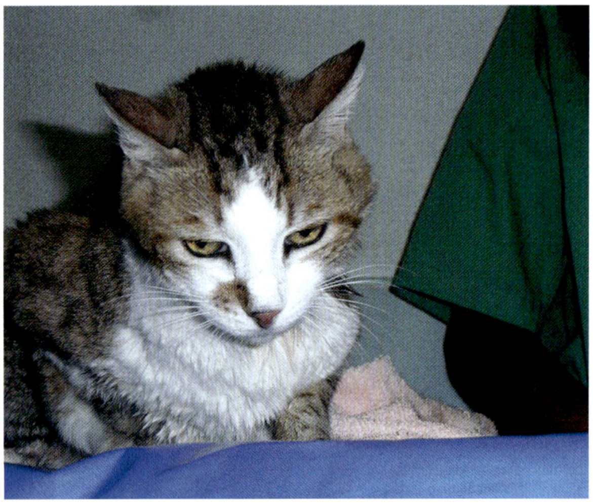

**Figure 6.28.** Cat with cervical ventroflexion due to hypokalaemia.

factors) should be taken into consideration. The prognosis should be based on the animal's clinical condition, the **speed of progression** of renal dysfunction, the **response to treatment**, the **cause** of the underlying kidney disease and **other risk factors**.

The **IRIS classification system** can be useful for providing a prognosis: in the more advanced stages, survival rates are lower. The **level of proteinuria** is an important prognostic factor.

**Cats with CKD survive longer than dogs** with CKD. It is possible that this difference can be explained by the higher prevalence of proteinuric disease and poorer control of arterial hypertension in the dog. However, disease in dogs with CKD due to congenital or familial nephropathies usually progresses more slowly than that in dogs with acquired kidney disease.

## Glomerular disease

### *Epidemiology*

**Glomerular diseases are more frequent in dogs** than in cats, with a prevalence around 43–90% in all dogs with CKD, 1.5% of which visited a veterinary practice.

### *Aetiopathogenesis*

Glomerular disease can present with different renal syndromes:

- CKD
- AKD
- nephrotic syndrome
- isolated proteinuria.

**The presence of proteinuria is a key factor for the diagnosis of glomerular disease**. Proteinuria is a marker of severity of kidney disease and is of prognostic value. It has also been suggested that proteinuria itself can be harmful and contributes to the progression of renal insufficiency. This is because the proximal tubular cells reabsorb proteins from the glomerular filtrate which, when present in excessive amounts, can accumulate in tubular cell lysosomes causing rupture of lysosomes and cell lesions. In addition, glomerular lesions allow the entry of substances into the renal tubules that can be reabsorbed and damage tubular cells (complement, lipoproteins, etc.). Therefore, it is possible that proteinuria leads to more severe renal lesions. An important question that remains to be answered is whether reduction in proteinuria definitely improves the prognosis in cases of chronic renal failure.

**Nephrotic syndrome is a consequence of severe proteinuria**. This results in the accumulation of fluid and tissue oedema, and is defined by the presence of proteinuria, hypalbuminaemia, hypercholesterolaemia and oedema or ascites.

The **glomerular filtration barrier** consists of a fenestrated endothelium, a basement membrane and visceral epithelium (podocytes) (Figure 6.29). All these components **determine the filtration selectivity** of the said barrier, limiting the passage of high-molecular-weight substances (60–70,000 Daltons) and negatively charged substances (which are repelled, such as proteins). Albumin has a molecular weight of 69 Daltons and a negative charge, and therefore it **does not usually appear in urine**. Low-molecular-weight proteins are filtered by the glomerulus but are reabsorbed into the proximal tubules. A small amount of protein in urine (30 mg/kg/day) in dogs and cats is considered normal.

**Angiotensin II** has an important role in the pathophysiology of proteinuric kidney disease. It is produced in the vascular endothelium due to the action of ACT, it has receptors in the kidney and exerts multiple actions in this organ. For example, angiotensin II produces **constriction of the efferent arterioles**

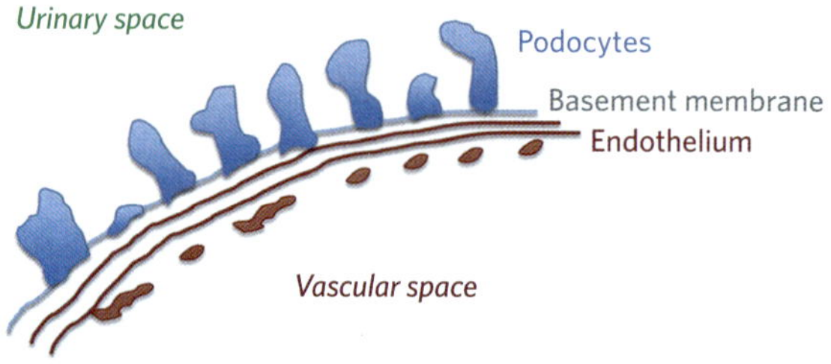


**Figure 6.29.** Diagram showing the glomerular filtration barrier.

thus **increasing intraglomerular pressure**. It also acts as a growth factor for vascular and tubular structures and **increases the production of vasoactive substances**.

Glomerular lesions are caused by:

- The formation or **deposition of immune complexes in the glomerulus** (e.g. membranous nephropathy, membranoproliferative glomerulonephritis, mesangioproliferative glomerulonephritis).
- **Systemic factors** that damage the glomerulus (amyloidosis, glomerulosclerosis, etc.).

Once the **glomerulus is damaged**, other processes contribute to the progression of glomerular disease such as activation of complement and coagulation, infiltration with inflammatory cells and the synthesis of growth factors. There are also hereditary nephropathies.

When faced with a patient with glomerulopathy, it is essential to **establish whether this is secondary** to a neoplastic, infectious or inflammatory systemic disease that may cause renal injury. Often **proteinuria is the first clinical sign of hidden systemic diseases**. It is important to evaluate the pet's **travel history** for exposure to infectious agents and the history of **medications** administered, since certain drugs are associated with the development of glomerular lesions (Table 6.12).

In 2013 the IRIS association and several authors published consensus guidelines for the diagnosis and management of glomerular disease, which are essential to understanding these pathologies.

Table 6.12. Conditions that can cause glomerular damage.

| Conditions associated with glomerular disease | |
|---|---|
| **Neoplasia**<br>Leukaemia, lymphoma, mastocytosis, primary erythrocytosis, systemic histiocytosis, others | |
| **Infectious** | |
| **Bacteria/Rickettsia**<br>Borreliosis, bartonellosis, brucellosis, ehrlichiosis, endocarditis, pyelonephritis, pyometra, pyoderma, chronic bacterial infections, polyarthritis due to Mycoplasmas, etc. | **Viruses**<br>Canine adenovirus type I, IVF, FeLV, FIP |
| **Protozoa**<br>*Babesia* spp., *Theileria* spp., leishmaniosis, hepatozoonosis | **Parasites**<br>Dirofilariasis |
| **Fungi** (blastomycosis, coccidiodomycosis) | |
| **Inflammatory**<br>Chronic dermatitis, IBD, pancreatitis, cholangiohepatitis, polyarthritis, periodontal disease, immune-mediated disease (SLE) | |
| **Miscellaneous**<br>Corticosteroids, trimethoprim-sulpha, hyperlipidaemia, mercury toxicity, acromegaly, C3 deficiency, Collie cyclic haematopoiesis, excessive vaccination, idiopathic | |

## Clinical signs

The variable clinical signs include:

- **Asymptomatic** (with proteinuria detected during a routine check-up).
- Associated with **underlying disease**.
- **Uraemia** in patients with CKD (anorexia, weight loss, polyuria/polydipsia, vomiting etc.).
- **Nephrotic syndrome**.
- Due to **thromboembolism** (respiratory difficulty due to pulmonary thromboembolism, lameness due to aortic thromboembolism etc.).
- **Sudden blindness** or other ocular changes due to the presence of **arterial hypertension**.

## Diagnosis

The **patient's signalment** should be taken into account, remembering that certain breeds have a predisposition to selected glomerulopathies (Table 6.7). Table 6.13 lists diagnostic tests for glomerular disease.

The objectives of the diagnostic protocol are:

- **Identify underlying diseases** or conditions that may be responsible for glomerular lesions (infectious, inflammatory, immune-mediated, vascular, neoplastic, endocrine, toxic or genetic).
- Detect and **assess the severity of the sequelae** of glomerular disease (hypertension, hypalbuminaemia, azotaemia, hypercoagulability, water balance, etc.) and determine whether they need medical treatment.
- Define **pathological renal changes** to obtain more accurate information about diagnosis, prognosis and therapeutic options.

**Hypoalbuminaemia** (with normal globulin concentrations) is common in animals with glomerular disease. Depending on the severity and extent of kidney disease, some will also have **azotaemia**. **Hypercholesterolaemia** is also frequent in animals with glomerular disease, due to the increase in lipoprotein synthesis and alterations in lipid metabolism.

Table 6.13. Diagnostic tests to be performed in patients where glomerular disease is suspected.

| In all patients |
|---|
| **Complete clinical history** |
| Signalment, history of similar problems in genetically related pets, environment, travel history, drugs, etc. |
| **Thorough physical examination** |
| Including body condition score, rectal and retinal examinations |
| **Measurement of arterial blood pressure** |
| **Blood and urine tests** |
| Complete blood count |
| Biochemistry |
| Urinalysis including urine sediment examination |
| UPC ratio |
| Urinary culture (in cases of microscopic pyuria, haematuria, bacteriuria, USG <1025, azotaemia, suspected hyperadrenocorticism, diabetes, etc.) |
| If there is an endemic infectious disease in the area, perform tests to rule it out |
| Storage of samples for possible future tests (whole blood in EDTA, serum, urine) is recommended |
| **In patients with severe proteinuria (>3.5), progressive proteinuria, hypertension, hypo-albuminaemia and/or azotaemia** |
| **Complete abdominal ultrasound** |
| **Thoracic** radiography |
| More extensive evaluation of **infectious diseases** |
| If there is hypertension |
| To assess non-renal causes of hypertension (hyperadrenocorticism, pheochromocytoma, hyperaldosteronism, drugs, fluid or salt overload, etc.) |
| Echocardiography to assess the presence of concentric hypertrophy of the left ventricle |
| If there is hypo-albuminaemia and/or azotaemia |
| Rule out neoplasia |
| Rule out other causes of hypo-albuminaemia |
| Characterize azotaemia as non-renal, AKD, CKD or exacerbation of CKD and classify according to the appropriate IRIS scheme |
| **In cases of severe proteinuria (UPC >3.5), which progresses despite treatment, in which immunosuppressive therapy has been administered or the option is contemplated, with CKD in the initial stages** |
| Renal biopsy |

**Nephrotic syndrome is pathognomonic of glomerular** disease, but only in 15% of animals with glomerular disease, and is characterized by a combination of:

- hypoalbuminaemia
- proteinuria
- hypercholesterolaemia
- oedema.

These animals may **retain the ability to concentrate urine** if the renal tubules are not affected, so they have **azotaemia and concentrated urine** (USG >1035), giving the false **impression that there is pre-renal azotaemia**. The urine sediment may contain cylinders (usually hyaline) and red blood cells.

### *Assessment of proteinuria*

A key point for **the diagnosis of a glomerular disease is the presence of proteinuria**. Proteinuria is not only a diagnostic marker of kidney disease, but also a **negative prognostic marker** (Figure 6.30).

To **evaluate proteinuria**, qualitative or semi-quantitative techniques are used initially, such as **urine test strips** (or the sulpha-salicylic acid test), and then more accurately **quantified with the UPC ratio.**

**USG should be taken into account** when evaluating proteinuria with test strips:

- With high protein values a UPC should be performed.
- If there are traces of protein, quantification is recommended depending on USG:
  - USG <1.012, UPC should be measured.
  - USG >1.012, the majority of these patients are not proteinuric (according to research published).

Numerous studies demonstrate **UPC can be evaluated** in samples taken during **spontaneous micturition**, provided no active sediment is observed.

It is important to confirm that proteinuria is of renal origin (Figure 6.30) and persists with time. Given the large temporary variation that may exist, **repetition of UPC** measurement at least twice on different days is recommended.

When the **UPC is only mildly elevated** it is best to confirm that there is persistent renal proteinuria (Table 6.14) and before determining that intrinsic glomerular disease is present. In patients with more marked proteinuria, obtain an average estimate of UPC with repeat sampling.

## *Treatment*

### *Non-specific therapy or standard treatment*

Regardless of the histological diagnosis, the following is recommended in all patients:

- **Monitor and treat** neoplastic, infectious and/or inflammatory diseases (which may appear long after detection of proteinuria).

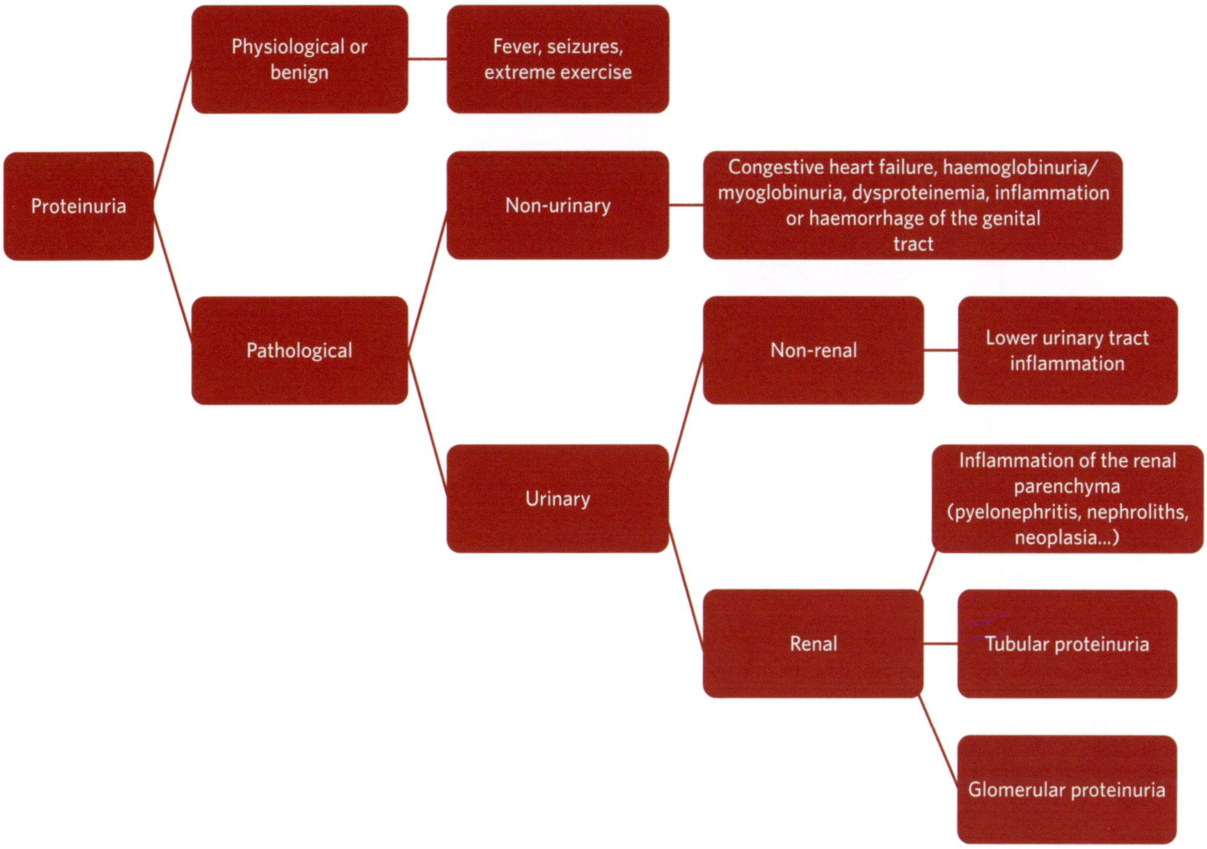


**Figure 6.30.** Origins of proteinuria.

Table 6.14. Implications of persistent renal proteinuria.

| | DOG | CAT |
|---|---|---|
| **UPC** | >2: glomerular disease | >1: uncommon |
| **Negative prognosis** | CKD + initial UPC >1 | CKD + progressive increase in UPC<br>In non-azotaemic cats, the greater the proteinuria the greater the risk of mortality from other causes |
| **Persistent renal proteinuria** | Yes | Yes |
| **UPC 2–3 times every 2–3 weeks** | UPC >0.5 | UPC >0.4 |

- **Address signs of uraemia** and other complications of kidney disease.
- Establish treatments for **reduction of proteinuria**.

Reduction of proteinuria is an important objective in the treatment of these diseases. There is evidence that **ACEIs reduce blood pressure and proteinuria and may slow the progression of kidney disease**. ACEIs reduce proteinuria through different mechanisms:

- Reducing the resistance of the efferent arterioles of the glomerulus.
- Reducing the size of the pores in the glomerular endothelium.
- Stopping proliferation of interstitial tissue.
- Inhibiting degradation of bradykinin, which dilates the afferent glomerular arterioles and increases the formation of nitric oxide and prostacyclin (both vasodilators).

Various drugs are available for the control of proteinuria that act on the renin–angiotensin–aldosterone axis (Figure 6.31).

Whenever **UPC >0.5 is recorded continuously, treatment with ACEI drugs is recommended** in order to achieve UPC <0.5 or at least 50% without renal function worsening. At the same time, a **protein-restricted diet should be fed**, supplemented with **omega-3 fatty acids** and with a low sodium content.

Patients with glomerular disease are at **increased risk of thromboembolism**, which is why thromboprophylactic measures such as the administration of **low-dose aspirin (1–5 mg/kg/day)** or **clopidogrel** are recommended (although there is no evidence that it is more effective than aspirin).

**Control of hypertension** is essential, with an individualized treatment for the patient and any concurrent

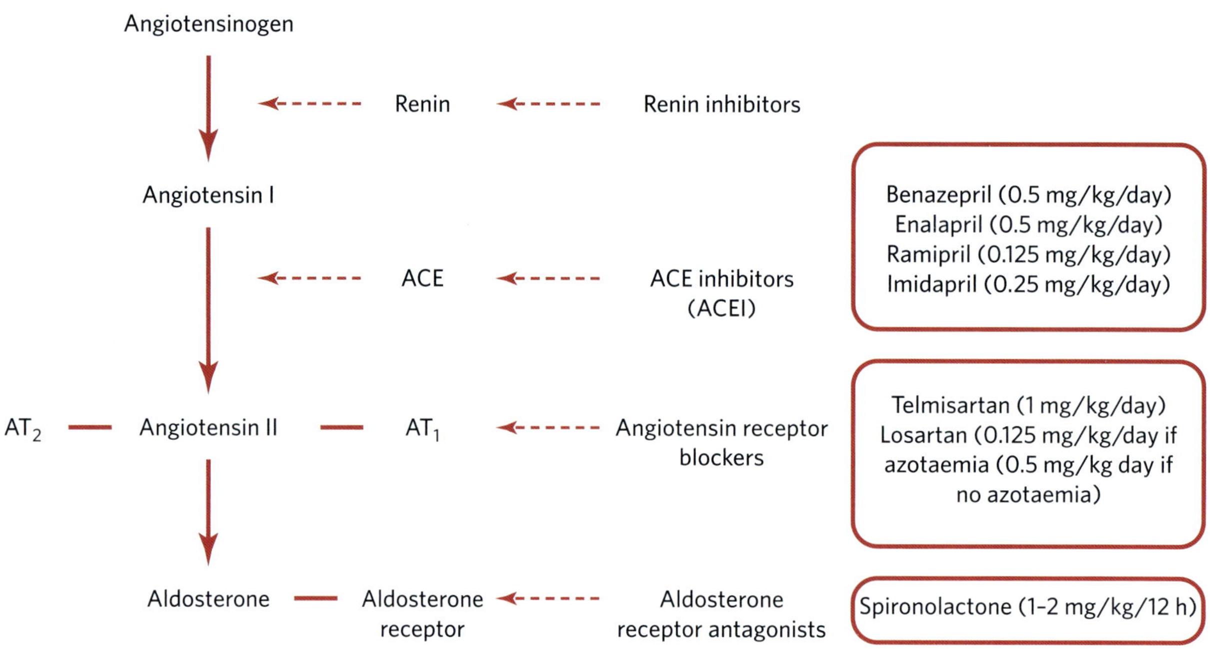


**Figure 6.31.** Renin–angiotensin–aldosterone system and mechanism of action of medications used to control proteinuria.

conditions. This is done through the use of **ACEIs alone or in combination with calcium blockers or angiotensin receptor blockers**.

In animals with **nephrotic syndrome**, administration of **diuretics should be limited** to situations in which the function of an organ is critically compromised (ascites or pleural effusion that makes breathing difficult), with the following medications being first choice:

- **Furosemide** in cases of pulmonary oedema.
- **Spironolactone** in cases of pleural and/or abdominal effusion.

**Fluid therapy should be administered only if necessary and with great caution**, since these patients are predisposed to volume overload. In some cases, when haemodynamic dysfunction has not been corrected with crystalloids only, the use of colloids should be considered.

### *Immunosuppressive therapy*

It is advisable to empirically **administer immune suppressants** (provided there are no contraindications) in dogs with severe, persistent and progressive glomerular disease in which there is **evidence of an active immune-mediated pathogenesis on renal biopsy**. In general, immunosuppressive therapy is recommended in cases of membranous glomerulopathy and, although there are fewer specific recommendations in these cases, also in patients with membranoproliferative or mesangioproliferative glomerulonephritis in which active deposits of immune complexes in the renal tissue are observed by electron microscopy or immunofluorescence.

Immunosuppressive drugs such as **mycophenolate, chlorambucil, cyclophosphamide, azathioprine and prednisone** are recommended.

The administration of immunosuppressants can be considered even without having a histopathological diagnosis in patients without a response to standard treatment, with progressive azotaemia and severe hypoalbuminaemia, but **these should not be used if proteinuria is of unknown origin**, if there are contraindications or if it is likely to be a familiar glomerulopathy or amyloidosis.

## *Prognosis*

The **prognosis is very variable** and depends on the underlying disease and the type of glomerular lesion. In some patients a spontaneous remission may be observed, while in others the stable disease can be maintained for months to years or progress to CKD more or less rapidly. **Negative prognostic factors** include:

- azotaemia
- severe proteinuria
- hypertension
- nephrotic syndrome.

Given the low frequency of glomerular disease in the cat, there is little information about its management, treatment and progression.

## Lower urinary tract pathologies

### General considerations

Animals with lower urinary tract diseases (LUTD) usually present with:

- Signs of inflammation and irritation of the bladder and/or urethra (such as dysuria, polyuria or stranguria).
- Changes in urine colour (due to haematuria).
- Urinary incontinence or inability to completely empty the bladder.

In cases of ascending infections of the ureters, the renal pelvis and parenchyma, the problem **may spread to the upper urinary tract**. In some patients with **urinary tract rupture**, signs of uraemia (anorexia, lethargy, diarrhoea, vomiting) and accumulation of fluid in the abdomen may be observed.

It should be noted that in many cases the **clinical signs are the same regardless of the cause** (infection, urolithiasis, neoplasms, etc.), so it is important to perform the appropriate tests to reach a diagnosis before starting treatment.

The minimum **initial assessment** should include:

- detailed clinical history
- thorough physical examination
- urinalysis.

And, depending on the situation:

- urine culture
- blood tests
- urogenital tract imaging techniques (radiography, ultrasound, cystoscopy, tomography, etc.).

The following should be asked when taking the clinical history:

- Frequency and volume of urine.
- Amount of water ingested daily.
- Urine colour.
- Presence of blood in the urine or independent of urination.
- Signs of discomfort or difficulty urinating.

In the case of incontinence:

- How long has it been present for?
- When does it occur (when the animal is awake, asleep, continuously, etc.)?

The **physical exam** should emphasize:

- Careful abdominal palpation.
- Rectal palpation.
- Examination of external genitalia.
- Neurological examination (hind limbs and perineal region).

## Urolithiasis

### Definition

**Uroliths are solid polycrystalline concretions** that are composed, in most cases, of substances found normally in urine, which for different reasons, concentrate and solidify forming fragments of variable size (Figure 6.32).

### Aetiopathogenesis

Calculi formation is the **consequence of the interaction of multiple organic abnormalities**, which should be identified to establish a correct long-term management of the problem (although this is not always possible).

- Some of these conditions **can be corrected**, such as the formation of struvite uroliths due to urinary infections.
- Others can be **identified but not corrected**, such as hyperuricosuria present in Dalmatians which is responsible for ammonium urate urolithiasis.
- With others the exact cause that leads to urolithiasis is **unknown**, as occurs with calcium oxalate urolithiasis in the Miniature Schnauzer.

### Epidemiology

In practice **urolithiasis is common**: it affects 1.5–3% of the canine population and accounts for 15–23% of cases of feline lower urinary tract pathologies (which affect 1% of the feline population).

The most frequent minerals are those which form **struvite and calcium oxalate**, but purines, cystine, silica and those associated with drug use (sulphonamides, ciprofloxacin, allopurinol, etc.) can also be found.

### Clinical signs

Clinical signs include **dysuria, stranguria, polyuria and/or haematuria**. There may also be obstructive anuria. Nephroliths/ureteroliths can cause acute renal

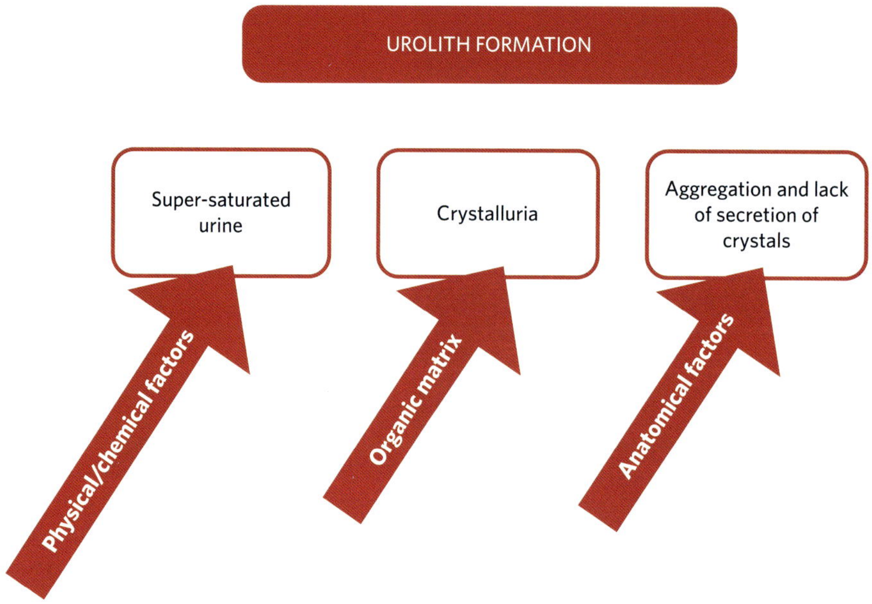


**Figure 6.32.** Factors that favour the formation of calculi. In some animals, over-saturation of normal crystals can be seen in urine, in addition to the presence of the organic matrix which may be abnormal in urine and the lack of inhibitors or anatomical factors that promote the aggregation of these crystals.

failure and **systemic symptoms**. Urethral obstruction can lead to **bladder atony or even rupture and peritonitis**.

The typical locations for obstruction are:

- The ischial arch and the penile bone, due to the low distention capacity of the urethra in this area in male dogs.
- In cats, the penile urethra.

## Diagnosis

Recommended initial tests include imaging techniques and urinalysis (Figure 6.33) in order to determine the location, size and type of calculi.

### Imaging techniques

Abdominal radiography is useful for detecting radiopaque calculi (Figure 6.34). It can be complemented with ultrasound and/or double-contrast cystography to detect radiolucent uroliths also.

Factors that can help predict the nature of calculi:

- radiographic density
- radiographic contour.

### Urinalysis

Urinalysis is an essential part of the diagnostic evaluation.

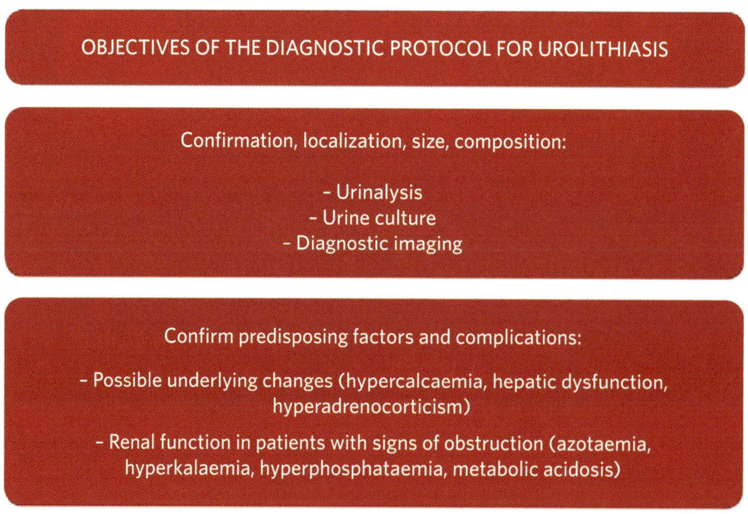


**Figure 6.33.** Diagnostic protocol in patients with urolithiasis.

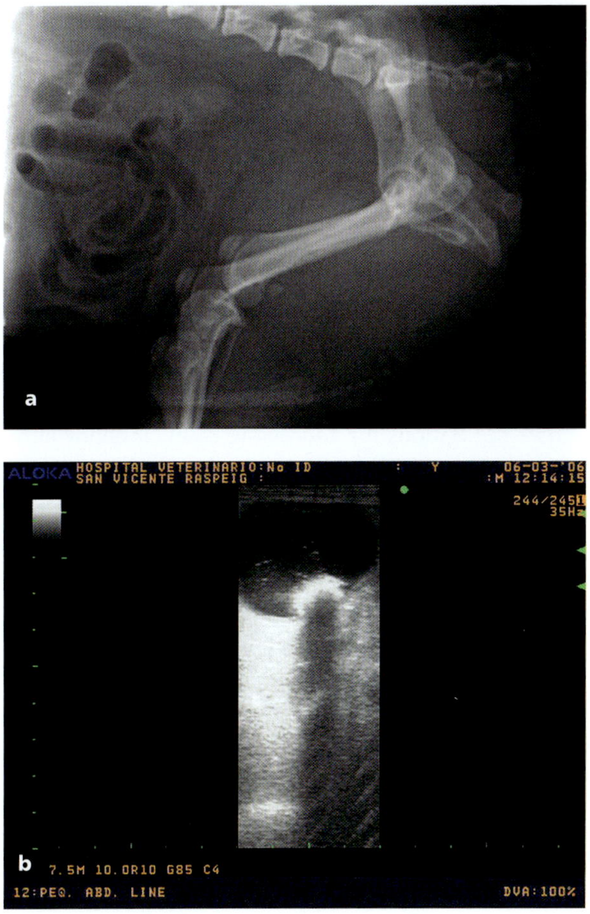


**Figure 6.34.** Urolithiasis in the penile urethra (a) and bladder (b) of a dog.

## Crystalluria

Crystalluria is an important finding. Although it suggests that there is crystalline super-saturation, the **presence of crystals in the urine is not synonymous with urolithiasis**. On the other hand, some patients with urolithiasis do not have crystalluria.

**Freshly collected urine** should be evaluated to avoid false positives due to crystal formation as a result of temperature changes. The type of crystals can be indicative in predicting the type of urolith (Figure 6.35), although factors such as recent dietary changes, presence of urine infection, etc. may also be influential.

Crystalluria in not synonymous with urolithiasis:

- It can occur without symptoms.
- Per se, it is not a cause of cystitis.
- It indicates that there is a risk of urolithiasis.
- It indicates the type of urolith, if they present.
- Crystalluria *in vitro*.

## Urinary specific gravity and pH

- Urinary specific gravity and pH help in evaluating the chemical characteristics of urine that promote urolith formation and hence **suggest the type of calculi** present:
  - Very concentrated urine leads to an increased concentration of urolith precursors.
- With regard to pH, **uroliths most commonly** occurring:
  - Calcium oxalate, purines and cystine in acidic urine (pH <7.0).
  - **Struvite in alkaline** urine (pH >7.0).

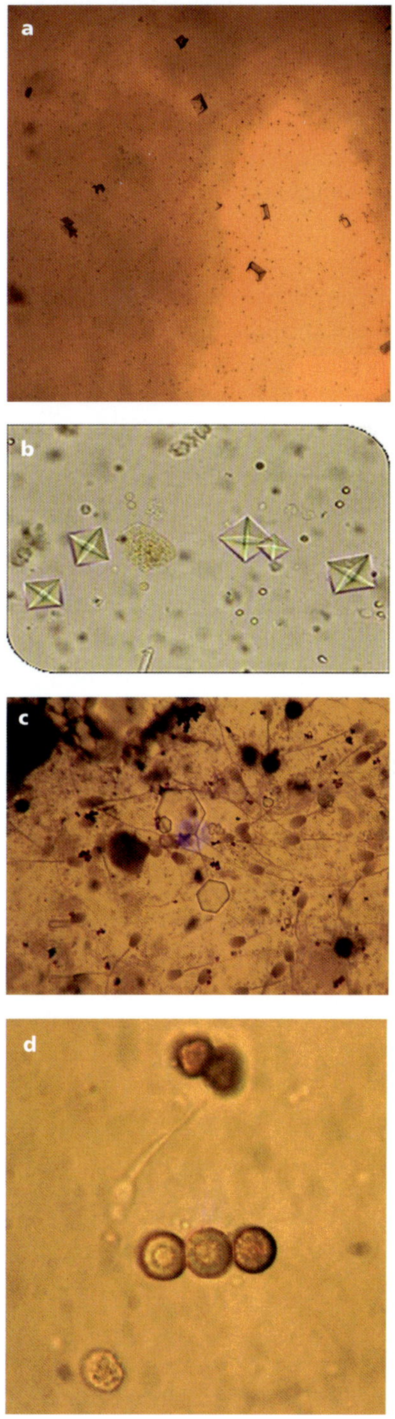


**Figures 6.35.** Images of different types of crystals found in urine sediment: struvite (a), cystine (b), calcium oxalate (c), xanthine (d).

### Urine culture and antibiogram

Urine culture and antibiogram are indicated because patients with urolithiasis may present with infections as a secondary complication, or an infection may be the cause of urolithiasis (e.g. infection-induced struvite). Urolithiasis contributes to the development of infection through:

- Mucosal injury due to calculi.
- Incomplete emptying of the bladder.
- Entrapment of microorganisms in calculi.

### *Blood tests*

Blood tests should be performed to detect underlying diseases and/or monitor renal function, especially if there is obstruction.

### *Identification of urolith composition*

**Uroliths** removed surgically, by other types of intervention or expelled naturally **should be analysed** even in cases of recurrence, since the composition may vary from one episode to another. However, even before uroliths are available for analysis, a prediction can be made as to their composition (Table 6.15). Many **uroliths are of mixed composition** and some are formed by layers of a different composition around a protein matrix. When urine is saturated with crystals they start to accumulate around the nidus, which is the central part and usually forms the main portion of the urolith on which the layers are deposited.

## *Treatment*

The following section focuses on the management of **urolithiasis of the lower urinary tract**. Table 6.16 shows the options for addressing cases of nephrolithiasis and ureterolithiasis.

Uroliths in the lower urinary tract are often associated with urethral obstruction. In these cases, an urgent approach is required, both to **relieve the obstruction** and to correct any **secondary metabolic imbalances** (azotaemia, hyperkalaemia, metabolic acidosis, dehydration) as soon as possible. In recurring cases of obstruction, perineal (cat) or scrotal (dog) urethrostomy can be considered, but these procedures are associated with an increased risk of urinary infections.

Table 6.15. Characteristics of the most frequent uroliths.

| Mineral type | Urine pH | Appearance of crystals | Urine culture | Radiographic density | Radiographic contours |
|---|---|---|---|---|---|
| **Struvite (magnesium ammonium phosphate)** | Neutral to alkaline | Colourless coffin-lid shape | Urease-positive bacteria (*Staphylococcus* spp. and *Proteus* spp.) Negative in the Cocker Spaniel | From moderately to notably radiopaque. Larger-sized uroliths have a more radio-dense impression | Can be smooth or spiculated and can take the shape of the bladder or urethra. If there are multiple stones in contact, pyramidal shapes are common |
| **Calcium oxalate** | Acid to neutral | Birefringent and colourless. Two octahedral shapes or in an envelope (dihydrate) and in dumbbell shape (monohydrate form) | Negative unless secondary infection with habitual uropathogens | Moderately to notably radiopaque | Rugged or smooth. Uroliths with sharp projections or blackberry shapes |
| **Urate** | Acid to neutral | Spiculated amorphous or spherical shapes with a yellow–brown hue | Negative unless secondary infection with habitual uropathogens | Radiolucent to slightly radiopaque | Multiple smooth, rounded or ovoid |
| **Cystine** | Acid to neutral | Flat, colourless hexagonal plaques | Negative unless secondary infection with habitual uropathogens | Slightly to moderately radiopaque | Multiple oval and smooth uroliths. If they settle in the kidney, they may look like a deer's antler |
| **Silica** | Acid to neutral | None | Negative unless secondary infection with habitual uropathogens | Moderately radiopaque | Round or ovoid-edged appearance |

Table 6.16. Approach to urolithiasis of the upper urinary tract.

| | Treatment options | Observations |
|---|---|---|
| **Nephrolithiasis** | Monitoring (inactive calculi) | If not associated with urinary obstruction or clinical signs, they should simply be monitored |
| | Surgery | If there is a risk of migration through the ureter |
| | Medical dissolution | Indications for nephrostomy: obstruction, recurrent infection, increase in renal size, reduced renal function |
| | Extracorporeal lithotripsy | |
| | Medical treatment to try to move the ureterolith to the bladder: fluid therapy, analgesia, mannitol, prazosin, amitriptyline, tamsulosin | Consider whether there is partial or complete obstruction |
| **Ureterolithiasis** | Surgery | Medical dissolution is difficult because there is not continuous contact of the stone with urine |
| | Interventional techniques (stents, lithotripsy, urethroscopy etc.) | |

## *Medical dissolution*

Fundamentally the efficacy of medical dissolution depends on:

- **Location**. Dissolution may be possible when uroliths reside in the bladder. Success depends on continuously surrounding the uroliths with hypo-satured urine that has been modified by diet and/or medications. This is not possible for uroliths in the urethra.
- **Type of calculi**. Struvite, urate and cystine are examples of uroliths composed of minerals amenable to dissolution.

The following are necessary in order to attempt dissolution of a urolith:

- **Reduce calculogenic substances** in urine.
- **Increase the solubility** of calculogenic components by changing the pH.
- **Increase the volume of urine** (through wet diets, improved access to water, etc.).

## *Surgical removal*

Through cystotomy, urethrotomy or urethrostomy (Figures 6.36 and 6.37).

It is important to perform imaging after surgery, to verify that no calculi remain. Studies show that, even in the hands of expert surgeons, stones were observed in 20% of cases post-cystotomy.

## *Removal with minimally invasive techniques*

If uroliths are small, **anterograde hydropropulsion** can be attempted. This technique is contraindicated if there is urethral obstruction. Currently, some centres perform extraction techniques with the help of cystoscopy, such as cystoscopy-assisted mini-laparotomy.

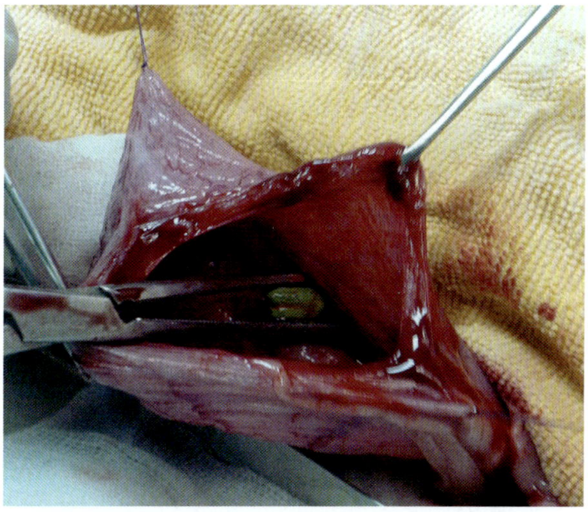

Figure 6.36. Extraction of a xanthine urolith via cystotomy in a dog.

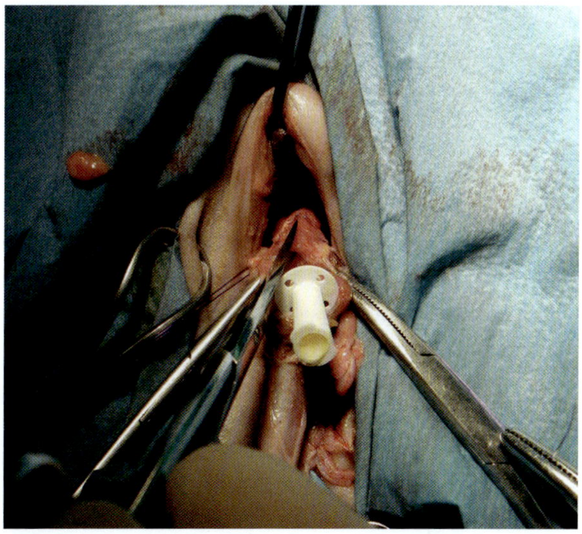

Figure 6.37. Urethrostomy in a cat with a urethral obstruction due to urolithiasis.

## Struvite urolithiasis (magnesium ammonium phosphate)

### Epidemiology

Struvite urolithiasis occurs **more frequently in females** than in males, due to an association with **bacterial infection**.

### Aetiopathogenesis

In dogs, these uroliths are formed primarily as a result of urinary infections caused by urease-producing microorganisms (*Proteus*, *Staphylococcus*, *Pseudomonas* and *Klebsiella*). Other risk factors, apart from urinary infections, include breed, urine concentration and pH, which can make the crystals more or less soluble (in which case, acidification of urine should be attempted for dissolution). In **cats, 95% of struvite uroliths are sterile** and not associated with urinary infection.

### Treatment

Medical dissolution can be achieved through **diet** and the administration of an **antibiotic** (if associated with infection) based on culture and antibiogram. The diets used have **reduced amounts of protein, phosphorus and magnesium**, in addition to a **urine acidifier**, and may be supplemented with sodium to favour diuresis. The administration of antibiotics should continue until the urolith is completely dissolved, since the bacteria can be encapsulated in the urolith and released as it dissolves.

Average dissolution time:

- Dog: about 3 months.
- Cat, with sterile struvite: about 36 days.

### Prophylaxis

Feeding a special diet in cases of struvite associated with infection is not necessary as a preventative measure, but rather the **adequate approach to urinary infection to prevent recurrence** (control of predisposing factors, diagnosis and adequate treatment of the infection, etc.). A struvite diet does not prevent the recurrence of urine infections and, therefore, urolithiasis.

In cases of **sterile struvite urolithiasis**, a preventative diet is indicated and aims to:

- Reduce urine pH to <6.8.
- Increase the volume of urine.
- Reduce the excretion of magnesium, ammonium and phosphorus.

## Calcium oxalate urolithiasis

### Aetiopathogenesis

**Calcium oxalate uroliths** (Figures 6.38 and 6.39) are among the **most frequent in dogs and cats** (Table 6.17).

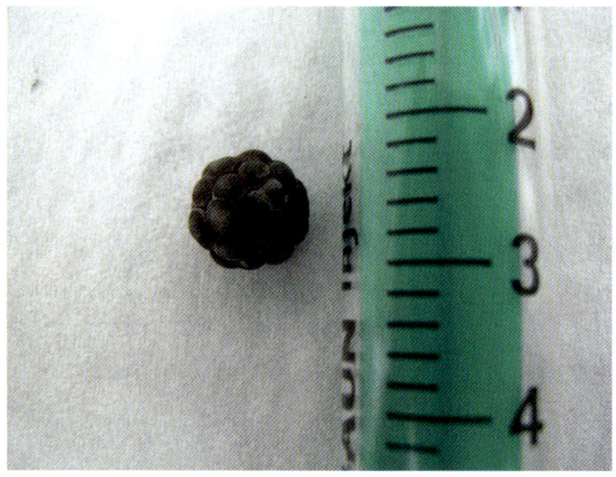

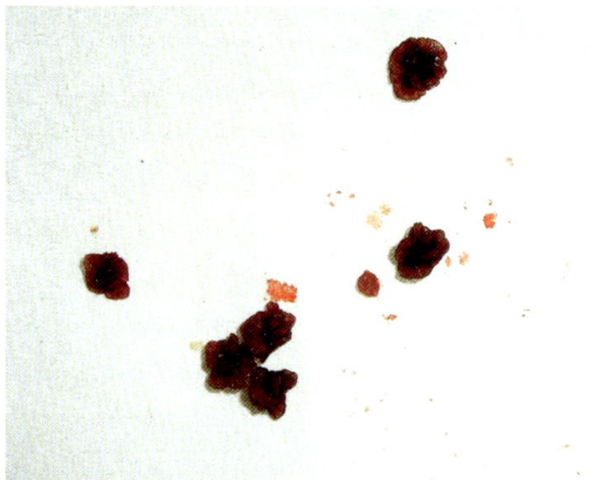

**Figures 6.38 and 6.39.** Images of calcium oxalate uroliths.

Table 6.17. Predisposing factors for calcium oxalate urolithiasis in small animals.

| | Breed | Age | Sex | Concurrent conditions |
|---|---|---|---|---|
| **Dog** | Miniature Schnauzer, Lhasa Apso, Cairn Terrier, Yorkshire Terrier, Cocker Spaniel, Bichon Frise, Shih-Tzu, Miniature Poodle | 5–11 years | Males, >70% | Obesity<br>Hypercalciuria (hyperparathyroidism, hyperadrenocorticism) |
| **Cat** | Persian, Burmese, Himalayan | 4–16 years | Equal risk in males and females | Obesity<br>Hypercalcaemia |

Oxalate is a derivative of amino acids and vitamin C. Urine calcium may increase due to **increased calcium absorption** in the intestine (for example, diets with excess vitamin D), **reabsorption of calcium** from the bones (hyperparathyroidism, metabolic acidosis, etc.)

or **tubular problems** that prevent the reabsorption of calcium filtered by the glomerulus.

This type of urolith occurs more frequently in the **male or neutered females**, perhaps because oestrogens reduce calcium concentrations in urine. Other risk factors common to all uroliths are **obesity and low activity** levels.

**Calcium oxalate formation inhibitors**:

- Citrate. Produces calcium complexes, making it more soluble.
- Magnesium pyrophosphate: magnesium and pyrophosphate complex with oxalate.
- Tamm–Horsfall mucoproteins.
- Glycosaminoglycans.
- Nephrocalcin.

The following have been linked with calcium oxalate urolith formation:

- Renal disease, especially of the upper urinary tract (nephroliths or ureteral uroliths), either due to metabolic acidosis, which promotes the excretion of calcium in the urine, or the lack of tubular reabsorption of calcium.
- Hypercalcaemia, especially in cats:
  - 35% of cats with calcium oxalate uroliths have calcaemia.
  - 35% of cats with idiopathic hypercalcaemia develop urolithiasis.

### *Treatment*

There are **no protocols for the dissolution** of calcium oxalate uroliths, so **physical removal** is the only treatment option.

### *Prognosis and prophylaxis*

**Recurrence is common**, with rates of up to 50% in the 3 years following the initial extraction. Therefore, it is important to **establish preventive measures** to reduce recurrence (Table 6.18) among these are:

- **Increase water intake** (with wet diets or by adding water).
- Use a **modified diet**. Available studies suggest that diet may play a role in reducing recurrence, however, more controlled studies are needed that validate these observations and indicate the ideal formulation in terms of composition.
- Add an **alkalizing agent** such as potassium citrate, if a neutral or slightly alkaline urine is not achieved with the diet.
- In the case of feeding a home-made diet, **supplement with vitamin B6** (vitamin B6 deficiency promotes the production and urinary excretion of oxalic acid).

Table 6.18. Preventive measures to reduce the recurrence of urolithiasis due to calcium oxalate.

| | Objective | Methods available to achieve the objective |
|---|---|---|
| **Diet** | Reduce recurrence, achieve an adequate pH | Use a non-acidifying diet with restricted calcium, oxalate and proteins, but not restricted in magnesium and phosphorus, without vitamin C/D supplementation<br>Avoid foods with excess oxalate (chocolate, spinach, peanut, tea, etc.) |
| **Urine specific gravity** | <1.020 (dog)<br><1.025 (cat) | Feed a wet diet<br>Add water to the diet<br>Make multiple drinking fountains available<br>Provide flavoured water<br>Increase dietary sodium |
| **Urine pH** | 7.0–7.5 | Give diet ± potassium citrate (initial dose 75 mg/kg/12 h) |
| **Crystalluria** | Minimize | Control hypercalcaemia; administer hydrochlorothiazide (2–4 mg/kg/12 h)<br>Supplement with vitamin B6 if a home-cooked diet is fed (2 mg/kg/24 h) |

- Administer **hydrochlorothiazide** in hypercalcaemic patients, although it can cause hypokalaemia.
- **Avoid the indiscriminate use of antibiotics** to prevent elimination of intestinal flora formed by *Oxalobacter formigenes*, which is **an intestinal bacterium that degrades dietary oxalate** and whose absence may be accompanied by increased intestinal absorption of oxalate.
- **Avoid medications that enhance the excretion of calcium in urine** (furosemide and glucocorticoids).
- Investigate the presence of **hyperadrenocorticism**, if there are compatible clinical or laboratory signs.

## *Purine urolithiasis*

### *Aetiopathogenesis*

The **metabolism of purines** leads to the formation of uric acid, which is converted to allantoin in the liver and then excreted in urine (Figure 6.40). Allantoin is soluble in the urine. The solubility of uric acid is much lower and, when urine is super-saturated with uric acid, urate crystals form.

The **Dalmatian** (Figure 6.41) and the **English Bulldog** suffer from a combination of factors that **predispose them to ammonium urate urolithiasis**, such

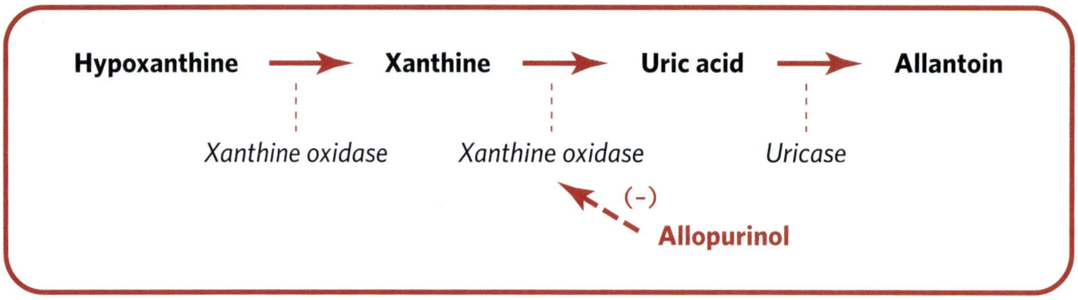


**Figure 6.40.** Purine metabolism.

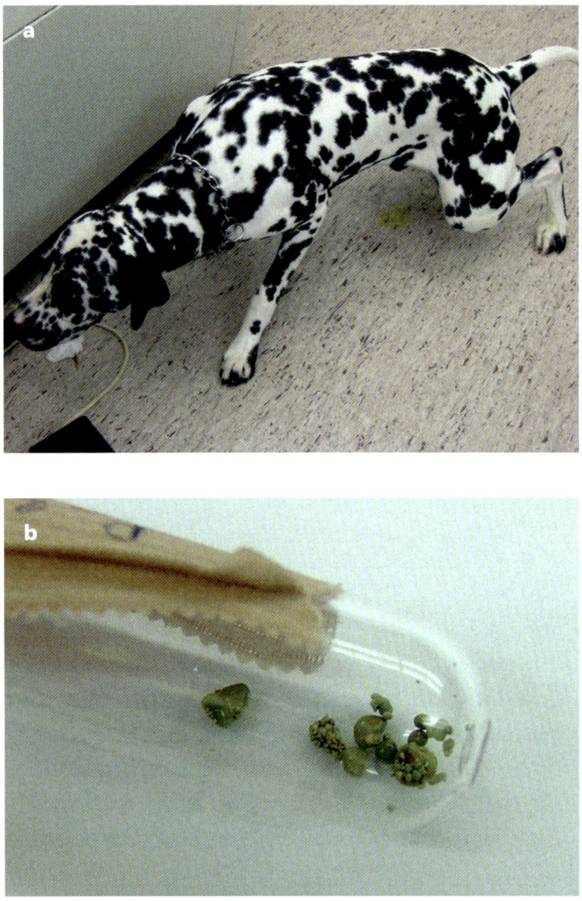


**Figures 6.41.** Dalmatian (a) with stranguria due to urethral urolithiasis (b) with urates.

as a decrease in tubular reabsorption of uric acid and uricase deficiency.

Because conversion of uric acid to allantoin occurs mainly in the liver, animals with **hepatic dysfunction or portovascular abnormalities** suffer a higher incidence of this type of urolith. High levels of blood ammonia and acidic urine are factors that predispose to the formation of these crystals.

### *Treatment*

Medical dissolution can be attempted by using an **alkaline diet restricted in purines**, accompanied by **allopurinol (15 mg/kg/12 h)**.

In animals with liver disease, the approach of choice is physical elimination of calculi and to treat the underlying disease where possible (portosystemic shunts).

### *Prophylaxis*

As a preventive measure, a **restricted purine diet** should continue to be fed and, only in cases where it is necessary, **allopurinol at lower doses (5–10 mg/kg/12 h)**.

## *Xanthine urolithiasis*

Xanthine uroliths (Figure 6.42) are **rare in animals that do not receive allopurinol**. However, there are some cases in cats and certain breeds of dogs (Cavalier King Charles Spaniels and Dachshunds).

## *Cystine urolithiasis*

### *Aetiopathogenesis*

**Cystinuria is a hereditary disease** due to changes in the tubular transport of dibasic amino acids (cystine, arginine, lysine, ornithine).

Certain breeds of dog, such as the **Newfoundland, Labrador, English Bulldog and Dachshund**, among others, are predisposed to cystinuria and, for some, there are **genetic tests** available for detection.

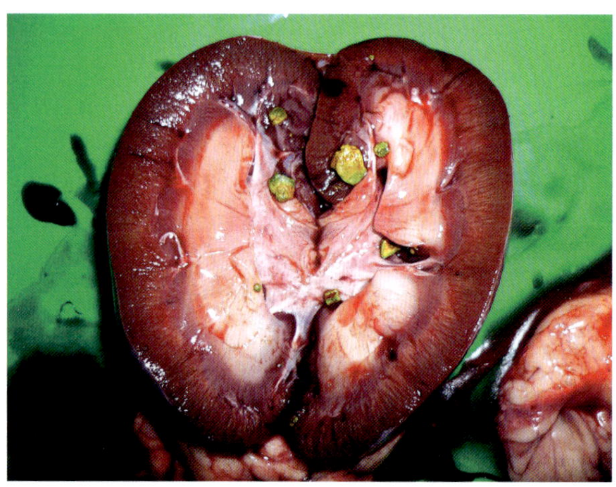

**Figure 6.42.** Xanthine nephrolithiasis in a dog receiving allopurinol as a treatment for leishmaniosis over several years.

The most important clinical manifestations are lithiasis, although not all patients with cystinuria develop this.

#### *Treatment*

**Medical dissolution** can be performed in the dog using a **low-protein, alkalizing diet** which induces diuresis (wet diet). This can be combined with either **alkalizing agents** or drugs that **solubilize cystine**, such as tiopronin (2-mercaptopropionylglycine, 15 mg/kg/12 h). However, tiopronin is **not advisable in the cat** due to its adverse effects (digestive upsets, liver disease, anaemia). Castration is recommended as a preventative treatment, which can be effective in some forms of cystinuria (non-type I cystinuria) in males, which can have a testosterone dependent molecular basis.

### *Silica urolithiasis*

#### *Aetiopathogenesis*

The aetiopathogenesis is not fully understood, although there some risk factors associated with silica urolithiasis such as (1) acidic urine, (2) ingestion of soil (pica), water or plants in areas with geothermal activity, (3) diets rich in silica (soya, maize gluten, rice husk) and (4) ingestion of medications containing silica salts.

#### *Treatment*

Medical dissolution is not possible, and uroliths require **surgical removal**.

#### *Prophylaxis*

Prophylaxis: avoid risk factors, such as ingestion of soil (and assess the causes of pica), avoid food and or treatments rich in silica, implement a balanced diet, including in some cases alkalinising diets and, as in other urolithiasis, increase water consumption.

### *Compound uroliths*

#### *Treatment*

Compound uroliths pose a **therapeutic and preventive challenge**. Most of these require removal by **surgical techniques** as it is almost impossible to predict the composition of each of the layers and dissolve all of them medically.

#### *Prophylaxis*

Post-extraction strategy is usually aimed at **preventing the mineral making up the nucleus from re-forming,** which has been the initial promoter that has resulted in the heterogeneous nucleation of the different minerals.

## Inflammatory conditions of the LUT

### *Clinical signs*

Most of the conditions that cause lower urinary tract inflammation affect both the bladder and the urethra, and the **clinical signs are the same regardless of the cause**.

### *Aetiology*

In dogs, the most frequent cause of inflammation of the LUT is **bacterial infection**. In cases of chronic bacterial infection, multiple follicles with lymphoid infiltrates can develop throughout the entire LUT, which spontaneously resolve after infection control. It is important to differentiate follicular cystitis from a polypoid cystitis or LUT neoplasms.

### *Polypoid cystitis*

Polypoid cystitis is a **rare disease** in dogs with inflammation, proliferation of the epithelium and development of **polypoid masses in the urinary bladder** without histological evidence of neoplasia.

#### *Aetiopathogenesis*

It is believed that it may be a **hyperplastic inflammatory reaction** in the presence of **chronic irritation of the bladder** from recurrent infections or urolithiasis (Figure 6.43). However, it is unknown whether this condition predisposes to the formation of polyps or vice versa. It is not clear whether it may be a pre-neoplastic lesion.

#### *Differential diagnosis*

The lesion's location can help differentiate polypoid cystitis from neoplasia, since polyps are usually located cranioventrally, unlike canine transitional cell carcinoma which is more common in the trigone.

#### *Treatment*

Although in **some cases polyps resolve spontaneously** after the management of urinary tract infections, in most cases **resection is necessary**; it is important for a biopsy to be performed in order to confirm the nature of the problem.

### *Sterile haemorrhagic cystitis*

In some dogs under **treatment with cyclophosphamide**, a sterile haemorrhagic cystitis can be triggered as a result of the urinary excretion of the metabolite **acrolein**. Treatment consists of **discontinuation of the**

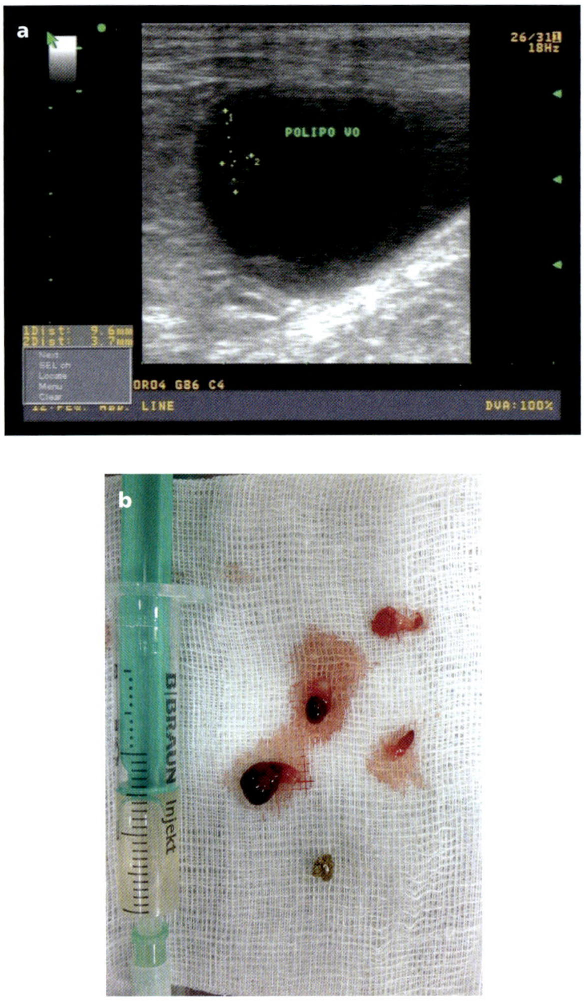


**Figure 6.43.** Dog with polypoid cystitis (a) and vesicle calcium oxalate calculi (b).

**cyclophosphamide therapy**, symptomatic short-term treatment as necessary (analgesics) and treatment of secondary infections that may occur.

## Proliferative or granulomatous urethritis

### Aetiopathogenesis

Proliferative or granulomatous urethritis is a rare infiltrative disease of the canine urethra, where thickening and proliferation of the urethral mucosa are observed. The term 'proliferative' is preferred since not all dogs have granulomatous infiltration.

Proliferative changes may be secondary to chronic bacterial infections or immune-mediated disease.

### Differential diagnosis

In many cases urethritis produces **symptoms of obstruction** and the presentation is similar to that of neoplastic conditions, so **biopsy is important** to differentiate the two conditions because treatment and prognosis are very different.

### Treatment

Treatment is aimed at **controlling urinary infection**: if the clinical signs are not resolved, **immunosuppressive therapy** (prednisone in combination or not with other immunosuppressants) may be indicated.

### Prognosis

The **prognosis is reserved**, especially if there is urethral obstruction, since not all dogs respond to treatment. In some cases, placement of urethral stents or cystotomy tubes, laser therapy or even, in specific cases, surgical resection may be necessary.

## Urinary infections

### Epidemiology

**Urinary infections are common** in daily practice, especially in dogs, with an estimated 15% of all dogs suffering from at least one episode of urinary infection during their lifetime.

### Aetiopathogenesis

Urinary tract infection (UTI) occurs when **normal defence mechanisms are compromised** and an infectious agent colonizes (adheres, multiplies and persists) in part of the urinary tract. Normal defences include the urination mechanism, anatomical structures, mucosal barrier, properties of urine and systemic immunocompetence. Generally, the origin of these infections is in the **distal urethra** (which is not sterile). Other sources of infection are the intestinal tract, the prostate and the genital tract.

### Important definitions

#### Bacteriuria

**The presence of bacteria in the urine** (due to UTI, asymptomatic bacteriuria, sample contamination or bacterial growth *in vitro*). Subclinical bacteriuria is defined as the presence of bacteria in urine as determined by positive bacterial culture from a properly collected urine specimen, in the absence of clinical evidence of infectious urinary tract disease. Bacteriuria can be found in patients without urinary signs and culture, and probably treatment, is not indicated, with spme exceptions (suspected pyelonephritis, investigation of the bladder as a source of septicemia, patients with surgical procedures that invove the transection of urinary tract, dogs with suspected struvite urolithiasis).

#### Pyuria

**The presence of leukocytes in urine** (>4 WBC/100x). This is indicative of **inflammation** but is not synonymous with infection.

## Resistance

An inherent or acquired mechanism in a microorganism that allows it to **resist a certain drug**.

## Simple infections

The presence of UTI with no suspicion of an underlying structural or functional abnormality. Recently these type of infection have been classified as sporadic bacterial cystitis. Diagnosis is based on the presence of lower urinary tract signs, ideally with concurrent evidence supporting bacterial cystitis (e.g. hematuria, pyuria, sytologically evident bacteriuria), and bacterial culture results. Include those patients with less than 3 UTI in 3 months.

## Complex infections

A UTI associated with **structural or functional abnormalities** of the urinary tract, with impaired immune competence or recurrent (if ≥3 UTIs occur in 1 year), or with involvement of the upper urinary tract and/or the prostate. This term has been actually substituted by "recurrent bacterial cystitis", and include recurring infections, reinfections, super-infection and refractory infections.

## Recurring infections

Recurrent UTI in which the **same organism reappears** weeks/months after treatment ceases (which implies failure to eradicate the pathogen).

## Reinfections

Recurrent UTI in which a **different organism** appears in a variable period of time (implies compromise of defence mechanisms).

## Super-infections

Infection with a **different pathogen during the treatment of the original infection** (in dogs with urinary catheterization, neoplasia, etc.).

## Refractory or persistent infections

Persistence of the original pathogen despite *in vitro* susceptibility to antibiotic therapy. It occurs because adequate antibacterial concentrations of the drug in the urine are not reached. It is unusual.

**Bacteria are the main agents involved in UTIs.** The majority of infections (75%) are caused by a single organism, Escherichia coli **being the most common uropathogen** in both cats and dogs (Figure 6.44).

**Fungal infections are rare** and usually appear when there are temporary or permanent deficiencies of systemic or local immunity of the urinary tract. They are usually associated with bacterial infections, the use of antibiotics or other urogenital diseases. The **most frequent organism is** Candida albicans (Figure 6.45), which is a commensal agent of the genital mucosa, upper respiratory tract and gastrointestinal tract. Other agents have been sporadically described in UTIs although they are of less clinical importance, such as some algae (*Prototheca zopfi*), protozoa (*Toxoplasma gondii*) and viral agents (*feline calicivirus)*.

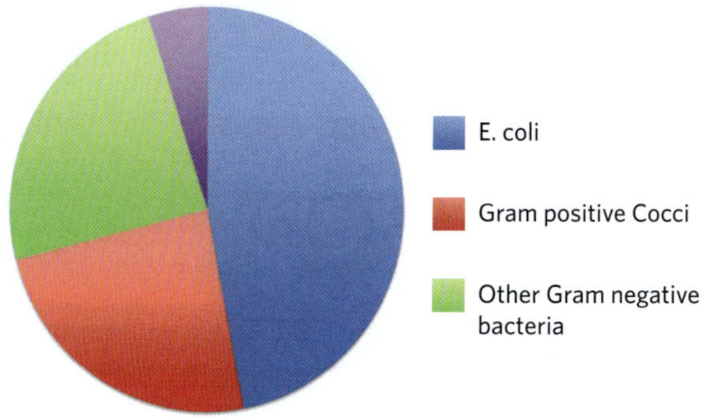


**Figure 6.44.** Prevalence of uropathogens.

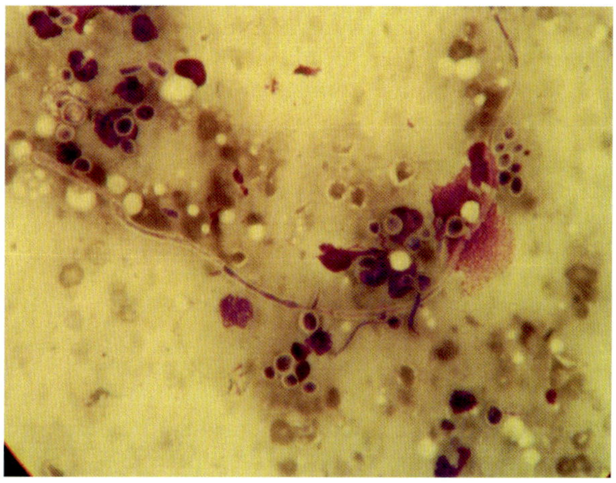

**Figure 6.45.** Urine sediment in a cat with a fungal infection caused by *Candida albicans*.

The **factors that predispose to UTIs** (Table 6.19) should be assessed since, where possible, these should be corrected for definitive control of the problem and avoidance of the occurrence of complex infections. Therefore, they should be detected by guiding diagnostic tests according to the animal's signalment (for example, suspicion of congenital diseases in young animals with UTI), clinical history and examination.

### *Clinical signs*

Clinical signs depend on:

- The **location** of the infection:
  - **Lower UTI**. Signs of irritative micturition: haematuria, polyuria, stranguria, dysuria and, in some cases, incontinence.
  - **Upper UTI** can present with systemic signs such as fever, uraemia, polyuria/polydipsia and kidney pain.

Table 6.19. Factors that predispose to UTIs.

| | | Comments |
|---|---|---|
| **Anatomical anomalies** | **Ectopic ureter** | Greater predisposition in females and certain breeds (Retriever, Husky, West Highland White Terrier, English Bulldog, Poodle)<br>The most common clinical sign is incontinence<br>UTI as a frequent secondary complication |
| | **Persistent urachus** | Associated with a reservoir of stagnant urine, which favours UTIs and, sometimes, micro-abscesses |
| | **Vulvar alterations** | In cases of ovariohysterectomy at a very early age, vulvar hypoplasia may remain favouring the presence of UTIs<br>In obese bitches, folds in the vulvar area can also be the cause of UTIs<br>Other alterations: urethral sphincter incompetence, ureterocoeles, etc. |
| **Metabolic and endocrine diseases** | **Hyperadrenocorticism or glucocorticoid (GC) administration** | UTIs in 40% of dogs with long-term GC use and in 46% of those with hyperadrenocorticism<br>GCs decrease urine density and the migration of neutrophils to the urinary system<br>UTIs can be asymptomatic, without the presence of inflammatory cells in sediment<br>Culture is necessary for diagnosis |
| | **Diabetes mellitus** | UTIs in 37% of dogs and 12% of cats<br>It can be asymptomatic and without inflammatory cells in sediment (culture needed) |
| | **Feline hyperthyroidism** | UTIs in 12% of hyperthyroid cats<br>May be asymptomatic |
| | **Chronic renal insufficiency** | It can be a factor in the progression of CKD |
| **Iatrogenic causes** | **Perineal urethrostomy** | |
| | **Urethral catheterization** | Higher risk with continuous catheterization in males (50%), but in females even with occasional catheterization (20%) |
| **Others** | **Urolithiasis** | Sometimes the culture can be negative and mucosal and urolith cultures are necessary (bacteria adhere to the bladder mucosa or uroliths) |
| | **Neoplasms** | |
| | **Micturition disorders** | Conditions that cause retention or incontinence |
| | **Chemotherapy administration** | |

- The **virulence** of the microorganism. Chronic infections may have fewer clinical symptoms and some are totally subclinical.
- The **spread of the infection** (discospondylitis, sepsis, prostatitis, etc.).
- **Underlying pathology**. For example, there may be signs of hyperadrenocorticism.

**Physical examination** must be comprehensive and includes:

- **Digital vaginal examination**: to detect anatomical abnormalities that may compromise defence mechanisms, such as the presence of changes in the vulva (Figure 6.46).
- **Rectal palpation**: palpate the prostate and identify changes in the urethra.
- **Neurological examination**: important in animals with urination disorders (incomplete and difficulty emptying of the bladder).

### *Diagnosis*

For diagnosis, a complete urine test is important, which includes:

- measurement of urine specific gravity
- urine test strip
- examination of sediment
- culture
- antibiogram.

It is important to remember that the **presence of pyuria or haematuria alone is not sufficient to diagnose an infection**. In addition, the measurement of white blood cells and nitrites using **test strips is not reliable** in the dog and cat, due to lack of sensitivity and specificity.

**Urine sediment**, especially when cyto-centrifuged and stained, is useful in the initial approach since it can give an approximation of the **most likely pathogen involved** (Table 6.20, Figure 6.47). However, in

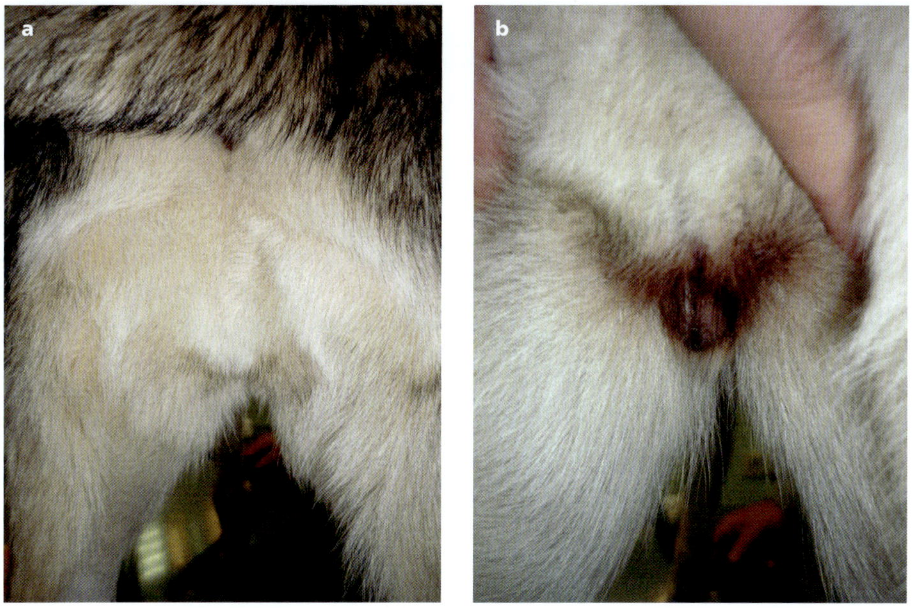

**Figure 6.46.** Vulvar hypoplasia in a bitch with recurrent urine infections.

Table 6.20. Most likely pathogen responsible for UTI according to urinary pH and sediment.

| | Cocci | Bacilli |
|---|---|---|
| **alkaline pH** | *Staphylococcus* | *Proteus* |
| **Acid pH** | *Streptococcus, Enterococcus* | *E. coli, Klebsiella, Pseudomonas, Enterobacter* |

cases with very dilute urine or low bacterial load, the sediment may be less sensitive **so culture** should be performed to completely rule out the presence of UTI.

The **method of choice to diagnose a UTI is culture of** urine from samples obtained by **cystocentesis** and where culture is **performed as soon as possible** after taking the sample (within 6 hours, at most 24 hours, keeping the sample refrigerated). Ideally, perform a **quantitative culture** that includes the isolation and identification of the organism and determines the bacterial load (colony-forming units). To minimize the effects of sample deterioration due to delay in sending to an external laboratory, **use a commercial culture medium** and incubate the sample in the practice laboratory for 24–72 hours. When using this method, always send the positives for culture so that an antibiogram can be performed.

In **complex UTI cases** follow a diagnostic protocol to **evaluate other concomitant conditions** or factors that predispose to the presence of UTI or a poor response to treatment (blood tests, imaging tests, endocrine tests, etc.).

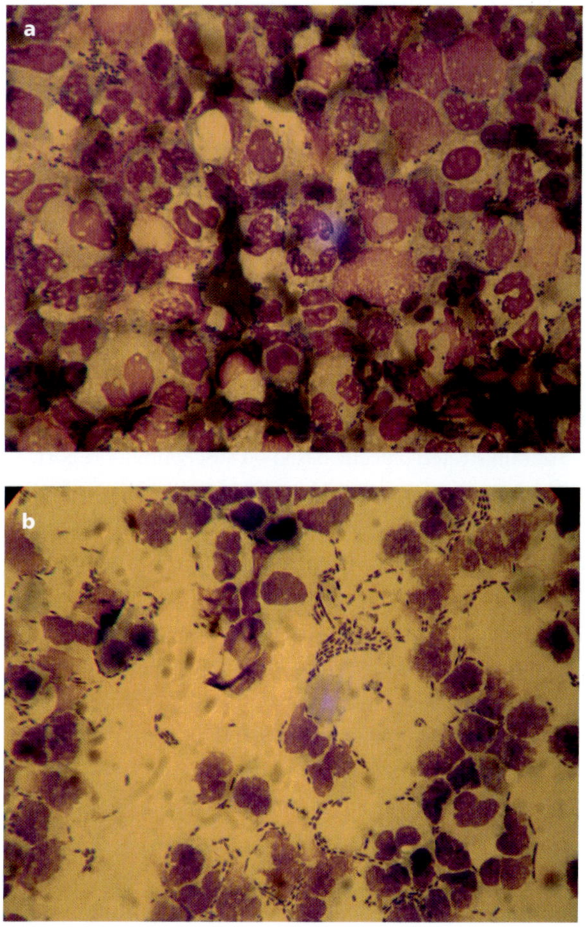

**Figure 6.47.** Urine sediments where phagocytosed cocci (a) and bacilli (b) can be seen.

### *Treatment*

Start treatment whenever there are **clinical signs associated with bacteriuria** (positive culture) or asymptomatic bacteriuria with **risk of ascending infection**. When deciding on treatment always **consider factors specific to the patient** (type of infection, predisposing factors, etc.) and **antibiotic characteristics**

Table 6.21. First-choice treatment options in UTI in the dog and cat.

| Type of infection | First-choice antibiotic |
|---|---|
| **Simple UTI** | Amoxicillin, trimethoprim/sulphamides |
| **Complicated UTI** | According to an antibiogram; until then, amoxicillin or trimethoprim/sulphamides |
| **Subclinical bacteriuria** | Antibiotic treatment is not recommended unless there is a risk of ascending infection, in which case it should be treated as a complicated UTI |
| **Pyelonephritis** | Start with fluoroquinolones, reassessing treatment according to antibiogram |
| **Prostatitis** | Trimethoprim/sulphonamides, enrofloxacin, chloramphenicol |

(concentration in the urine, penetration into tissues such as renal parenchyma or prostate, toxicity, etc.). Bacterial resistance is increasingly common, and prevention depends on **responsible use of the appropriate antimicrobial** (Table 6.21).

The **duration of treatment is controversial**, with little real evidence for the optimum length of antibiotic therapy. However, as a consensus, administration of antibiotics:

- Previously, in uncomplicated infection (sporadic bacterial cystitis), a 7-10 days course of antibiotic was recommended. However, now analgesia is recommended and only if clinical signs persist after 3-4 days, a short course of 3-4 days of antibiotic can be administrated , ideally based on susceptibility report.
- In the case of recurrent bacterial cystitis, it is important to complete a diagnostic work up to find risk factors and comorbidities. Analgesia is again recommended to improve clinical discomfort of the patient. In case of reinfection, a 3-5 days course of antibiotic is enough. If tisular penetration must be obtained e.g pyelonephritis), longer duration is suggested, until 7-15 days. In acute or chronic prostatitis, 4 or 4-6 weeks, respectively, can be needed.

Select the antibiotic based on the results of culture and sensitivity. Until these are available, start treatment according to sediment findings:

- **Cocci**: administer cefalexin or trimethoprim/sulpha drugs.
- **Bacilli**: administer amoxicillin-clavulanic or cefalexin.

**Do not use trimethoprim/sulpha drugs along with a calculolytic medical treatment**, as these may precipitate on the surface of the stone and make dissolution more difficult. **Quinolones** should be reserved for **infections resistant to other antibiotics** or when prostate involvement is suspected.

**Antibiograms** are a useful tool in the treatment of urinary infections but, when interpreting the results, remember that sensitivity discs reflect the **serum concentration of antibiotics** and so it is important to know the **urine diffusion level of each antibiotic**. For example, a bacterium that shows resistance to a particular antibiotic on an antibiogram may be eliminated *in vivo* by the same antibiotic if it is well concentrated in urine.

In some situations **antibiotic use is controversial**, such as in patients with a urinary catheter, which should not be treated if no clinical signs are present. When signs are present, ideally remove the catheter and, if this is not possible, change the catheter and culture a urine sample obtained via cystocentesis.

**Complications** can occur in UTI patients, resulting in **infections that are difficult to eradicate**. These special situations include:

- Polypoid cystitis.
- Emphysematous cystitis (presence of gas in the bladder wall or renal pelvis, common in diabetic patients because glycosuria provides a fermentable substrate) (Figure 6.48).
- Struvite urolithiasis.
- Pyelonephritis (due to ascending infection).
- Prostatitis.

Sporadic infections by *Corynebacterium urealyticum* have been described. This bacterium has urease activity and favours the precipitation of struvite and calcium phosphate which form **encrusted plaques on the bladder mucosa** (Figure 6.49). This makes treatment

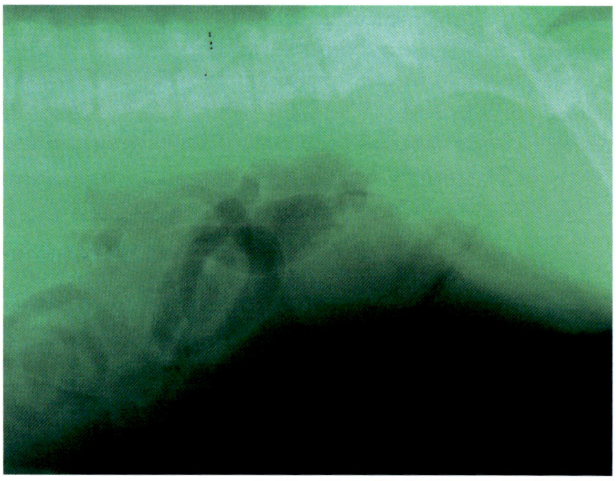

Figure 6.48. Lineal gas inclusions in the ventral wall of the bladder of a diabetic bitch with emphysematous cystitis.

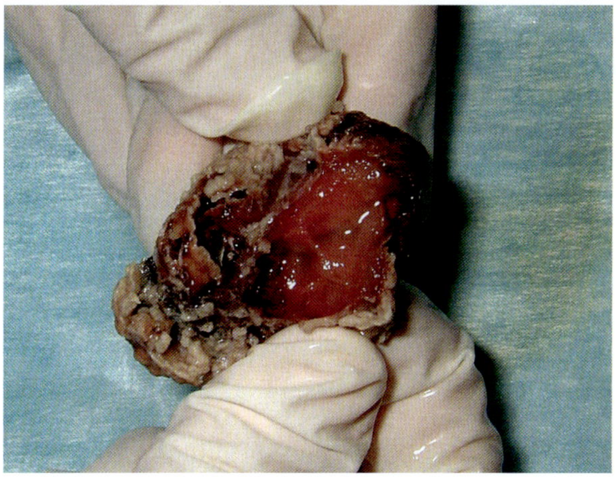

**Figure 6.49.** Encrusted plaques in the vesicular mucosa of a cat with an infection due to *Corynebacterium urealyticum*.

difficult without using a **surgical approach to debride** these lesions on the bladder wall.

**Following antibiotic treatment, resolution of the UTI should be monitored by a culture 5–7 days after treatment is discontinued**. With complex infections, this culture can also be carried out 4–5 days after the start of the treatment, to check effectiveness.

## FLUTD

### *Aetiopathogenesis*

The lower urinary tract (LUT) responds similarly in the face of different stimuli, so different **urinary conditions present with the same clinical signs**:

- dysuria
- stranguria
- periuria (urination in inappropriate places, out of and around the litter tray)
- polyuria (increased frequency of urination, small quantities)
- haematuria.

The terms '**Feline urologic syndrome**' (**FUS**) and '**feline lower urinary tract disease**' (**FLUTD**) refer to urinary disorders that occur with this symptomatology, and are in turn divided into **obstructive and non-obstructive uropathy** depending on the presence or absence of urethral obstruction.

### *Causes of FLUTD*

- unknown (50–70%); idiopathic feline cystitis or feline interstitial cystitis (FIC)
- urolithiasis (15–21%)
- urethral plugs (10–21%)
- anatomical defects (10%)
- behavioural problems (9%)
- neoplasia (1–2%)
- UTI (1–8%).

Many therapeutic measures have been recommended for the management of these patients, although many are not based on randomized, controlled scientific studies, and in patients with spontaneous disease.

**Different causes of FLUTD can occur in isolation or in combination** – for example, the formation of urethral plugs may be a consequence of inflammation of the urinary tract and crystalluria.

### *Epidemiology*

The overall incidence of FLUTD in cats is around 1%, and the **significance of this condition increases in parallel with the increase in the number of indoor cats**.

Several studies have evaluated the effects of dietary, environmental and behavioural factors on the development of FLUTD. Most cats with FLUTD are between **2 and 6 years old**, and it is **rare in cats under 1 or over 10 years old**. **Idiopathic forms are more frequent in young cats**, while UTIs, neoplasms and urolithiasis are more common in the elderly.

**Obstructive forms occur mainly in males**, and very sporadically in females. Although the diameter of the urethra does not vary between castrated and uncastrated cats, it seems that urethral obstruction occurs more frequently in castrated animals. Non-obstructive forms occur with the same frequency in males and females.

The influence of diet and lifestyle have been the subject of discussion for a long time. It seems that **dry diets and indoor lifestyle are important risk factors**. Although some authors have also found a **predisposition in obese cats** (Figure 6.50), obesity does not seem

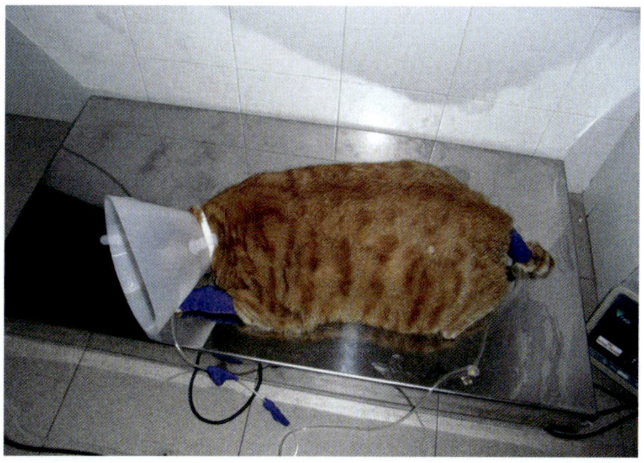

**Figure 6.50.** Obese cat with urinary obstruction due to feline idiopathic cystitis (FIC).

to be decisive in other studies, probably due to the superposition of other internal and/or environmental factors.

Various **environmental factors**, such as interaction with the owners, living with other cats and changes in routine habits, have also been related to the presence of signs of FLUTD, and are discussed later.

With regard to breed, it seems to be **more frequent in the Persian** and less common in the Siamese.

## *Feline idiopathic cystitis (FIC)*

### *Clinical signs*

**Feline idiopathic cystitis** (also known as idiopathic FLUTD, interstitial cystitis and feline idiopathic cystitis) is characterized by episodes with signs of UTI which (in the non-obstructive form) **resolve spontaneously**, with or without treatment, **after 4–7 days**.

However, signs may precede the obstructive form.

These **episodes recur with variable frequency**, decreasing with age. Approximately 15% of patients may have a chronic form, with clinical signs that persist for weeks to months, or have constant recurrences.

The FIC syndrome is similar to that described in humans called '**chronic pelvic pain**' or 'interstitial cystitis', in which it is thought there are changes outside the urinary tract and for which other nomenclatures such as '**unexplained medical syndrome**' are suggested, or 'functional somatic syndrome'. Therefore, Buffington (2011) suggests the term '**Pandora syndrome**', **referring to the concomitant presence of changes or problems outside the urinary system**. Regardless of the denomination, it is essential to fully evaluate these cats to determine whether there are other somatic or behavioural problems.

**Pandora syndrome**

1. Signs in other organs besides chronic idiopathic urinary signs.
2. Severity of alternating and intermittent clinical signs.
3. Resolution with environmental enrichment.

Recently, certain **changes in the bladder, nervous system and hypothalamic–pituitary–adrenal axis (HPA)** have been observed in cats with FIC, but the aetiopathogenesis of these changes is still unknown. FIC is similar to human interstitial cystitis, with certain differences such as the predisposition in women. In the human there are two forms of interstitial cystitis, **ulcerative and non-ulcerative**. Cats usually have a non-ulcerative form (in some cases, haemorrhages in the form of petechiae in the bladder submucosa can be seen on cystoscopy).

### *Epidemiology*

FIC is more frequent in **young and middle-aged, overweight cats**, with **low levels of physical activity**, **limited outdoor access**, fed on a **dry diet** and that live in a **multi-cat** household. There is an even distribution between males and females, although castrated cats are more susceptible.

### *Aetiopathogenesis*

The aetiopathogenesis of the disease is **multifactorial** (Figure 6.51). Various **stress factors** cause central changes, as well as changes in the permeability of the urothelium and the interaction of inflammatory mediators with nerve fibres locally in the bladder.

It seems in patients with interstitial cystitis that there is **dysfunction of the bladder's epithelial barrier**. On its luminal surface there is normally a **layer of glycosaminoglycans** (**GAG**) that **inhibits the adhesion of bacteria** and protects against urine constituents that can damage the mucosa. People and cats with interstitial cystitis excrete lower amounts of GAG in urine. This **defect in the GAG layer leads to increased permeability**, which allows urine particles to contact nerve endings causing **neurogenic inflammation**. This neurogenic inflammation can be initiated by the stimulation of nerve endings by either urine compounds or central factors (such as stress). Both **central and local mechanisms are involved**, producing stimulation of afferent sensory fibres (C fibres) that cause the release of various inflammatory mediators and neuropeptides (substance P and others), which are responsible for the appearance of pain, vasodilation of the intramural blood vessels, increased vascular permeability of the bladder wall, oedema of the submucosa, contraction of the smooth muscle of the bladder and activation of the mast cell population located around these nerve fibres.

In people with interstitial cystitis, **an antiproliferative factor** has also been found that leads to a defect in the proliferation and differentiation of superficial epithelial cells, so in cases of injury the normal mechanisms for replacement of these damaged layers by new epithelial cells are delayed.

**Stress is an important factor** in the appearance of FIC. Chronic stress (environmental, psychological, concurrent diseases, etc.) **activates tyrosine hydroxylase (TH) centrally**, in the locus coeruleus (LC, an area of the brain that is responsible for surveillance and autonomic activity) and, when activated, **increases the influx of catecholamines** that travel by descending excitatory pathways to the bladder. The connection of the LC with the bladder is **bidirectional**, so bladder distension also stimulates the LC (the micturition centre is located close to the LC and there are fibres connecting both points). Activation of the LC and the

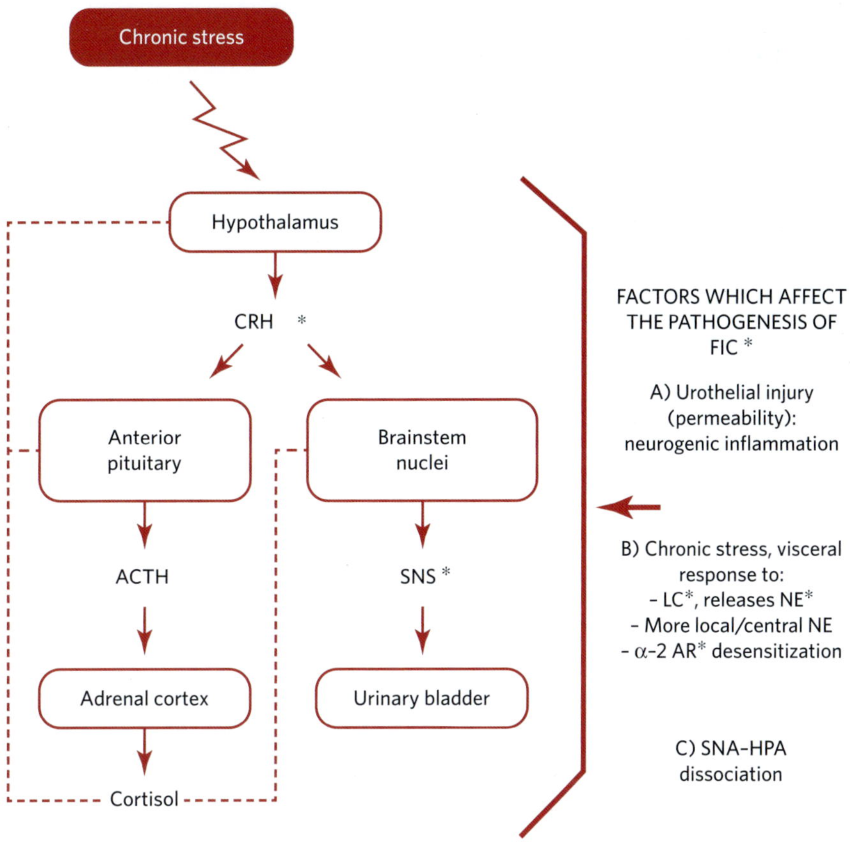


* CRH: corticotropin-releasing hormone ; **SNS:** sympathetic nervous system

FIC: feline idiopathic cystitis ; **LC:** locus coeruleus; **NE:** norepinephrine

**α-2 AR**: α-2 adrenergic receptor agonists ; **HPA:** hypothalamic-pituitary axis

**Figure 6.51.** Pathogenesis of feline idiopathic cystitis.

sympathetic system is thus an important response to stress; however, it is unknown whether this response is the cause or consequence of bladder abnormalities.

**Stress also activates the HPA axis**, but in cats with FIC it has been shown that they have a lower cortisol secretion response after administration of ACTH than in healthy cats. This HPA axis deficiency has also been found in other chronic pain syndromes in humans and is believed to be the result of desensitization of α-2 adrenergic agonist receptors secondary to chronic stimulation. Thus, it seems that there is a dissociation between the responses of the HPA axis and the sympathetic nervous system to stress in cats with chronic FIC.

Although it is believed that this **neurogenic inflammation** is essential in the development of the clinical signs of FIC, it is **not known whether it is a primary factor or secondary** to other factors not yet been identified. The role of infectious agents, such as certain viruses, is subject to debate and research, but to date the involvement of any bacterial, fungal or viral organism in FIC has not been demonstrated.

In some cats with FIC, the presence of a **vesiculourethral diverticulum** is observed, which, unlike congenital diverticula, almost always disappears after the remission of clinical signs.

## *Diagnosis*

A diagnosis of FIC is made by excluding other conditions, in combination or not with the presence of characteristic findings on cystoscopy. Therefore, diagnostic tests are performed to detect pathologies that require specific treatments (urolithiasis, urine infections, neoplasms, trauma, etc.) and other concomitant conditions or diseases (Figures 6.52–6.55).

Most important tests:

- Imaging (simple radiography, contrast radiography, ultrasound, etc.).
- Urinalysis.

If these **tests are normal**, the clinical signs are probably **due to the presence of FIC**.

**Cystoscopy is not recommended** for the diagnosis of FIC, but it may be useful to exclude other less common conditions (small uroliths, urachal diverticula, ectopic ureter, polyps, etc.).

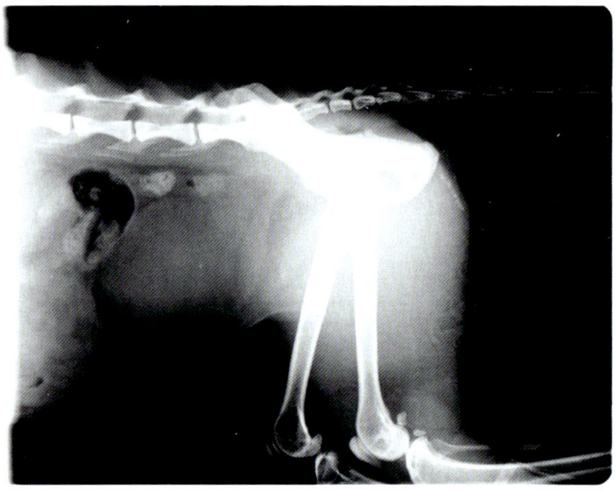

**Figure 6.52.** Urolithiasis in a cat with LUT signs and urethral obstruction.

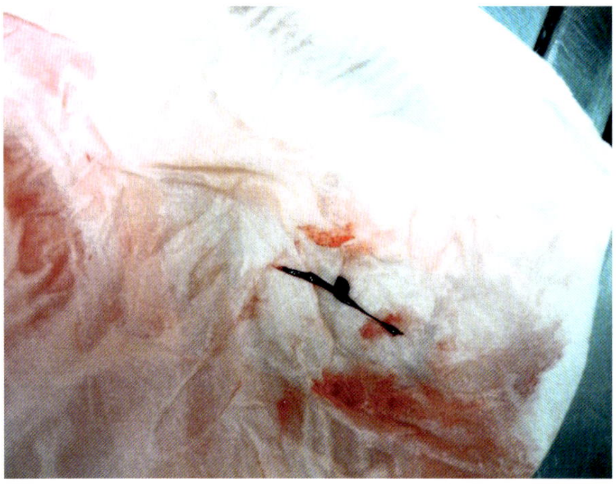

**Figure 6.53.** Urethral plug in a cat with LUT signs and urethral obstruction.

In patients where the **obstructive form** occurs, **blood tests are important** to detect changes such as azotaemia, hyperkalaemia and metabolic acidosis.

### *Treatment*

Most cases of **idiopathic FLUTD resolve spontaneously within a few days**, regardless of the treatment used. Therefore, it is difficult to assess the response to treatment since improvement may be spontaneous.

The **obstructive form is a medical emergency** in which the obstruction and secondary metabolic disorders (azotaemia, hyperkalaemia, metabolic acidosis) must be quickly resolved. Prior to catheterization a **careful penile massage should be performed** (Figure 6.56), as this is often enough to resolve the obstruction.

In cases with azotaemia, poor urine stream and/or bladder atony, severe haematuria and/or very difficult and traumatic catheterization, it is advisable to **leave a catheter in place (with a closed urine collection system) for a maximum period of 1–3 days**. In most cases there is no urine infection, so **antibiotics are not indicated** (especially in cats with urinary catheterization).

For the **long-term treatment of FIC, diet is one of the main therapeutic measures**. Cats fed a **wet diet have fewer recurrences** than those fed on a dry diet. The benefit of wet diets is because more dilute urine is formed. It is also important to take different measures to **increase water consumption**. Similarly, the type of diet fed should aim to maintain a **neutral urinary pH**, avoiding extreme levels. One of the main objectives is to maintain a urine specific gravity of 1.035 or less.

It is also essential to consider different aspects of the cat's habits and environment to **minimize stress factors** (handling of litter trays, playing time and patterns, interaction with other pets and owners, moving house etc.).

It should be remembered that **FIC is a painful condition**, so the **administration of analgesics** is advised to reduce the severity of clinical signs.

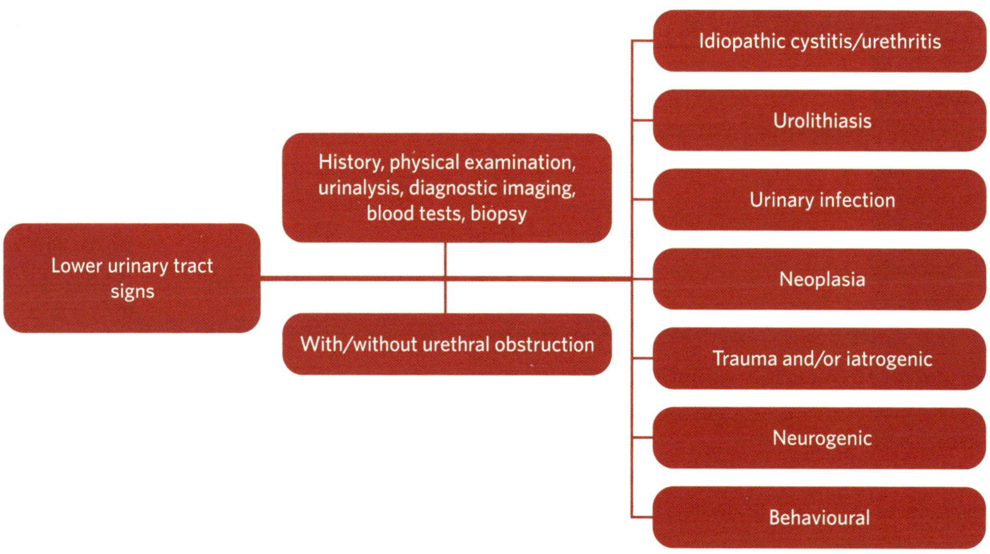


**Figure 6.54.** Causes of lower urinary tract signs in cats.

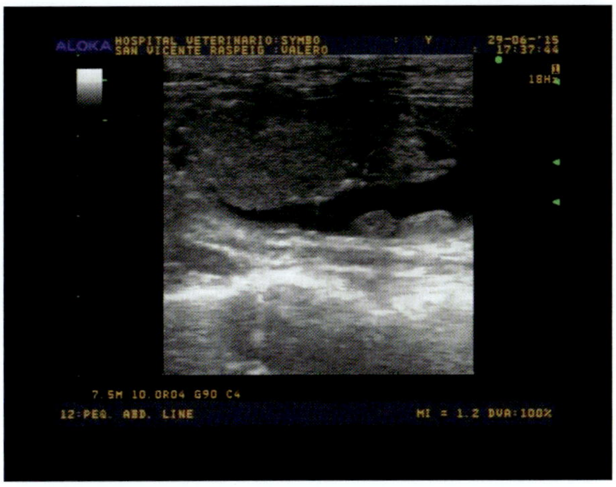

**Figure 6.55.** Transitional cell carcinoma in the bladder of a cat with LUT signs and urethral obstruction.

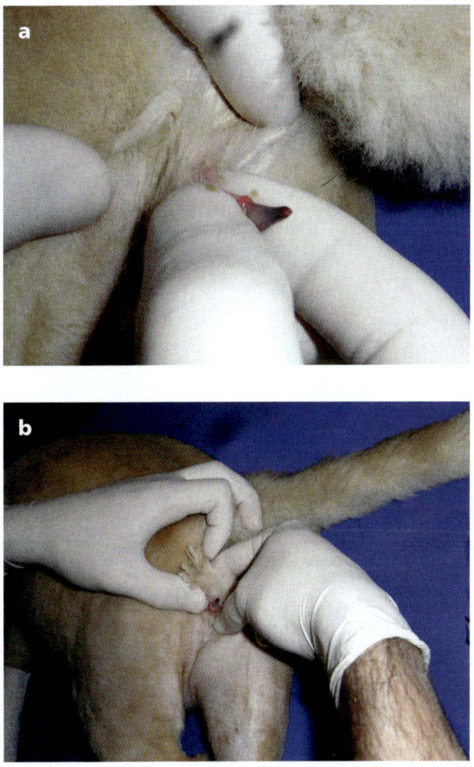


**Figure 6.56.** Penile (a) and urethral (b) massage to dislodge a urethral obstruction.

In more complicated or refractory cases, the administration of complementary treatments such as **antispasmodic drugs, amitriptyline, glycosaminoglycans, feline pheromones**, etc. can be considered. As mentioned before, their **efficacy has not been proven** and recommendations are based on either uncontrolled studies or expert opinions. Some studies have evaluated the use of corticosteroids and antibiotics, but none have shown them to have a positive effect. In addition, certain products, such as certain urinary antiseptics (methylene blue) and analgesics (phenazopyridine), should never be used in cats because of the risk of severe anaemia due to Heinz body formation.

Tables 6.22 and 6.23 cite some of the drugs used in FIC, as well as recommended measures for control and management and the degree of evidence available for each.

**Table 6.22.** Treatments used to manage FIC.

| | Dose | Use |
|---|---|---|
| **N-Acetylglucosamine** | 125 mg/cat/24 h VO | Possible adjuvant therapy in chronic refractory cases |
| **Prazosin** | 0.25–1 mg/cat/8–24 h VO | Antispasmodic (smooth muscle) |
| **Phenoxybenzamine** | 0.5–1.0 mg/kg/12 h VO | Antispasmodic (smooth muscle) |
| **Acepromazine** | 0.05–0.2 mg/kg IV, IM or SC<br>1–3 mg/kg VO | Antispasmodic (smooth muscle) |
| **Diazepam** | 0.2–0.5 mg/kg IV | Antispasmodic (striated musculature) |
| **Dantrolene** | 0.–2.0 mg/kg/12 h VO | Antispasmodic (striated musculature) |
| **Amitriptyline** | 2.5–10 mg/cat VO at night | Various behavioural and organic effects |
| **Clomipramine** | 0.25–0.5 mg/kg/24 h VO at night | Behavioural effects |
| **Buprenorphine** | 10–30 µg/kg/8–12 h VO, SC, IM or IV | Analgesic |
| **Atracurium besylate** | Administer a total of 4 ml of the final solution made up of 0.2 ml of the 10 mg/ml solution diluted in 3.8 ml of sterile physiological saline (0.5 g/ml) as intra-urethral bolus | Antispasmodic (striated musculature) |
| **Meloxicam** | 0.1 mg/kg/24 h VO for 4 days, and then 0.05 mg/kg/24 h VO | Anti-inflammatory |

Table 6.23. Summary of the treatment for FIC according to evidence-based medicine.

| Recommendation | Level of proof |
|---|---|
| Enriches the environment | III |
| Wet diets and UG <1.040 | III |
| Salt-rich diets in cats without CKD | IV |
| Boosts water intake | IV |
| Amitriptyline in the long term | III |
| Analgesics and NSAIDs | IV |
| Pheromones | III/IV |
| GAG | IV |
| Routine antibiotics not useful | I and IV |

I. ≥1 double-blind study on patients of the same species in question.
II. Double-blind study in experimental animals of the same species in question.
III. Controlled but not double-blind studies, epidemiological studies, dramatic results in uncontrolled studies, simulations.
IV. Opinion of reputable experts or expert committees, studies in other species, descriptive studies, pathophysiological justification.

### *Conclusions*

- Although a cause is often never found, if idiopathic cystitis is suspected (diagnosis by exclusion) a **cause should be sought**.
- Obstructive and non-obstructive forms are **different forms of the same disease**.
- The **obstruction must be treated as an emergency** since, if it is not resolved in time, it can cause the death of the cat.
- **Treatment must be appropriate to the cause**. The administration of antibiotics and glucocorticoids should be avoided, acidifying diets in cases indicating suitability, environmental changes should be considered and the client should be educated, and a clear communication should be maintained with them.

## Prostatic pathologies

The prostate contributes to the first and third fractions of the ejaculate. **Testosterone maintains the size of the prostate** and therefore the latter is significantly reduced in neutered animals. Therefore, prostate diseases (except tumours) mainly occur in **adult male uncastrated dogs**. In cats isolated cases of prostatic pathologies have been described, but these are rare.

The main types of prostate disease include:

- benign prostatic hyperplasia
- prostatitis
- cystic lesions (prostatic and paraprostatic)
- neoplasia.

The most frequent signs of prostate disease are:

- tenesmus
- haematuria
- urethral discharge
- anorexia
- lethargy.

The **enlarged prostate can compress the rectum, causing tenesmus and even constipation. Prostate infections can cause secondary urinary tract infections**, which is why it is assumed that the prostate may be involved in any uncastrated male dog with a UTI. Other less specific symptoms include:

- fever
- abdominal pain
- abnormalities in pelvic limb function (Figure 6.57)
- weight loss; hyperplasia and prostatic cysts may not cause symptoms.

The combination of **abdominal and rectal palpation** is useful for assessing the size, shape and symmetry of the prostate. The **sublumbar lymph nodes** can be palpated if they are enlarged. **Radiographs of the caudal abdomen** can help assess the location, size and shape of the prostate; it is considered to be enlarged if on a lateral radiograph it has a diameter >70% of the distance between the sacral promontory and the pubis (Figure 6.58a). It is also possible to detect mineralization in the prostate and metastatic lesions in the lumbar vertebrae and pelvis. **Contrast media** can be used to better determine the position of the prostate and the location of the bladder, urethral size and mucosal contour (Figure 6.58b). **Ultrasound** allows evaluation of the **structure and echogenicity of the prostate** (Figures 6.61b, 6.62 and 6.64), which may be increased

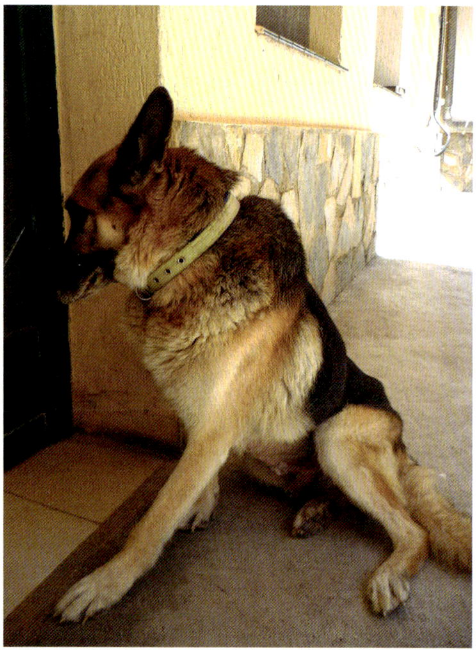

Figure 6.57. Hind-end weakness in a dog with a prostatic abscess.

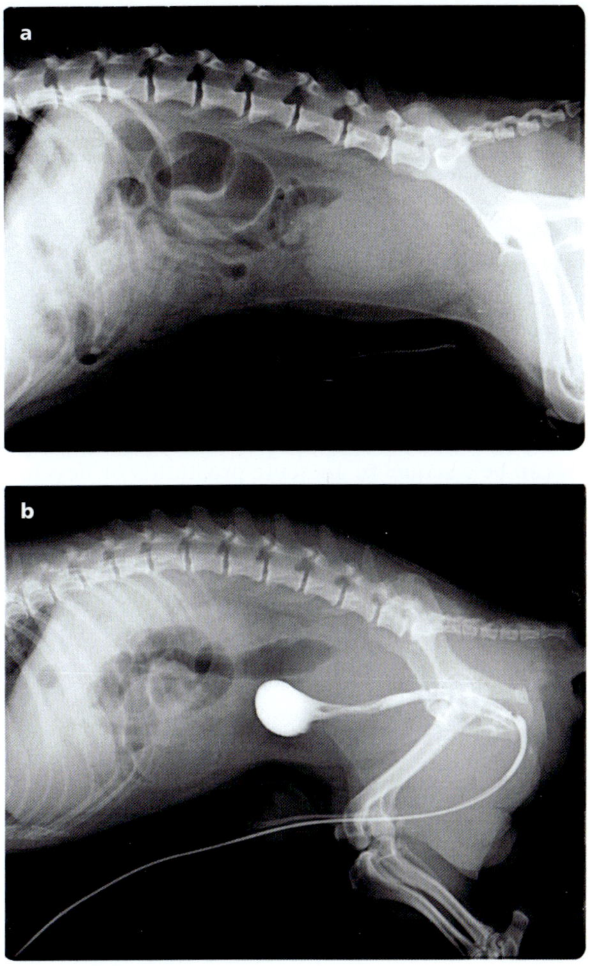


**Figure 6.58.** Prostatic hyperplasia and prostatitis in a dog. Plain radiograph (a) and with retrograde contrast (b).

in cases of hypertrophy, inflammation, infection and neoplasia. Prostatic cysts increase the size of lymph nodes and other abdominal abnormalities (uroliths, metastases, etc.) can also be detected.

A useful diagnostic test is the **examination of prostatic secretions** (Figure 6.59). These can be obtained by placing a catheter in the urethra at the height of the prostate and aspirating the secretions while performing **prostatic massage**. Percutaneous aspiration of the prostate can also be performed, but it can cause complications especially in cases of bacterial prostatitis, abscesses, coagulopathies and neoplasia. When aspirates do not lead to a definitive diagnosis, percutaneous or surgical biopsies are necessary.

## Benign prostatic hyperplasia (BPH)

### Aetiopathogenesis

BPH occurs in elderly dogs resulting from increase in the density of androgen receptors due to hormonal changes. These animals develop glandular hyperplasia and prostatic cysts that can favour secondary infections.

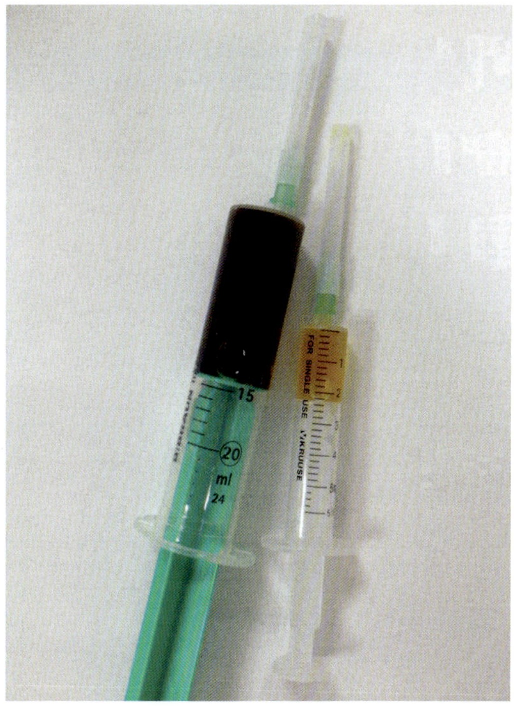


**Figure 6.59.** Secretions obtained from a paraprostatic cyst, and urine from the same patient.

### Clinical signs

Symptoms include:

- haematuria
- discharge
- dysuria
- faecal tenesmus.

On rectal palpation the prostate shows:

- increased size
- a uniform contour
- no pain.

### Diagnosis

The diagnosis is made according to signalment, radiography (Figure 6.60), ultrasound and analysis of prostate fluid.

### Treatment

The most effective treatment in animals that are not going to be used for breeding is castration. Clinical signs usually improve 7–10 days after castration, and full involution usually occurs at 12 weeks.

If castration is not an option, medical treatment based on anti-androgenic drugs can be used (Table 6.24), although it is less effective and the disease recurs if treatment is stopped. Oestrogens are not currently recommended due to their side effects (appearance of cysts and abscesses, myelosuppression).

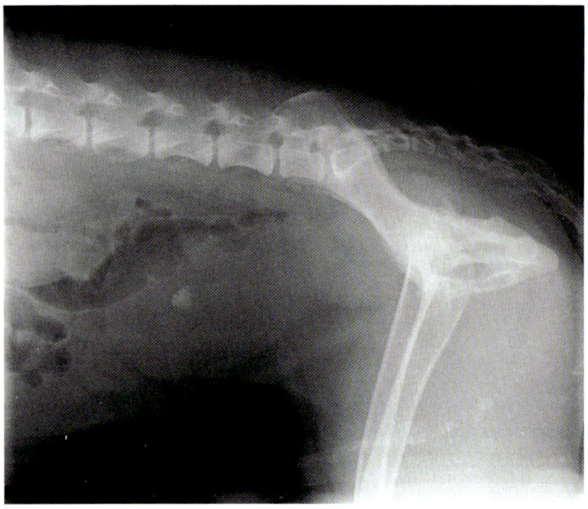

**Figure 6.60.** Lateral radiograph of a prostate enlarged due to BPH in the pelvic canal, where compression and dorsal deviation of the rectum can be seen in addition to vesicular urolithiasis.

Table 6.24. Anti-androgenic pharmacological treatment.

| Antiandrogenic treatments for BPH | Comments |
|---|---|
| **Delmadinone Acetate (Tardak®)** | Progestogen with anti-androgenic and anti-oestrogenic effects; can affect semen quality and inhibit adrenal gland function |
| **Cyproterone (Androcur®)** | Anti-androgenic; can affect semen quality and inhibit adrenal gland function |
| **Osaterone acetate (Ypozane®)**<br>**0.25–0.5 mg/kg/24 h VO for 7 days** | Blocks the entry of testosterone into the prostate and is a competitive androgen receptor antagonist. Reduces the size of the prostate up to 40% in 2 weeks. Can reduce cortisol levels (interference with ACTH test) and increase appetite. Does not alter fertility or semen quality<br>Pregnant women should avoid contact. |
| **Finasteride**<br>**0.1–1 mg/kg/24 h VO** | 5-α-reductase enzyme inhibitor, blocks the conversion of testosterone to its active metabolite. Does not affect semen quality. Continuous treatment is necessary and the prostate regains its volume at 4–8 weeks after treatment is suspended. Possible teratogenic effects |
| **Deslorelin (Suprelorin®)** | GnRH agonist that inhibits the gonadal pituitary axis when a low dose is applied continuously (subcutaneous implant). Effect in 4–6 weeks. Minimum duration: 6 months. Causes infertility and lower semen quality, until the implant is removed |

## Prostatitis

### *Aetiopathogenesis*

Prostatitis can **coexist with other prostate diseases** and is the **second most common prostate** pathology in dogs. **Changes** in the secretion of prostatic fluid, as in the case of squamous metaplasia and cystic hyperplasia, may **predispose to prostatic infection**. Infection can reach the prostate via the urethra or haematogenously. **Urine infections can cause prostatitis and vice versa.**

As prostatitis progresses, **micro-abscesses** may form and, if these join together, this leads to the **development of larger abscesses. Chronic bacterial prostatitis can be a sequel to an acute prostatitis or develop from an insidious onset.**

### *Clinical signs*

#### Acute prostatitis

Animals with acute bacterial prostatitis have systemic signs such as fever, depression, vomiting and inappetence. The physical examination shows:

- pain on abdominal palpation
- purulent urethral secretion
- asymmetric, painful prostate.

#### Chronic prostatitis

Animals with chronic prostatitis usually have less severe signs:

- signs of recurrent UTI
- haematuria
- urethral discharge
- tenesmus.

### *Diagnosis*

#### Acute prostatitis

Diagnostic tests may show:

Blood tests: **leucocytosis.**

Examination of **urine sediment: intracellular bacteria.**

Ultrasound: **enlarged prostate** with changes in echogenicity.

**Cytology and prostate fluid culture confirm** the diagnosis and are useful when selecting the most appropriate antibiotic.

#### Chronic prostatitis

There are no specific radiographic changes associated with chronic prostatitis, although ultrasound may reveal **changes in echogenicity**. Prostatic biopsy provides a definitive diagnosis for prostatitis, but is not usually necessary unless another concomitant prostate disease (neoplasia) must be ruled out.

### *Treatment*

#### Acute prostatitis

**Antibiotics that penetrate the prostate** should be administered, such as sulpha drugs and enrofloxacin, and **treatment continued for 4–6 weeks**. Cases of acute prostatitis may respond to other antibiotics since the blood–prostate barrier is altered, but this barrier may already be restored once the initial active inflammation subsides.

BPH is a risk factor for prostatitis, and so **castration is recommended** to minimize possible recurrence, and as an adjuvant therapy to reduce prostate size and accelerate healing. However, in the presence of acute infection, immediate castration is not advised as the patient should first be stabilized with medical treatment.

Some dogs with acute prostatitis develop **prostatic abscesses** (Figure 6.61), which require surgery for drainage (through omentalization of the prostate), performing castration at the same time.

#### Chronic prostatitis

With chronic prostatitis, the prostate–blood barrier is usually intact and therefore it is essential to select an antibiotic with good prostatic penetration (fat-soluble and basic), administered for 4–6 weeks, alongside castration.

## *Prostatic and paraprostatic cysts*

### *Aetiopathogenesis*

This not fully understood. Prostatic cysts may present as multiple cavitated areas within the parenchyma (Figure 6.62) and can be the result of ductal occlusion due to squamous metaplasia of the prostate (retention cysts). **Prostatic cysts may evolve into abscesses**.

Paraprostatic cysts present as fluid-filled structures that extend into the interior of the abdomen or pelvic canal, and may be secondary to remnants of the paramesonephric duct (Figure 6.63). **Paraprostatic cysts are less likely to become secondarily infected, since they do not communicate with the urogenital tract**.

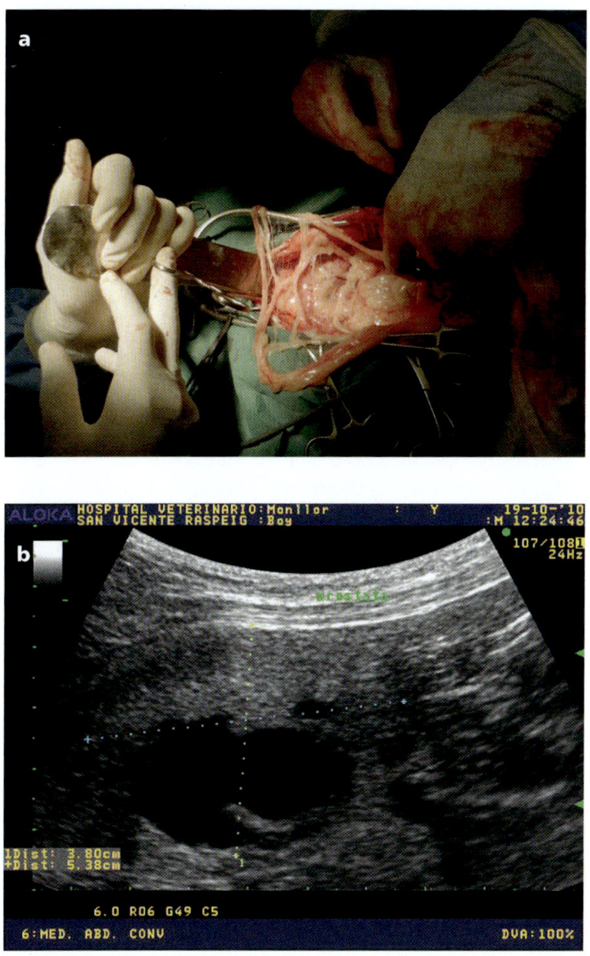


**Figure 6.61.** Canine prostatic abscess: surgery (omentalization of the prostate (a) and ultrasound (b).

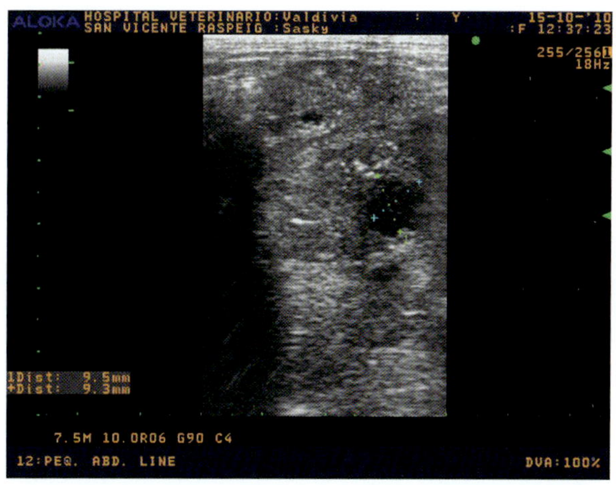


**Figure 6.62.** Prostatic cyst.

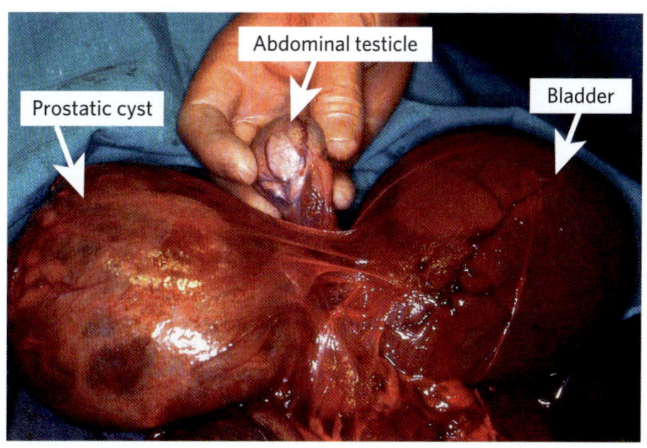


**Figure 6.63.** Paraprostatic cyst.

### *Clinical signs*

Animals may be asymptomatic or suffer from dysuria, haematuria or compression of abdominal structures.

### *Treatment*

**Treatment is surgical** (excision, omentalization and castration).

## *Prostatic neoplasia*

**Prostatic adenocarcinoma** is the most common prostatic tumour, with others including transitional cell carcinoma and haemangiosarcoma. **Metastasis** can occur in sublumbar lymph nodes, the pelvis, lumbar vertebrae and lungs.

### *Clinical signs*

Symptoms include:

- tenesmus
- haematuria
- dysuria
- urinary obstruction
- others related to the presence of metastases.

On physical examination the prostate can be described as:

- hard
- immobile
- asymmetric.

**Enlargement of the prostate in a neutered animal is typical of neoplasia.**

### *Diagnosis*

On ultrasound, the prostate appears **enlarged with changes in echogenicity** and, in some cases, **mineralization or local metastases** (Figure 6.64). Diagnosis is confirmed by **biopsy**, although the ultrasound appearance of the prostate and the presence of metastases are often sufficient.

### *Treatment*

Treatment includes **surgical resection, radiotherapy**, piroxicam (0.3 mg/kg/24 h PO) or **chemotherapy** (mitoxantrone or carboplatin). All these **treatments are palliative**, of limited efficacy, with an average survival time of 1–12 months and carry risks.

If the patient has concurrent infections, treatment of UTIs can relieve symptoms.

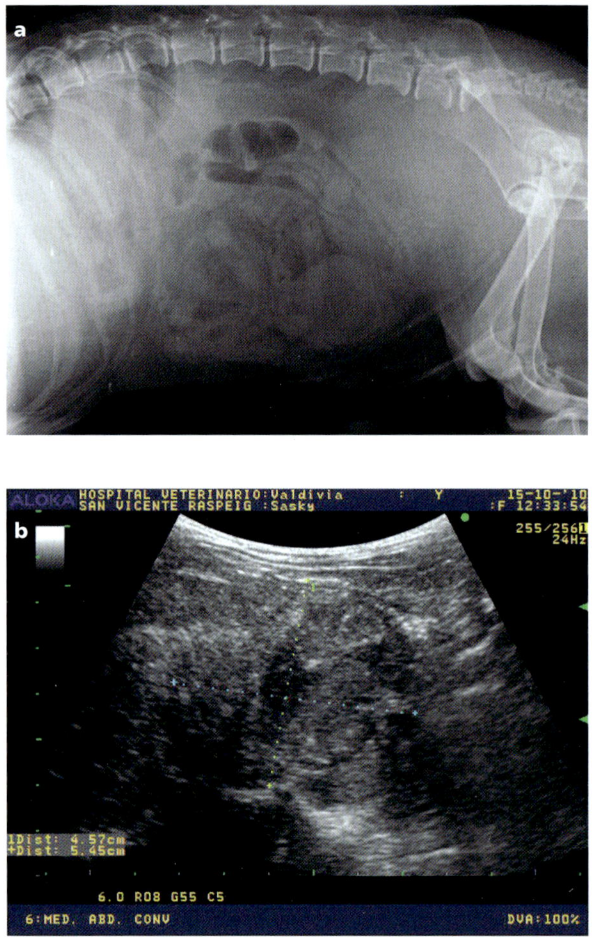


**Figure 6.64.** Radiograph (a) and ultrasound (b) of a dog with prostatic carcinoma.

## Changes in micturition: retention and urinary incontinence

## *Aetiopathogenesis*

Micturition is a complex process which requires the **central nervous system plus the autonomic and somatic nervous systems to interact**, together with the proper functioning of the organs involved.

The **lower urinary tract** is composed of the **detrusor muscle (smooth muscle)** and two muscular sphincters:

- The external sphincter (**smooth muscle**) that begins in the bladder neck and extends to the proximal urethra (is a continuation of the detrusor muscle).
- External sphincter (**skeletal muscle**).

Its functions are to **store urine** (99% of the time) and **empty the bladder** (1% of the time).

Although urination is a fully automatic spinal process, the central nervous system provides voluntary control. In this way, urination can be initiated or inhibited by centres in the brain.

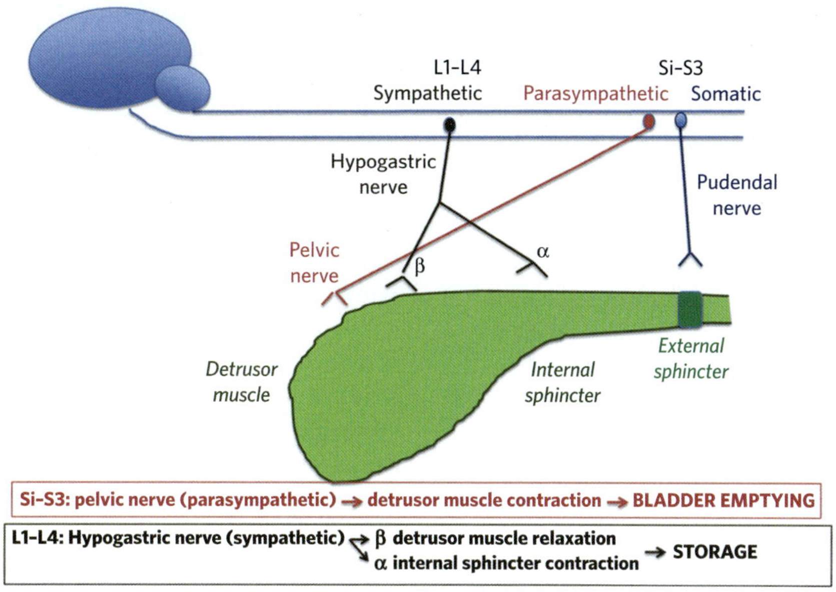


**Figure 6.65.** Innervation of the muscular structures involved in the process of micturition.

The three components of the peripheral nervous system are involved in micturition:

1. **Sympathetic** via the hypogastric nerve.
2. **Parasympathetic** via the pelvic nerve.
3. **Somatic** via the pudendal nerves.

In addition, conscious emptying requires the involvement of the **lumbar and sacral spinal** segments, as well as the **cerebral cortex and the brainstem**.

**Important nerves for the control of micturition** (see also Figure 6.65):

- **Hypogastric nerve**. Originates in L1–L4 and provides **sympathetic innervation** to the **detrusor muscle and urinary sphincter**. Promotes detrusor muscle relaxation by β-adrenergic receptors and urinary sphincter contraction by adrenergic receptors.
- **Pelvic nerve**. Originates from S1–S3 and provides **parasympathetic innervation** to the bladder causing **contraction of the detrusor muscle of the bladder**. It also has a sensory function: it transmits the sensation of a full bladder to the central nervous system.
- **Pudendal nerve**. Originates from S1–S3 and innervates the peri-urethral skeletal muscle, causing **urinary sphincter contraction**. In addition, it carries motor and nervous impulses to the perineum. Therefore, **perineal and bulbo-urethral reflexes** can be used to assess the integrity of this nerve.

The **sympathetic nervous system facilitates the storage of urine** and **the parasympathetic nervous system facilitates the emptying of the bladder**.

When there is a spinal cord injury:

- Between L5 and S3 the pudendal and pelvic nerves are affected, with consequent hypotonia of the sphincter and detrusor muscle. The bladder has a large residual volume, but emptying it manually is simple.
- Between S1 and S3 the perineal and bulbo-urethral reflexes can be affected. This symptomatology occurs with:
  - traumatic spinal injuries
  - disc herniation
  - cauda equina syndrome
  - dysautonomia.
- **Cranial to L7**, the **urinary sphincter remains contracted** due to a lack of inhibitory impulses. Thus, the bladder is **difficult to empty manually** and, in the long term, atony of the detrusor muscle develops due to constant distention of the bladder.

Various conditions, whether neurogenic or not, **cause changes in normal micturition leading to problems emptying the bladder (urinary retention)** or in its storage ability (**urinary incontinence**) depending on the aetiology (Table 6.25).

## *Clinical signs*

Signalment and clinical history can help determine the most likely cause.

- In very **young animals** with urinary incontinence, **congenital problems** such as urethral sphincter incompetence and ectopic ureter should be suspected, among others.

Table 6.25. Conditions or diseases that cause changes in micturition.

| | | |
|---|---|---|
| **Micturition disorders** | Problems related to urine **storage** | Urethral sphincter **incompetence** and other congenital anomalies<br>Lower motor neuron disease<br>Detrusor muscle hyper-reflexia |
| | Problems with **emptying** of the urinary bladder | Physical obstruction (urolithiasis, urethral plug, neoplasia, urethral stenosis, urethritis, prostate disease)<br>Detrusor muscle atony<br>Reflex dys-synergia (detrusor–urethral)<br>Upper motor neuron disease<br>Dysautonomia |

- If the animal also has **polyuria, dysuria**, etc. the **incontinence may be secondary** (or the primary problem has been complicated by an inflammatory cause, such as a urine infection).

Information about the **circumstances and/or timing** of the urinary issues is important. In patients with incontinence, owners should be asked whether **it occurs when animals are relaxed (lying down), while walking or after urinating**, etc. For example, animals with vaginal stenosis have urinary retention in the bladder and lose urine when they change position. This also occurs when there is urinary sphincter incompetence. Ideally, the animal should be observed while urinating (outside consulting room, or with videos taken by the owner, etc.).

A **thorough physical and neurological examination** of the patient is essential. The **bladder should be palpated** and its **size observed** (large or small), evaluating the residual volume after urination and, if a full bladder is detected, it should be assessed as to **whether it is easy to empty** by pressure or not (flaccid or spastic bladder).

The residual volume after urination can be estimated by palpating the bladder, abdominal ultrasound or catheterization.

In general, **small bladder is seen** in cases of:

- urethral sphincter incompetence
- incontinence due to inflammation of the urinary tract
- congenital problems such as ectopic ureters.

**Large bladders are observed in the presence of**:

- urinary obstruction
- neurological problems
- dys-synergia.

The urethra (via rectal palpation) must be palpated and the **genitals examined** for:

- dermatitis
- malformations.

The **neurological exam** should include:

- evaluation of anal tone
- movement of the tail.

**Clinical history and physical examination** are essential for formulating a diagnostic plan. An adult animal with symptoms of inflammation of the lower urinary tract will require a different diagnostic approach to a very young animal presenting with incontinence from birth. It is important to remember that an animal may have **several concurrent problems**. For example, a neutered female with urinary sphincter incompetence may not have any symptoms until she develops a urinary infection and, if the infection is not diagnosed and treated, the animal will remain incontinent despite receiving treatment for urinary sphincter incompetence. Likewise, an animal may have **several congenital problems** (for example, ectopic ureters, vesical urachus and intra-pelvic bladder), and treatment will fail if each one of these is not addressed.

## *Diagnosis*

Diagnostic tests include those to diagnose underlying diseases, **urine analysis and culture** and **imaging** (ultrasound and contrast radiography). More specialized tests include cystoscopy and urethral pressure studies. Obviously, not all cases require the same level of investigation and each one must be evaluated based on history and physical examination.

## *Urethral sphincter mechanism incompetence (USMI)*

### *Aetiopathogenesis*

Animals with USMI usually urinate normally but **lose urine when they are lying down or sleeping**, or when they are nervous or excited.

Structures involved in the urethral sphincter mechanism are the:

- **smooth muscle** of the urethra and surrounding tissues
- **blood vessels** of the submucosa and the urothelium.

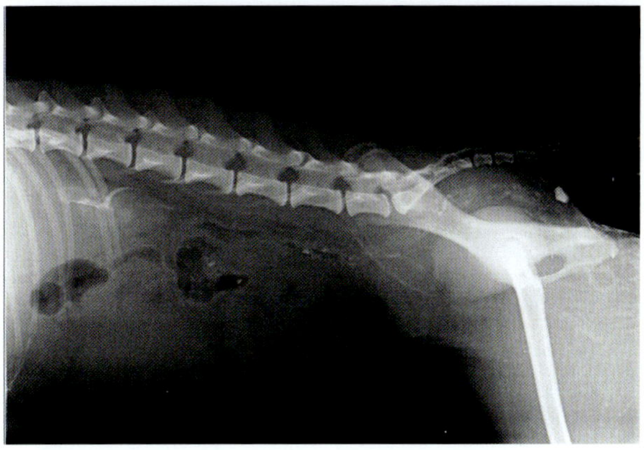

**Figure 6.66.** Bladder in intra-pelvic position in a bitch with urinary incontinence.

USMI occurs when **changes affect any of these components**, causing lack of response, change of muscle tone and/or structural alterations in the peri-urethral tissues. An abnormal position or morphology of the bladder or urethra may contribute to failures in sphincter functionality, such as when the urethra is very short or when the bladder is positioned intra-pelvically (Figure 6.66).

USMI occurs more frequently in **spayed females** as a result of the lack of hormones after spaying ('incontinence associated with spaying'). **Lack of oestrogen** can decrease the response of the α-adrenergic receptors in the urethra, leading to lower muscle tone. Some studies show that it can affect **20–30%** of spayed female dogs, especially in **medium–large breeds** and, although it can appear at any time after sterilization, it is more frequent in the first few years.

Sporadically, **USMI responds to hormonal treatments in male dogs and in cats**. The pathophysiology in these cases is not fully known. In male dogs with suspected USMI, **evaluation of the residual urine volume** is essential to **differentiate from reflex dys-synergia** (which is a problem in urinary retention due to incomplete emptying of the bladder).

**USMI can also be congenital**, most often associated with other congenital urinary tract abnormalities. In some congenital cases, incontinence resolves after puberty when urinary tract development is complete. In patients with congenital USMI, sterilization is discouraged, especially until they reach puberty.

### *Diagnosis*

This can be confirmed by **urethral pressure studies** but, unfortunately, they are not widely available or practical in day-to-day practice. The signalment, clinical history, physical examination and protocol to rule out other causes depending on clinical suspicions, as well as the response to the treatment, all help to make the diagnosis.

### *Treatment*

The recommended treatment in patients with **USMI is hormonal supplementation** with α-adrenergic agonist drugs, which increase activity of the urethral smooth musculature (Table 6.26). The most commonly used is **phenylpropanolamine**, which is effective in 85% of affected bitches and 50% of affected males. Weight should be controlled since **obesity is a factor that can contribute to USMI**.

In cases **refractory to medical treatment, surgery** (colposuspension or urethropexy, particularly in the bladder in an intra-pelvic position) can be considered. Other options include endoscopic injection of collagen into the wall of the urethra (an improvement in incontinence can be obtained, but it usually recurs over time and, in addition, many manufacturers have stopped producing these agents which currently makes it difficult to find them) or the use of **artificial urethral sphincters**, which have recently allowed significant improvements in incontinent male

**Table 6.26.** Pharmacological treatment of USMI.

| | Dose | Comments |
|---|---|---|
| **Phenylpropane-lamina** | 1–1.5 mg/kg/8–12 h VO | α-Adrenergic agonist. Use with caution if there is hypertension, hyperadrenocorticism or kidney disease: may cause hypertension, gastrointestinal signs, anxiety |
| **Oestriol** | 1 mg/dog/24 h VO and adjust treatment according to response | Natural short-acting oestrogen, which is why it does not cause myelosuppression. Can cause nausea and mild oestrogenic effects, such as vulvar and mammary swelling and/or attraction to males |
| **DES (diethyl-stilbestrol)** | 0.1–1 mg/dog/24 hours 5–7 days, then weekly or as nee ded | Oestrogen. May cause myelosuppression, attraction to males, vulvar and mammary swelling, behavioural changes and prostatic metaplasia (in males) |
| **Testosterone cypionate** | 2.2 mg/kg IM every 4–8 weeks | Androgen (used in some males with USMI). It can produce behavioural changes, aggressiveness, perianal adenomas and prostatic hyperplasia |

and female dogs that had not responded to medical treatments.

## Ectopic ureters

### Aetiopathogenesis

Ectopic ureters are a frequent **congenital cause of urinary incontinence in young animals**. The incontinence is due to the abnormal position of the ureters that empty in the vagina or distal urethra.

Ectopic ureters can be **unilateral or bilateral**, and **intramural** (they enter the bladder at the right point but pass through the submucosa eventually leading to the urethra) or **extramural** (connecting directly to the urethra or genital tract).

Patients with ectopic ureters may have other **concurrent congenital urinary abnormalities** and are **predisposed to recurrent UTIs**.

### Epidemiology

Ectopic ureters are more common in **females of certain breeds** such as the Golden Retriever and Labrador Retriever, Siberian Husky, Newfoundland, English Bulldog, Poodle and West Highland White Terrier, amongst others.

### Diagnosis

A diagnosis is made using **diagnostic imaging techniques**. Traditionally this involves excretory urography and ultrasound and, more recently, more advanced procedures such as tomography and cystoscopy (Figure 6.67).

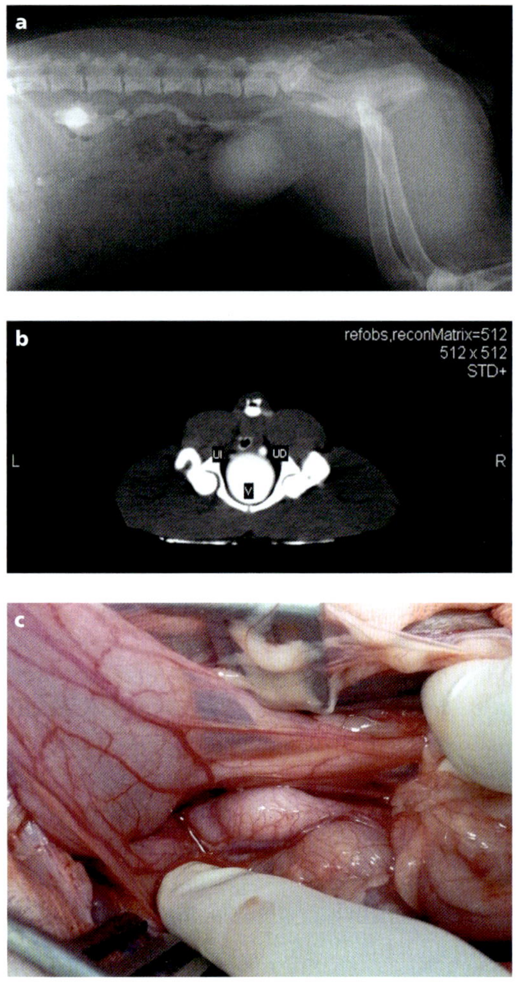


Figure 6.67. Ectopic ureter. Excretory urography (a), CT (b) and visualization of the ectopic ureter during surgery (c).

### Treatment

**Correction is surgical**. In certain centres, cystoscopy-guided laser ablation of the ureter is performed. In some patients, partial improvement may be observed but incontinence persists, usually due to the concomitant presence of functional disorders of the bladder and urethra (congenital USMI).

## Persistent urachus

Persistent urachus is another **anatomical change** observed in **young patients with urinary incontinence** and/or a history of recurrent urinary infections (Figure 6.68). The solution is surgical.

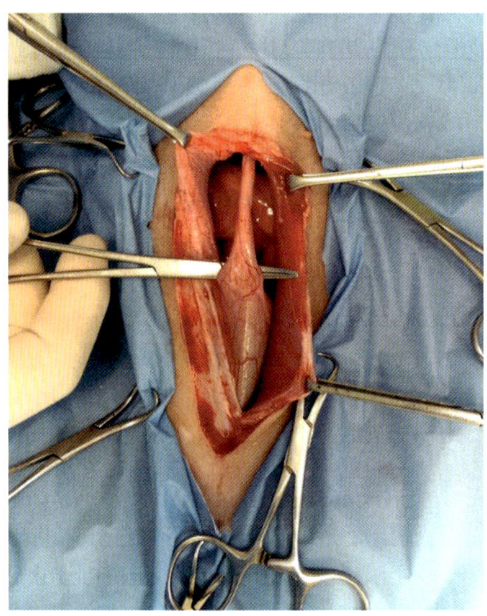

Figure 6.68. Persistent urachus.

## Ureterocoele

Ureterocoele is a **cystic dilation of the terminal portion of the ureter** that forms cavities that often protrude into the bladder (Figure 6.69). It usually occurs in dogs with other **congenital** changes such as ectopic ureters, and is also a cause of UTI. Treatment consists of its **resection** together with the correction of concurrent anomalies.

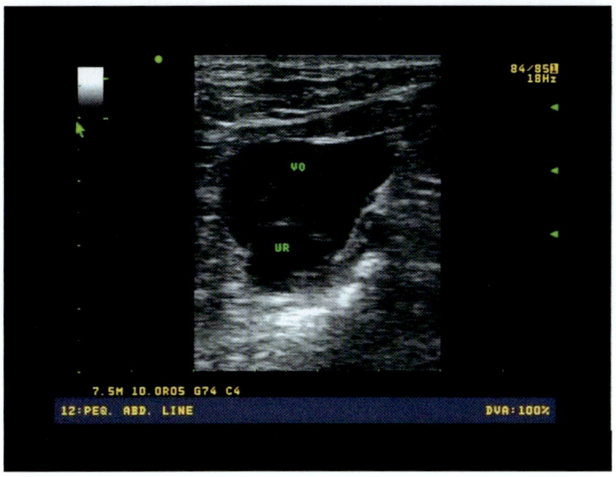


**Figure 6.69.** Focal cystic dilatation protruding towards the lumen of the bladder, and is compatible with a ureterocoele.

## Lower motor neuron (LMN) lesions

### Aetiopathogenesis

Conditions affecting the **spinal segments of the sacral area** cause areflexia of the detrusor muscle and sphincter reflexes, resulting in **urine retention** (because the detrusor muscle does not contract) and **incontinence due to overflow** of urine and lack of sphincter muscle function.

**Causes can be traumatic** (fractures / sacro-coccygeal dislocations, tail avulsion injury), inflammatory **compressive lesions** of the cauda equina, neoplasms, fibrocartilaginous embolism, etc. These types of urinary problem may also be due to certain peripheral neuropathies.

### Clinical signs

Affected animals have a **large bladder that is easy to empty by manual compression, and an absence of anal tone and perineal reflex**.

### Treatment

Correction of the inciting cause may improve urinary function in some cases. Many of these animals need to have their bladder intermittently emptied by manual expression or catheterization. **Bethanechol** can be used to increase detrusor contraction, although the evidence behind it is controversial. Treatment with **adrenergic antagonists** can be accompanied to reduce the urethral tone and favour emptying of the bladder (Table 6.26).

## Hyper-reflexia or detrusor muscle instability

### Clinical signs

Characterized by **involuntary contractions of the bladder** that result in frequent emptying of small amounts of urine.

### Aetiopathogenesis

It may be due to:

- UTI
- neoplasia
- urolithiasis.

Idiopathic, as it occurs in some cats with idiopathic cystitis. Although it is common in people, in dogs the idiopathic form is not fully understood. These could be dogs that lose the ability to store urine through the bladder and need to urinate more frequently in the absence of polyuria or an inflammatory cause.

### Treatment

Treatment with smooth muscle relaxants or α-adrenergic agonists can be attempted (Table 6.27).

## Detrusor atony

### Aetiopathogenesis

As a result of a **functional or mechanical obstruction**, **bladder over-tension** can occur, injuring the muscle fibres of the detrusor muscle.

Detrusor atony may also result from **LMN injury** from sacral or pelvic nerve lesions.

### Clinical signs

The animal has a **history of obstruction** followed by reflux and overflow incontinence. On palpation, a large bladder which is easily compressed is observed.

### Treatment

In some cases, detrusor muscle function can be restored by **keeping the bladder small (by catheterization) for a long period (about 2 weeks). Bethanechol** is indicated to stimulate detrusor muscle contraction, provided that the obstruction has been resolved beforehand. Other medications used for this purpose but with varying efficacy include cisapride and metoclopramide (Table 6.27).

## Reflex dys-synergia (detrusor–urethral dys-synergia)

### Aetiopathogenesis

In this condition there is a **lack of coordination** of the activating mechanisms for bladder emptying, so that when the detrusor muscle contracts, involuntary contraction of the external urethral sphincter or smooth muscle of the bladder neck and urethra occurs proximally.

The aetiology is not entirely clear, although it is believed to be caused by **lesions in the reticulospinal**

Table 6.27. Medications used in the management of urination disorders.

| Effect | Medication | Dose | Comments |
|---|---|---|---|
| **Increases urethral tone** | Phenylpropanol-amine | 1–1.5 mg/kg/8–12 h VO | α-Adrenergic agonist. Use with caution if there is hypertension, hyperadrenocorticism or kidney disease: may cause hypertension, gastrointestinal signs, anxiety |
| | Oestriol | 1 mg/dog/24 h VO and adjust treatment according to response | Natural short-acting oestrogen, which is why it does not cause myelosuppression. It can cause nausea and mild oestrogenic effects such as vulvar and mammary swelling and/or attraction to males |
| | DES (diethylstil-bestrol) | 0.1–1 mg/dog/24 hours 5–7 days, then weekly or as needed | Oestrogen. May cause myelosuppression, attraction to males, vulvar and mammary swelling, behavioural changes and prostatic metaplasia (in males) |
| | Testosterone cypionate | 2.2 mg/kg IM every 4–8 weeks | Androgen (used in some males with USMI). Can produce behavioural changes, aggressiveness, perianal adenomas and prostatic hyperplasia |
| **Reduces detrusor muscle contraction** | Propantheline | 0.25–0.5 mg/kg/8–12 h VO | Anticholinergic, antispasmodic |
| | Oxybutynin | 2–5 mg/8–12 h VO | Antispasmodic |
| **Stimulates detrusor muscle contraction** | Bethanechol | 2.5–15 mg/dog/8 h o 1.25–5 mg/cat/8 h VO | Parasympathomimetic. Use with a relaxed urethral sphincter. May cause vomiting |
| | Cisapride | **Dog**: 0.1–0.5 mg/kg/8–12 h VO **Cat**: 2.5–5 mg/cat/8–12 h VO | Increases the release of acetylcholine. May cause ataxia, gastrointestinal signs |
| **Decreases urethral tone (relaxant)** | Phenoxy-benzamine | **Dog**: 0.25 mg/kg/8–12 h VO **Cat**: 1.25–7.5 mg/cat/8–12 h VO | α-Adrenergic antagonist, relaxes smooth muscle. May cause hypotension and gastrointestinal signs |
| | Prazosin | **Dog**: 1 mg/15 kg/12–24 h VO or 0.03 mg/kg/8 h VO **Cat**: 0.25–0.5 mg/12–24 h VO | α-Adrenergic antagonist, relaxes smooth muscle. May cause hypotension |
| | Tamsulosin | 0.01–0.2 mg/kg/24 h VO (up to 1 mg/dog/24 h) | α-Adrenergic antagonist, relaxes smooth muscle. May cause hypotension |
| | Diazepam | **Dog**: 2–10 mg/dog/8 h VO or 30 min before urinating | Relaxes skeletal muscle. May cause sedation and ataxia. Do not use in cats because of risk of liver necrosis |
| | Dantrolene | **Dog**: 1–5 mg/kg/8 h VO Cat: 0.5–2 mg/kg/8 h VO | Relaxes skeletal muscle. Do not use in animals with liver dysfunction |

**tract** or in the caudal mesenteric nodes, which alter the inhibitory signals that allow the urethral sphincter to relax.

### Epidemiology

It is more frequent in large-breed male dogs.

### Clinical signs

These patients begin to urinate and **flow of urine is interrupted**, with several attempts without completely emptying the bladder. Neurological examination is normal, unlike those with UMN lesions.

### Diagnosis

Presumptive diagnosis can be made by observing the said pattern of urination, large residual volumes of urine, catheterizations without difficulty and ruling out a mechanical obstruction.

### Treatment

**α-Adrenergic antagonists** can be administered to decrease sympathetic tone, as well as skeletal muscle relaxants (Table 6.26).

## UMN injury

### Aetiopathogenesis

**Spinal lesions above the sacral** segments can produce detrusor areflexia and hypertonia of the urethral sphincter, impeding bladder emptying, which appears **large, spastic and difficult to compress**.

### Clinical signs

Urethral tone and sacral reflexes are normal, but paralysis or **paralysis of the hind limbs** is frequently observed.

### Treatment

When managing these cases the cause must be corrected, which usually leads to partial or complete resolution of urinary retention in days to weeks, during which time intermittent bladder catheterization and medical treatment to relax the urethra may be necessary (Table 6.26).

### Dysautonomia

Dysautonomia is a **rare disease of unknown aetiology** (neurotoxicity is suspected) in which there is an autonomic nervous system (ANS) dysfunction. Affected animals have various changes in autonomic ANS-dependent functions, including **urinary retention** due to bladder atony and **overflow incontinence**. The **prognosis is reserved**, although mild cases may improve with cholinergic drugs.

## Bibliography

### Upper urinary tract pathologies

Bexfield, N.H., Heiene, R., Gerritsen, R.J., Risøen, U., Eliassen, K.E., Herrtage, M.H. et al. (2008) Glomerular filtration rate estimated by 3-sample plasma clearance of iohexol in 118 healthy dogs. *Journal of Veterinary Internal Medicine* 22, 66–73.

Braff, J., Obare, E., Yerramilli, M., Elliott, J. and Yerramilli, M. (2014) Relationship between serum symmetric dimethylarginine concentration and glomerular filtration rate in cats. *Journal of Veterinary Internal Medicine* 28(6), 1699–1701.

Brown, N., Segev, G., Francey, T., Kass, P. and Cowgill, L.D. (2015) Glomerular filtration rate, urine production, and fractional clearance of electrolytes in acute kidney injury in dogs and their association with survival. *Journal of Veterinary Internal Medicine* 29, 28–34.

Brown, S., Atkins, C., Bagley, R., Carr, A., Cowgill, L., Davidson, M. et al. (2007) Guidelines for the identification, evaluation and management of systemic hypertension in dogs and cats. *Journal of Veterinary Internal Medicine* 21, 542–558.

Callens, A.J. and Bartges, J.W. (2015) Urinalysis. *Veterinary Clinics of North America Small Animal Practice* 45, 621–637.

Cianciolo, R.E., Brown, C.A., Mohr, F.C., Spangler, W.L., Aresu, L., van der Lugt, J.J. et al. (2013) Pathologic evaluation of canine renal biopsies: methods for identifying features that differentiate immune-mediated glomerulonephritides from other categories of glomerular diseases. *Journal of Veterinary Internal Medicine* 27 (Suppl. 1), S10–18.

Cianciolo, R.E., Mohr, F.C. and Aresu, L. (2016) World Small Animal Veterinary Association Renal Pathology Initiative: classification of glomerular diseases in dogs. *Veterinary Pathology* 53(1), 113–135.

Cowgill, L.D. and Segev, G. (2014) What biomarkers are useful with acute kidney injury, if any? *Proceedings of Advanced Renal Therapies Symposium*.

DiBartola, S.P. (2010) Clinical approach and laboratory evaluation of renal disease. In: Ettinger, S.J. and Feldman, E.C. (eds) *Textbook of Veterinary Internal Medicine*, 7th edn. Saunders Elsevier, Missouri, pp. 1955–1968.

Elliot, J. and Watson, D.J. (2014) Chronic kidney disease: International Renal Interest Society staging and management. In: Bonagura, J.D. and Twedt, D.C. (eds) *Kirk's Current Veterinary Therapy XV*. Saunders Elsevier, Missouri, pp. 857–863.

Finch, N.C., Heiene, R., Elliott, J., Syme, H.M. and Peters, A.M. (2013) A single sample method for estimating glomerular filtration rate in cats. *Journal of Veterinary Internal Medicine* 27(4), 782–790.

Ghys, L., Paepe, D., Smets, P., Lefebvre, H., Delanghe, J., Daminet, S. and Cystatin, C. (2014) A new renal marker and its potential use in small animal medicine. *Journal of Veterinary Internal Medicine* 28(4), 1152–1164.

Hall, J.A., Yerramilli, M., Obare, E., Yerramilli, M. and Jewell, D.E. (2014) Comparison of serum concentrations of symmetric dimethylarginine and creatinine as kidney function biomarkers in cats with chronic kidney disease. *Journal of Veterinary Internal Medicine* 28(6), 1676–1683.

Hecht, S. (2014) Applications of ultrasound in diagnosis and management of urinary disease. In: Bonagura, J.D. and Twedt, D.C. (eds) *Kirk's Current Veterinary Therapy XV*. Saunders Elsevier, Missouri, pp. 840–845.

IRIS Canine GN Study Group Diagnosis Subgroup, Littman, M.P., Daminet, S., Grauer, G.F., Lees, G.E. and van Dongen, A.M. (2013) Consensus recommendations for the diagnostic investigation of dogs with suspected glomerular disease. *Journal of Veterinary Internal Medicine* 27(S1), S19–26.

IRIS Canine GN Study Group Standard Therapy Subgroup, Brown, S., Elliott, J., Francey, T., Polzin, D. and Vaden, S. (2013) Consensus recommendations for standard therapy of glomerular disease in dogs. *Journal of Veterinary Internal Medicine* 27(S1), S27–43.

IRIS Canine GN Study Group Established Pathology Subgroup, Segev, G., Cowgill, L.D., Heiene, R., Labato, M.A. and Polzin, D.J. (2013) Consensus recommendations for immunosuppressive treatment of dogs with glomerular disease based on established pathology. *Journal of Veterinary Internal Medicine* 27(S1), S44–54.

IRIS Canine GN Study Subgroup on Immunosuppressive Therapy Absent a Pathologic Diagnosis, Pressler, B., Vaden, S., Gerber, B., Langston, C. and Polzin, D. (2013) Consensus guidelines for immunosuppressive treatment of dogs with glomerular disease absent a pathologic diagnosis. *Journal of Veterinary Internal Medicine* 27(S1), S55–59.

IRIS Glomerular Disease Study Group, Goldstein, R.E., Brovida, C., Fernández-Del Palacio, M.J., Littman, M.P., Polzin, D.J., Zatelli, A. and Cowgill, L.D. (2013) Consensus recommendations for treatment for dogs with serology positive glomerular disease. *Journal of Veterinary Internal Medicine* 27(S1), S60–66.

Jacob, F., Polzin, D.J., Osborne, C.A. et al. (2005) Evaluation of the association between initial proteinuria and morbidity rate or death in dogs with naturally occurring chronic renal failure. *Journal of the American Veterinary Medical Association* 226(3), 393–400.

Keir, I. and Kellum, J.A. (2015) Acute kidney injury in severe sepsis: Pathophysiology, diagnosis, and treatment recommendations. State of the art review. *Journal of Veterinary Emergency and Critical Care (San Antonio)* 25(2), 200–209.

Klosterman, E.S., Moore, G.E., de Brito Galvao, J.F., DiBartola, S.P., Groman, R.P., Whittemore, J.C. et al. (2011) Comparison of signalment, clinicopathologic findings, histologic diagnosis, and prognosis in dogs with glomerular disease with or without nephrotic syndrome. *Journal of Veterinary Internal Medicine* 25, 206–214.

Korman, R. and White, J. (2013) Feline CKD. Current therapies – what is achievable? *Journal of Feline Medicine and Surgery* 15(S1), 29–44.

Langston, C. (2010) Acute uremia. In: Ettinger, S.J. and Feldman, E.C. (eds) *Textbook of Veterinary Internal Medicine*, 7th edn. Saunders Elsevier, Missouri, pp. 1968–1984.

Langston, C. (2012) Managing fluid and electrolyte disorders in renal failure. In: DiBartola, S.P. (ed.) *Fluid, Electrolyte, and Acid–Base Disorders*. Saunders Elsevier, Missouri, pp. 544–556.

Lees, G.E., Brown, A., Elliot, J. et al. (2005) Assessment and management of proteinuria in dogs and cats: 2005 ACVIM Forum Consensus Statement (Small Animal). *Journal of Veterinary Internal Medicine* 19, 377–385.

Monaghan, K., Nolan, B. and Labato, M. (2012) *Feline acute kidney injury. Pathophysiology, etiology and etiology-specific management considerations. Journal of Feline Medicine and Surgery* 14, 775–784.

Monaghan, K., Nolan, B. and Labato, M. (2012) Feline acute kidney injury. 2. Approach to diagnosis, treatment and prognosis. *Journal of Feline Medicine and Surgery* 14, 785–793.

Nielsen, L.K., Bracker, K. and Price, L.L. (2015) Administration of fenoldopam in critically ill small animal patients with acute kidney injury: 28 dogs and 34 cats (2008–2012). *Journal of Veterinary Emergency and Critical Care (San Antonio)* 25(3), 396–404.

Polzin, D.J. (2010) Chronic kidney disease. In: Ettinger, S.J. and Feldman, E.C. (eds). *Textbook of Veterinary Internal Medicine*, 7th edn. Saunders Elsevier, Missouri, pp. 1990–2020.

Polzin, D.J. and Cowgill, L.D. (2013) Development of clinical guidelines for management of glomerular disease in dog. *Journal of Veterinary Internal Medicine* 27, S2–S4.

Pressler, B.M. (2013) Clinical approach to advanced renal function in dogs and cats. *Veterinary Clinics of North America Small Animal Practice* 43(6), 1193–1208.

Quimby, J. (2015) Evidence-based treatment of chronic renal disease in cats. *ACVIM Forum Proceedings, June 3–6, Indianapolis.*

Ross, L. (2014) Medical management of acute kidney injury. In: Bonagura, J.D. and Twedt, D.C. (eds) *Kirk's Current Veterinary Therapy XV*. Saunders Elsevier, Missouri, pp. 868–871.

Schneider, S.M., Cianciolo, R.E., Nabity, M.B., Clubb, F.J. Jr, Brown, C.A. and Lees, G.E. (2013) Prevalence of immune-complex glomerulonephritides in dogs biopsied for suspected glomerular disease: 501 cases (2007–2012). *Journal of Veterinary Internal Medicine* 27(S1), S67–75.

Vaden, S.L., Levine, J. and Breitschwerdt, E.B. (1997) A retrospective case-control of acute renal failure in 99 dogs. *Journal of Veterinary Internal Medicine* 11, 58–64.

Vaden, S.L. (2010) Glomerular diseases. In: Ettinger, S.J. and Feldman, E.C. (eds) *Textbook of Veterinary Internal Medicine*, 7th edn. Saunders Elsevier, Missouri, pp. 2021–2035.

Vaden, S.J. and Pressler, B.M. (2014) Glomerular disease and nephrotic syndrome. In: Bonagura, J.D. and Twedt, D.C. (eds) *Kirk's Current Veterinary Therapy XV*. Saunders Elsevier, Missouri, pp. 853–857.

http://www.iris-kidney.com

## *Lower urinary tract pathologies*

Adams, L.G. and Syme, H.M. (2010) Canine ureteral and lower urinary tract diseases. In: Ettinger, S.J. and Feldman, E.C. (eds) *Textbook of Veterinary Internal Medicine*, 7th edn. Elsevier Saunders, Missouri, pp. 2086–2115.

Allen, H.S., Swecker, W.S., Becvarova, I., Weeth, L.P. and werre, S.R. (2015) Associations of diet and breed with recurrence of calcium oxalate cystic calculi in dogs. *Journal of the American Veterinary Medical Association* 246(10), 1098–1103.

Bailiff, N.L., Westropp, J.L., Jang, S.S. et al. (2005) *Corynebacterium urealyticum* urinary tract infection in dogs and cats: 7 cases (1996–2003). *Journal of the American Veterinary Medical Association* 226, 1676–1680.

Bartges, J.W. and Callens, A.J. (2015) Congenital diseases of the lower urinary tract. *Veterinary Clinics of North America Small Animal Practice* 45, 703–720.

Bartges, J.W. and Callens, A.J. (2015) Urolithiasis. *Veterinary Clinics of North America Small Animal Practice* 45, 747–768.

Buffington, CA. (2011) Idiopathic cystitis in domestic cats – beyond the lower urinary tract. *Journal of Veterinary Internal Medicine* 25(4), 784–796.

Byron, J.K. (2015) Micturition disorders. *Veterinary Clinics of North America Small Animal Practice* 45(4), 769–782.

Carney, H.C., Little, S., Brownlee-Tomasso, D., Harvey, A.M., Mattox, E., Robertson, S., Rucinsky, R. and Manley, D.S. (2012) AAFP and ISFM Feline-Friendly Nursing Care Guidelines. *Journal of Feline Medicine and Surgery* 14, 337.

Chew, D.J., Buffington, C.A.T., Kendall, M.S. et al. (1998) Amitriptyline treatment for severe recurrent idiopathic cystitis in cats. *Journal of the American Veterinary Medical Association* 213, 1282–1286.

Coates, J.R. (2004) Neurogenic micturition disorders. *Proceedings of the ACVIM Forum Congress 2004, Minneapolis.*

Defarges, A., Dunn, M. and Berent, A. (2013) New alternatives for minimally invasive management of uroliths: lower urinary tract uroliths. *Compendium of Continuing Education in Veterinary Medicine* 35(1), E1.

Defauw, P.A.M., Van de Maele, I., Ducateau, L., Polis, I.E., Saunders, J.H. and Daminet, S. (2011) Risk factors and clinical presentation of cats with feline idiopathic cystitis. *Journal of Feline Medicine and Surgery* 13, 967–975.

Drobatz, K.J. (2009) Urethral obstruction in cats. In: Bonagura, J.D., David, C. and Twedt, D.C. (eds) *Current Veterinary Therapy XIV*. Saunders Elsevier, Missouri, pp. 951–954.

Forrester, S.D. and Roudebush, P. (2007) Evidence-based management of feline lower urinary tract disease. *Veterinary Clinics of North America Small Animal Practice* 37, 533–558.

Francey, T. (2010) Prostatic diseases. In: Ettinger, S.J. and Feldman, E.C. (eds) *Textbook of Veterinary Internal Medicine*, 7th edn. Elsevier, Missouri, pp. 2047–2058.

Galluzzi, F., De Rensis, F., Menozzi, A. and Spattini, G. (2012) Effect of intraurethral administration of atracurium besylate in male cats with urethral plugs. *Journal of Small Animal Practice* 53(7), 411–415.

Gerber, B., Boretti, F.S., Kley, S., Laluha, P., Müller, C., Sieber, N. et al. (2005) Evaluation of clinical signs and causes of lower urinary tract disease in European cats. *Journal of Small Animal Practice* 46, 571–577.

Grant, D.C., Harper, T.A. and Werre, S.R. (2010) Frequency of incomplete urolith removal, complications, and diagnostic imaging following cystotomy for removal of uroliths from the lower urinary in dogs: 128 cases (1994–2006). *Journal of the American Veterinary Medical Association* 236, 763–766.

Gunn-Moore, D.A. (2003) Proceedings of the ESFM Feline Congress, Stockholm, September 2002, feline lower urinary tract disease. *Journal of Feline Medicine and Surgery* 5, 133–138.

Hamaide, A. (2014) Medical management of urinary incontinence and retention disorders. In: Bonagura, J.D. and Twedt, D.C. (eds) *Kirk's Current Veterinary Therapy XV*. Saunders Elsevier, Missouri, pp. 915–919.

Hostutler, R.A., Chew, D.J., Eaton, K.A. and DiBartola, S.P. (2004) Cystoscopic appearance of proliferative urethritis in 2 dogs before and after treatment. *Journal of Veterinary Internal Medicine* 18, 113–116.

Hostutler, R.A., Chew, D.J. and DiBartola, S.P. (2005) Recent concepts in feline lower urinary tract disease. *Veterinary Clinics of North America Small Animal Practice* 35, 147–170.

Kirck, C.A., Jewell, D.E. and Lowry, S.R. (2006) Effect of sodium chloride on selected parameters in cats. *Veterinary Therapeutics* 7, 333–336.

Kruger, J.M., Osborne, C.A. and Lulich, J.P. (2009) Changing paradigms of feline idiopathic cystitis. *Veterinary Clinics of North America Small Animal Practice* 39, 15–40.

Labato, M.A. and Acierno, M.J. (2010) Micturition disorders and urinary incontinence. In: Ettinger, S.J. and Feldman, E.C. (eds) *Textbook of Veterinary Internal Medicine*, 7th edn. Saunders Elsevier, Missouri, pp. 160–164.

Lulich, J. and Osborne, C. (2009) Incomplete urolith removal: prevention, detection, and correction. In: Bonagura, J.D. and Twedt, D.C. (eds) *Kirk's Current Veterinary Therapy XIV*. Saunders Elsevier, Missouri, pp. 936–939.

Lulich, J.P. and Osborne, C.A. (2009) Changing paradigms in the diagnosis of urolithiasis. *Veterinary Clinics of North America Small Animal Practice* 39, 79–91.

Lulich, J.P., Berent, A.C., Adams, L.G., Westropp, J.L., Bartges, J.W. and Osborne, C.A. (2016) ACVIM Small Animal Consensus Recommendations on the Treatment and Prevention of Uroliths in Dogs and Cats. *Journal of Veterinary Internal Medicine* 30, 1564–1574.

Martinez, I., Mattoon, J.S., Eaton, K.A., Chew, D.J. and DiBartola, S.P. (2003) Polypoid cystitis in 17 dogs (1978–2001). *Journal of Veterinary Internal Medicine* 17, 499–509.

Neilson, J.C. (2003) Feline house soiling: elimination and marking behaviours. *Veterinary Clinics of North America Small Animal Practice* 33, 287–301.

Nizanski, W., Levy, X., Ochota, M. and Pasikowska, J. (2014) Pharmacological treatment for common prostatic condition in dogs – benign prostatic hyperplasia and prostatitis: an andate. *Reproduction in Domestic Animals* 49(S2), 8–15.

Olin, S.J. and Bartges, J.W. (2015) Urinary tract infections: treatment/comparative therapeutics. *Veterinary Clinics of North America Small Animal Practice* 45(4), 721–746.

Osborne, C.A., Kruger, J.M., Lulich, J.P., Johnston, G.R., Polzin, D.J., Ulrich, L.K. et al. (1996) Prednisolone therapy of idiopathic feline lower urinary tract disease: a double-blind clinical study. *Veterinary Clinics of North America Small Animal Practice* 26, 563–569.

Osborne, C.A., Lulich, J.P., Swanson, L.L. and Albasan, H. (2009) Drug-induced urolithiasis. *Veterinary Clinics of North America Small Animal Practice* 39(1), 55–63.

Pressler, B. and Bartges, W. (2010) Urinary tract infections. In: Ettinger, S.J. and Feldman, E.C. (eds) *Textbook of Veterinary Internal Medicine*, 7th edn. Saunders Elsevier, Missouri, pp. 2036–2046.

Sirinarumitr, K. (2014) Benign prostatic hypertrophy and prostatitis in dogs. In: Bonagura, J.D. and Twedt, D.C. (eds) *Kirk's Current Veterinary Therapy XV*. Saunders Elsevier, Missouri, pp. 1012–1015.

Smee, N., Loyd, K. and Grauer, G. (2013) UTIs in small animal patients: Part 1: Etiology and pathogenesis. *Journal of the American Veterinary Medical Association* 49(1), 1–7.

Smee, N., Loyd, K. and Grauer, G. (2013) UTIs in small animal patients: Part 2: Diagnosis, treatment and complications. *Journal of the American Veterinary Medical Association* 49(2), 83–94.

Stella, J.L., Lord, L.K. and Buffington, C.A. (2011) Sickness behaviors in response to unusual external events in healthy cats and cats with feline interstitial cystitis. *Journal of the American Veterinary Medical Association* 238(1), 67–73.

Suarez, M. (2013) Urolitiasis en perros y gatos: cómo acabar con la cantera. *Proceedings de Formación Continuada Medicina Interna AVEPA, 2013.*

Weese, J.S., Blondeau, J., Boothe, D., Guardabassi, L.G., Gumley, N., Papich, M., Jessen, L.R., Lappin, M., Rankin, S., Westropp, J.L., Sykes, J. (2019) International Society for Companion Animal Infectious Diseases (ISCAID) guidelines for the diagnosis and management of bacterial urinary tract infections in dogs and cats. *The Veterinary Journal* 247, 8–25.

Weese, J.S., Blondeau, J.M., Boothe, D., Breitschwerdt, E.B., Guardabassi, L., Hillier, A. et al. (2011) Antimicrobial use guideline for treatment of urinary tract disease in dogs and cats: Antimicrobial Guidelines Working Group of the International Society for Companion Animal Infectious Diseases. *Veterinary Medicine International* 263768. https://doi.org/10.4061/2011/263768.

Westropp, J.L., Welk, K.A. and Buffington, C.A. (2003) Small adrenal glands in cats with feline interstitial cystitis. *Journal of Urology* 170, 2494–2497.

Westropp, J.L., Kass, P.H. and Buffington, CA. (2007) In vivo evaluation of alpha (2)-adrenoceptors in cats with idiopathic cystitis. *American Journal of Veterinary Research* 68, 203–207.

Zezza, L., Reusch, C.E. and Gerber, B. (2012) Intravesical application of lidocaine and sodium bicarbonate in the treatment of obstructive idiopathic lower urinary tract disease in cats. *Journal of Veterinary Internal Medicine* 26(3), 526–531.

The indoor cat initiative. www.vet.ohio-state.edu/indoorcat.

## Test

### Upper urinary tract pathologies

1. **Which answer is incorrect?**
   A) Urine density may be low when there is post-renal azotaemia.
   B) Hypo-adrenocorticism can cause post-renal azotaemia.
   C) Response to fluid therapy and urine density can help differentiate between pre-renal and renal azotaemia.
   D) Urine density is low in cases of renal azotaemia.
2. **Azotaemia is:**
   A) The combination of clinical signs presented by patients with kidney disease.
   B) A change seen on laboratory tests that implies a primary renal dysfunction.
   C) Elevated levels of urea and creatinine in blood.
   D) The change that indicates glomerular injury.
3. **Which statement is correct?**
   A) Urea comes from the catabolism of proteins.
   B) Creatinine comes from the catabolism of proteins.
   C) The relationship between creatinine and the glomerular filtration rate is curvilinear.
   D) Urea levels may be affected by factors which are non-renal in origin.
4. **Which statement is correct?**
   A) In a dehydrated patient a UD of 1.015 indicates a good ability to concentrate urine.
   B) A patient with a UD <1.008 has renal failure.
   C) A patient with a UD of 1.010 may have renal failure.
   D) A UD >1.035 indicates azotaemia of renal origin.
5. **Which statement is correct?**
   A) The normal UPC in the cat is <1.
   B) The normal UPC in the cat is <0.5.
   C) The normal UPC in the dog is <0.5.
   D) The normal UPC in the dog is <0.4.
6. **What statement with regards to SDMA is incorrect?**
   A) It comes from amino acid metabolism.
   B) Muscle mass interferes with SDMA values.
   C) It has recently been added to the IRIS classification for CKD.
   D) It is specific for kidney disease and increases before creatinine.
7. **Which of these tests is the most accurate for estimation of GFR?**
   A) Creatinine.
   B) SDMA.
   C) Urine specific gravity.
   D) Plasma clearance of iohexol.
8. **Renal biopsy is contraindicated in:**
   A) Advanced IRIS stage IV kidney disease in a uraemic patient.
   B) Acute renal failure.
   C) Severe persistent proteinuria in a non-azotaemic patient.
   D) Chronic renal disease in a young patient.
9. **Which statement is false?**
   A) Animals with AKD are classified by IRIS stages I, II, III and IV.
   B) The classification of AKD represents a specific moment in the course of the disease.
   C) Ethylene glycol can produce AKD.
   D) Aminoglycosides can produce AKD.
10. **Which statement is true?**
    A) Leptospirosis with kidney involvement always presents with azotaemia.
    B) The bacteria most frequently involved in pyelonephritis are Gram-positive.
    C) Ischaemia is the most frequent cause of AKD.
    D) Patients with AKD never recover renal function.

**11. Which statement is correct?**

A) Chronic kidney disease is the most frequent cause of hypercalcaemia.

B) Fluoroquinolones have good penetration in renal tissue.

C) A negative urinary culture excludes the possibility of pyelonephritis.

D) In ethylene glycol poisoning, hypercalcaemia can be detected.

**12. Which of the following relationships is incorrect?**

A) Ethylene glycol/hypo-echogenic corticomedullary band in kidney on ultrasound.

B) Renal asymmetry/ureteral obstruction.

C) Leucocytosis/hypo-adrenocorticism.

D) Hyperkalaemia/anuria.

**13. Which of the following relationships is incorrect?**

A) Shar Pei/renal amyloidosis.

B) West Highland White Terrier/polycystic kidney disease.

C) Persian cat/polycystic kidney disease.

D) Acute kidney disease/secondary renal hyperparathyroidism.

**14. Which statement is true?**

A) A renal diet is indicated in all patients with CKD.

B) The first choice of drug for the control of systemic hypertension in cats is benazepril.

C) ACEIs are contraindicated in dehydrated patients.

D) ACEIs are not indicated as the first choice of antihypertensives in dogs.

**15. Which statement is false?**

A) Fever can cause proteinuria.

B) The proteinuria of renal origin is always glomerular.

C) Selectivity of the glomerular filtration barrier is determined by molecular size and electrical charge.

D) Proteinuria is a marker of prognosis and severity in CKD.

**16. Which statement is false?**

A) ACEIs reduce the pressure in the afferent arterioles of the glomerulus.

B) Telmisartan inhibits angiotensin receptors.

C) Clopidogrel can be used in the prevention of thromboembolism.

D) Amlodipine is a calcium channel blocker used as an antihypertensive agent in cats.

### Lower urinary tract pathologies

**1. Which statement is true?**

A) The presence of crystalluria indicates urolithiasis.

B) The presence of pyuria indicates urinary tract infection.

C) The most common uroliths are cystine and silica.

D) In stored urine crystals can form *in vitro*.

**2. Point out which relationship is incorrect**

A) Hyperuricosuria/Dalmatian.

B) Urine infection/struvite urolithiasis.

C) Portosystemic shunt/purine urolithiasis.

D) Hypokalaemia/urinary obstruction.

**3. Which statement is true?**

A) Calcium oxalate uroliths can be dissolved with dietary treatment.

B) Antegrade hydropropulsion is indicated in cases of urethral obstruction.

C) In cats, 95% of struvite uroliths are sterile.

D) Dietary control is indicated for the prevention of urolithiasis due to struvite associated with UTI.

**4. What relationship is incorrect?**

A) Calcium oxalate/alkaline urine.

B) Purine/acid urine.

C) Struvite/alkaline urine.

D) Cystine/acidic urine.

**5. Which statement is false?**

A) Tiopronin is indicated in cystine urolithiasis.
B) Allopurinol can cause cystine urolithiasis.
C) Allopurinol is indicated in purine urolithiasis.
D) Sulphonamides can cause urolithiasis.

**6. Which statement is false?**

A) Canine transitional cell carcinoma locates preferentially in the trigone of the bladder.
B) Bladder polyps are more frequently located in the cranioventral area of the bladder.
C) The clinical presentation is sufficient to differentiate between proliferative urethritis and neoplasia, since urinary obstruction is rare in the former.
D) Cyclophosphamide can cause haemorrhagic cystitis.

**7. Which statement is false?**

A) *Escherichia coli* is the bacterial species most frequently involved in UTI.
B) The presence of an ectopic ureter may predispose to UTI.
C) Urinary infections caused by *Candida albicans* are very frequent in dogs.
D) An inactive urinary sediment does not rule out the presence of UTI.

**8. Which statement is true?**

A) All animals with UTI show signs of urination due to irritation.
B) In the physical examination of a patient with UTI, digital vaginal examination is important.
C) The presence of nitrites on the urine strip confirms the presence of a UTI.
D) To perform a urine culture, it is best to collect the urine sample using spontaneous urination.

**9. Which statement is false?**

A) Quinolones are indicated as the first choice of antibiotic in a simple UTI.
B) The use of urinary catheters may favour the appearance of UTIs.
C) Quinolones are indicated in UTIs in non-neutered males.
D) In cases of complicated UTIs, 30–60 days of antibiotic treatment is recommended.

**10. Which statement is true with regard to a cat with signs of lower urinary tract problems?**

A) Antibiotics are always indicated, since UTIs are very common in the cat.
B) Idiopathic cystitis is a very rare cause of signs of irritative urination in the cat.
C) The diagnosis of feline idiopathic cystitis should always be made by cystoscopy and biopsy.
D) 15% of cats with idiopathic cystitis may have a chronic form, with longer duration of signs and/or continuous recurrences.

**11. Which option is not indicated in the treatment of prostatic hyperplasia?**

A) Osaterone acetate.
B) Deslorelin.
C) Aglepristone.
D) Castration.

**12. Which statement is false?**

A) The sympathetic system facilitates storage of urine.
B) The parasympathetic system facilitates storage in the bladder.
C) The pelvic, pudendal and hypogastric nerves are important for controlling urination.
D) In a cranial spinal lesion at L7, a spastic bladder which is difficult to empty by manual pressure will be seen.

**13. Which statement is false?**

A) A dog with USMI usually urinates normally but has urinary incontinence especially while lying down.
B) Oestrogens such as diethylstilboestrol can cause myelosuppression.
C) In patients with urinary incontinence and an intra-pelvic bladder, a colposuspension may be performed to help manage it.
D) In a dog castrated with USMI, treatment with β-adrenergic drugs can be attempted.

**14. Which statement is false?**

A) Bethanechol may be indicated in animals with detrusor muscle injury.
B) With a detrusor muscle injury, a small bladder can be felt on palpation.
C) Reflex dys-synergia is more common in large-breed male dogs.
D) Severe bladder distention may result in detrusor muscle injury.

**15. Which statement is false?**

A) With an upper motor neuron lesion, a large bladder which is difficult to empty using manual pressure will be seen.
B) With a lower motor neuron lesion, a large bladder which is easy to empty using manual pressure will be seen.
C) A patient with a lumbar disc herniation may have urinary retention.
D) Detrusor muscle atony can occur as a result of an upper motor neuron injury.

**16. What relationship is incorrect?**

A) Prazosin/increases urethral tone.
B) Propantheline/reduces detrusor muscle contraction.
C) Phenylpropanolamine/increases urethral tone.
D) Diazepam/decreases urethral tone.

## Clinical case 1

**Signalment**: 6-year-old cross-breed dog, 8.1 kg.

**Reason for consultation**: Progressive weight loss in recent months. PU/PD. Intermittent bilious vomiting and loss of appetite 3 weeks ago. Last few days, weaker, barely moves.

**Physical examination**: Body condition 2/9 (8.1 kg); 37.8°C. Pale, somewhat dry mucous membranes. Cardiopulmonary auscultation normal (180 bpm). Discomfort on abdominal palpation (probable splenomegaly). Mild generalized lymphadenopathy.

Table Case 1.1 Complete blood count and biochemistry

| Parameter | Value | Reference range |
|---|---|---|
| RBC × 106/μl | 1.94 | 5.65–8.87 |
| HGB (g/dl) | 4.1 | 13.1–20.5 |
| HCT (%) | 11.6 | 37.3–61.7 |
| MCV (fl) | 59.8 | 61.6–73.5 |
| MCHC (g/dl) | 35.3 | 32.0–37.9 |
| MCH (pg) | 21.1 | 21.2–25.9 |
| % RETIC | 0.7 | |
| RETIC (K/μl) | 13.0 | 10.0–110 |
| WBC /μl | 6.63 | 5.05–16.76 |
| LYM /μl | 2.03 | 1.05–5.10 |
| MONO /μl | 0.46 | 0.16–1.12 |
| NEU /μl | 4.02 | 2.95–11.64 |
| EOS /μl | 0.12 | 0.06–1.23 |
| BASO /μl | 0.00 | 0.00–0.10 |
| PLT × 103 /μl | 44 | 148–484 |

| Parameter | Value | Reference range |
|---|---|---|
| Chol (mg/dl) | 153 | 110–320 |
| Alb (g/dl) | 2.9 | 2.3–4.0 |
| TP (g/dl) | >12 | 5.2–8.2 |
| Ca (mg/dl) | 10.7 | 67.9–12.0 |
| Phos (mg/dl) | 15.2 | 2.5–6.8 |
| Crea (mg/dl) | 2.8 | 0.5–1.8 |
| BUN (mg/dl) | >130 | 7–27 |
| Glu (mg/dl) | 7 | 70–143 |
| ALT (UI/l) | 37 | <50 |
| AST (UI/l) | 65 | <50 |
| GGT (UI/l) | 1.2 | 1–6.5 |
| FAL (UI/l) | 190 | 30–120 |
| Cl (mmol/l) | 109 | 109–122 |
| K (mmol/l) | 5.1 | 3.5–5.8 |
| Na (mmol/l) | 151 | 144–160 |

### Urinalysis

Urinary density: 1.022.

Urine test strip: pH (5.5), protein (++++), leukocytes (negative), glucose (negative), ketones (negative), bilirubin (negative), erythrocytes (+).

Urine sediment: inactive.

Urine culture: negative.

**Blood pressure** (Doppler technique): 155 mmHg

### Abdominal ultrasound

Diffuse splenomegaly with normal to reduced echogenicity.

Increased renal cortical echogenicity, conservation of renal structure.

Rest of the abdomen without noticeable changes.

1. **What is the most accurate interpretation of the tests carried out based on the results and information from the medical history and physical examination?**
   A) The dog has azotaemia of pre-renal origin.
   B) The dog has azotaemia of postrenal origin.
   C) The dog has a urinary obstruction.
   D) The dog has azotaemia of renal origin.
2. **From the results of the urinalysis, which statement is true?**
   A) Proteinuria is not significant.
   B) The urine is adequately concentrated.
   C) Proteinuria should be quantified with a urine protein/creatinine ratio.
   D) Evaluation of urinary sediment is not necessary once proteinuria has been evaluated.
3. **Regarding the classification for kidney disease in this patient, which statement is true?**
   A) The patient has chronic kidney disease which is IRIS stage IV.
   B) The patient has chronic non-proteinuric IRIS stage III kidney disease.
   C) The patient should be hydrated, before defining the renal stage, with creatinine levels already stabilized.
   D) If the UPC ratio was 4, this patient is considered non-proteinuric.
4. **Indicate the correct statement regarding blood pressure in this patient:**
   A) Patient is hypertensive:
   B) The blood pressure measurement should be repeated later.
   C) Treatment with aldosterone-converting enzyme inhibitor drugs should be initiated.
   D) Treatment with aldosterone and amlodipine-converting enzyme inhibitor drugs should be initiated.
5. **What tests would be indicated in this patient?**
   A) Renal biopsy as soon as possible.
   B) Serology for leishmaniasis and bone marrow and/or lymph node biopsy.
   C) Dexamethasone suppression test to rule out hyperadrenocorticism.
   D) Digestive endoscopy.
6. **Which of these treatments is not indicated in this patient?**
   A) Furosemide and dopamine infusion.
   B) Initial stabilization (monitored fluid therapy, assessment of need for blood transfusion).
   C) Supportive therapy (antiemetics, antacids). Subsequently, renal diet and ACEIs, adding phosphorus chelates later according to serum phosphorus levels in successive check-ups.
   D) Treatment of the cause of kidney disease (leishmanicidal treatment since amastigotes of leishmania in bone marrow and elevated serum antibody titre) are identified.

## Clinical case 2

**Signalment**: 7-month-old, female, un-neutered Golden Retriever.

**Reason for consultation**: Less active over the last few weeks and, over the last few days, is urinating small amounts frequently, sometimes with some blood.

She is now smaller than the rest of the litter. She has an appetite although she is not very 'greedy'. Since they have had the puppy, she dribbles urine all the time and stains the bed where she sleeps. When taken out for a walk she adopts a normal position and urinates normally. The owners do not know how much she drinks because she shares a drinking fountain with another dog. She was prescribed a syrup with phenylpropanolamine, but the owners did not notice any difference in the urine and they are no longer administering it. When she was younger the owners were told that she had a urine infection. Has not appeared to be in season yet.

Lives in a flat with a balcony, with another dog. Bought in a pet shop. First vaccinated 2 months before. Periodic internal and external parasite treatments. Eats dry dog food.

**Physical exam**: Body condition 4/9 (16 kg), 37.8°C. Vital signs and cardiopulmonary auscultation without changes. Rear area around the vulva, wet with traces of urine. No changes to the vulva. Abdominal palpation normal (distended bladder cannot be palpated).

Table Case 2.1 Complete blood count

| Parameter | Value | Reference range |
|---|---|---|
| RBC x 106/µl | 4.72 | 5.65–8.87 |
| HGB (g/dl) | 10.8 | 13.1–20.5 |
| HCT (%) | 31.1 | 37.3–61.7 |
| MCV (fl) | 65.9 | 61.6–73.5 |
| MCHC (g/dl) | 34.7 | 32.0–37.9 |
| MCH (pg) | 22.9 | 21.2–25.9 |
| % RETIC | 1.7 | |
| RETIC (K/µl) | 79.8 | 10.0–110 |
| WBC /µl | 19.333 | 5.05–16.76 |
| LYM /µl | 6.60 | 1.05–5.10 |
| MONO /µl | 0.99 | 0.16–1.12 |
| NEU /µl | 10.36 | 2.95–11.64 |
| EOS /µl | 1.23 | 0.06–1.23 |
| BASO /µl | 0.15 | 0.00–0.10 |
| PLT x 103 /µl | 466 | 148–484 |

| Parameter | Value | Reference range |
|---|---|---|
| Alb (g/dl) | 2.4 | 2.3–4.0 |
| TP (g/dl) | 5.5 | 5.2–8.2 |
| Crea (mg/dl) | 1.5 | 0.5–1.8 |
| BUN (mg/dl) | 17 | 7–27 |
| Glu (mg/dl) | 109 | 70–143 |
| ALT (UI/l) | <10 | <50 |
| FAL (UI/l) | 157 | 30–120 |
| Cl (mmol/l) | 112 | 109–122 |
| K (mmol/l) | 4.1 | 3.5–5.8 |
| Na (mmol/l) | 153 | 144–160 |

### Urinalysis

Urinary density: 1.038.

Urine test strip: pH (9.0), leukocytes (25 leu/µl), protein (traces), glucose (negative), ketone bodies (negative), bilirubin (negative), erythrocytes (negative).

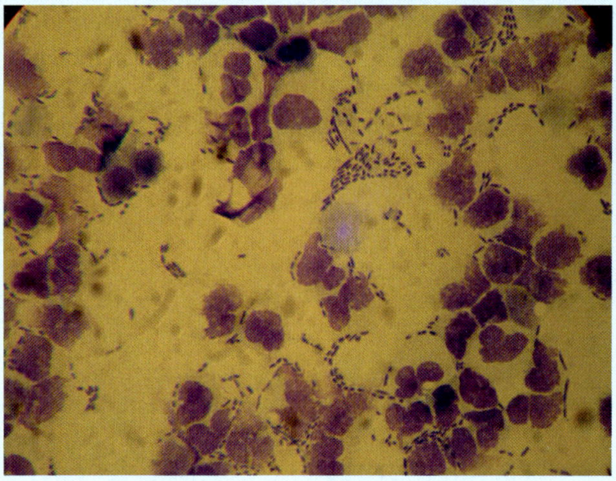

**Figure case 2.1** Urine cytology

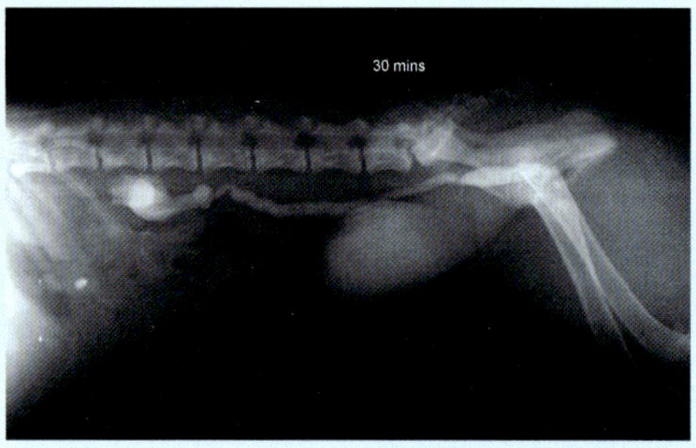


**Figure case 2.2** Abdominal radiography with contrast (IV pyelogram)

1. **Of the clinical signs that you would describe in this patient, which one is not present?**
   A) Urinary incontinence.
   B) Dysuria.
   C) Polyurea.
   D) Haematuria.
2. **From the results of the urinalysis, which statement is false?**
   A) Urine concentration mechanisms appear to be adequate.
   B) Proteinuria in this situation is probably not significant.
   C) Polymorphonuclear and phagocytosed bacteria are observed on cytology.
   D) The patient probably has a urinary infection due to *Streptococcus*.
3. **In a 7-month-old dog with a history of recurrent urinary infections, which statement is false?**
   A) There is no need to investigate, because causes that predispose to urinary infections are rare in young animals.
   B) Diagnostic imaging tests are advisable.
   C) Performing a urine culture and antibiogram is advised.
   D) It is advisable to evaluate renal function.
4. **What would be your diagnosis in this patient?**
   A) Persistent urachus and secondary urinary infection.
   B) Ectopic ureter and secondary urinary infection.
   C) Urethral sphincter incompetence due to lack of oestrogen and urinary infection.
   D) Dysautonomia and urinary infection.
5. **What medication is indicated in this patient?**
   A) Cefovecin, pending the result of the antibiogram.
   B) Pradofloxacin, regardless of the result of the antibiogram, because it is very strong.
   C) Amoxicillin-clavulanic acid, awaiting the results of the antibiogram.
   D) Clindamycin, pending the results of the antibiogram.

**6. What is the most appropriate approach in this patient?**

A) Treatment with phenoxybenzamine and antibiotics.
B) Initial stabilization of the urine infection and subsequently a surgical approach.
C) Emergency surgical approach.
D) Treatment with bethanechol and antibiotics.

## Correct answers

### Test: Upper urinary tract pathologies

| | | |
|---|---|---|
| 1. B | 7. D | 13. D |
| 2. C | 8. A | 14. C |
| 3. B | 9. A | 15. B |
| 4. C | 10. C | 16. A |
| 5. C | 11. B | |
| 6. B | 12. C | |

### Lower urinary tract pathologies

| | | |
|---|---|---|
| 1. D | 7. C | 13. D |
| 2. D | 8. B | 14. B |
| 3. C | 9. A | 15. D |
| 4. A | 10. D | 16. A |
| 5. B | 11. C | |
| 6. C | 12. B | |

### Clinical case 1

| | | |
|---|---|---|
| 1. D | 3. C | 5. B |
| 2. C | 4. B | 6. A |

### Clinical case 2

| | | |
|---|---|---|
| 1. C | 3. A | 5. C |
| 2. D | 4. B | 6. B |

# 7

# Infectious diseases

Albert Lloret Roca

## Chapter summary



## Introduction

Change is all around us, including the technology, climate change, and indeed the infectious diseases threatening our small animal patients. From the emergence of new *Leptospira* serovar to a wider geographical distribution of arthropod vectors, new threats are constantly developing. This chapter aims to give the clinician practical information about the symptoms, diagnosis, treatment and prevention of the prevalent infectious diseases they are likely to encounter in first-opinion practice.

While it is true that widespread vaccination has reduced the numbers of patients presenting from day to day with certain infections, this doesn't mean that veterinarians can be blasé about them. In real terms the clinician may be faced with a patient suffering disease, such as babesiosis or leishmaniosis, not endemic to their area, or the evolution of a new strain of parvovirus means that vaccinated pets are not adequately protected, both of which illustrate the importance of the veterinarian remaining well informed so as to make the best clinical decisions for the animals in their care.

In a changing world, another area of advancement is the development of diagnostic tests to detect specific pathogens. However, this raises a new set of diagnostic challenges in that the clinician must now understand how much emphasis to place on, for example, a titre result. A low titre result for *Borrelia* in a sick animal does not necessarily mean their symptoms are due to this organism. One of the aims of this chapter is to put diagnostic tests in context, and help the clinician decide which option is most helpful when making a diagnosis.

## Key learning points

- Vaccines and vaccination protocols.
- A practical overview of the infectious diseases most likely to be encountered in first-opinion clinical practice.
- The symptoms, diagnosis and treatment of the above infectious diseases.
- The management of FeLV-, FIV- or FIP-infected animals in multi-cat households.
- Appropriate advice to pet owners regarding various zoonotic diseases.
- Use of vaccination to maintain 'herd health' in the pet population, without compromising the best interests of the individual patient.

## Feline infectious diseases

### *Respiratory infections*

#### *General considerations*

**Upper respiratory tract infections (URTI) are common in cats.** In the majority of cases, cats with an acute URTI present with general, non-specific signs that give no clue as to the exact pathogen involved. Indeed, identifying the causative pathogen requires specific diagnostic tests and often has little impact on treatment choices.

**Symptoms** of acute URTI include:

- sneezing
- nasal discharge
- coughing
- aphonia
- conjunctivitis
- keratitis.

In practice, acute cases are often given **symptomatic and supportive treatment** based on a presumptive diagnosis.

- If the condition is accompanied by **ocular signs** (conjunctivitis, keratitis or corneal ulcers), the most likely diagnosis is **feline herpesvirus infection (FHV-1)**.
- If it is accompanied by **superficial ulcers on the tongue or oral mucosa**, the diagnosis is **feline calicivirus** (FCV).

Table 7.1. Causes of URTI in cats.

| Causes |
|---|
| **Infectious** |
| Viral (FHV-1, FCV, poxvirus) |
| Bacterial (Bordetella, Mycoplasma, Chlamydophila, Streptococcus) |
| Fungal (Cryptococcus, Aspergillus) |
| **Anatomical/congenital** |
| Nasopharyngeal polyps |
| Brachiocephalic syndrome |
| Nasopharyngeal stenosis |
| **Inflammatory/immune-mediated** |
| Idiopathic chronic rhinosinusitis |
| Lymphoplasmacytic rhinitis |
| **Neoplasms** |
| Nasal lymphoma |
| Epithelial neoplasms |
| Sarcomas |

Table 7.1 lists the main causes of feline URTI. Viral or **viral and bacterial co-infections are common** in many cats that present with URTI, since commensal bacteria of the URT colonise and infect tissues affected by the primary viral infection (Figure 7.1). Leaving aside the usual bacteria found in the respiratory tract, the most frequent primary bacteria in URTI are:

- *Chlamydophila felis*
- *Mycoplasma felis*
- *M. gateae.*

Recurrent or chronic infections may occur when the **animal is predisposed by an underlying anatomical or congenital anomaly**, or by an idiopathic inflammatory disease.

However, other causes of URTI should be included on the **list of differential diagnoses**, especially in

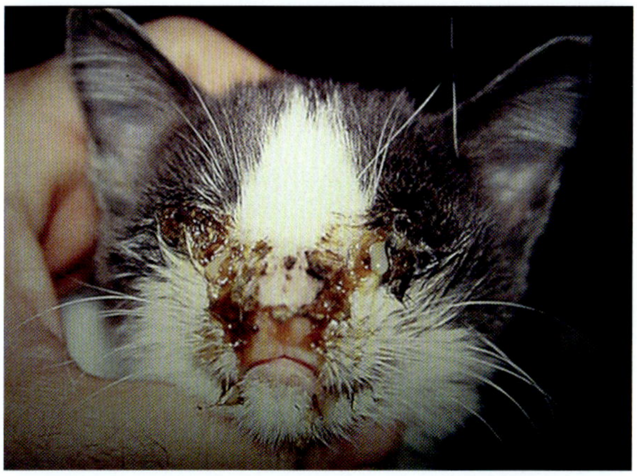

Figure 7.1. Kitten with severe respiratory and eye infection; frequently caused by viral co-infections (FHV-1, FCV) with bacteria (*Chlamydia*, *Mycoplasma*, *Bordetella* and other secondary bacteria).

**atypical or chronic cases**. When there are signs of respiratory obstruction and/or inspiratory wheezing or stridor, then **obstructive anatomical abnormalities** of the upper respiratory tract should also be considered.

### *Diagnostic tests*

The **diagnosis of acute URTIs is essentially clinical**, but the causative organism can be confirmed via the polymerase chain reaction (PCR) techniques offered by commercial laboratories. **Understanding the sensitivity and specificity of each of these PCRs is important for correct interpretation**, since in some cases the presence of the pathogen does not necessarily mean this is the cause of the disease.

In cases with **chronic URT signs**, tests to **rule out other diseases or abnormalities** should be performed, in addition to tests to detect pathogens:

- diagnostic imaging tests:
  - computerised tomography (CT)
  - flexible endoscopy.
- tests under anaesthesia:
  - visual examination (Figure 7.2)
  - nasal lavage.

## *Feline herpesvirus infections*

### *Aetiopathogenesis*

FHV-1 is a **DNA virus** of the Herpesviridae family. This shows little genetic variability and is relatively **unstable in the environment**, remaining infective for a few hours at most. It is also **sensitive to most disinfectants** (for example, sodium hypochlorite).

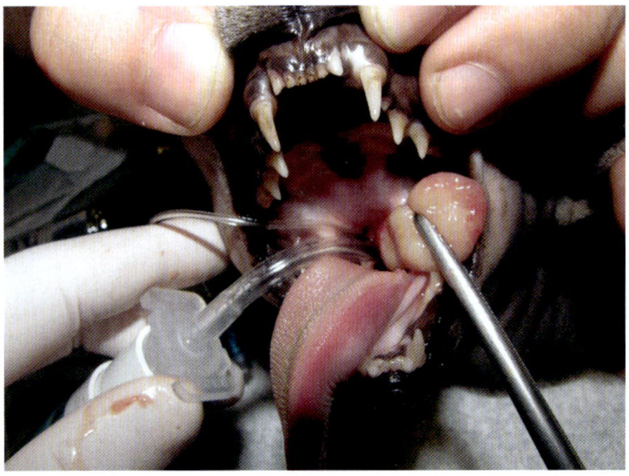

**Figure 7.2.** A frequent cause of persistent nasal and nasopharyngeal symptoms is the presence of nasopharyngeal polyps. These generally appear in cats that have previously been suffering from respiratory infections, and may lead to the false idea that the infection or inflammation has become chronic. Removal of the polyp is curative and causes resolution of clinical signs.

FHV-1 has a special **tropism for the nasal, oropharyngeal, conjunctival and corneal mucous membranes**. Most cats are infected by **direct contact** with an infected cat (indirect contagion is less frequent) and, after a **2–6-day incubation period**, the virus produces necrotic and inflammatory lesions in epithelia with associated acute clinical signs (nasal, ocular). Less frequently, FHV-1 can cause **skin lesions**, especially in the facial area near the nasal cavity and mouth, to produce ulcerative lesions (herpetic dermatitis) with an eosinophilic inflammatory component in the dermis.

In most cases the disease goes into **spontaneous remission** and the mortality rate is low. However, the virus is **excreted in respiratory and ocular secretions for 2–3 weeks** and, during this time, poses a risk to in-contact cats.

**Viraemia and pneumonia are rare**, although in some weak, malnourished or immunosuppressed cats this can occur, in which case mortality can be high. On some occasions the virus has been isolated in the central nervous system (CNS), but this has been documented in only one case of meningoencephalitis caused by FHV-1. Unlike herpesviruses in other species (e.g. dog), FHV-1 does not cause abortions in the cat as a result of direct viral replication in the genital organs.

After acute infection and clinical cure, in the vast majority of cats the **virus remains dormant** in the **trigeminal nerve** ganglion without producing clinical signs or prolonged excretion in secretions. However, **stress and other immunosuppressive factors can reactivate viral replication** with or without clinical signs, which can cause virus excretion to occur again. This phenomenon of reactivation and new virus outflow keeps it present in communities, despite the herpesvirus being fragile in the environment.

The exact pathogenesis of **chronic herpesvirus disease** is not known. The chronic nasal and ocular disease conditions associated with the presence of herpesviruses are mainly **immune-mediated inflammatory conditions** in which the virus is not actively detected:

- **Stromal ulcers**. The immune-mediated response causes serious inflammatory lesions in the cornea, leading to blindness.
- **Chronic rhinosinusitis**. A similar mechanism of action is suspected.

There are most likely conditions in which inflammation and destruction persist when the virus has stopped replicating. **Destruction of the nasal turbinates** and the presence of **secondary bacterial infections** that worsen and maintain inflammation are frequent. **Corneal necrosis and eosinophilic keratitis** may also be related to FHV-1, although the **mechanism is unclear** and the **virus cannot be identified** in all cats with these diseases. Likewise, some cases of uveitis associated with the presence of FHV-1 have been documented, although the cause–effect association has yet to be demonstrated.

### *Epidemiology*

The prevalence of feline herpesvirus infections is **high in feline communities** (20–50% according to the study consulted). In groups, **latent carrier cats** that **undergo periods of viral reactivation and excretion can infect young kittens**, which perpetuates herpesvirus in that population. The prevalence of herpesvirus in cats that live in isolation or live indoors is low (<5%), but it is important to note that a cat living alone may show signs of herpesvirus if reactivation is associated with clinical symptoms.

### *Clinical signs*

Most commonly the clinical signs are those of an **acute condition**:

- sneezing
- nasal discharge:
  - serous, if the condition is solely viral
  - purulent, due to bacterial coinfection, which is common
- coughing
- accompanied or not by signs of conjunctivitis and ocular secretion
- superficial corneal ulcers; very frequent, especially dendritic ulcers.

**Herpetic dermatitis** consists of **ulcerative lesions** in the nasal septum area or around the lips in cats with a history of respiratory signs, but which have not always been recognised. Often, there is **secondary bacterial infection** of the lesions, which can be acute or chronic, and histologically an eosinophilic inflammatory component can be seen which sometimes causes them to be mistakenly diagnosed as of allergic inflammatory origin (Figure 7.3).

The most frequent **chronic symptoms** are:

- **Chronic rhinosinusitis**, with sneezing and chronic or recurrent purulent nasal discharge in cats that show no signs of systemic disease.
- **Keratitis or stromal corneal ulcers**, deep ulcers that are difficult to cure and that sometimes cause corneal perforation and loss of vision.

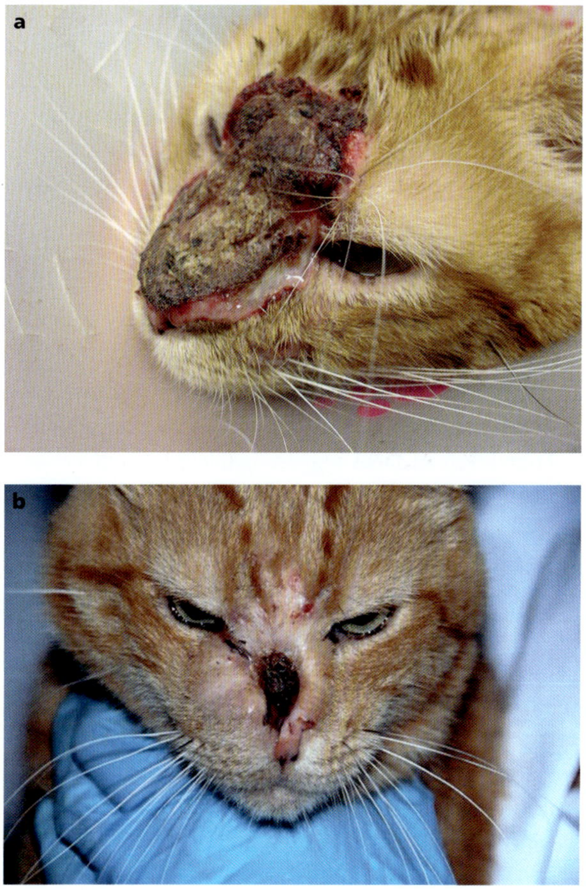


**Figure 7.3.** Cat with extremely severe herpetic dermatitis (a) that was initially diagnosed as eosinophilic dermatitis and treated with high-dose corticosteroids. The herpetic lesion deteriorated due to the immunosuppression and the nasal septum necrosed (b). It is important to remember that inflammatory herpetic lesions can have an eosinophilic component. The lesion improved after treatment with famciclovir, but permanent sequelae remain due the nasal septal defect.

### *Diagnosis*

The clinical **diagnosis** of acute conditions is usually **based on the typical clinical signs** and the response to symptomatic or supportive treatment. However, nowadays it is easy to confirm the presence of the virus using **PCR** techniques. These represent significant advances in virus detection in the day-to-day practice compared to other, less practical, techniques such as immunofluorescence or virus isolation. Any veterinarian can confirm the presence of FHV-1 **through nasal, conjunctival, oropharyngeal or corneal swabs** sent to laboratories capable of performing good-quality PCR techniques. In cases of herpetic dermatitis, PCR can also be done on biopsies or skin swabs.

There are, however, some limitations in the interpretation of PCR for FHV-1:

- The presence of viral DNA **does not mean that the virus is replicating** and, therefore the cause of the cat's disease. PCR can detect DNA from the virus in a

sample because there is replication of the virus (**latent carrier**), even if the clinical signs are caused by another disease.
- **DNA detection of the vaccine virus**. Herpesvirus vaccines are attenuated and produce a subclinical infection, especially in the weeks following vaccination.

Although there are currently no clinical studies to prove it, **quantitative real-time PCR** (RT-PCR) techniques could be extremely helpful:

- A **small amount of DNA** suggests latency or low levels of replication and no involvement in the clinical signs.
- **High levels of DNA** suggest high levels of replication and a greater involvement in the clinical signs.

**Serological antibody detection techniques are not useful for diagnosis** of herpesvirus, since the presence of antibodies has no correlation with the disease and active infection. Given the high prevalence of natural infection and vaccination, a large number of cats are seropositive. Consequently, serology can be useful for seroprevalence studies or to assess the humoral immune response against the virus, but not for clinical diagnosis.

### Treatment

The treatment of herpesvirus is based on:

- **Supportive** treatment (hydration, nutritional, mucolytics).
- **Antibiotics** suitable for respiratory infections (doxycycline, amoxicillin, azithromycin, fluoroquinolones).
- In some cases, **antiviral drugs**.

Numerous antiviral drugs against FHV-1 have been tested, all of them with good activity against the virus in ***in vitro* studies**, but this does not always correspond to efficacy *in vivo*. Because most studies are case series or clinical cases, treatment recommendations are not based on controlled studies. There is a wide range of anti-herpetic drugs (nucleoside analogues).

As a general rule, **topical ocular anti-herpetic agents** should be administered **every 2–4 hours** as these have a virostatic action, and sufficient continuous concentrations must be administered continuously to inhibit viral replication. In the past the most commonly used were **trifluridine and idoxuridine** (whose efficacy *in vivo* has not been demonstrated). **Ganciclovir is currently used more frequently in ophthalmic ointment** (2 or 3 times per day, although there are no clinical studies), or **0.5% cidofovir** (there is a clinical study that proves its efficacy when applied twice a day). However, cidofovir is a preparation for intravenous use and is very expensive; for topical ocular use the intravenous format must be reformulated.

In recent years the use of **systemic antiherpetic agents** such as **famciclovir** (pro-drug of penciclovir) has become widespread. Studies in experimentally infected cats and in groups of naturally infected cats show that tolerance is good and clinical improvement is significant. The dose for **famciclovir is 40–90 mg/kg/8–12 h for 3–4** weeks, and should never be <40 mg/kg/8–12 h as it may not be effective.

Other treatments used for herpesvirus are **L-lysine** and **interferon**. Lysine (amino acid) is widely used at doses of **500 mg/12 h**. Its mechanism of action is based on competition and displacement of arginine, an essential amino acid for herpesvirus replication. A systematic review of experimental and clinical studies on lysine has recently been published, with the conclusion that there are **no clinical benefits** with the use of lysine. Even an *in vitro* study did not observe the inhibition of feline herpesvirus replication against various concentrations of lysine.

There are some publications on the use of interferon, human alpha and feline omega, systemically or topically in FHV-1 infections. The results are inconclusive, but in general these **reduce the intensity of clinical signs**.

### Prognosis

The prognosis for herpesvirus is:

- **Good** in the vast **majority** of cases.
- **Bad** in some weakened or **immunosuppressed kittens** in which systemic dissemination or pneumonia occurs.
- **Reserved in chronic cases**, as many do not respond to anti-herpetic treatments and should be treated continuously with combinations of antibiotics and anti-inflammatory drugs (non-steroidals and, sometimes, steroids).

### Prevention

The prevention of herpesvirus is difficult in groups of felines, due to the existence of latent carriers which undergo reactivation and excretion phases of the virus. **Cats that recover from herpesvirus are not immunised** and can manifest the disease again. For many years there have been attenuated vaccines available against feline herpesvirus that prevent the appearance of clinical signs and **decrease their intensity**. However, they do not produce a robust or sterilising immunity that prevents infection or latency. Consequently, vaccinated cats can become infected or be latent carriers but they will not show clinical signs. Although the **revaccination programme (Table 7.2)** recommended

Table 7.2. Vaccination programme for herpesvirus.

| Essential vaccines recommended in all cats | | |
|---|---|---|
| **Primary vaccination** | **Booster vaccination** | **Annual vaccination** |
| 3 doses: 8, 12 and 16 weeks | One year after the last dose | Annual in cats at risk of exposure<br>Every 3 years in low-risk cats |

by vaccine manufacturers is annual, there are studies on immunity duration (ID) and experimental infection that show that ID is **at least 3 years**.

## Chlamydia infections

### Aetiopathogenesis

*Chlamydia felis* is a bacterium from the Chlamydiaceae family. Infection is by **direct contact** between cats, as this organism is **fragile in the environment**. The main **tropism** of *C. felis* is the eye, specifically the **conjunctiva**, causing inflammation and ocular secretions. *C. felis* does not cause corneal involvement. For a long time it was thought that *C. felis* is capable of producing infection and clinical signs in the URT, but nowadays it is thought that it is **only a conjunctival pathogen**. There are **chronic carriers**.

### Epidemiology

The **prevalence of *C. felis* is high in groups** of felines and low in cats that live in isolation. Sick cats and chronic carriers are the main source of infection for those susceptible to infection.

### Clinical signs

**Signs of acute or chronic conjunctivitis**. Initially the signs are of **serous conjunctivitis** (inflammation and serous secretion) that begin unilaterally, become bilateral and worsen to manifest as **blepharospasm**, purulent secretions and a marked conjunctival inflammation and **chemosis**. Chemosis is a clinical feature of this infection (Figure 7.4).

Generally, there are **no systemic or respiratory** signs and if they exist, they are likely to be caused by **co-infection with respiratory pathogens**. **Chronic carrier cats can be asymptomatic** or suffer chronic conjunctivitis. Up to 30% of cases of chronic feline conjunctivitis are due to *C. felis*.

### Diagnosis

Clinical suspicions should be raised in cats with **acute or chronic conjunctivitis**, especially those with a marked **chemosis**. Diagnosis can be confirmed by observing inclusion bodies in **conjunctival cytology**

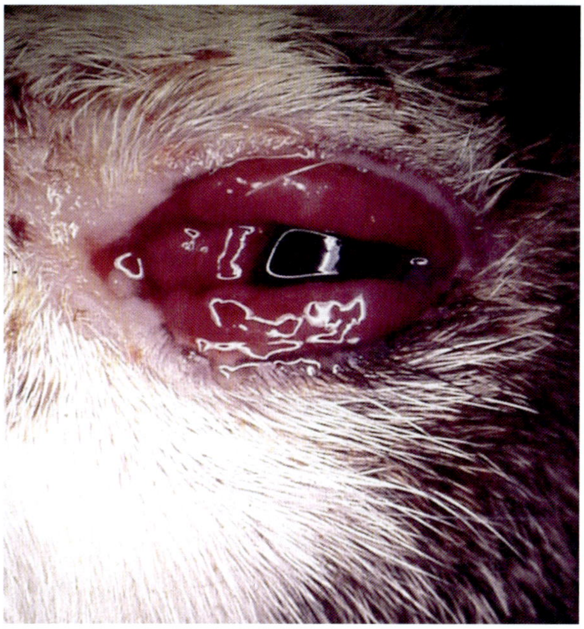

Figure 7.4. Infectious conjunctivitis is very common in cats and is generally caused by FHV-1, *C. felis* or *Mycoplasma* spp. Clinically they are indistinguishable, although the presence of a marked chemosis is most compatible with *C. felis* infection. PCR techniques on conjunctival swabs allow aetiological diagnosis if considered necessary.

(low sensitivity) or **PCR of a conjunctival swab** (high sensitivity). **PCR is the technique of choice** for confirmation of diagnosis and detection of chronic carriers.

### Treatment

The **treatment of choice is tetracyclines**, either in the form of eye drops or ophthalmic ointment. However, it is preferable to **administer doxycycline (10 mg/kg/24 h for 3–4 weeks)** systemically to completely eliminate bacteria from the conjunctiva and prevent the animal becoming a chronic carrier. It is important to treat all in-contact cats even if they have no clinical signs. Quinolones can also be effective, especially pradofloxacin.

### Prognosis

The **prognosis is good**. This is not an infection that causes death and, if treated properly, is **curable**. It may be more difficult to eliminate or eradicate *C. felis* in a community where it is endemic, since all cats should be treated, systematic vaccination initiated and the cat population reduced.

### Prevention

Prevention is based on the **treatment of affected cats** and those that have been in contact. There are **vaccines** against *C. felis* which, in general, are not considered essential or core for all cats (Table 7.3). These vaccines

Table 7.3. Vaccination programme for *Chlamydia*.

| Non-essential vaccine, recommended in colonies and groups in which the infection is endemic and in cats at risk of exposure | | |
|---|---|---|
| **Primary vaccination** | **Booster vaccination** | **Annual vaccination** |
| 2 doses: 8 and 12 weeks | One year after the last dose | Annual |

do **not prevent infection** but do decrease the appearance or intensity of clinical signs. Vaccination should be considered as part of a broader plan to eradicate *C. felis* from a community (consisting of doxycycline treatment, systematic vaccination and improvements to the community's environmental conditions).

## *Feline calicivirus (FCV) infections*

### *Aetiopathogenesis*

**FCV** is an RNA virus belonging to the Caliciviridae family, with **high genetic variability** and is **resistant in the environment** (it can be infective for several days), and it can be **transmitted indirectly**.

There are numerous calicivirus variants that arise as a result of genetic mutation in the course of infections in different cat populations. Different genetic variants exhibit different virulence, and consequently clinical signs of varying severity. In addition, the evolutionary ability of the virus allows it to adapt its genome to evade the cat's immune response.

FCV has a special **tropism** for the **nasal, oropharyngeal and oral mucous membranes**. When **a cat is infected by direct or indirect contact**, after a **few days of incubation** the virus produces necrotic and inflammatory lesions in the epithelia with associated acute clinical signs (nasal and oral). Less frequently, it replicates in synovial tissue and causes **polyarthritis** (on rare occasions this is an adverse effect of attenuated vaccines). Variants with higher virulence can produce **systemic signs, fever and pneumonia**. FCV spreads in blood producing a significant viraemia, and is **excreted in saliva, respiratory secretions, faeces and urine**.

Infected cats usually manifest the **acute clinical condition**, and the disease **remits spontaneously** without causing death while the virus is excreted for a month or more, infecting other in-contact animals. Around 20% of cats remain **chronic carriers** of FCV without showing clinical signs, but they excrete and spread the virus continuously, a mechanism by which the virus remains in the environment.

Several outbreaks of a severe systemic disease caused by virulent variants of FCV (**virulent systemic calicivirosis, VS-FCV**) have been described in the last decade. These outbreaks described in the US, UK and other countries in Europe have similar characteristics:

- **Systemic inflammation syndrome**, vasculitis, involvement of the liver and pancreas, disseminated intravascular coagulation and **multi-organ failure**.
- Clinical signs are most serious in adult and older cats.
- **High mortality**, close to 50%.
- It also affects cats vaccinated against FCV.
- Transmission of the virus to other cats is very effective, even when indirectly through fomites.

### *Epidemiology*

The prevalence of feline FCV infections is **high in communities (20–50%)**. Cats that are chronic carriers of FCV in the oral mucosa infect young kittens and perpetuate the presence of the virus in the environment. The prevalence of FCV is lower in isolated indoor cats.

### *Clinical signs*

Most characteristic acute clinical signs:

- sneezing
- nasal discharge
- ocular discharge
- superficial ulcers on tongue and palate (anorexia, sialorrhoea and odynophagia) (Figure 7.5).

Some cases presenting with **fever and apathy** may be accompanied by joint or generalised pain (**polyarthritis**) (Figure 7.6). Recently corneal ulcers caused by FCV have been described, although this lesion is poorly documented.

Given the diversity of genomes and genetic variants of FCV, clinical conditions vary from **mild to severe** and, in some cases, mortality can be very high.

The clinical signs associated with virulent systemic calicivirus include:

- oedema of extremities
- ulcerated pads
- mouth ulcers
- fever
- jaundice
- vomiting
- diarrhoea
- respiratory distress
- bleeding, hepatitis, pancreatitis, pneumonia, disseminated intravascular coagulation and multi-organ failure.

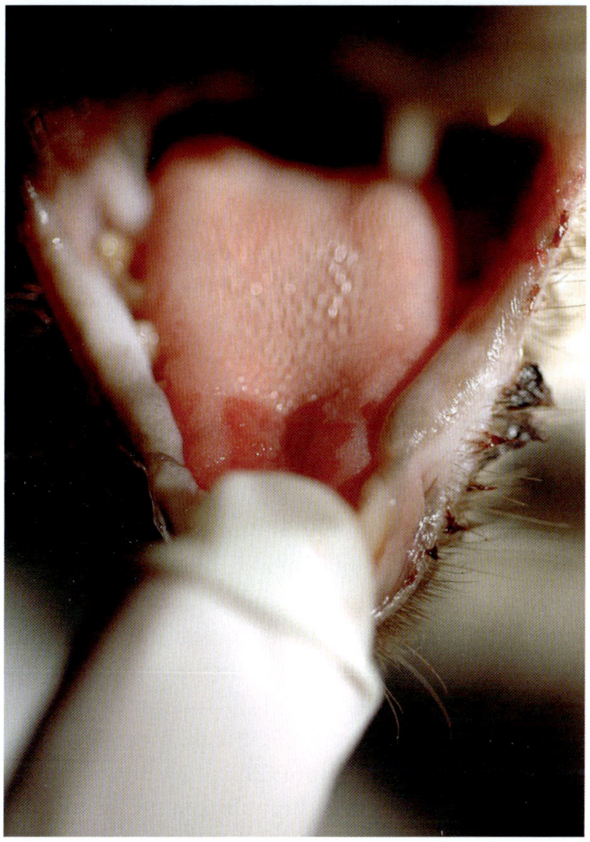

**Figure 7.5.** Superficial ulcers on the tongue and palate are typical of acute infections caused by FCV. They should be differentiated from toxic or caustic lesions following the ingestion of plants or toxic substances. Treatment is based on analgesics and antibiotics, which are used to treat the secondary bacterial infection which can complicate healing of the ulcers.

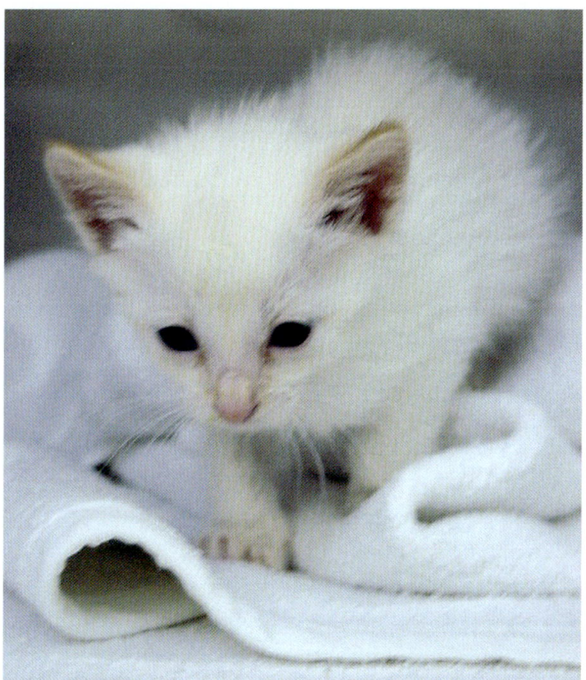

**Figure 7.6.** FCV infections can cause polyarthritis and generalised pain through the course of the viraemia. The signs present over 4–6 days and then improve. In some cases, they have been seen after vaccination with attenuated vaccines.

### Diagnosis

Diagnosis of acute cases is usually based on the typical clinical signs. However, it is easy to confirm the presence of the virus through **PCR techniques**: this can be done by any veterinarian with oral, conjunctival or blood swabs sent to laboratories capable of performing good-quality PCR techniques.

Given the wide variability in the genome of the different strains and variants, **the sensitivity of FCV PCR can be reduced, giving false negatives**. On the other hand, as with FHV-1, the presence of viral RNA does not necessarily mean that the virus is the cause of the disease, since many cats can carry the virus without it being the cause.

Diagnosis by **immunohistochemistry on biopsies** from oral lesions to detect virus antigens within cells is also feasible. This diagnostic technique is especially useful for confirmation in cases of VS-FCV and sequencing of FCV variants.

### Treatment

There is **no known specific antiviral treatment against FCV**. Some antivirals that are useful in RNA viruses such as ribavirin or vidarabine are toxic in cats and cannot be safely administered. The approach to acute calicivirosis is based on supportive treatment (hydration, nutritional, antibiotics and analgesics). In experimental studies, **feline omega interferon** is able to inhibit *in vitro* replication although its efficacy in diseased cats is unknown. However, in the most severe cases its use is worthwhile in attempting to increase the chances of cure, given its non-specific antiviral action.

To date there is no specific treatment for virulent systemic calicivirosis, but **the use of feline omega interferon is logical**. Given the immune-mediated component of vasculitis and the lesions caused by this condition, corticosteroids may be indicated, even at the risk of immunosuppression, but there are no clinical studies.

### Prognosis

With mild and moderate calicivirus the prognosis is good. With severe calicivirus involving the presence of **systemic signs, the prognosis is poor**. With virulent systemic calicivirus, mortality is very high.

### Prevention

The prevention of calicivirosis is difficult in feline communities due to the presence of **chronic carriers**. Cats that are cured are not immunised and can manifest the disease again in the future. For many years **attenuated and inactivated vaccines** against FCV have been available and which are generally effective at preventing it, either by preventing the appearance of clinical signs or

Table 7.4. Vaccination programme for FCV.

| Essential vaccine, recommended in all cats | | |
|---|---|---|
| **Primary vaccination** | **Booster vaccination** | **Annual vaccination** |
| 3 doses: 8, 12 and 16 weeks | One year after the last dose | Annual in cats at risk of exposure<br>Every 3 years in low-risk cats |

by **decreasing their intensity**. However, they do not produce a robust or sterilising immunity that prevents infection or latency (Table 7.4).

Consequently, **vaccinated cats can become infected** and be latent carriers with no clinical manifestation. On the other hand, given the great diversity of genomic variants of FCV and their ability to evolve within cat colonies, **vaccines may not fully immunise against all existing FCV variants**. To try to improve the prevention capacity of FCV vaccines, new variants (G1 and 431) have been added to those already included (F9 and 255). If clinical signs of calicivirosis are observed in previously vaccinated cats, it is advisable to **vary the type of vaccine**. Although the revaccination schedule recommended in the vaccine prospectus is annual, there are studies of ID and experimental infection showing that the ID is at least 3 years.

## Chronic feline gingivostomatitis (CFGS)

### General considerations

**CFGS** is a relatively common disease, characterised by diffuse and widespread proliferative and **ulcerative inflammation of the gums and oral mucosa**, that appears mainly in **adult cats**. Although it is often considered to be associated with a **chronic FCV infection**, it does not fulfil Koch's postulates of infectious disease and it has never been possible to reproduce the disease experimentally.

### Aetiopathogenesis

Although the exact cause is unknown, the most widely accepted hypothesis is that CFGS is a **multifactorial immune-mediated disease** in the cat, due to a loss of immune system tolerance to antigens frequently present in the oral mucosa, mainly bacteria from plaque and calicivirus.

Numerous oral and systemic immunological abnormalities have been demonstrated in cats with CFGS. Early studies showed abnormal levels of **immunoglobulins A and G** in saliva and serum when compared to healthy cats. More recent studies have evaluated the inflammatory response using **cytokine patterns** and observed that, in the mouth of healthy cats, a Th1 pattern predominates whilst in cats suffering from CFGS there is a mixed pattern of Th1 and Th2. The **immune-mediated basis** for the disease is also supported by the inflammatory histological pattern with predominant lymphocytes and plasma cells without the presence of pathogens and the clinical response to anti-inflammatory / immunosuppressive treatments.

A variable percentage of cats with CFGS (according to studies, from 0 to 70%) is FCV positive using PCR techniques on oral samples. However, the presence of FCV in the oral mucosa does not demonstrate the cause–effect relationship since a variable but **significant percentage of healthy cats are positive for FCV** in the oral mucosa, and in addition a significant group of cats with the disease are negative for FCV. It is likely that the presence of **FCV is one of the factors** that contributes to inflammation in CFGS, but it is not the direct cause. In addition, in general, treatments with an antiviral mechanism, such as high-dose interferons, are not effective. In a recent study, immunohistochemistry (IHC) techniques specific to FCV were performed on biopsies from 26 cats with CFGS and all were negative, as well as with the PCR for FCV.

The disease has also been **linked to retrovirus, FeLV and FIV infections**. Co-infections by retrovirus and calicivirus could increase the pro-inflammatory response and predispose to CFGS. Cats with FIV infection have a high prevalence of chronic gingivitis and stomatitis, although no direct relationship with the virus has been shown. Rather, they are related to **immunodeficiency**, the presence of **chronic bacterial infections** or the **pro-inflammatory state** associated with FIV infection. In a recent study, IHC detected FeLV antigens in oral lesions, which suggests they have a direct influence on inflammation.

Recent studies have evaluated the **type of oral bacteria** in cats with CFGS. Some of these studies are based on the detection of bacteria by traditional techniques such as bacteriological cultures, but the most recent ones are based on detection by **PCR** of bacteria that cannot be cultured. In general, these studies show that there are important differences in the oral bacterial flora of cats with CFGS compared to that of healthy cats. Specifically:

- Less bacterial diversity.
- Predominance of *Pasteurella multocida*.
- Increased presence of *Pseudomonas* spp., *Tannerella forsythia* and *Porphyromonas circumdentaria*.

The hypothesis for **bacterial antigenic influence** is reinforced by the clinical improvement observed with antibiotic administration (especially with effects on *Pasteurella* and anaerobes) and the large percentage of total cure or remission of inflammation after complete dental extraction. Years ago, some studies associated this disease with *Bartonella henselae* infection, but more recently it has been shown that the prevalence of *B. henselae* is no different from that observed in healthy cats.

## Epidemiology

CFGS usually **occurs in young adult cats**, although in some cats inflammation begins at an early age. Among the risk factors that predispose to the disease are:

- presence of FCV
- cats that live in communities
- elements of environmental stress.

## Clinical signs

The main **external clinical signs** are:

- odynophagia
- pseudo-anorexia
- submandibular lymphadenopathy
- sialorrhoea, sometimes with the presence of blood.

There may also be **systemic signs** such as:

- weight loss
- poor hair quality.

And, in some serious cases, even:

- hyperglobulinaemia
- polyclonal gammopathy
- proteinuria
- chronic kidney disease.

On examination of the mouth the following may be seen:

- **Intense 360° gingivitis** around the teeth.
- Alveolitis.
- **Caudal stomatitis** (glossopalatine angle). Inflammation can be more or less intense, from erythema to intense proliferative inflammation with the existence of **ulcerated areas** (Figure 7.7). Lesions may be covered with purulent secretion and bleed easily, and in some cases they extend to the oropharynx and/or present as deep ulcers on the tongue, although this is unusual.

The disease can be mild, moderate or intense, depending on:

- degree of pain
- proliferation (Figure 7.8)

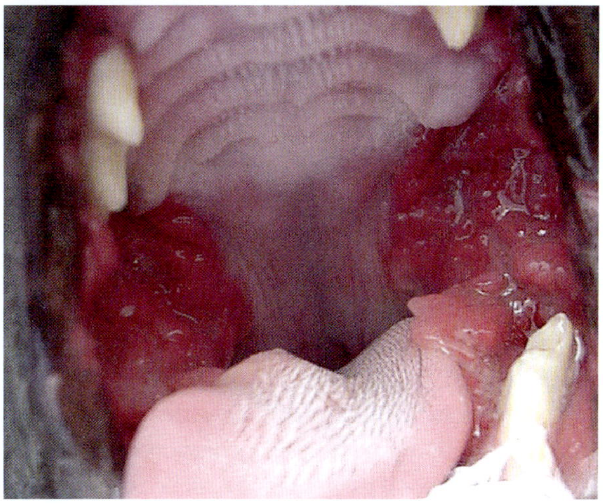

**Figure 7.7.** Typical lesions caused by moderate CFGS: intense gingivitis and alveolitis 360° around all teeth and proliferative caudal stomatitis with some areas of erosion and ulceration. The clinical signs had been established for months and partially responded to antibiotics and corticosteroids, but did not resolve completely.

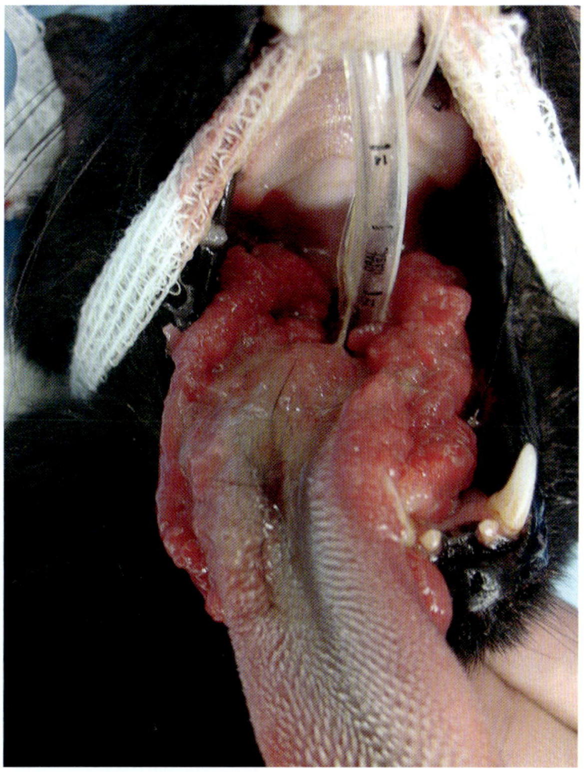

**Figure 7.8.** Extremely severe CFGS that developed over several years without showing any response to medical treatment or complete exodontics.

- ulceration
- chronicity.

## Diagnosis

The diagnosis is based on several criteria, the main one being the **type and distribution** of the lesions. The presence of **inflammation in the caudal part of the** mouth and caudal stomatitis determines the clinical diagnosis and helps to differentiate from other oral or dental pathologies such as periodontal disease, dental resorption or juvenile hyperplastic gingivitis. **Lesions are diffuse and symmetrical**, which allows them to be distinguished from proliferative lesions that are not necessarily symmetrical, such as eosinophilic granulomas or oral neoplasms.

In case of doubt about the diagnosis, or if a histological diagnosis is desired, **biopsies of the lesions** should be performed. The histological pattern of CFGS is a lymphoplasmacytic inflammation, although it is possible that there is a neutrophilic component especially in ulcerated areas. IHC techniques can be applied to the same samples to detect the presence of pathogens such as FCV or FeLV.

Although subsequent decisions about treatment are not influenced by the results, since there are no effective antiviral treatments for FCV, in many cases an FCV PCR is performed. It is also necessary to know the retrovirus status, because the presence of **FeLV or FIV can influence the choice of treatment** – for example, whether to use immunosuppressive treatments. In addition, there may be other diseases associated with retroviruses.

Normally, in first-opinion clinical practice, bacterial microbiological cultures of the secretions are not performed except in cases where resistance to the usual antibiotics is suspected.

To assess whether there are **systemic abnormalities associated with oral disease**, the following tests should be performed:

- complete blood count
- serum biochemistry
- proteinogram
- urinalysis.

### *Treatment*

There is currently no known treatment that can 100% cure cats with CFGS.

**Milder cases usually respond to medical treatment**:

- antibiotics (amoxicillin-clavulanic, clindamycin, spiramycin-metronidazole)
- dental hygiene
- non-steroidal anti-inflammatories and analgesics.

Over time, the response to antibiotics and analgesics is usually reduced. In moderate states, to relieve inflammation and pain, **corticosteroids** are necessary at anti-inflammatory doses, and possibly even **immunosuppressants**. Occasionally a temporary remission of the signs and inflammation is achieved, but many cats do not respond or soon stop responding to treatment.

In 1994 a first series of cases was published in which it was demonstrated **that complete exodontics** of all teeth (except, in some cases, the canines) allowed **complete healing in approximately 70%** of cats (Figure 7.9). In the remaining 30%, although the disease was not cured there was a partial improvement with the usual treatments and better control of pain and inflammation. In the last 20 years, many cats have been treated using exodontics (carefully performed by experienced surgeons and avoiding leaving any tooth roots) and the same phenomenon is observed: a large number are slowly and gradually cured in 4–6 months after teeth removal and a smaller group is not cured but can be more easily controlled with corticosteroids, **oral feline omega interferon at low doses or cyclosporine** (Figure 7.10). One study showed how those which did not fully respond to exodontics could

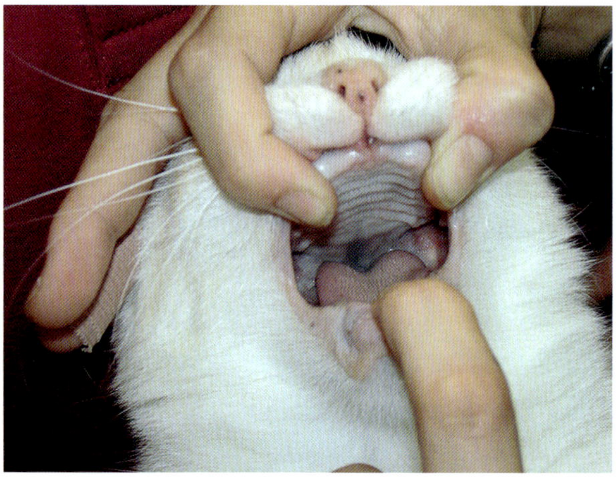

**Figure 7.9.** Oral cavity free from lesions 6 months after complete exodontics in a cat with CFGS. The reduction in bacterial plaque after exodontics seems to be the most important factor for a favourable clinical response, which occurs in approximately 80% of cats.

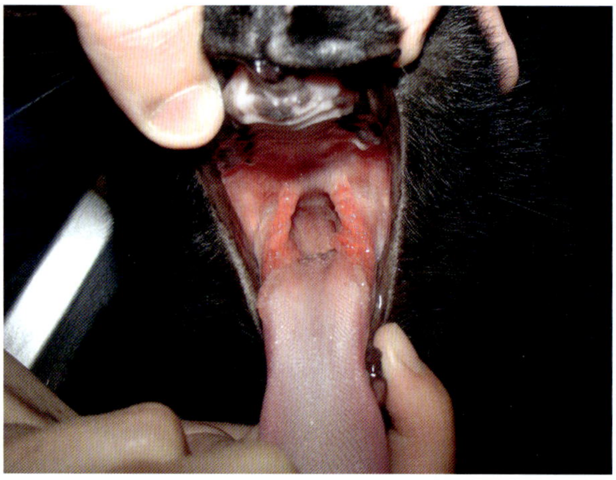

**Figure 7.10.** Partial remission of lesions after exodontics. This cat was not cured, but inflammation response was enhanced and was better controlled with feline interferon omega at low doses and/or prednisolone at anti-inflammatory doses.

be controlled **with oral feline omega interferon at a continuous dose of 0.1 MU/24 h PO**. The response to interferon was similar to that of prednisolone regarding the control of pain and inflammation.

Other treatments, documented in a small number of cats, are natural or **hypo-allergenic diets**, the use of a **$CO_2$ laser** (to remove proliferative lesions) and stem cell treatments, but further studies are required before these can be recommended.

Two studies using stem cells in cat's refractory to the usual treatments have been published so far. In one of them, autologous mesenchymal stem cells of adipose tissue origin were used. Of 7 cats treated, only 2 did not respond and in the remaining 5 the inflammation subsided completely or partially.

In addition, the change in immune response in the mouth of these cats was demonstrated by the study of cytokines and other parameters. Therefore, the treatment produced a normalization of the immune response or pattern and the remission of inflammatory lesions. A second study with allogeneic stem cells did not show the same beneficial results.

### Prognosis

The prognosis for cure is **reserved or poor** unless the removal of all teeth is attempted. Some owners are reluctant to use such an aggressive technique that does not guarantee total healing. However, the quality of life of cats with moderate and intense CFGS is very poor and sometimes they are not even able to eat without high, continuous doses of corticosteroids that end up causing serious adverse systemic effects (diabetes mellitus, urine infections, hypercortisolism). In addition, over time, **corticosteroids become less effective** and, in some cats, the lack of response to treatment can be a reason for opting for euthanasia.

The prognosis after **exodontics is good, with 70–80%** of cats completely cured and **20–30% showing partial improvement**. Cats without teeth that are not cured are more easily manageable with regular medical treatments.

### Prevention

There are currently no preventive measures. However, given the involvement or association with FCV in a significant percentage of cats, prevention of FCV infection may be useful.

Ensuring optimal living conditions, without overcrowding and **avoiding environmental stress** as much as possible, can also show good results. In any case, some affected animals are indoor cats and in these no obvious stress factors or environment deficits are identified.

## Gastrointestinal infections

### General considerations

**Diarrhoea of infectious origin is common** in cats, especially in kittens and young cats. There are several pathogens that can cause acute and, in some cases, chronic diarrhoea (Table 7.5).

In any case of diarrhoea it is essential to identify whether it is of **small or large intestinal** origin, as in some infectious or parasitic causes the differential diagnoses vary. For example, in a large intestinal diarrhoea *Tritrichomonas* should be suspected but not in cases of small intestinal diarrhoea.

The **general condition of the cat** is also important. Sometimes there are additional **systemic signs or involvement of other organs**, while in others the only clinical sign is diarrhoea. For example, cats with feline panleukopenia usually have other systemic signs such as fever, anorexia and dehydration.

### Diagnostic tests

The diagnosis of infectious or parasitic causes of diarrhoea is based on **detection of the pathogen** in faeces, microscopy, detection of antigens using serological techniques or detection of the pathogen's genome by PCR.

#### Microscopic appearance

Microscopic observation can be by **direct observation** in fresh stool samples, rectal cytology or after **flotation techniques** with zinc sulphate. The sensitivity depends mainly on the type of pathogen involved, but in some

Table 7.5. Main causes of infectious/parasitic diarrhoea in cats.

| Causes |
|---|
| **Viral** |
| Feline panleucopenia virus |
| Feline coronavirus |
| Other viruses (rotavirus, torovirus) |
| **Bacterial** |
| *Campylobacter* |
| *Clostridium* |
| *Salmonella* |
| *E. coli* |
| **Helminth parasites** |
| *Toxocara* |
| *Ancylostoma* |
| *Strongyloides* |
| **Protozoan parasites** |
| *Giardia* |
| *Tritrichomonas* |
| *Isospora* |
| *Cryptosporidium* |
| *Toxoplasma* |

cases it is zero (virus) or low (bacteria or certain parasites that are excreted intermittently or in very low numbers). Stools should be analysed as quickly as possible to increase sensitivity in the detection of parasites. In general, **flotation techniques** with zinc sulphate improve sensitivity for the detection of **parasites**, especially if several samples are taken on different days.

### Serological tests

Antigen detection using serological tests exists for some pathogens, such as panleukopenia virus, and some parasites such as *Giardia* and *Cryptosporidium*. These are **sensitive techniques** that can be done rapidly with diagnostic kits, although they have their limitations.

### PCR techniques

Because PCR techniques are useful for the diagnosis of pathogens and bacteria toxins that are otherwise difficult to detect, they increase the sensitivity in the diagnosis of certain infections. It should be kept in mind that, on the one hand, faeces contain DNase enzymes that degrade DNA and decrease the sensitivity of the test in some cases and, on the other, genetic material may be detected from pathogens that are present in faeces but are not the cause of diarrhoea. Therefore, the **clinical interpretation of the results is very important**. Currently some commercial laboratories offer complete PCR panels from a single stool sample for detection of the main intestinal pathogens.

## Feline parvovirus/feline panleukopenia virus

### *Aetiopathogenesis*

Feline panleukopenia is a disease caused by infection with **feline parvovirus (FPV)**, a single-stranded DNA virus that is **highly resistant** in the environment, where it can persist for months. This virus has long been recognised as infecting cats and other felines. Canine parvovirus appeared in the late 1970s from a mutation of FPV. The new variants of canine parvovirus (2b, 2c) can re-infect cats, although it seems that this does not cause disease.

The virus enters the cat **orally** causing a rapid viraemia, providing it with access to all organs. FPV has a special **tropism for cells with a high replication rate**, particularly those in the S phase of cell growth, where it replicates and subsequently destroys them. **Enterocytes and myeloid cells** are particularly affected, so the infection causes **haemorrhagic enteritis** and **marked neutropenia**. Cats with severe panleukopenia usually have **sepsis** due to the bacterial translocation phenomenon. In some cases it can cause septic shock, disseminated intravascular coagulation and multi-organ failure. The **virus is present in large amounts in blood and faeces**.

**Purkinje cells of the cerebellum** can also be attacked by the virus in foetuses and neonates. Consequently, infection or application of attenuated vaccines in pregnant cats can lead to the birth of kittens with **cerebellar hypoplasia** and with signs of **non-progressive ataxia**.

It has not been fully demonstrated whether FPV has a myocardial tropism as can occur with canine parvovirus.

Feline parvovirus infection is an **acute infection** that can be subclinical if the cat develops a good immune response. The **incubation time is about 7 days** and, a week after the clinical signs have appeared, the animal is cured or dies due to associated complications.

### *Epidemiology*

**Oro-faecal transmission** is possible by **direct contact** with sick or infected cats, and also by **indirect infection** in contaminated environments given the virus's high level of environmental resistance. The disease is **very common in young cats** under 1 year of age, but it is not unheard of even in older cats, adults or elderly animals who have poor natural or vaccination immunity and are then exposed to the virus.

The prevalence of infection is high, especially in feline communities where the virus can circulate and is frequently present in the environment. The prevalence of infection is low in cats living indoors and that are not in contact with other cats, although infection is not impossible since the virus can enter the house through fomites, especially if the owner has regular contact with cats or environments where cats live.

### *Clinical signs*

Panleukopenia may present with a **wide spectrum of clinical signs** of acute onset. Especially in kittens living in communities, the clinical symptoms can be very acute, with sudden death unaccompanied by presenting digestive or other clinical signs.

However, the most common clinical signs are:

- anorexia
- apathy
- fever
- vomiting
- diarrhoea; sometimes it is not very profuse and may be undetectable (Figure 7.11)
- dehydration.

The clinico-pathological abnormalities that may be found include:

- **leucopenia** due to marked neutropenia (often <1000/mcl)
- thrombocytopenia

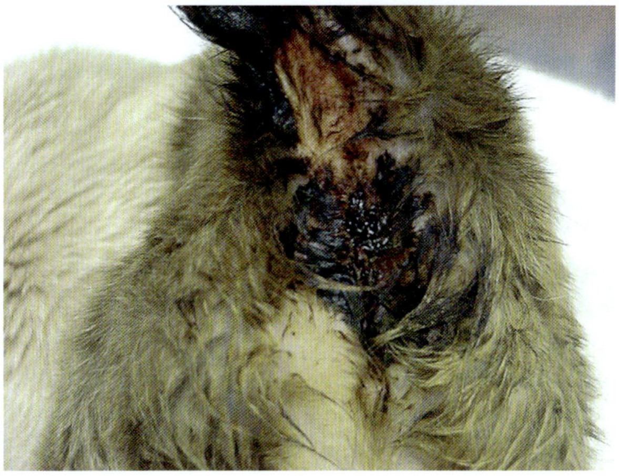

**Figure 7.11.** Diarrhoeic faeces stuck to the perineal area on a cat with feline panleukopenia. Sometimes the diarrhoea is not particularly profuse or may not even be clearly seen.

- mild anaemia
- prerenal azotaemia
- electrolyte abnormalities (due to serious dehydration)
- increase in bilirubin (associated with septicaemia).

Clinical signs in kittens with **cerebellar hypoplasia** include:

- ataxia, non-progressive (Video 7.1)
- intention tremors
- hypermetric gait, with no abnormalities in mental state or other neurological signs
- good general condition.

### *Diagnosis*

Clinical diagnosis is based on the characteristic clinico-pathological appearance, but it can be confirmed by tests that detect the virus in faeces or blood.

#### ELISA

There are ELISA tests with **good sensitivity and specificity** for the detection of **virus antigens in faeces**. They can be done in the practice and are useful for a quick diagnosis. However, it is important to take into account the possibility of **false negatives**, especially in the initial stages of infection when the antigenic load may be below test detection limit. But also, and more importantly, false negatives occur during the course of the disease if the viral antigens are blocked by antibodies that have already been formed. In short, a negative result does not rule out panleukopenia in a cat where this disease is suspected.

#### PCR

In recent years the use of feline parvovirus PCR has also become widespread. It is a **highly sensitive test in faeces and blood**. It is not affected by the presence of antibodies. The only related problem is false positives due to poor-quality laboratory technique.

> **Video 7.1.** Kitten with cerebellar hypoplasia showing ataxia and intention tremors. This neurological condition is diagnosed after a thorough neurological examination demonstrating cerebellar neuro-localisation with no other neurological signs and non-progressive history. http://publication.improveinternational.com.

#### Electron microscopy

Electron microscopy on faeces has also been used in a research setting, but it is not a test for day-to-day use in practice.

#### Antibody detection

Diagnosis by **antibody detection is not useful**, since there are no antibody titres that differentiate between disease, subclinical infection, exposure and previous vaccination. The technique can be used for epidemiological studies or to assess the immune response, but not for disease diagnosis.

#### Post-mortem

In cases of death in communities, post-mortem is very useful since histological intestinal lesions are characteristic and allow confirmation that it is due to panleukopenia.

### *Treatment*

There are no controlled clinical studies looking at treatment of feline panleukopenia. However, it is mainly supportive:

- Adequate **fluid therapy** to correct dehydration and continuous losses due to vomiting and diarrhoea (crystalloids and colloids).
- **Broad-spectrum antibiotic** therapy (e.g. -lactams plus quinolones or aminoglycosides).
- **Anti-emetics** (e.g. maropitant).
- **Analgesics** (e.g. buprenorphine).

In the most severe cases, and in very young or weakened kittens, some clinicians administer **fresh plasma** from either vaccinated cats or those that have recovered from panleukopenia, for rapid, **passive transfer of antibodies (5 ml/kg/day for 2–3 days)**. Alternatively, whole blood transfusions can be used to transfer antibodies or if the animal is suspected of having disseminated intravascular coagulation (DIC).

There are **no studies** on the use of **feline interferon omega** in cats with panleukopenia, but there are in canine parvovirus in dogs. Adding it to treatment is an option to try to enhance the non-specific immune response, and it may also have some antiviral action.

It is essential to **start feeding** an enteral or micro-enteral diet as soon as possible; when the most intense vomiting subsides, the necrotised intestine that is in the process of repairing itself should receive nutrients in order to recover as soon as possible. Enteral nutrition is probably beneficial for the prevention of sepsis due to bacterial translocation, although this has not yet been proven.

### Prognosis

**Prognosis is reserved** but depends entirely on the severity of the condition, the age and nutritional status of the cat and the treatment possibilities that can be accessed. The prognosis is poor in kittens in communities and rehoming centres, with mortality close to 80% if there is not access to intensive hospital treatment. On the contrary, if the animal can be treated thoroughly and intensively, depending on the severity of the condition, survival is >80%.

### Prevention

Prevention is based on the control of infections in communities and a thorough **disinfection of the environment with bleach**.

There have been **attenuated vaccines** available against feline parvovirus for many years (Table 7.6). These are very effective and produce robust or sterilising immunity. A well-immunised cat will not be infected even if it is exposed to the virus.

However, it is common to see infected cats during the primary vaccination process or shortly thereafter. These cases occur due to the fact that immunisation has not been done correctly or sufficiently, or due to interference with antibodies or maternal immunity. Many cats between 8 and 16 weeks old still have sufficient levels of maternal antibodies (especially from well-immunised mothers) to block subclinical infection by the vaccine. In contrast, these antibody levels are not sufficient to protect against natural infection by a pathogenic virus. Due to this phenomenon, **three doses of vaccine** are recommended for **primary vaccination** and **one revaccination per year**. In the latest WSAVA vaccination guides, revaccination before 1 year is proposed, around 6 months.

Table 7.6. Vaccination programme for feline panleukopenia.

| Essential vaccine, recommended in all cats | | |
|---|---|---|
| **Primary vaccination** | **Booster vaccination** | **Annual vaccination** |
| 3 doses: 8, 12 and 16 weeks | One year after the last dose | Annual in cats at risk of exposure<br>Every 3 years in low-risk cats |

## Giardia *infections*

### Aetiopathogenesis

***Giardia*** (*G. duodenalis*, *G. lamblia*, *G. intestinalis*) is a **flagellated protozoan** that can infect numerous mammalian species, including the cat. Several variants have been identified (A, B, C, D, E, F and G):

- F and G mainly affect the cat.
- Recent studies have identified variant A in cats.

The ***Giardia* cycle is direct**, with **oro-faecal infection**. It has two different stages:

- Mobile forms or trophozoites.
- Oocysts, which are formed by binary division.

Both forms can be identified in faeces. It is a **parasite with a small intestinal tropism**, where it produces lesions in enterocytes, and an **inflammatory response and atrophy** of the intestinal villi, resulting in acute or chronic diarrhoea with nutrient malabsorption.

### Epidemiology

Oocysts excreted in faeces are a form of resistance and remain **infective in the environment for months**, so consequently **infection can be direct or indirect**. The prevalence is generally high in cats with diarrhoea as well as in those without, although often there are no differences between prevalence in one or the other. Most of those with diarrhoea are kittens or young **cats under one year old**. There are numerous studies in different countries with a variable prevalence of up to 20%. **Co-infection with other parasites** is frequent.

### Clinical signs

Although **diarrhoea is small intestinal**, with malabsorption and weight loss, some cases show signs of large intestinal diarrhoea such as mucus and fresh blood.

### Diagnosis

#### Direct observation of faeces

Direct observation of faeces for the detection of **trophozoites** (Z-type movement) or oocysts is **not very sensitive** but very specific (if observation is positive, no further tests are needed).

#### Flotation with zinc sulphate

Since oocyst excretion is erratic – **several samples** are required on different days so that the sensitivity of zinc sulphate flotation is good (better than that of direct stool observation).

### ELISA

The sensitivity of a single ELISA test is similar to that of three flotations on alternate days.

### PCR

***Giardia* PCR** has a high sensitivity and allows different variants to be distinguished, which may be important for determining the zoonotic potential but gives a large number of positives in which the cause of diarrhoea is not *Giardia*.

### Response to treatment

This is used as a diagnostic test because it is **common to treat cats** with chronic diarrhoea with **antiparasitic agents with anti-*Giardia*** action in the initial stages of the diagnostic protocol, even if tests are negative.

### *Treatment*

The treatment of choice is **fenbendazole at 50 mg/kg/24 h for 5 days**, which has a response rate >90%. If a cat with chronic diarrhoea and *Giardia* does not respond to correct treatment with fenbendazole, it is very likely that this is not the cause of diarrhoea.

Alternative treatments:

- **Metronidazole (15–25 mg/kg/12 h for 7 days)**.
- Combination of febantel pyrantel pamoate and praziquantel at the standard dose for 3 consecutive days.

### *Prognosis*

**Prognosis is good** – no treatment resistant giardiasis has been identified.

Re-infection indicates that there is a source of environmental infection, although persistent diarrhoea in a cat that has been treated suggests that another disease is the cause of the diarrhoea.

### *Prevention*

There is no vaccine or preventive treatment. Years ago, in the United States, an inactivated vaccine was marketed that was used both as prevention and treatment, but in Europe it was not commercialised and is not currently available.

**Hygiene standards are important** to avoid infection and re-infection.

## Tritrichomonas *infestations*

### *Aetiopathogenesis*

The first description of *Tritrichomonas* diarrhoea in cats dates back to 2003. *Tritrichomonas foetus* is a **flagellated protozoan** parasite of cattle that is increasingly diagnosed in cats. Currently, research is being undertaken into whether the species that causes disease in cats is different from that in cattle, and *T. blagburni* has been proposed as a name (pending confirmation).

The parasite **cycle is direct**: trophozoites are excreted in faeces and spread to other cats by **oro-faecal contact**, either directly or by contamination of food or water. Unlike *Giardia*, there are no oocysts in the faeces. They have a special **tropism for the colon** and the distal part of the ileum, where they cause an **intense inflammatory response** (neutrophilic and lymphoplasmacytic) and the parasite lingers. They may be present in the colon without causing clinical signs, but in some cats the inflammation is very intense.

### *Epidemiology*

The disease has been documented globally worldwide, from the appearance of the first cases. Tritrichomoniasis usually occurs in pure-bred cats that come from a breeder or an **environment where there are a large number of animals**, especially in young cats less than one year old. Adults and the elderly can be subclinical carriers. **Co-infections** with other protozoa are frequent, especially with *Giardia* and *Isospora*.

### *Clinical signs*

Typical clinical signs include chronic large intestinal diarrhoea with:

- foul-smelling stools
- large amount of mucus (Figure 7.12)
- presence of fresh blood.

Sometimes there is a **marked proctitis** that can occur with faecal incontinence and even **rectal prolapse**. The

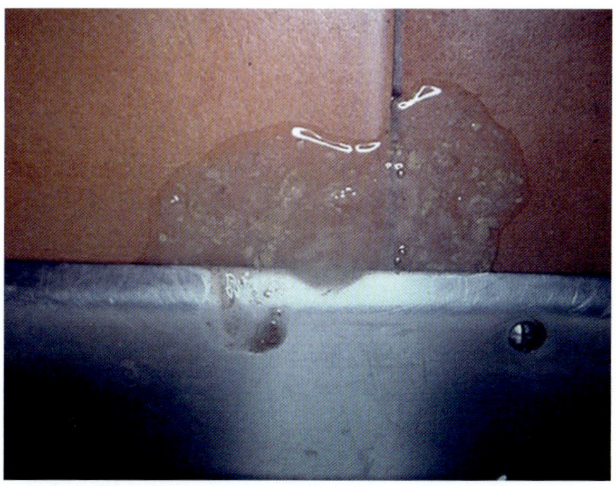

**Figure 7.12.** *Tritrichomonas* can cause severe, extremely intense, colitis and proctitis in cats, with high levels of mucus in the faeces and even some faecal incontinence.

> **Video 7.2.** Rectilinear movement of *Tritrichomonas* in fresh stools. The sensitivity of this test is low but it is improved if mucus samples are obtained, which are better than stools. http://publication.improveinternational.com.

presence of systemic signs is rare, but in some cases (<25%) there may be **anorexia and apathy**. Affected cats have no abnormalities on blood tests.

### *Diagnosis*

Diagnostic confirmation of tritrichomoniasis is important, otherwise cats with chronic colitis may end up being treated with immunosuppressants.

#### Direct observation of faeces

Direct **observation of trophozoites** in fresh stool samples is easy, immediate and cheap, but sensitivity is <20%. Samples should be examined immediately and should be observed in mucus samples. Trophozoites move rectilinearly, unlike *Giardia*. A negative result does not rule out the disease (Video 7.2).

#### Specific cultures

Faeces are incubated for a few days in a special culture medium (In-pouch TF) so that the parasites proliferate and it is possible to observe them under a microscope. The sensitivity is 60% but, at a technical level, specific cultures are more complex.

#### PCR

**PCR** is currently considered the **technique of choice**, although it is more expensive and requires a few days for results to be obtained.

#### Other

Sometimes the parasite can also be observed on histology of colonic biopsies, although the sensitivity is not very high.

### *Treatment*

Firstly, it is essential to **treat any coinfections** that exist, since sometimes diarrhoea is caused by other pathogens. Tritrichomoniasis heals spontaneously in most cases but, as it may take time (from 5 months to 2 years), the diarrhoea must be treated to improve the quality of life of the animal, in addition to correcting the inconvenience caused around the house due to large intestinal diarrhoea with faecal incontinence.

There is **no effective commercially registered treatment** for this disease, but the drug that provides the best results is **ronidazole**, with approximately 70% efficacy at a **dose of 30 mg/kg/12–24 h for 2 weeks** (at higher doses it frequently causes **neurological (vestibular) toxicity**). Many cats remain infected after treatment, but diarrhoea disappears or improves.

Cats that recover spontaneously may remain asymptomatic chronic carriers and are a source of infection for other cats that are in contact.

### *Prognosis*

The **prognosis is good**, although some cats do not respond to safe doses of ronidazole and diarrhoea persists, or they relapse shortly after treatment.

### *Prevention*

At the time of writing there is **no vaccine** or preventive treatment for this parasitosis. The implementation of good hygienic and sanitary standards to reduce the possibility of infection is essential at breeders' premises and amongst cat communities. It is important to treat cats that manifest diarrhoea to reduce the parasitic burden in the environment.

## *Coronavirus infections*

### *General considerations*

Over the past two decades **opinions have changed** considerably on the **relationship between coronavirus infections and infectious peritonitis**. Nowadays it is clear that the previous distinction between coronavirus and feline infectious peritonitis was inadequate In reality, many cats are **temporarily or permanently infected** with feline coronavirus (FCoV), especially if they live in groups. However, the **majority have no clinical signs** and will never be sick, with a small number, perhaps **<10%, developing the disease** known as feline infectious peritonitis(FIP).

## *Feline infectious peritonitis (FIP)*

### *Aetiopathogenesis*

Feline coronaviruses are **RNA viruses** with an **extraordinary mutational capacity** and genetic variability. They are widely distributed in groups of animals and in the environment where they are **extremely resistant**.

Many cats acquire infection from contact with faeces from carrier cats or in contaminated FCoV environments. FCoVs show a predominant **tropism for enterocytes** and produce a **transient or permanent intestinal infection** that may or may not cause mild clinical signs. They can also produce viraemia and systemic infection, although without clinical consequences.

Continuous virus mutations that occur during intestinal replication can lead to **variants of the virus** with different tropisms and an ability to enter the systemic circulation and infect monocytes/macrophages to escape the defence mechanisms of the immune system. If the cellular immune response is not adequate, the cat can develop the disease known as FIP, **in which lesions are immune mediated**. The virus does not produce direct cytolysis of cells or epithelia, but **hides in monocytes and tissue macrophages** avoiding the cellular immune response. This triggers an exaggerated and ineffective humoral immune response with immune complex deposition and complement activation that can cause different forms:

- **Wet form**. In the most **severe and acute form**, vasculitis occurs in serosa, especially in the peritoneum and pleurae, with extravasation of a **protein-rich exudate** into cavities.
- **Dry form**. In the most **chronic forms**, a perivascular pyogranulomatous inflammatory **infiltrate occurs in solid organs** (lymph nodes, spleen, central nervous system, eyes).

These two clinical forms are not exclusive – rather they **represent the extremes** of a dynamic process influenced by the cat's immune response. Both types of lesion can co-exist in the same animal suffering from FIP.

The probability that a FCoV carrier develops FIP is higher if it is **young** and lives with other cats, especially if the environmental or nutritional conditions are not optimal. Therefore, **environmental stress** is an important factor in the development of FIP.

In general, FIP does not spread from one sick cat to another. **Mutant viruses do not usually replicate in the intestines**, and consequently they are **neither excreted in faeces** nor spread in the environment. Cats suffering from FIP generally continue to **spread FCoV in their faeces** (virus not responsible for causing FIP). However, there are **exceptions** to this model since in some rare cases outbreaks of FIP have been described in cats in contact with natural infection. This phenomenon has also been described in experimental infections – that is, there are **variants of the virus capable of producing FIP and maintaining intestinal replication and contaminating the environment** or other cats.

## Epidemiology

**FCoV infections are prevalent** in cat populations due to the **high environmental resistance** of these viruses and the large number of cats that suffer from transient or permanent intestinal infections. Most felines originating from **group situations** suffer from FCoV infections from an early age, especially if the mother is infected. The **percentage of cats that suffer from FIP is low in relation to the large number of coronavirus carriers**.

The main **risk factors**, as a result of the inability of the immune system to control mutated pathogenic variants capable of producing systemic infection in monocytes, meaning that the cat becomes affected by FIP, include:

- Age (<2 years old and old cats).
- Poor environmental conditions (overcrowding, poor nutrition).
- Breed.
- Stress.
- Immunosuppression (other diseases, surgery, feline leukaemia virus infection).

## Clinical signs

Cats with intestinal infection due to FCoV do not show clinical signs or, at most, suffer from **acute diarrhoea that remits spontaneously** after a few days. Persistent FCoV infections have not been shown to be a cause of chronic diarrhoea (Figure 7.13).

Cats with FIP usually show **systemic signs of illness** such as anorexia, apathy, fever and weight loss.

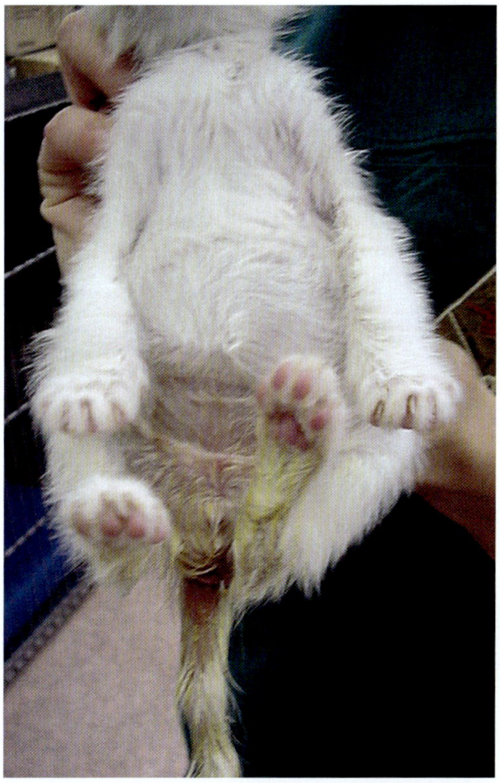

**Figure 7.13.** Kitten with acute signs of diarrhoea without systemic signs of disease. Coronavirus infections are a common cause, with many cats seropositive to coronavirus and positive to coronavirus RNA PCR on faeces.

If they have the **wet form** of the disease they may have:

- Abdominal distention (peritoneal effusion) (Figure 7.14).
- Respiratory distress (pleural effusion) (Figures 7.15 and 7.16).
- Eye disease (keratitis, keratic precipitates, exudative uveitis, hyphaema).
- Signs of CNS disease (ataxia, depression, seizures, compatible with vestibular syndrome or multifocal disease). Many cats only present with CNS signs.

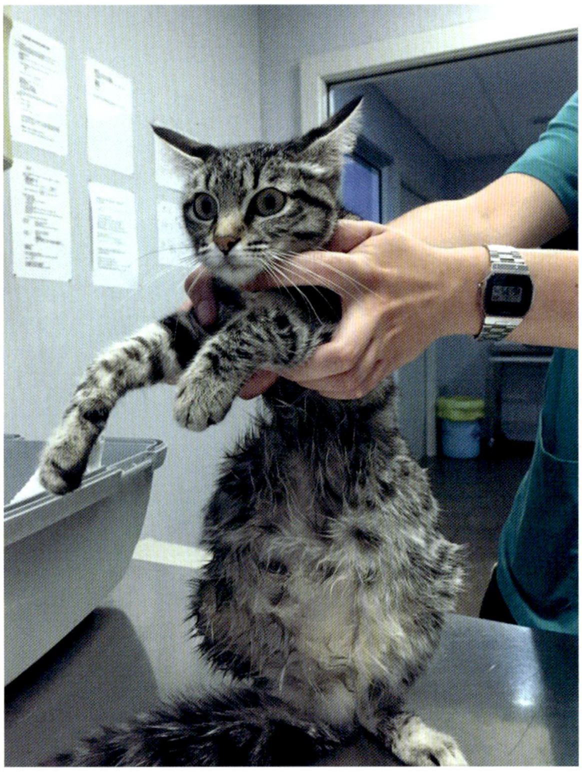

**Figure 7.14.** Kitten with marked abdominal distension due to an abdominal effusion. Complete testing of abdominal fluid confirms the diagnosis of wet-form FIP.

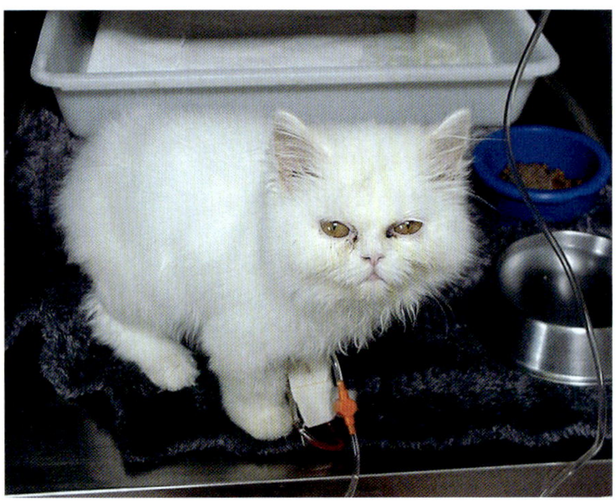

**Figure 7.15.** Persian kitten with respiratory distress and fever just a few weeks after being bought from a kitten farm.

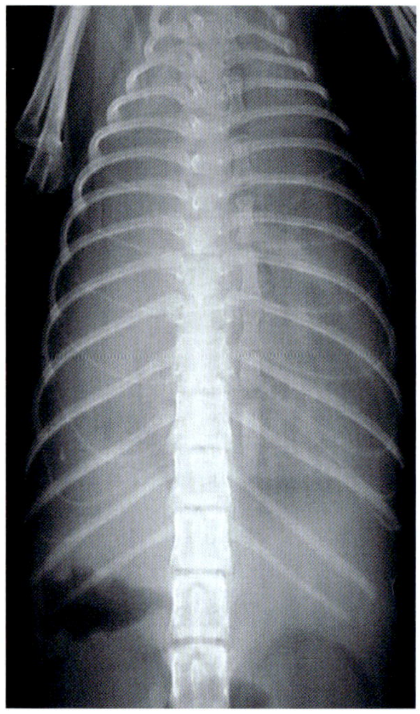

**Figure 7.16.** Radiography of the previous cat, where abundant pleural fluid is seen. Complete testing on pleural fluid confirmed a diagnosis of wet-form FIP.

If the **dry form** predominates the **clinical signs are less specific** and depend on which organ is most affected. Apart from the systemic signs that develop over months, other symptoms may appearincluding:

- Kidney disease (Figure 7.17).
- Palpable or visible mesenteric lymphadenopathy on abdominal ultrasound.
- High bilirubin.
- Ocular and/or neurological lesions (more frequent in the dry or granulomatous form).

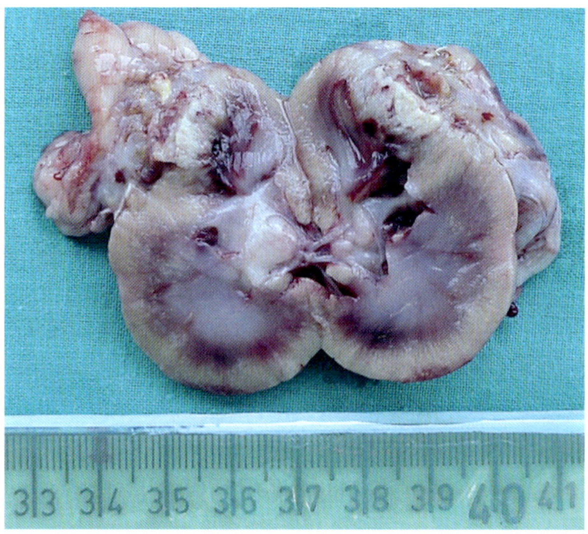

**Figure 7.17.** Macroscopic lesions due to granulomatous nephritis caused by FIP, confirmed histologically using immunohistochemistry. The cat improved clinically but died 7 months after starting treatment with prednisolone.

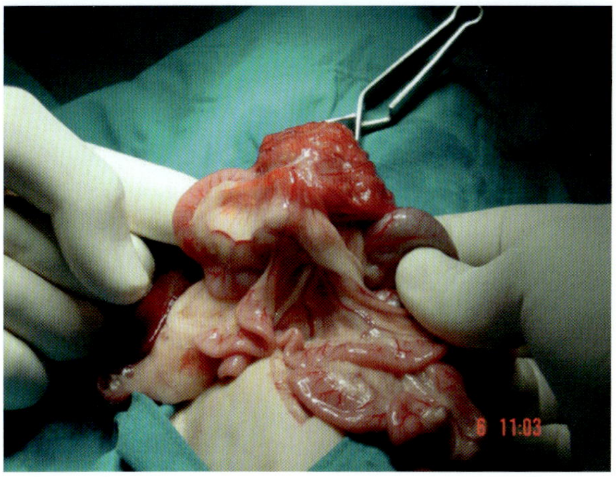


**Figure 7.18.** Intestinal granuloma found on exploratory laparotomy. Histology and immunohistochemistry confirmed intestinal granuloma due to FIP. This is an atypical form which can be confused clinically with intestinal neoplasia.

**Atypical forms** have also been described with the following symptoms:

- cutaneous granulomas
- joint effusion
- pericardial effusion
- scrotal effusion
- intestinal granulomas (Figure 7.18).
- cutaneous fragility.

### *Diagnosis*

**Diagnosis of FIP is difficult**, especially in most chronic cases with the formation of pyogranulomas in different organs.

#### FCoV antibody titre

**Serological techniques that detect anti-FCoV antibodies do not discriminate between antibodies and the virus causing FIP**. A diagnosis of FIP based solely on an antibody titre is incorrect, however high it may be. It is also incorrect to think that a healthy FIP-positive cat that does not currently present with FIP will go on to develop the disease sooner or later. A **high percentage of healthy cats are seropositive** and most will never develop FIP.

To the contrary, there are documented cases of cats with FIP that were seronegative (antibodies are bound in antigen–antibody complexes and are not detected by the test). Consequently, antibody titres against FCoV should always be interpreted alongside the clinical signs. The maximum titre from a laboratory, together with highly suggestive clinical-analytical signs of FIP and having ruled out other diseases that may also cause similar signs, helps to lead to suspicions of FIP, but it never constitutes a definitive diagnostic confirmatory test. On the other hand, a negative antibody titre makes it less likely, though not impossible, for it to be FIP. In addition, there is wide variability between laboratories with regard to the serological techniques used for FCoV identification, which implies that the results are not very reliable.

#### PCR

Neither are PCR tests that detect the FCoV genome the definitive solution in the diagnosis of FIP, since **conventional PCR does not discriminate between FCoV and the FIP virus**. Changes in the genome between the two variants are minimal, the result of deletions in the genome, which has made it difficult to design a PCR that differentiates pathogenic from non-pathogenic forms. However, in recent years it has been possible to detect at least two mutations in the spike protein associated with variants with a greater tropism to produce systemic infections by means of a pyrosequencing technique.

In general, PCR techniques on **blood samples have low sensitivity** and most cats with FIP have negative results. On the contrary, **PCR sensitivity increases considerably in effusion samples**, cerebrospinal fluid (CSF) and biopsies from organs in which there is a granulomatous lesion. Currently, if a good real-time RT–PCR of one of these samples is positive and one of the two mutations associated with systemic infection is detected in pyrosequencing, a diagnosis can be confirmed. However, even in samples such as these, RT–PCR can be negative and even if FIP is the final diagnosis.

On the other hand, blood PCR is positive in certain cats infected with FCoV but not suffering from FIP since, although in small quantities, the virus is present and replicating in the intestine, and also in circulating monocytes. In these cases, the mutations associated with FIP may even be detected since these variants acquire the capacity to produce systemic infection, but do not necessarily cause FIP.

#### Diagnostic suspicions

**Diagnostic suspicion**: In summary, diagnosis of FIP is complex, clinical and clinico-pathological aspects must always be **interpreted together** with results of specific tests (serological or molecular).

The **wet form**, characterised by vasculitis in serosal membranes, is easier to diagnose. Effusions caused by FIP have specific characteristics that allow a clinical diagnosis to be reached with a reliable prognostic value (Figure 7.19). These **effusions are characterised by**:

- low or moderate cellularity
- presence of neutrophils and macrophages
- high levels of globulins
- albumin/globulin ratio <0.8
- positive Rivalta test

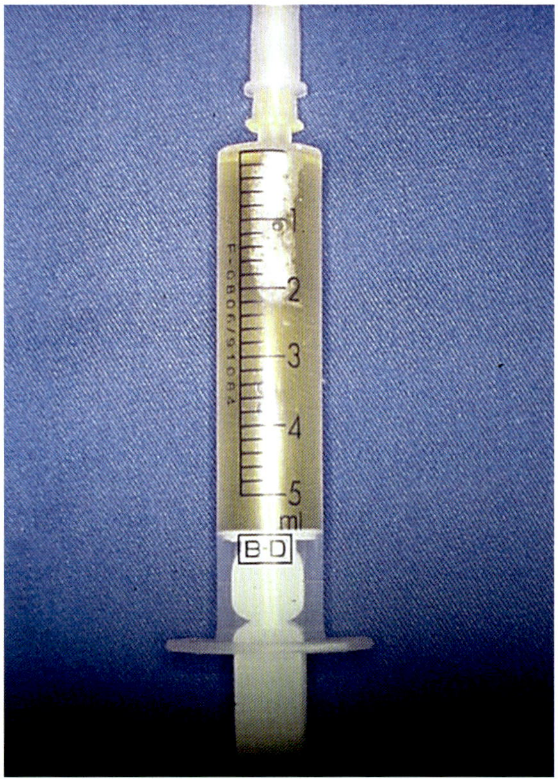


Figure 7.19. Fluid from the abdominal or pleural cavity with the typical appearance of an FIP effusion: yellow, ochre in colour with a dense, viscous appearance. Complete analysis of the fluid includes counting and cytology, electrophoresis (or the Rivalta test), techniques for antigen detection (IFA) or detection of genetic material from coronavirus (PCR).

- FCoV detection using the following techniques:
  - immunofluorescence
  - RT–PCR
  - pyrosequencing.

The **effusive form is typical**, although not exclusive, to **young cats** (<2 years of age), pure-bred cats and those from breeders.

Cases without effusions are harder to confirm, and ruling out other diseases and correct interpretation of laboratory tests are very important. The organs that most frequently present with **lesions due to dry FIP** are:

- liver
- kidneys
- eyes
- CNS.

Most cats with non-effusive FIP have:

- **fever**
- **weight loss**
- abnormalities or clinical signs related to the involvement of one or more of these organs.

The most frequent laboratory abnormalities are:

- lymphopenia
- non-regenerative anaemia
- microcytosis
- hyperbilirubinaemia
- hyperglobulinaemia or decreased albumin/globulin ratio
- high levels of $\alpha\alpha$-1 glycoprotein
- high antibody titres against FCoV.

If a cat has several of these abnormalities and other diseases are ruled out, a diagnosis of FIP is highly probable although not definitive.

### Diagnostic confirmation

The only way to fully confirm the diagnosis is to demonstrate typical histological lesions (pyogranulomas) in the affected organs, and to test for the **presence of FCoV within macrophages** (Figure 7.20) by means of immunohistochemical techniques (or RT–PCR).

### *Treatment*

FIP is considered a deadly disease with, to date, no curative treatment available. Veterinarians who say that they have cured cases of FIP, or who have observed abnormally high survival with different treatments, probably start from erroneous diagnoses given the complexity involved in confirmation of the diagnosis and the existence of other diseases (lymphoma, lymphocytic cholangitis, pyothorax) with similar clinical presentations. However, there are well-documented cases of FIP with longer survival times than usual, even for several years or with complete recovery, although these are exceptional.

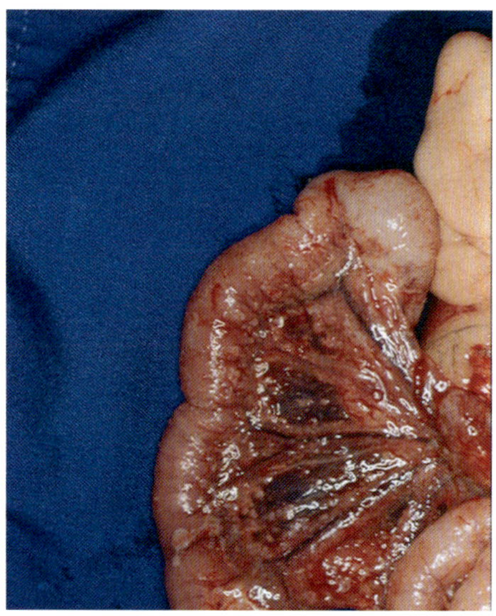

Figure 7.20. Nodular lesions in the mesentery found on postmortem of a cat with confirmed FIP.

**Palliative or symptomatic treatment** for FIP is based on **suppression of the inflammatory/immune-mediated cause** of the lesions. The most widely accepted is the use of **high-dose corticosteroids (prednisolone 2–3 mg/kg/day)** through systemic or intra-cavitary routes, although there are no controlled studies. Other drugs that have been tested include **pentoxifylline** (vasculitis), **ozagrel** (thromboxane synthesis inhibitor) and **aspirin** (inflammation and vasculitis).

There are two clinical studies on the treatment of FIP with **feline omega interferon**, at high doses of **106 MUI/kg/24 h SC for 7 days and then every 7 days**. The first gave promising results, since the survival rate of some cats was very high. In some cases, the diagnosis of FIP was not fully confirmed.

Only cats with confirmed FIP were included in the second, and two groups were compared: those treated with interferon and cortisone and those treated with cortisone and placebo. No statistically significant differences were observed between groups, but one of the cats treated with interferon had a survival time longer than expected.

Studies with a greater number of cats are needed.

Although there are no prospective studies, at low doses human alpha-interferon used as an immunostimulant is contraindicated, since with FIP **non-specific stimulation of the immune system should be avoided**.

There are also some case series of dry FIP treated with the immune stimulator **Polyprenil Immunostimulant**, marketed in the United States. In a first series of three cases of confirmed FIP, survival was unexpectedly high, more than 2 years in two cats and 14 months in another. In a second series, looking at 58 cats, the results were not so good: 20% of cats survived >6 months and only one cat exceeded a survival time of one year.

Recently, studies have been carried out with the use of protease inhibitor antiviral drugs in cats suffering from FIP. So far, the results of a study in experimentally infected cats and a series of 20 cats with natural infection have been published. In both the results are good in a high percentage of cases, so that remission of the clinical signs occurs temporarily or even long term. This drug (3c-*like* protease inhibitor, 15 mg/kg/12 h SC) is not yet commercially available, but the results of these first studies are promising so in the future there is the possibility of effectively treating cats with FIP.

Another new promising treatment approach is the use of nucleoside analogues that act as an alternative substrate for viral RNA synthesis. The compound GS-441524, was shown to be non-toxic in vitro and effectively inhibited replication of FIP-associated FCoV strains and field isolates in two different cell culture systems. In ten young cats with experimentally induced FIP, GS-441524 (applied SQ q 12 h) caused a rapid reversal of clinical signs and return to a clinically healthy status within two weeks of treatment in all ten cats. Two of the ten treated cats had recurrences of clinical signs at four and six weeks post treatment, respectively. These two cats were treated a second time with GS-441524 for two weeks and they responded again, identically to the response seen with the first treatment. All ten cats remained clinically healthy 8 eight months post infection with no signs of toxicity.

GS-441524 treatment has recently also been evaluated in a field non-controlled study of 31 cats with FIP. The cats were started with a primary treatment course of GS-441524 at a dosage of 2 mg/kg SQ q 24 h for at least 12 weeks. The dosage was increased to 4 mg/kg SQ q 24 h for later treatments in the trial when cats showed a relapse or when a treatment course of longer than 12 weeks was deemed necessary. Five of the 31 cats died or were euthanized within 26 days of the first treatment. The remaining 26 cats completed 12 or more weeks of GS-441524 treatment and showed rapid clinical improvement within two weeks. Of these 26 cats, 18 remained healthy, while eight others showed FIP relapses (six cats non-neurological FIP and two cats neurological FIP) at a mean of 23 days following treatment. Three of the eight cats with relapses were treated again with GS-441524 at 2 mg/kg SQ q 24 h; one of these three cats relapsed with neurological FIP and was euthanized whilst the two remaining cats responded well but relapsed with FIP again and were treated again with GS-441524 but at a higher dosage of 4 mg/kg SQ q 24 h. Of the original 31 cats, 25 were classified as long-time survivors after successful treatment. Neither GC376 nor GS-441524 are currently commercially available.

### Prognosis

The **prognosis is poor** for cats with FIP, except for rare cases with a survival time longer than normal. Those suffering from effusive or **wet forms die within a few weeks** after diagnosis, while those affected by dry forms can survive a few months.

In a study of cats with wet forms, the average survival was 9 days (50% of cats) and only one cat lived more than 6 months (200 days).

### Prevention

Prevention of FIP is based on the **management of feline communities** and on avoiding large numbers of in-contact cats carrying FCoV, which is difficult to put into practice.

An **intranasal vaccine** is available, based on thermosensitive variants of the virus that replicate only in the nasal mucosa, which induces a local humoral

Table 7.7. Vaccination programme for FIP.

| Non-essential vaccine, consider its use in seronegative cats at risk of exposure to FCoV | | |
|---|---|---|
| **Primary vaccination** | **Booster vaccination** | **Annual vaccination** |
| 2 doses: 16 and 19 weeks | One year after the last dose | Annual |

response (Table 7.7). It has been shown that while the vaccine is safe, it **does not protect cats that are already seropositive** or FCoV carriers from FIP. However, it can protect cats that are seronegative but that have not yet been exposed to FCoV from FCoV infection and that will enter an environment where the virus is the present. However, this situation is unlikely in real life since many cats have contact with FCoV before the age at which the vaccine can be used (4 months), so it is considered a **non-essential vaccine** in committee guides by experts such as those of the AAFP, ABCD and WSAVA.

## Retrovirus infections

### General considerations

There are several retroviruses, both pathogenic and non-pathogenic, that can infect the cat. The most important are:

- feline leukaemia virus (FeLV)
- feline immunodeficiency virus (FIV).

FeLV and FIV infections have some **points in common** – for example, both viruses may be **present for a time in clinically healthy cats** and both can **produce an acquired immunodeficiency syndrome**. However, they have many epidemiological, pathogenic and diagnostic differences. In any healthy or sick cat, knowing the status of retrovirus infection is essential so that diagnostic tests for both viruses are performed frequently.

Retroviruses have a characteristic and unique infection mechanism: they are single-stranded RNA viruses that have a reverse transcriptase enzyme through which they are able to copy their own genome to double-stranded DNA and integrate it into the genome of the cell they infect.

**Depending on the virus and host immunity**, the infection is more or less active and **may or may not cause disease**. However, even when illness is not caused by the virus genome, the latter may become integrated and **latent in the genome of some cells**. This fact may not have clinical consequences, but sometimes it is at the origin of the reactivation of the infection or of the neoplastic transformation of infected cells.

## Feline leukaemia virus (FeLV) infection

### Aetiopathogenesis

FeLV is an oncogenic gamma retrovirus with the ability to transform the cells it infects into neoplastic ones. It is a **very fragile RNA virus in the environment**, which is easily inactivated with common disinfectants. Indirect contagion by fomites is unlikely, unless it is immediate.

Because FeLV is **transmitted both horizontally** (saliva, urine, faeces, milk) and **vertically** (intrauterine), any positive cat that eliminates virus in saliva or other secretions is a source of infection for other cats in direct contact, and to their own offspring, and it can even spread to cats that are not in direct contact if they **share food and water bowls**.

Adults are more resistant to infection even if they are not vaccinated, but they may be infected if the viral load is high or the animal's immune status is not good.

When a cat becomes infected, a **viraemia** occurs which may be:

- **Transitory**. Presence of free and lymphocyte-associated virus. If the cat develops good immunity, infection is blocked.
- **Persistent**. If immunity is not sufficient to stop the infection, the virus infects and replicates in the bone marrow progenitor cells. It causes a neutrophil- and platelet-associated viraemia. Subsequently, epithelia and glands are infected and the virus spreads throughout the body.

Sometimes the immune response contains virus already present in the bone marrow, and prevents persistent viraemia from developing. Consequently, the **interaction between the virus and the immune response determines the course of the infection**, which may be one of the following:

- **Abortive**. There is no viraemia after exposure to the virus.
- **Regressive**. Transient viraemia that is blocked by the immune response, although some cells may remain with DNA provirus integrated into their genome.
- **Progressive**. Persistent viraemia and infection of epithelia and glands; clinical disease develops within months or a few years.

### Epidemiology

Retrovirus infections in cats have a **variable prevalence** depending on the geographical area and lifestyle of the animal. In fact, in many countries the prevalence of FeLV infection has decreased considerably thanks to good management programmes and vaccination.

At-risk cats are those that may have **continued direct intimate contact with persistently viraemic cats** excreting virus in bodily secretions.

Given the vertical mode of transmission, **cats used for breeding must be negative**. Blood donor cats must also be negative, so performing provirus PCR on potential donor cats is advisable. If they are positive, the blood should be rejected even if they are not viral (ELISA-negative).

### *Clinical signs*

Cats may remain healthy for a relatively long time (up to 3–4 years). In a healthy cat, or one with mild signs of illness, a positive FeLV result does not necessarily imply that it suffers from a progressive infection – it may be suffering from a transient viraemia or regressive infection. In these cases, **tests should be repeated after 6–8 weeks**.

**Progressive infections** manifest with a wide variety of diseases, including:

- neoplasms (lymphoma, leukaemia, others)
- non-neoplastic haematological diseases (myelodysplastic syndromes, medullary aplasias)
- immunodeficiency syndrome (opportunistic diseases, chronic or recurrent oral, respiratory, skin or gastrointestinal infections)
- immune-mediated diseases (glomerulonephritis, uveitis, polyarthritis, haemolytic anaemia)
- peripheral neuropathies (anisocoria, urinary incontinence)
- reproductive disorders (abortion, neonatal mortality)
- lymphoid hyperplasia
- virus-associated dermatosis.

The **most frequent clinico-pathological abnormalities** in cats with progressive infections are:

- anaemia (regenerative or non-regenerative)
- macrocytosis
- cytopenias (neutropenia, lymphopenia, thrombocytopenia) or pancytopenia
- lymphocytosis or extreme monocytosis with immature neoplastic forms (in cases of neutrophilic leukaemia).

### *Diagnosis*

There are several diagnostic tests for FeLV that should be **interpreted together**, and always depending on whether the cat is **sick or healthy**.

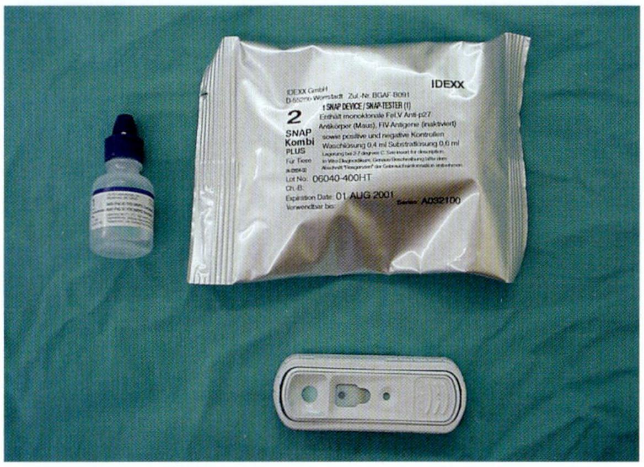


**Figure 7.21.** Numerous diagnostic kits are available for the rapid detection of FLV antigens (p27) and antibodies against FIV. The sensitivity and specificity of snap tests are good, although there is a small percentage of false positives.

#### ELISA or immunochromatographic (IC) tests

These tests **detect a virus circulating antigen**, specifically p27, whose presence in blood or serum (antigenaemia) means that there is infection and viraemia. The sensitivity and specificity are good (> 90%), although not perfect, which is of vital importance when interpreting results in healthy or low-risk cats (Figure 7.21).

Because these tests are positive with both transient viraemia (regressive infection from which the cat can recover) and persistent viraemia (progressive infection), in a healthy animal or with clinical signs attributable to other diseases a **positive result is not definitive** and should not lead to euthanasia.

Both techniques have a small percentage of false positives associated with the technique itself. In populations with a low prevalence, or in healthy cats on which the test is performed for epidemiological reasons or prior to vaccination, a confirmatory test should be performed.

In a **sick cat**, especially with abnormalities or diseases typically associated with FeLV (anaemia, lymphoma, immunosuppression, myeloproliferative diseases), a positive ELISA result is sufficient to **establish a diagnosis**.

In a **healthy cat**, or one with abnormalities or clinical signs that can be attributed to other causes, a positive ELISA result must be confirmed by **provirus PCR** (to rule out false positives) and by **repeated ELISA** (or IFA if available) weeks or months later (to differentiate regressive infection from progressive).

#### Immunofluorescence (IFA)

This test is not widely used. In the UK this is considered a good method for differentiating between transient and persistent viraemia in the face of a positive ELISA result. It is based on the **detection of intracellular p27**, not that which is soluble or circulating in blood, so it **confirms persistent viraemia** (progressive infection).

On the other hand, it can give false positives (eosinophils) or false negatives (leucopenia).

### DNA PCR and PCR provirus

In the past decade, numerous laboratories have begun to offer DNA PCR tests. A positive result means that the **virus genome has already been integrated into some cat cells** – that is, confirms FeLV infection (regressive or progressive).

Provirus PCR must always be interpreted in conjunction with the ELISA/IC result: it should **never be used as the only test**. Its main utility is to confirm the presence of infection in cases of doubtful or inconclusive ELISA results (Table 7.8).

Provirus PCR is positive in transient and persistent viraemia.

### PCR for virus RNA detection

This is a new test not yet used routinely in diagnostic laboratories. It allows the detection and **quantification of free virus** in the absence of cells: for example, for a negative-ELISA cat, positive on provirus PCR and negative on RNA, PCR is not viral. Another utility of RNA PCR could be to detect virus genome in ELISA-negative cats given its greater sensitivity. The test has been shown to have good sensitivity in whole blood, serum and plasma, saliva and faeces.

### Detection of neutralising antibodies

This is generally not used in diagnosis, and **results are difficult to interpret**. Many cats develop antibodies against endogenous retroviruses that are integrated into their cells. Few laboratories offer this test routinely.

Table 7.8. Joint evaluation of provirus PCR and ELISA/IC.

| PCR provirus | ELISA/IC | Evaluation |
|---|---|---|
| Positive | Negative | Cats with good immunity in which the virus did not reach the bone marrow, but that have cells into which the virus genome has integrated<br>They do not pose a risk of infection to other cats, and the infection will rarely reactivate |
| Positive | Persistent positive (two positive tests 2–3 months apart) | The cat is infected |
| Negative | Positive or doubtful | ELISA/IC positives are false positives |

## *Treatment*

The first measure should be to **isolate cats**, to avoid infecting other cats and decrease the likelihood of them acquiring other infections.

If the cat has an opportunistic disease or chronic infection, it should be treated as normal; if suffering from lymphoma, it can be treated with chemotherapy in the same way as cats with virus-negative lymphomas, although the prognosis is generally worse (Figure 7.22).

Retrovirus infections can be treated with **antiretroviral drugs** and/or **immunostimulatory or immunomodulatory drugs** such as interferons, amongst others.

Anti-retroviral studies in infected cats: a controlled clinical study with several treatment groups showed **no benefits in the use of AZT (zidovudine)** in cats with progressive infection.

Recent experimental and clinical studies with **raltegravir** (integrase inhibitor) demonstrate beneficial effects in FeLV-positive cats. Tolerance of raltegravir is good at a **dose of 20 mg/kg/12 h PO**, and has shown

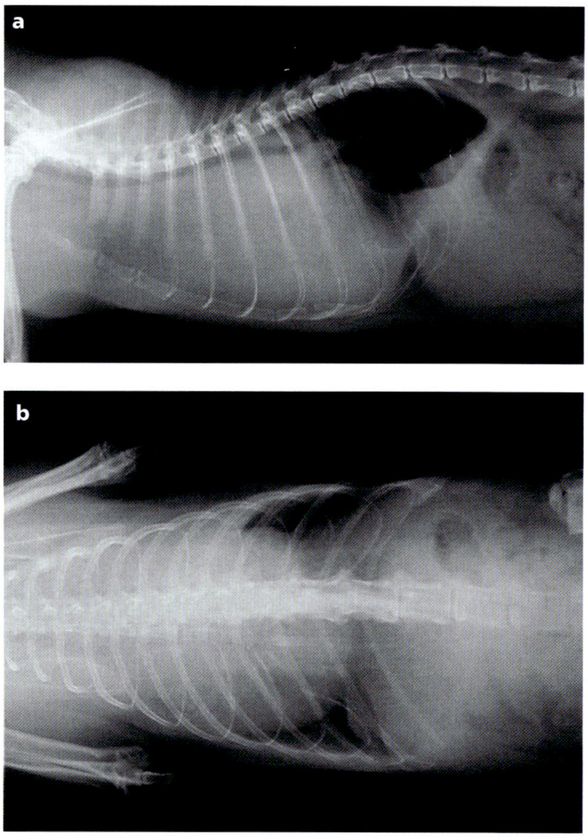


Figure 7.22. Lateral (a) and dorsoventral (b) radiographs of a pyrexic, 2-year old cat in respiratory distress, which tested positive to feline leukaemia antigen. A cranio-ventral mediastinal mass can be seen, confirmed using ultrasound-guided aspiration and cytology as a high-grade lymphoma.

a beneficial effect both in clinico-pathological aspects and infection parameters as well as viral load. Because viraemia did not remiss in any of the cats, treatment should be continuous.

One controlled study showed that the use of **feline omega interferon in positive cats improves clinical status and survival**. It was not evaluated whether the positive effect was due to antiviral action or the immunological effect on infections or opportunistic diseases.

In a subsequent study, with the same treatment regime, the viral load (RNA PCR) was evaluated and no decreases were observed, so it follows that interferon acts as an **immunomodulator** rather than as an antiviral.

### *Prognosis*

For sick cats with progressive viraemia the **prognosis is poor**, and this is considered a deadly disease. The life expectancy of FeLV-positive cats is variable:

- If the cat is healthy without any serious associated illness, 1–3 years, but cases with longer survival times have even been documented.
- If the cat has lymphoma, around 6 months.
- If the cat lives in a group, <3 years although a small percentage may live longer.

### *Prevention*

**Infection prevention is based on isolation and vaccination.** Since the virus is not transmitted via aerosol and fomites, if the cat lives at home alone or with other negative cats, and no contact with unknown cats, the risk of acquiring the infection is nil. This is why vaccination recommendations established by some expert committees (AAFP, ABCD, WSAVA) do not consider feline leukaemia vaccination as essential in indoor cats (Table 7.9). On the contrary, it is strongly recommended for those that may have contact with uncontrolled cats because of their lifestyle. Sometimes this recommendation is clarified by advising that, although it is considered that the cat is at low risk, it is better to administer **the annual vaccination and revaccination since it is not possible to guarantee 100% that the cat does not come into contact with uncontrolled cats**.

Table 7.9. Vaccination programme for FeLV.

| **Vaccine highly recommended in outdoor cats or in possible contact with other cats, and not essential in indoor cats which do not come into contact with other cats** | | |
|---|---|---|
| **Primary vaccination** | **Booster vaccination** | **Annual vaccination** |
| 2 doses: 9 and 12 weeks | One year after the last dose | Annual until 3 years old<br>Cats >3 years old, every 2 or 3 years |

Current vaccines against feline leukaemia are very effective overall. They induce a good cellular immunity that does not protect from infection, but from clinical disease and p27 antigenaemia. A vaccinated cat may be provirus PCR positive if it is subsequently infected, but it will be ELISA negative and is not a source of infection for others.

**Cats at risk of being in contact with unknown cats should be vaccinated.** Primary vaccination at **9 and 12 weeks** is very important given the greater susceptibility in kittens, and annual revaccination is also essential; and, if the risk of infection persists, annual revaccination is recommended, although with age the risk of infection decreases. A recent study of duration of immunity showed that the vaccine is effective for at least 2 years, and consequently the revaccination in cats >3 years of age, in which the natural immunity is greater, could be every 2 years.

It is important to know whether the cat is positive before vaccinating. Vaccination of an already positive cat is not dangerous and does not accelerate the infection or disease, but will lead to a 'vaccine failure' in the opinion of the owner, or even for them to think that the infection has been caused by the vaccine. **Inactivated FeLV vaccines are epidemiologically associated with the development of sarcomas at injection sites**, because they are vaccines with adjuvant and produce an inflammatory reaction that, in some predisposed cats, is the trigger for the appearance of such sarcomas. The new recombinant vaccines that use a canarypox viral vector do not carry adjuvant and produce less inflammation in the area, which should reduce the risk of sarcomas in susceptible cats, although this has not yet been proven.

## Feline immunodeficiency virus (FIV) infection

### *Aetiopathogenesis*

**FIV is a lentivirus** that produces **chronic and persistent infections in cats**. It is a **fragile** virus, of which there are up to six different variants that can have **different levels of virulence**, and does not last long in the environment. **Infection by direct or intimate contact** between a positive and a negative cat is inefficient and not a common cause of disease.

The most common route of transmission is natural **infection through bites between a positive** and a negative cat, since contact with saliva and/or blood is necessary for effective infection. Although the transmission of positive mothers to kittens has been demonstrated under experimental conditions, it seems to be ineffective under natural infection unless the cat is infected near or during pregnancy, since the viral load is higher in the early stages of the infection.

When a cat becomes infected, FIV replicates in lymphoid tissue and **produces viraemia**, initially with a considerable viral load. At this point humoral and cellular immune responses develop that reduce, but do not eliminate, the viraemia. In this first phase of acute infection, the cat may manifest **non-specific clinical signs** of viraemia (fever, discomfort, neutropenia, diarrhoea and lymphadenopathy).

The condition then progresses to a **subclinical or asymptomatic phase**. This can last for months or years, during which time the cat has no clinical signs but is seropositive.

During this phase, FIV progressively **destroys CD4$^+$ lymphocytes**, which is the main direct action of the virus. When CD4$^+$ levels are **very low, serious dysfunction** of cellular immunity occurs and an acquired immunodeficiency syndrome appears, with **chronic infections**, opportunistic diseases and certain neoplasms. Many cats also have **chronic oral and respiratory infections**. Immune-mediated diseases associated with the deposition of immune complexes (uveitis, glomerulonephritis) may also appear – in fact a significant number of cats that become ill may develop chronic proteinuric kidney disease.

It is common for old, seropositive cats living in good environmental and nutritional conditions to die of other age-related conditions without developing immunodeficiency syndrome.

**Blood transfusions are another route of infection**; therefore, donor cats must be seronegative.

## *Epidemiology*

The prevalence of FIV varies mainly according to the lifestyle of the cat:

- Among un-neutered outdoor cats that manifest territorial aggressiveness and fight with other cats, it stands at ≥20%.
- In indoor cats and in some geographical areas, <5%.

## *Clinical signs*

There are a wide variety of diseases that can manifest in cats in the advanced stages of FIV infection.

However, if they live indoors in good environmental and nutritional conditions they do not develop the disease and, although seropositive, the majority die of diseases unrelated to the infection. Therefore, in a healthy cat or with slight signs of disease, a positive FIV result does not imply that it is getting worse or entering the immunodeficiency stage.

Cats that enter a state of immunodeficiency or pre-immunodeficiency generally suffer from the following:

- **Chronic inflammatory or infectious diseases in the oral, gastrointestinal or respiratory tract mucosa** (Figure 7.23).
- **Immunodeficiency syndrome** (opportunistic diseases, and chronic or recurrent oral, respiratory, cutaneous or gastrointestinal infections) (Figure 7.24).
- **Neurological signs** of meningoencephalitis (associated with opportunistic diseases or the virus itself).
- **Immune-mediated** diseases (glomerulonephritis, uveitis), especially chronic kidney disease (Figure 7.25).

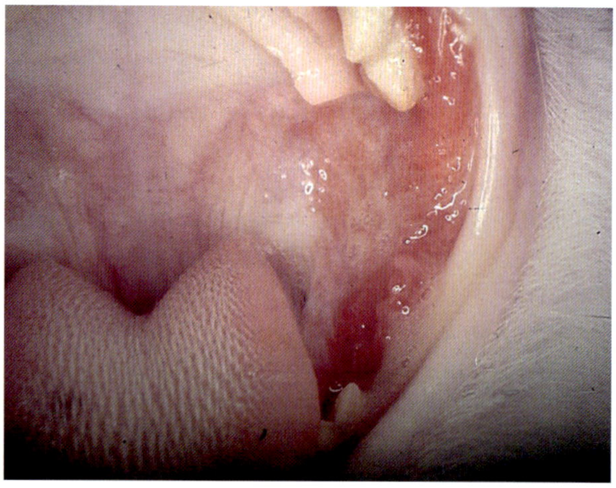

**Figure 7.23.** Stomatitis in a FIV-seropositive cat. This is one of the diseases most frequently associated with FIV-positive cats and reflects a pro-inflammatory state or immunodeficiency. These cats should be treated with antibiotics and interferons and, in some, partial or complete exodontics can be considered.

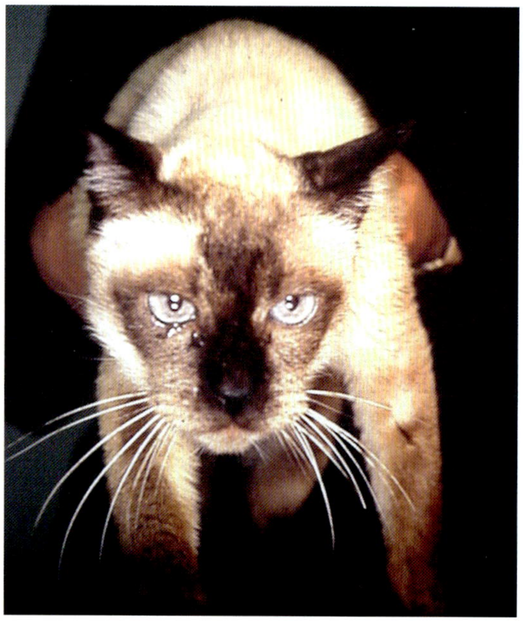

**Figure 7.24.** Cats in an advanced stage of immunodeficiency can show signs of fever or unknown origin, opportunistic diseases and neoplasia.

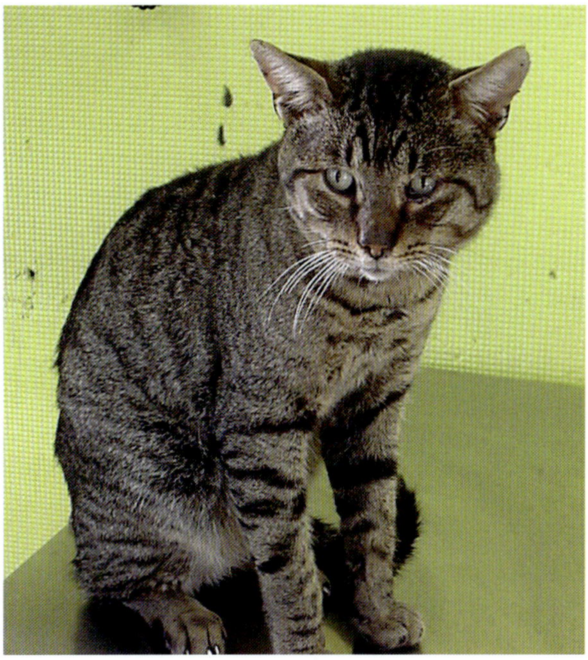

Figure 7.25. Cats positive for immunodeficiency can develop chronic proteinuric renal disease years after being infected. Infection with FIV is one of the most common causes of chronic renal disease and proteinuria in young adult cats.

The most frequent clinico-pathological abnormalities in cats are:

- anaemia (non-regenerative)
- different cytopenias (neutropenia, lymphopenia, thrombocytopenia)
- hyperglobulinaemia
- polyclonal gammopathy
- proteinuria
- azotaemia.

## *Diagnosis*

Diagnosis of FIV infection is based on the **detection of antibodies**, which appear within a few weeks of infection and correlate with the permanent presence of the virus.

### ELISA or IC

Antibodies are detected by ELISA or IC tests, using kits either in the clinic or in the laboratory. These tests have **good sensitivity and specificity** (> **90%**).

However, there may be some false positives, which is important when testing healthy or low-risk cats. Another type of false positive is due to the detection of maternal antibodies, from an infected mother, in a kitten <6 months old. Intra-uterine virus transmission is ineffective and occurs only if the cat is infected during pregnancy, so a young seropositive kitten is most likely to have antibodies that will disappear after 6 months but will not be a carrier of the virus.

False negatives can occur if the test is performed in the early stages of infection prior to seroconversion – for example, in a cat with signs of viraemia or in a terminal stage in the immunodeficiency phase in which antibody production has been depleted, situations both possible but unlikely in practice.

### Western blot assay

In dubious cases or in **healthy cats with positive ELISA tests, it is advisable to perform a Western blot assay**, which detects several specific antibodies against the virus rather than just one. This is considered a confirmation test and is currently offered by some laboratories.

### PCR

PCR tests for FIV genome detection are not as well developed as those for FeLV. Their sensitivity and specificity are not well established, and there is **great variability and discrepancies in the results**, as demonstrated in some studies. Detection of the A variant of the virus is good, but for detection of the other variants of the virus this test does not seem to work as well. Consequently, it is not considered the test of choice. However, some commercial laboratories are beginning to perform some new PCR tests with improved sensitivity and specificity. The use of PCR in the diagnosis of FIV infection is especially important in countries where the FIV vaccine is marketed, since in vaccinated cats the diagnosis for antibody detection is unreliable.

### Flow cytometry

Flow cytometry techniques allow **quantification of $CD4^+$ T lymphocytes**, the main targets of FIV. In humans, values <200 $CD4^+$ lymphocytes are associated with the onset of immunodeficiency syndrome. In cats, different studies have unsuccessfully tried to demonstrate the relationship between the numbers of $CD4^+$ and the clinical signs. Some cats with normal values are very sick, while others with low values have no signs of disease. What has been shown to be of interest is the monitoring of $CD4^+$ values in the same patient: a marked decrease in $CD4^+$ levels is associated with clinical deterioration while stable values are not.

## *Treatment*

The first measure with seropositive cats is to keep them **isolated**, to avoid infecting other cats and decrease the likelihood of acquiring other infections. The life expectancy of a healthy positive cat can be many years, and it may not even develop into disease.

If the cat has an opportunistic disease or chronic infection, it must be treated properly. A poor response to treatment may indicate that the cat is in an advanced stage of immunodeficiency.

Numerous studies of the treatment of seropositive cats with antiretroviral drugs have been published:

**AZT (zidovudine) at a dose of 5–10 mg/kg/12 h PO or SC** improved chronic stomatitis, increased survival, decreased viral load and increased $CD4^+$ levels. However, as in humans, resistance appears around 6 months and the effect diminishes or disappears.

With other **anti-retrovirals** (PMEA, FPMPA, tenofovir analogue, plerixafor), the clinical and virologic results are good and there is a good tolerance in cats. Their use is not widespread because they are not readily available and are expensive.

For many years, FIV-seropositive cats have been treated with immunomodulatory drugs, mainly interferons, with the intention of restoring immune function and promoting non-specific antiviral action.

High-dose treatments with **human interferon alpha** (105 IU/kg/24 h SC) have not proven to be effective. In addition, antibodies are produced within a few months.

The use of **human interferon alpha at low doses (30–50 IU/24 h PO)** generally delivered clinical improvement and, in some cases, increased survival, but with no effect on viral load or immunological parameters such as $CD4^+$ levels.

**Feline interferon omega** was marketed in 1992, and studies have been published in seropositive cats using protocols at **high doses (106 IU/kg/24 h for 5 days SC, three rounds) and at low doses (104 IU/24 h PO for 6 weeks)** in both symptomatic and asymptomatic cats.

Asymptomatic changes in viral load and immunological parameters were not demonstrated.

In recent studies with low doses, 0.1 MU/24 h PO has shown improvement in both clinical signs and the quality of life of cats, without changes in viral load.

In a controlled study, survival rates did not improve compared to the placebo group.

Other studies series of cases treated with human interferon-alpha at low doses showed an improvement in clinical signs and survival time.

### Prognosis

The **prognosis of healthy seropositive cats is good**. At least two studies and numerous clinical experiences have shown that, if living conditions are satisfactory and controlled, life expectancy can be relatively long and the disease may not even develop, with cats dying from unrelated geriatric pathologies. Moreover, in feline communities it has been shown that seropositive cats do not have a lower life expectancy than the seronegative cats that live with them.

However, for **seropositive cats with diseases associated with an immunodeficiency syndrome the prognosis is poor**, since in general inflammatory or opportunistic diseases, or even the development of neoplasms such as lymphomas, respond poorly to treatment and can cause death in a relatively short time.

### Prevention

Infection prevention is mainly based on **avoiding fights** between cats through **indoor life or castration**. The risk of infection by direct or intimate contact between cats that do not fight is low, but not unheard of.

In the USA and Japan, since 2002 an inactivated vaccine has been marketed that has created some division of opinion, since vaccinated cats test positive on diagnostic tests and it is impossible to differentiate an infected from a vaccinated cat. On the other hand, this vaccine mainly protects against infections by the A-variant of FIV, so it would probably not be very effective in Europe where most of the viruses identified are from other variants, mainly B-variants.

## Haemoplasmosis

### Aetiopathogenesis

**Haemotropic mycoplasmas or haemoplasmas** are small bacteria that parasitise the periphery of red blood cells and can trigger an **immune-mediated haemolytic anaemia**. Initially they were classified within the Rickettsiae and denominated *Haemobartonella* spp., but genetic studies showed that they were mycoplasmas.

**Routes of infection**:

- **Fleas**, *Ctenocephalides felis*. The presence of haemoplasmic DNA has been demonstrated. This was considered the most important route of infection, but recent studies contradict this hypothesis and it is not currently considered an important route.
- **Saliva**. Fights are considered the most effective route of infection (Figure 7.26).

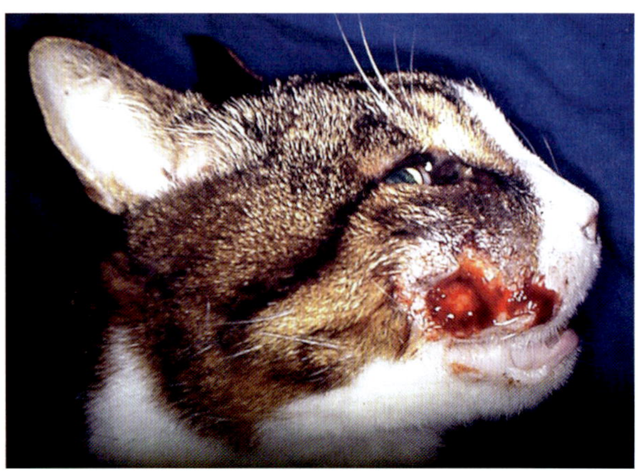

**Figure 7.26.** Fights between cats are the most likely route of infection for haemoplasma infections.

- **Vertical transmission**.
- **Blood transfusions**.

It is suspected that some **arthropods could act as vectors**, but this has not been confirmed in controlled studies. Molecular studies have confirmed the existence of different haemoplasma species with different pathogenicities:

- *Mycoplasma haemofelis* (*Mh*). It is suspected that **acute infection** causes **severe haemolytic anaemia**, but chronic infection does not cause anaemia. The prevalence varies greatly depending on whether the cats studied are healthy or suspected of being infected, and the geographical area.
- *Candidatus Mycoplasma haemominutum* (*CMh*). It is less pathogenic, but it can cause **anaemia** in some circumstances, especially in acute infections which usually produce a decrease in erythrocytes without being sufficient to cause anaemia. It causes signs of anaemia in immunosuppressed cats or those with concurrent diseases, in particular FeLV infections or co-infected by FeLV and FIV. In one study an association was found between the presence of CMh and chronic kidney disease, although this association could be purely coincidental given the age of the cats. It is the most prevalent species according to some studies, although there are large differences between studies.
- *Candidatus Mycoplasma turicensis* (*CMt*). This species was described a few years ago. It is thought that in some cases it can induce **mild to severe anaemia**, especially in immunosuppressed cats. Its presence is frequently associated with **co-infection** with one or both other haemoplasmas, especially CMh.
  Haemoplasma infections cause:
  - **Haemolytic anaemia**, mainly extravascular, although sometimes it is intravascular. Coombs' tests may be positive, sometimes self-agglutination is observed and the presence of anti-erythrocyte antibodies has been demonstrated. Recently the importance of these anti-erythrocyte antibodies has been questioned, since it has been observed that in some cases they appear once haemolysis has begun and, in addition, the response to treatment can be very good with the use of antibiotics without corticosteroids.
  - **Erythrocyte sequestration** in the spleen and decreased haematocrit.
  - Increase in **osmotic fragility** (Mh and CMt).

## *Epidemiology*

There are numerous epidemiological studies on the prevalence of haemoplasmic DNA in the blood of healthy and diseased cats in numerous countries. The **prevalence is generally high**, with CMh being the most frequent followed by Mh and CMt. The prevalence is high in healthy animals and those with other diseases, which means that many cats are asymptomatic carriers.

## *Clinical signs*

The disease that occurs after **infection depends on**:

- The haemoplasma species involved.
- Whether the infection is acute or chronic.
- The presence of concurrent diseases and/or state of immunity.

The most frequent clinical and **pathological clinical signs** are:

- Dehydration.
- Anorexia.
- Depression.
- Weight loss.
- Intermittent fever.
- Anaemia. Typically, this is regenerative hypochromic macrocytic anaemia, although these animals do not always have a marked reticulocytosis.
- Splenomegaly. Sometimes obvious.
- Jaundice. It is possible, but not consistent.

Some studies have shown that retrovirus infection increases the risk of CMh and Mh co-infection, but the influence of retrovirus infection status on haemoplasmosis is not fully understood. However, performing **retrovirus tests on cats with haemoplasmosis is advisable**.

Some cats are **chronic carriers of haemoplasmas**, especially those infected with CMh. Although it has been shown that many cats infected with Mh and CMt completely eliminate the infection after a few months, a general rule cannot be established because there is wide variability in the course and evolution of infection in chronic carriers. Generally, chronic carriers are subclinical although in some cases the infection can be reactivated.

## *Diagnosis*

### Peripheral blood smear

Diagnosis by examination of peripheral blood smears has a **low sensitivity** and variable specificity. **Haemoplasmas are visible cyclically** and usually for a short period of time that coincides with the peak of bacteraemia after acute infection. In addition, smears do not allow differentiation between species. Haemoplasmas located on the periphery of erythrocytes can also be confused with other basophilic corpuscles.

### PCR

**PCR, performed in a reliable laboratory, is the test of choice** for the diagnosis of haemoplasmosis. It is extremely sensitive and specific, allowing diagnosis of the infection, in addition to differentiating between different species and quantification of the DNA of haemoplasmas, which can be useful for:

- Determining the significance of the infection.
- Monitoring the course of the infection.
- Monitoring the response to treatment.

However, the interpretation of quantitative PCR can be complicated given the large fluctuation in the number of haemoplasmas demonstrated in studies on experimental Mh infection. The reason for this large fluctuation is not fully understood, although the possibility of infections sequestered in organs such as the spleen has been investigated, and antigenic variability has been suggested as another possible cause. Results should be interpreted taking this factor into account and, to classify a cat as having completely eliminated the infection, a single negative PCR is not enough – several PCRs must be performed over a period of time. This fluctuation is characteristic of Mh infection but has not been seen in CMh and CMt infections.

### *Treatment*

Administration of any of the following antibiotics resolves the clinical signs, but the infection is not always eliminated completely and permanently:

- **Tetracyclines**, especially **doxycycline (10 mg/kg/24 h for 1 month)**, are the drug of choice to treat feline haemoplasmosis. Although only controlled studies of Mh treatment are available, it has also been found to be effective in CMh and CMt infections.
- **Quinolones** (enrofloxacin and marbofloxacin) are also clinically effective, although there may be variability in response depending on the haemoplasma species. Recent studies show that a sequential treatment of 1 month of doxycycline followed by 2 weeks of a quinolone (marbofloxacin) could be more effective in eradicating haemoplasmas and preventing the cat from becoming a chronic carrier.
- **Imidocarb (5 mg/kg/14 days IM)** is used in difficult cases or in those that do not respond to the usual treatment, but controlled studies of its efficacy are lacking.

In severe cases of haemolytic anaemia, especially if the Coombs' test is positive or the response to the antibiotic is not considered adequate, the use of **prednisolone is indicated (2–4 mg/kg/24 h)**. There is clinical evidence that the use of cortisone is not necessary in all cases – many respond well to doxycycline without the need for administration of corticosteroids.

Supportive treatment consists of fluid therapy and, in the most severe cases, blood transfusion.

### *Prognosis*

The **prognosis is good** providing the cat does not reach the practice in a critical condition with hypovolaemic shock. Even in these severe cases, if supportive treatment is started and doxycycline is administered quickly, the cat is very likely to survive.

### *Prevention*

Prevention is based on the **control of external parasites** (fleas and ticks). There are no vaccines or other types of preventive measures available.

## Canine infectious diseases

## *Viral infections in puppies*

### *Canine parvovirus infection*

### Aetiopathogenesis

Parvovirus is a disease caused by a **single-stranded DNA parvovirus**, canine parvovirus (CPV), which appeared in the 1970s from a persistent **mutation of feline parvovirus**. From there, it evolved into a pathogenic variant, CPV-2, which has subsequently produced three variants: CPV-2a, CPV-2b and CPV-2c.

After **oral exposure and ingestion** of the virus, CPV replicates in tonsillar, pharyngeal and intestinal lymphoid tissue. **Viraemia occurs approximately 3 days after infection**. Between 5 and 7 days after exposure, the virus **replicates in cells at a high replication rate**, such as intestinal crypts and bone marrow. This produces characteristic clinical signs such as **leucopenia** associated with neutropenia and lymphopenia, and **haemorrhagic gastroenteritis**. In addition, **sepsis** often occurs, due to intestinal bacteria. The virus is **excreted in faeces in large quantities** during infection and in the days following clinical resolution (2 weeks maximum). CPV can also manifest a **tropism for the myocardium**, causing inflammation and necrosis.

### Epidemiology

Parvoviruses are **extremely resistant** in the environment and to disinfection. They are **transmitted via the oro-faecal route**. **Indirect infection is frequent**, so dogs that have not had direct contact with other dogs can become ill.

## Clinical signs

Digestive tract signs usually begin with **anorexia and vomiting** and progress rapidly to **haemorrhagic diarrhoea**, which is abundant and profuse (Figure 7.27).

Other common signs are **fever and severe dehydration**. Animals can also arrive with **hypovolaemic shock**. During the course of the disease, some dogs show severe symptoms of sepsis, systemic inflammation syndrome (SIRS), DIC and **multi-organ failure** leading to death (Figure 7.28).

Occasionally during the disease, **intestinal intussusception** occurs due to abnormal intestinal motility. Rarely, sudden deaths from myocarditis occur.

**Clinico-pathological abnormalities** include:

- leucopenia
- neutropenia
- lymphopenia
- anaemia
- thrombocytopenia
- hypoglycaemia
- hypokalaemia
- hyponatremia
- hypochloraemia
- hypoproteinaemia
- hypo-albuminaemia
- metabolic acidosis
- elevated bilirubin (in some cases).

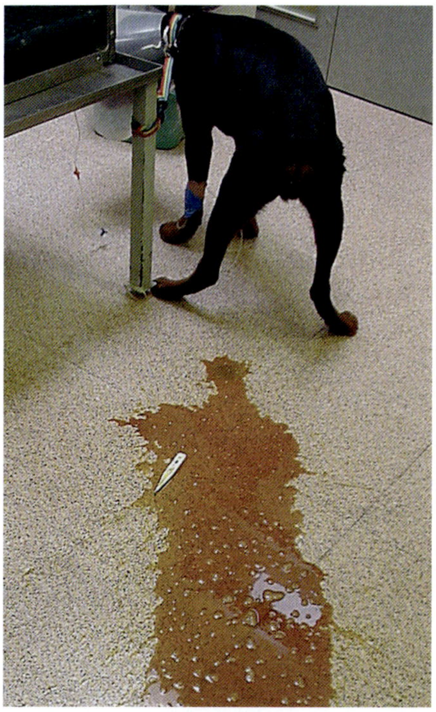

**Figure 7.27.** The majority of dogs with parvovirus present with signs of profuse, high-volume diarrhoea. This should be taken into account when calculating fluid requirements, which should be sufficient to offset the large volume lost through diarrhoea and vomiting.

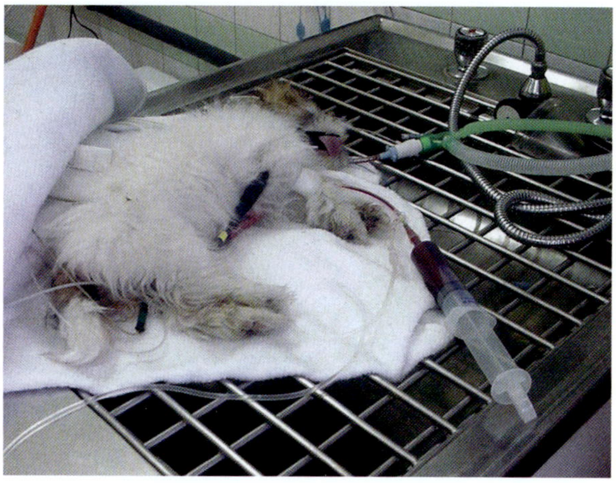

**Figure 7.28.** Puppy in septic shock and multi-organ failure associated with parvovirus and septicaemia, receiving a fresh blood transfusion and intensive care.

## Diagnosis

Diagnosis is based on **gastrointestinal signs** and the characteristic **neutropenia**, along with presentation in puppies or **young dogs that are not vaccinated** or undergoing the vaccination process.

However, confirmation of the presence of CPV using the following is common:

- **ELISA serological tests for faecal antigen detection**. These can be done quickly in practice and are relatively **sensitive and specific**, but the following should be kept in mind:
  - **False negatives**, due to low antigen levels or antigens blocked by antibodies.
  - **False positives**, due to recent vaccination with attenuated vaccines.
- **PCR techniques, both on blood and faeces**. Results are not immediate since they must be sent to external commercial laboratories. **Very sensitive**.

## Treatment

Treatment is based on **supportive and symptomatic measures**, since there is currently **no effective antiviral drug** for parvovirus treatment.

The fundamental treatment is **fluid therapy** for the correction of dehydration (intravenous crystalloids, replacement and maintenance, calculating losses due to vomiting and diarrhoea that can be extremely high), electrolyte abnormalities, especially **hypokalaemia** (sometimes supplementation with 30 or 40 mEq/l or even more), and **hypoglycaemia**, frequent due to fasting and sepsis (2.5 or 5% glucose supplementation in fluids) (Figure 7.29).

**Colloid treatment** is also common, due to the high protein loss that occurs with diarrhoea. **Synthetic colloids (hetastarch, 20 ml/kg/24 h)** are generally administered, since they are the ones that produce the

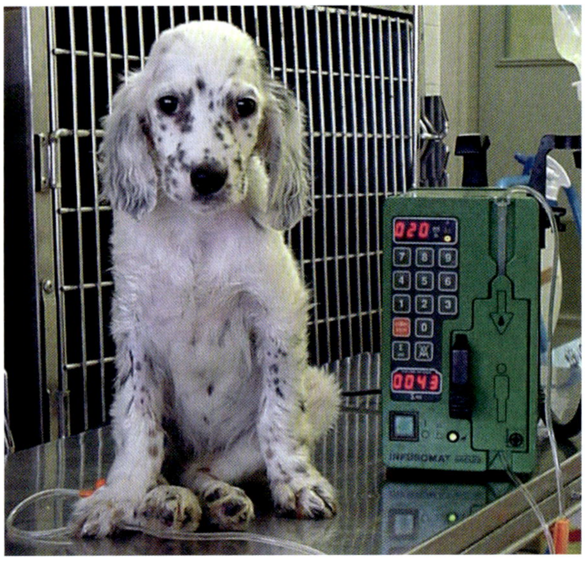

**Figure 7.29.** Continuous fluid therapy and monitoring of hydration and electrolytes are essential for survival in dogs with parvovirus.

greatest oncotic support by volume; however, depending on each case, 25% human albumin, fresh plasma or whole blood are also options.

One of the most effective support measures is **establishing enteral nutrition** as soon as possible, even if the dog is manifesting vomiting: enteral nutrition improves the integrity and repair of the intestinal epithelium and can increase survival and reduce the risk of bacterial translocation.

Generally, treatment is based on the use of **naso-oesophageal tubes** and the administration of **liquid diets in small doses**, often or continuously by means of an infusion pump. This should be accompanied by an **anti-emetic drug** that is effective as possible, such as **maropitant (1 mg/kg/24 h)** or ondansetron.

In addition, **broad-spectrum antibiotic therapy** is used to treat sepsis. There are different antibiotic protocols, but in general the following are administered:

- In less severe cases, first- or second-generation **cephalosporins administered intravenously**.
- In the most severe cases, when looking for a broader spectrum, combinations of **beta-lactams (ampicillin or amoxicillin-clavulanic) with quinolones** or aminoglycosides.

Other frequently used medications, according to the clinician's judgement, but whose utility is not proven, include antacids, analgesics and gastrointestinal protectors.

Occasionally passive immunity is used, administering **plasma (2.2 ml/kg IV, in one dose) from vaccinated dogs** or those that have overcome parvovirus to provide antibodies. Its effectiveness has not been fully demonstrated in prospective studies but, if there is a possibility it works and a higher dose is administered, it also allows provision of oncotic support.

**Feline interferon omega (25 MU/kg/24 h SC)** has been shown to reduce morbidity and mortality in canine parvovirus in two studies. However, experiences with clinical cases are scarce due to the high cost of complete treatment. There is also a clinical study using oseltamivir (Tamiflu) but, compared to placebo, it has not shown an improvement in survival or clinical signs.

### Prognosis

The prognosis for parvovirus is variable:

- **Good**. In dogs that can be hospitalised and receive intensive high-quality treatment, including early enteral nutrition. Even so, a low percentage (10–15%) may die as a result of sepsis and SIRS.
- **Reserved or poor**. In dogs that do not receive intensive hospital treatment or broad-spectrum antibiotics.

In any case, prognosis is based on the clinical severity of parvovirus, which depends on the vaccination status, age, weight and breed of the animal.

### Prevention

Parvovirus prevention is based on **disinfection of the environment** (where dogs live in groups) and **vaccination** (Table 7.10). This is an **essential or core vaccine**, which all dogs living in the same environment should receive. Several doses must be administered at **primary vaccination (6, 8, 12 and 16 weeks)**, for proper immunisation and to avoid interference with maternal immunity. Some breeds (Rottweiler, Dobermann) show a lesser response to vaccines so should receive more doses (6 months).

## *Distemper virus infection*

### Aetiopathogenesis

Canine distemper is caused by a **paramyxovirus, a single-stranded RNA virus that is poorly resistant in the environment and sensitive to most disinfectants**.

**Table 7.10.** Vaccination programme for canine parvovirus infection.

| Essential vaccine recommended in all dogs | | |
|---|---|---|
| **Primary vaccination** | **Booster vaccination** | **Annual vaccination** |
| 3 or 4 doses: 6, 8, 12 and 16 weeks | At one year or 6 months of age (if the risk is high for the breed or lifestyle) | Every 3 years |

The virus replicates in the lymphatic tissue of the respiratory tract and causes a lymphoid cell-associated viraemia until it reaches the respiratory, gastrointestinal and urogenital epithelia, the CNS and the optic nerve, to replicate in these tissues. The **incubation period can vary from 2 to 6 weeks**. The viral load and severity of the disease depend on the dog's humoral and cellular immune response during the viraemic phase. The interaction between the immune response and virus determines whether the infection is asymptomatic or progressive, and whether the dog recovers or dies.

## Epidemiology

**Infection is via the respiratory route** through contact with respiratory secretions, after sneezing and coughing. Some dogs act as reservoirs and can excrete the virus for several months. **The infection is highly contagious** after contact between infected and susceptible dogs.

In recent years the prevalence of distemper has increased, probably due to the appearance of antigenic variants, some of which seem to manifest a special neurological tropism.

## Clinical signs

The clinical signs can be **acute (10 days) or chronic (for weeks or even months)**. **The most common clinical signs** are:

- Fever (intermittent or persistent).
- Anorexia.
- Gastroenteritis (vomiting and diarrhoea).
- Respiratory and eye infection (sneezing, nasal and ocular secretions, coughing) (Figure 7.30).

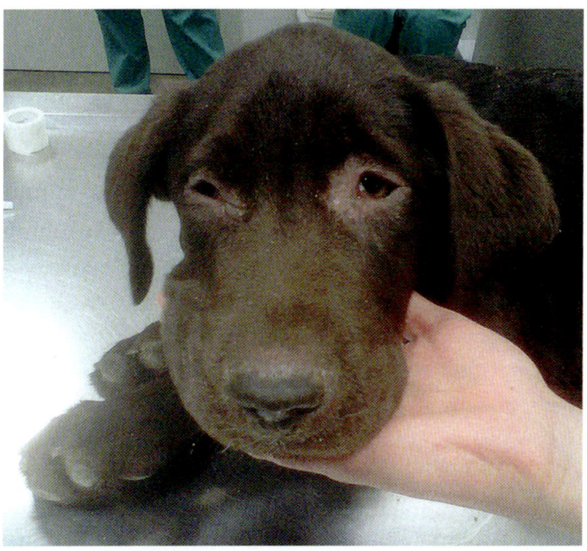

**Figure 7.30.** A 4-month-old puppy with respiratory and eye infections and fever, which has been present for several days, and is suspected of being infected with distemper. A few days later it starts to show myoclonus and a diagnosis of distemper is confirmed.

- Pneumonia (cough, respiratory distress).
- Secondary respiratory bacterial infections.

Less frequently:

- Pustular dermatitis in the abdominal ventral area.
- Hyperkeratosis of the plantar pads and/or nasal plane (Figure 7.31).

These symptoms can **present sequentially or simultaneously**. Some dogs get better and then deteriorate for several weeks.

The most severe cases may present with symptoms of **encephalomyelitis** (generalised seizures, vestibular signs, paresis or paralysis, fasciculations and myoclonus, and partial seizures that affect the musculature of the mouth) after manifesting either gastrointestinal or respiratory symptoms or as a single condition (Video 7.3). Surviving dogs may have tooth enamel hypoplasia.

The most common clinico-pathological abnormalities are:

- lymphopenia
- thrombocytopenia.

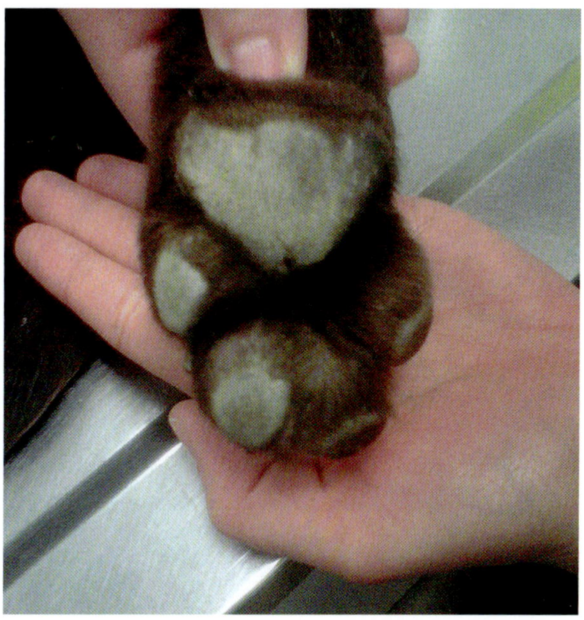

**Figure 7.31.** Pads from the same dog showing a degree of hyperkeratosis. This lesion (hardpad disease) in a puppy is highly suggestive of distemper if it is also showing other compatible signs.

**Video 7.3.** A 4-month-old puppy with fasciculations and myoclonus suggestive of distemper. A few days later a picture of generalised seizures was triggered. http://publication.improveinternational.com.

Other alterations are associated with secondary bacterial infections (leucocytosis, neutrophilia) and even septicaemia. Occasionally, viral inclusion bodies are detected in the cytoplasm of circulating leukocytes.

In dogs with respiratory signs, a typical interstitial radiological pattern of viral pneumonia can be observed, sometimes complicated by bacterial pneumonia.

### Diagnosis

Diagnosis is based on the characteristic clinical signs of systemic infection with a **gastrointestinal and/or respiratory focus**, and the exclusion of other infections or diseases with similar signs. Suspicions of distemper should be raised with the appearance of **characteristic neurological signs**, especially in young dogs.

Confirmation of the diagnosis can be made by **immunofluorescence techniques on conjunctival or respiratory smears** (low or moderate sensitivity), although today the use of **PCR is preferred for the detection of the virus genome**. PCR can be performed on samples of respiratory or ocular secretions, faeces, urine, CSF and blood. In order to distinguish natural from vaccine virus RNA, the laboratory must be informed of the brand and date of the last vaccination.

Diagnosis by evaluation of antibody titres is difficult and, although IgM titres (associated with active infection) can be measured, the cut-off value between exposure and disease is not clear.

Immunohistochemistry techniques are performed on tissues to detect virus antigens from lesions.

### Treatment

Currently there are no specific antiviral drugs, so **treatment is basically supportive and symptomatic**. This includes:

- broad-spectrum antibiotics
- fluid therapy
- enteral nutrition
- anti-pyretics
- analgesics
- anticonvulsants, including corticosteroids (chronic forms), if necessary, for neurological conditions.

### Prognosis

Prognosis is good in infections that are controlled before they can infect the CNS. However, most dogs with neurological signs die or must be euthanised. Those that survive a CNS infection may have permanent sequelae.

### Prevention

Prevention is based on **good hygiene** and management of puppies and young dogs, and the use of **attenuated vaccines** (Table 7.11). The distemper vaccine is an **essential vaccine** and should be administered to all dogs regardless of their lifestyle. Primary vaccination is most effective if **three doses (8, 12 and 16 weeks)** or even four (if started at 6 weeks) are administered to avoid interference with maternal immunity. Revaccination should be performed one year or 6 months after the last dose, and subsequently every three years is enough to maintain good immunity.

Table 7.11. Vaccination programme for distemper virus infection.

| **Essential vaccine recommended in all dogs** | | |
|---|---|---|
| **Primary vaccination** | **Booster vaccination** | **Annual vaccination** |
| 3 or 4 doses: 6, 8, 12 and 16 weeks | At one year or at 6 months of age | Every 3 years |

## *Coronavirus infections*

### Aetiopathogenesis

These infections are frequent. Three different types of canine coronavirus have been described:

- **Enteric**, the best known and diagnosed, with intestinal tropism. Does not produce a systemic infection.
- **Respiratory**, with respiratory tropism. Type 2.
- **Pantropic**, capable of producing a serious and even fatal systemic infection in puppies. Recently described in some countries. Type 1.

### Epidemiology

**Enteric coronavirus is a highly contagious virus spread by oro-faecal contact.**

In adult dogs, the **infection is usually subclinical**. Some may be carriers for months or years and excrete the virus into the environment during that time.

### Clinical signs

Enteric coronavirus usually produces symptoms of **mild and self-limiting non-haemorrhagic gastroenteritis**, without the presence of abnormalities on blood tests or signs of systemic disease after a **short incubation period (1–3 days)**. However, sometimes it can occur concurrently with parvovirus.

Dogs with respiratory coronaviruses have symptoms of respiratory infection, usually in the **upper airways**.

Dogs documented with **pantropic or systemic coronavirus** have symptoms of systemic, respiratory, gastrointestinal and neurological disease similar to that of distemper, with **high mortality**.

In enteric or respiratory forms there are not usually any clinico-pathological alterations.

## Diagnosis

Confirmation is based on the detection of **coronavirus faecal antigens** or, preferably, by **coronavirus PCR on faeces**. In general, in cases affecting the intestine diagnosis is not confirmed aetiologically. In cases where pantropic coronavirus is suspected, diagnosis by PCR and sequencing is important.

## Treatment

There are no specific antiviral drugs, and **treatment is supportive and symptomatic**.

## Prognosis

The prognosis is:

- Good for intestinal and respiratory infections.
- Poor for pantropic systemic infections.

## Prevention

Prevention is based on good management and application of **hygienic and sanitary measures** in puppies, especially in situations where there are groups of animals or they are being transported. There is a vaccine against intestinal coronavirus that is not considered essential but can be useful in show dogs or those attending competitions. **Routine use of the vaccine is not advised** in all dogs and most probably does not confer protection against the newly described pantropic variants.

# *Canine infectious tracheobronchitis*

## General considerations

Canine infectious tracheobronchitis, canine infectious respiratory complex or, as it is popularly known, '**kennel cough**' are terms used to describe the clinical signs associated with **infectious-contagious respiratory infection** in dogs. This problem has a widespread distribution and is especially important in **groups of dogs** at breeding kennels, boarding kennels and rehoming centres, although it can also affect individuals.

## Aetiopathogenesis

It is a **multifactorial disease**. In recent years, thanks to PCR techniques, knowledge of the number of pathogens involved has been expanded. In most cases the main pathogen is a virus, and the following have been identified:

- canine adenovirus type 2 (CAV-2)
- distemper virus (CDV)
- canine parainfluenza virus (CpiV)
- canine respiratory coronavirus (CRCoV)
- canine influenza virus (CIV)
- canine herpesvirus (CHV).

**Co-infections** with viruses and the presence of bacterial infections are frequent, mainly by *Bordetella bronchiseptica*, *Mycoplasma* spp. and *Streptococcus equi* subsp. *zooepidemicus*, either as secondary infection or as the primary pathogen.

These pathogens **colonise the respiratory tract** and may not cause signs of disease, whilst some cases are affected by necrotic and inflammatory lesions in the respiratory epithelium and corresponding clinical signs.

## Epidemiology

The **distribution of pathogens varies** with geographical area and from one group of dogs to another. Most viruses and *Mycoplasma* are **poorly resistant** in the environment and susceptible to most disinfectants. Despite this, the capacity for infection is high by direct contact through aerosolisation of respiratory secretions. However, CAV-2, *B. bronchiseptica* and *S. equi* are **highly resistant** in the environment and can also be transmitted indirectly.

***B. bronchiseptica* is a commensal** bacterium of the respiratory tract, and **both dogs and cats can be carriers**. However, different variants express greater or lesser virulence and, depending on the interaction between the pathogen and the dog's immune response, clinical signs may or may not be manifested. Some dogs excrete *B. bronchiseptica* for weeks or months without presenting respiratory clinical signs.

All the pathogens involved can be isolated in healthy dogs.

## Clinical signs

Most dogs have **acute and self-limiting clinical signs** (maximum duration of 10 days) of **paroxysmal coughing and/or sneezing and nasal discharge**, without systemic signs. If these persist for more than 10 days, the diagnosis should be reconsidered and other causes should be ruled out. In some cases, especially in young dogs, these can be complicated by **secondary bacterial pneumonia** and fever, anorexia, apathy and purulent nasal and/or ocular secretions may be seen (Figure 7.32).

***B. bronchiseptica*** is the primary pathogen most frequently implicated in bacterial pneumonia in dogs less than 1 year old, and can also cause epidemic outbreaks without a concurrent viral infection. Septicaemia and bacterial endocarditis due to *B. bronchiseptica* are rarely described.

## Diagnosis

The clinical diagnosis is based on the typical clinical signs, especially if several dogs are affected.

The aetiological diagnosis is based on **PCR tests** and/or **bacteriological cultures** of oro-pharyngeal,

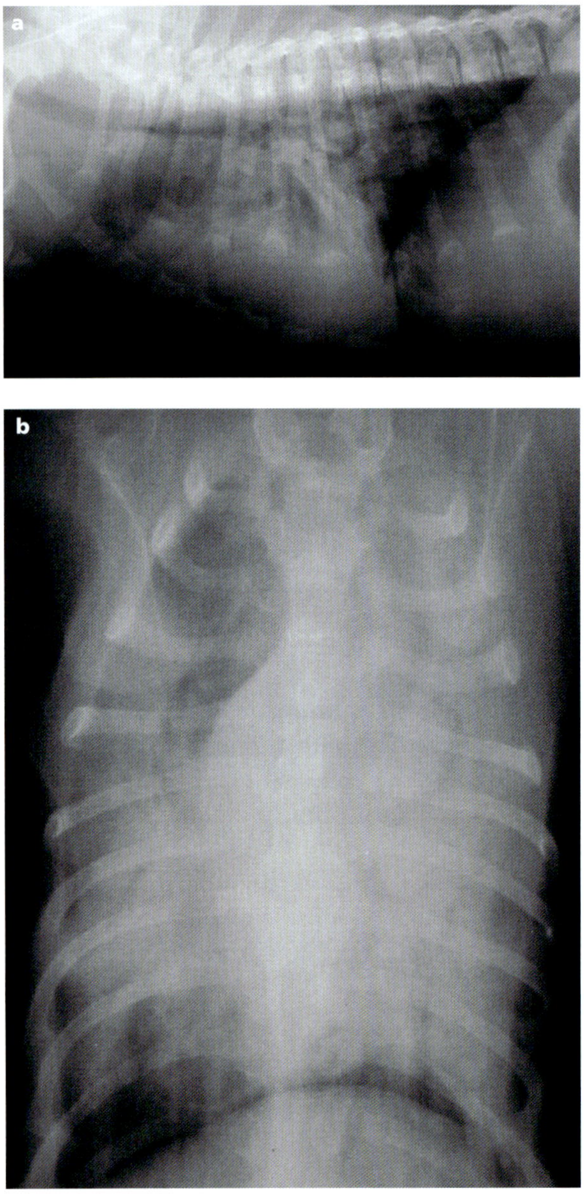


Figure 7.32. Lateral (a) and dorsoventral (b) radiographs of a dog with coughing and fever which show an alveolar pattern in all lung lobes. Analysis of samples from bronchoalveolar lavage confirmed bronchopneumonia due to *Bordetella bronchiseptica*.

conjunctival, nasal or respiratory samples. *B. bronchiseptica* and *S. equi* can be grown in conventional media. The presence of all other pathogens, including *Mycoplasma* spp., must be confirmed by PCR techniques. Usually these tests are performed only in complicated cases, those that do not respond to conventional treatment or for epidemiological studies of the prevalence of pathogens in a given area.

## Treatment

In the adult dog the vast majority of uncomplicated cases without systemic signs **resolve without treatment** regardless of the pathogen involved. Antiviral drugs are not indicated since, in general, none of the viruses involved (except canine influenza and herpesvirus) respond to commonly used antiviral drugs. Occasionally, antibiotics that are effective against the most frequently implicated bacteria (*Bordetella*, *Mycoplasma*) are prescribed to avoid complications, the drug of first choice being **doxycycline (10 mg/kg/day for 7–10 days)**.

Antibiotics such as doxycycline should be administered only in cases with clear signs of secondary or **systemic bacterial infection**. **Puppies with respiratory signs should also be treated** with antibiotics, even if they show no signs of secondary bacterial infection. **Amoxicillin-clavulanic acid and potentiated sulpha drugs** are other empirical options, although *Bordetella* frequently exhibits resistance to both and *Mycoplasma* is not sensitive to lactams. Other options for treatment are fluoroquinolones, or macrolides such as azithromycin.

In **severe cases with pneumonia, ideally antibiotics should be chosen based on culture** and antibiogram of samples from tracheal or bronchial secretions obtained by tracheal or bronchoalveolar lavage, especially if there has been no response to a good baseline antibiotic such as doxycycline.

In young dogs with **severe bronchopneumonia** that require hospitalisation, treatment with parenteral antibiotics with good diffusion into the respiratory tract should be initiated. For example, pending the results of culture and antibiogram, the combination of **quinolones and clindamycin** is a good choice. These severe cases require a 4-week course of antibiotic.

Symptomatic treatment of dogs with non-productive paroxysmal cough without systemic signs is based on the use of **cough suppressants** (codeine, butorphanol). Some clinicians use low doses of corticosteroids during the first few days. In severe cases of bronchopneumonia, fluid therapy, nebulisation, oxygen therapy and nutritional support may be required.

## Prognosis

The **prognosis is variable** depending on the pathogen(s) present and factors that may imply a poor immune response:

- **Very good in uncomplicated cases** in adult dogs even without treatment.
- It can be **poor in documented cases of canine influenza**, with some mortality, although it is not currently a very frequent cause.
- **Reserved or poor in young dogs with severe bronchopneumonia**, especially if there is no initial response to antibiotics. Bronchopneumonia associated with *B. bronchiseptica* may be more severe than that associated with other bacterial agents.

### Prevention

**High standards of routine hygiene and sanitation** are essential to avoid infection in packs and groups of dogs. In addition, vaccines against some the relevant pathogens are available. **Vaccination is advised in dogs at risk of infection**, or those that are going to boarding kennels, shows, rehoming centres and other places where there is a concentration of dogs. Specifically, there are vaccines against:

- *B. bronchiseptica*
- distemper
- Type 2 adenovirus
- parainfluenza virus
- influenza (available only in certain countries).

With the exception of distemper vaccine, non-essential vaccines prevent or minimise clinical signs but do not protect against infection, and even vaccinated dogs may excrete virus. The **duration of immunity is not more than one year**, and therefore vaccinated dogs should be revaccinated annually.

## Vector-borne diseases

### *Leishmaniosis*

#### *Aetiopathogenesis*

Leishmaniasis is a **vector-borne disease** caused by *Leishmania infantum* and transmitted by the sandfly genus, *Phlebotomus*.

The parasite cycle has been well studied.

Promastigotes (flagellated) multiply in the digestive system of female *Phlebotomus* and undergo changes into the infective form, which is deposited in the dermis of the host after a bite. This process of change and multiplication lasts about **10–14 days**. Macrophages in the dermis phagocytose the promastigotes, which lose their flagella to become amastigotes with a different morphology. If the immune system fails to control the infection they replicate, destroying macrophages and infecting more macrophages.

**Following infection by the sandfly bite** the following outcomes may occur:

- **Subclinical infections without signs of disease**. Dogs show a very effective cellular immune response (Th1) and control the infection without progressing to disease.
- **Mild signs of disease** (papular or nodular skin lesions) which, in some cases, can be self-limiting. Dogs show a mixed cellular (Th1) and humoral (Th2) immune response but with a Th1 predominance that controls the disease.
- **Progressive disease**, with lesions produced by the parasite itself (granulomatous inflammation) and by a type III hypersensitivity reaction with immune complex deposition due to a marked Th2 humoral immune response unable to eliminate the parasite. The patient may suffer from the following:
  - arthritis
  - uveitis
  - glomerulonephritis
  - vasculitis
  - meningitis.

**Other forms of parasite transmission** have been demonstrated, but these are less likely or less effective at transmitting disease: blood transfusions, vertical transmission, venereal contact or by direct contact between dogs, and even transmission via ticks has been investigated.

With leishmaniasis, **the relationship between the pathogen and the immune response determines the clinical signs and progression of the disease**:

- A greater cellular immune response and Th1 cytokine profile, leading to greater resistance to disease.
- The greater the humoral response and Th2 cytokine profile, the more likely the disease is to progressively develop and disseminate with a significant component due to immune-mediated lesions.

The immune response profile is not always fixed. Some dogs are subclinically infected for a while and control the infection, then suffer a sudden change in their immune response and succumb to illness. Alternatively, after treatment a sick dog with a decrease in parasitic load can undergo an improved immune response pattern with a higher Th1 profile, control the infection and may not suffer recurrences. However, in most dogs that have shown clinical signs of the disease, the infection is chronically latent and can recur.

In summary, in an endemic area there are:

- Dogs that never become infected (either because of their lifestyle or because of preventive anti-*Phlebotomus* measures).
- Dogs that are ill.
- Infected dogs resistant to the clinical effects of the disease.
- Infected dogs in which at some point the infection may progress and lead to signs of disease.

#### *Epidemiology*

Leishmaniasis is **endemic in some areas of the world**, including the Mediterranean basin. However, due to the mobility of people and their pets, cases are often diagnosed in non-endemic areas months after visiting an endemic area where they became infected. A new phenomenon being observed, perhaps related to **climate change**, is that certain vector-borne diseases (such as leishmaniasis) are being diagnosed as autochthonous in areas where they were not previously diagnosed. In **endemic areas** the prevalence of infection is very high: seroprevalence studies indicate a **large percentage of seropositive dogs, up to 40%**. The prevalence of disease is lower, between 3 and 10%.

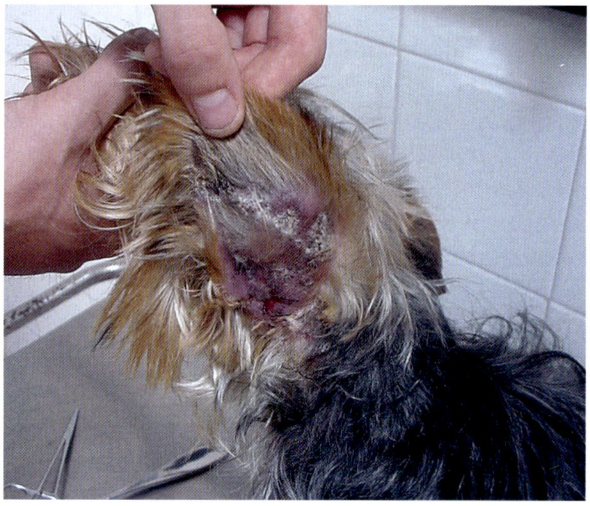

Figure 7.34. Desquamative and ulcerative skin lesions on the pinna of a Yorkshire Terrier infected with leishmaniosis.

## *Clinical signs*

Leishmaniasis manifests with a **diverse array of clinical signs** affecting practically **any organ or system**. This is due to the complex interaction between pathogen and immune response, the lesions caused by the parasite and immune-mediated-type problems.

**Cutaneous signs are common** and are generally the result of granulomatous inflammation by the parasite itself, but many dogs do not present with skin lesions. The most frequent skin lesions are:

- non-pruritic exfoliative dermatitis (Figures 7.33 and 7.34)
- ulcerative dermatitis (localised)
- nodular dermatitis
- mucocutaneous proliferative dermatitis
- papular dermatitis
- onychogryphosis (Figure 7.35)
- atypical signs:
  - depigmentation
  - hyperkeratosis

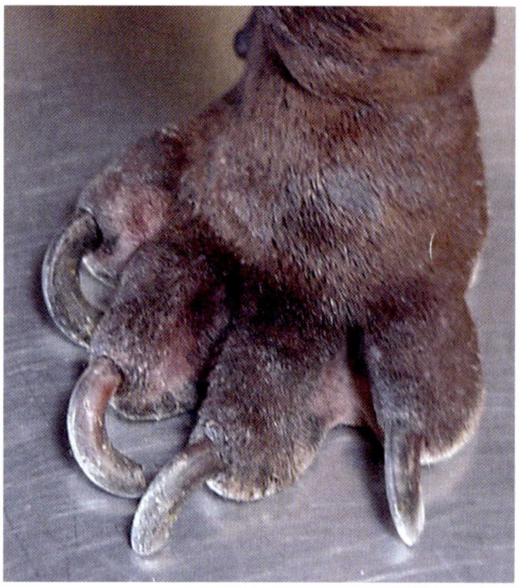

Figure 7.35. Long, curved nails (onychogryphosis) typical of dogs with leishmaniosis.

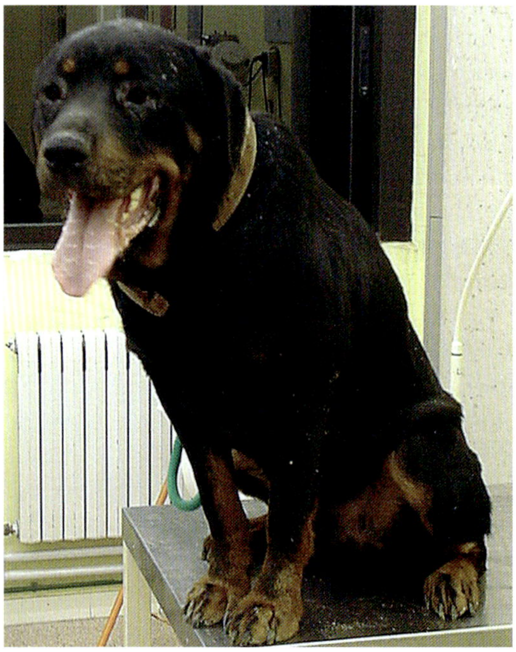

Figure 7.33. Rottweiler with temporal muscle atrophy, generalised desquamation and bilateral blepharitis. The results of diagnostic tests confirm the clinical suspicion of leishmaniosis.

  - panniculitis
  - autoimmune diseases (pemphigus, lupus)
  - with all the above there may also be secondary bacterial pyoderma.

The most frequent **systemic signs**:

- lymphadenopathy (not always present)
- fever
- anorexia
- apathy
- weight loss (Figure 7.36)
- muscle atrophy
- epistaxis (multifactorial pathogenesis).

**Kidney disease** and its clinical consequences are common in leishmaniosis. The most common cause of nephropathy is **glomerulonephritis due to immune**

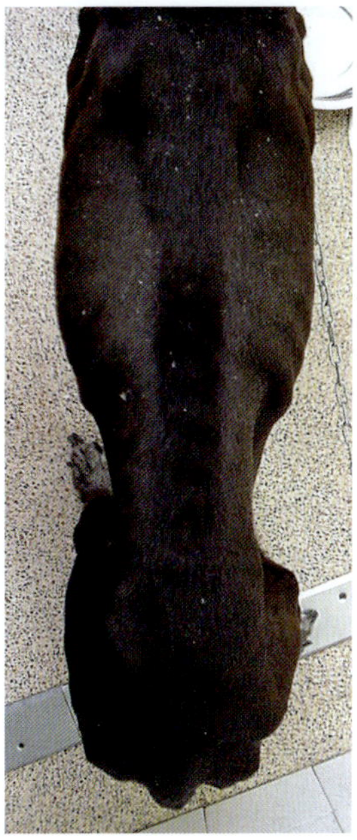

**Figure 7.36.** In many dogs with absence of cutaneous lesions, weight loss with loss of body condition is the predominant clinical sign of leishmaniosis.

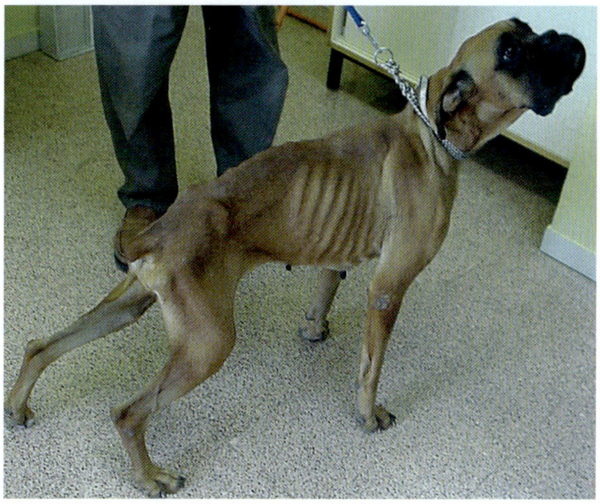

**Figure 7.37.** Once of the most serious consequences of leishmaniosis is renal lesions which, if undiagnosed in the early stages can be irreversible. Renal functionality (urine density, urea, creatinine, symmetric dimethylarginine and proteinuria (urine protein/creatinine ratio) should be monitored in all dogs with leishmaniosis.

**complex deposition**, and consequently more or less severe proteinuria and, in some cases, nephrotic syndrome and chronic kidney disease (CKD). **Interstitial renal lesions** caused by the parasite itself have also been documented and also **amyloidosis**, but these are less frequent. Dogs with kidney disease may not present any other typical sign of leishmaniosis and can sometimes arrive in advanced stages of CKD (Figure 7.37).

**Eye disease** is also frequent. Dogs with leishmaniasis can present with a wide variety of eye lesions and effects in all eye structures:

- conjunctivitis
- keratoconjunctivitis sicca
- corneal lesions (Figure 7.38)
- uveitis
- chorioretinitis.

**Less frequent signs** include:

- polyarthritis
- chronic colitis
- hepatitis
- mucosal granulomas (Figure 7.39)
- neurological signs
- symptoms of systemic vasculitis
- coagulopathies
- thromboembolism
- pericarditis
- osteomyelitis
- osteolytic lesions
- polymyositis.

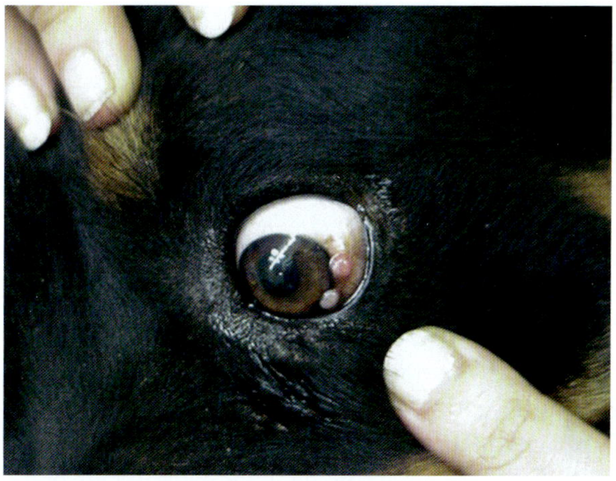

**Figure 7.38.** Episcleral nodules in a dog with leishmaniosis (an atypical lesion that is uncommon but very suggestive of leishmaniosis). It is not uncommon for leishmaniosis to cause eye lesions affecting all of the structures and layers of the eyes.

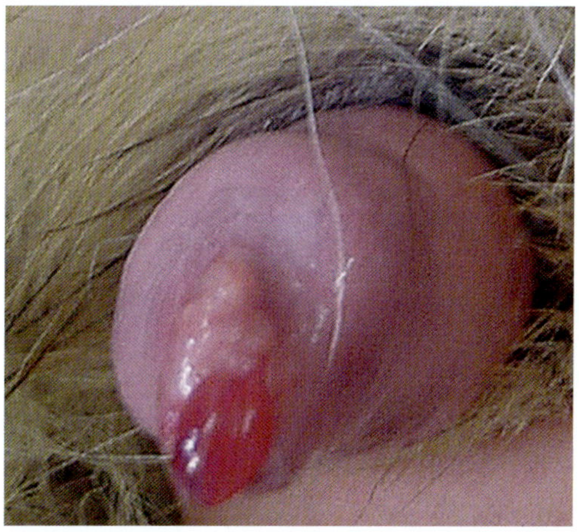

**Figure 7.39.** Granuloma in the mucosa of the prepuce of a dog due to leishmaniosis. These mucosal lesions have mainly been described in the oral mucosa and on the tongue.

Age: 2 years old

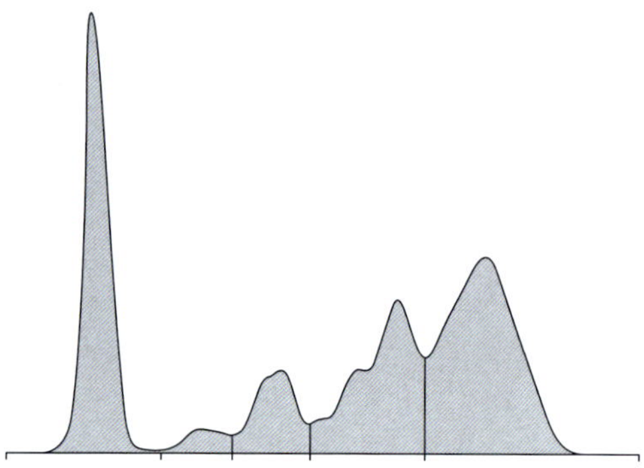

Serum protein electrophoresis

Total protein = 8.67 g/dl

A/G = 0.40

| Name | % | Normal % | Normal g/dl |
|---|---|---|---|
| Albumin | 28.61 | 2.48 | 2.6 |
| $Alpha_1$ | 2.70 | 0.23 | 0.2 |
| $Alpha_2$ | 9.59 | 0.83 | 0.3 |
| Beta | 22.54 | 1.95 | 0.9 |
| Gamma | 36.56 | 3.17 | 0.3 |

**Figure 7.40.** Electrophoresis of serum proteins from a dog suffering from leishmaniosis, showing a classic polyclonal gammopathy (wide-based). This abnormality can also be caused by other infectious or inflammatory diseases and neoplasia, but is very characteristic of leishmaniosis.

There are many general symptoms in dogs for which leishmaniosis should be on the list of **differential diagnoses**. This is problematic since in an endemic area many dogs are subclinically infected, making it difficult to determine whether the dog's disease (especially if seropositive) is caused by *Leishmania*.

Once the **diagnosis is confirmed**, it is advisable to **classify** the animal according to the clinical stage of the disease. Two groups of experts in leishmaniasis have proposed two different classifications, based on similar criteria:

- The severity of clinical signs.
- The serological response.
- The presence of kidney disease and/or immune-mediated lesions.

These classifications have great clinical value, especially for issuing a prognosis and deciding on the type of treatment.

## *Diagnosis*

The **diagnosis of leishmaniosis** should be based on the joint interpretation of:

- The clinico-pathological picture.
- Serological tests that detect antibody titres.
- Tests that detect the parasite or its DNA.

**Dogs suffering from leishmaniasis** (unlike those infected) usually have clinico-pathological abnormalities. Mainly:

- **Polyclonal hypergammaglobulinaemia** (rarely monoclonal) (Figure 7.40).

Frequently:

- Non-regenerative **anaemia** (of chronic disease).
- **Hypo-albuminaemia** (due to inflammation or glomerulopathy).
- **Proteinuria**.

Rarely:

- Azotaemia, if CKD is advanced.
- Elevated levels of liver enzymes.
- Leucopenia or leucocytosis.

Suspicions should be high if:

- **Clinical signs** are compatible with leishmaniosis.
- Other diseases have been **ruled out**.
- **Compatible abnormalities** found on blood tests.

### Serological tests

To confirm the disease, **antibody titres** are used as an accurate **quantitative test**. Diagnostic tests that indicate only positive or negative, without quantification, are not useful in the diagnosis of leishmaniasis since they indicate only whether antibodies are present, but not the level. The more sensitive a serological technique is in the quantification of antibodies, the greater predictive value its result will have.

A high, or very high, antibody titre in a dog with typical clinico-pathological signs of leishmaniosis is a diagnosis of the pathology. **A high antibody titre indicates an exaggerated Th2 response typical of a sick dog**.

However, in some cases the antibody titre in sick dogs can be medium or low positive and therefore does not always allow confirmation of leishmaniosis as the cause of symptomatic disease. **Positive antibody titres in healthy dogs or with other diseases do not confirm leishmaniasis**, and care should be taken interpreting serology.

### Parasite detection: direct observation

The ideal diagnosis is based on **visualisation of the parasite within macrophages**, either in bone marrow, lymph nodes, skin lesions or other organs by cytology or histology. If in any sample amastigotes are observed within macrophages, this confirms a diagnosis of leishmaniosis (Figure 7.41).

The main problem with this diagnostic test is its **moderate sensitivity**, because there are not always sufficient macrophages or parasites in the samples under observation. Therefore, if the diagnosis is based solely on samples from bone marrow or lymph nodes, there may be **false negatives**. On the contrary, there will be false positives only if *Leishmania* amastigotes are confused with other pathogens or macrophage inclusions.

### Immunohistochemistry

In **tissue biopsies** (skin or others), immunohistochemistry techniques can be requested to demonstrate the **presence of parasites within macrophages** (Figure 7.42). This may be useful if direct observation of peripheral samples proves negative.

### PCR

To increase sensitivity in parasite detection, **PCR techniques** for DNA detection can be used. There are **highly sensitive** and quantitative PCRs that allow measurement of very low levels of parasite in any sample. However, the detection of *Leishmania* DNA does not always indicate that the dog is ill with leishmaniasis because the illness may have another cause, with the coincidental presence of concurrent subclinical leishmaniasis. Therefore, PCR may be helpful but should be used in cases where the diagnosis could not be confirmed by other, simpler, techniques, and the results should be interpreted with care. The interpretation must be adapted to the sample or tissue being analysed.

In conclusion, a **diagnosis of leishmaniosis can be very simple in some cases and very complex in others**, requiring several sequential tests to confirm or rule out the disease.

## *Treatment*

Leishmaniasis experts believe **the treatment of choice is a combination of methyl-meglumine (Glucantime) 50 mg/kg/12 h SC or 75–100 mg/kg/24 h SC for 30–60 days, plus allopurinol 10 mg/kg/12 h VO for 6–12 months**.

Depending on the clinico-pathological response and antibody levels, allopurinol should be withdrawn or

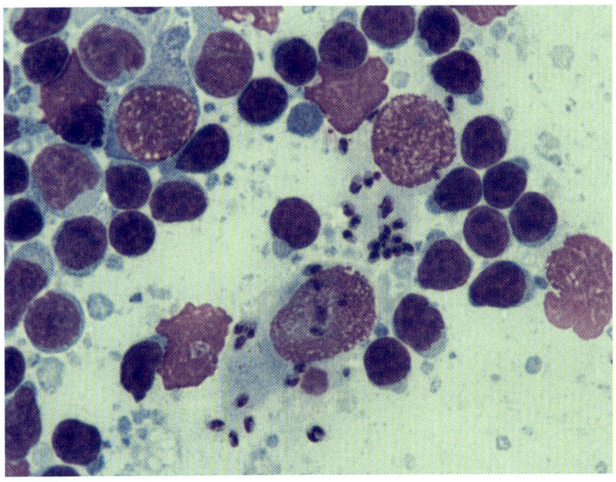

**Figure 7.41.** *Leishmania* amastigotes within macrophages in a sample obtained by aspiration of a cutaneous nodule lesion. The presence of *Leishmania* on cytology from a cutaneous lesion, lymph node or bone marrow confirms the disease. However, its absence does not completely rule out the possibility that the dog has leishmaniosis.

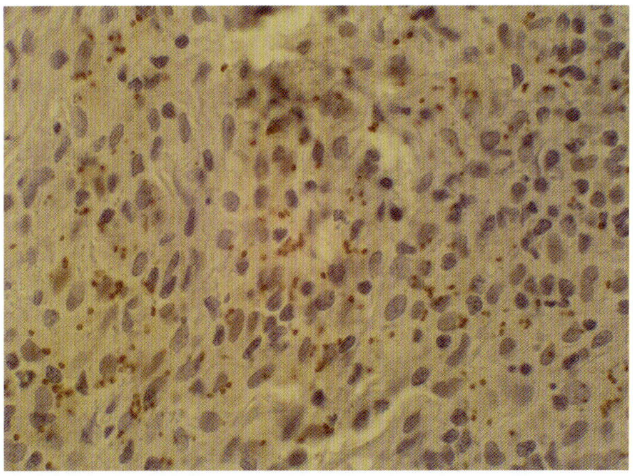

**Figure 7.42.** Specific immunohistochemical staining for *Leishmania* of a skin biopsy, which shows a positive result. Sometimes a granulomatous histological pattern suggests leishmaniosis but amastigotes not observed in the sample. Immunohistochemistry techniques allow the presence of parasites to be confirmed or ruled out in these cases.

continued for longer, sometimes indefinitely. In these cases, it is important to monitor the **possible occurrence of xanthine stones in the bladder** and even in the kidneys.

Alternative or second-line treatment: combination of **miltefosine 2 mg/kg/24 h for 4 weeks plus allopurinol**. There is evidence that this combination is as effective as the classic one, but there are veterinarians with clinical experience who believe the combination with meglumine produces better results. This combination is frequently used in dogs in the following circumstances:

- With CKD in advanced stages.
- In those that do not tolerate antimonials.
- Those whose owners cannot administer injectable treatments.

Other treatment alternatives: allopurinol as the sole drug, aminosidine, amphotericin B, metronidazole plus spiramycin, marbofloxacin and domperidone. However, none of these has proven superior to the two suggested combinations, and are not recommended as first-choice treatments.

Dogs with proteinuria and/or CKD should be treated according to their clinical state and the IRIS guidelines for kidney disease. Kidney disease associated with leishmaniasis is a frequent cause of progressive disease and death in dogs, so it is essential to determine the clinical stage early in the diagnostic process. Dogs with proteinuria that are not diagnosed or treated properly have a worse prognosis and lower survival rate. Therefore, determining whether proteinuria is present from the moment of diagnosis is essential.

Monitoring and check-ups on dogs undergoing treatment are based on routine testing of:

- renal function
- proteinuria (UPC)
- proteinogram
- antibody titres every 3 months initially and every 6–12 months thereafter.

Dogs with kidney disease at the point of diagnosis should be monitored more frequently, especially in the first weeks and months of treatment.

### *Prognosis*

The **prognosis is variable** depending on the stage of the disease at the time of diagnosis:

- Dogs with mild disease and a low humoral response (papular or nodular lesions with low or negative antibody titres) have an excellent prognosis.
- Dogs with kidney disease from the beginning or that maintain a high humoral response, despite treatment, have a worse prognosis.

**Decrease in antibody titres and normalisation of gammopathy are considered good prognostic factors** of adequate disease control, since they mean that the immune response is orientated towards a Th1 pattern and there is a lower Th2 response.

Some relapses are really re-infections, so it is also difficult to establish a specific prognosis in many cases.

### *Prevention*

Prevention of leishmaniosis is based on the use of **preventive and repellent treatments towards sandflies**. There is a wide variety of presentations (collars, pipettes) and substances with demonstrated good efficacy in preventing sandfly bites, especially during the first 3–4 weeks of treatment. These should always be applied to susceptible dogs in endemic areas or to dogs travelling to them. There are studies demonstrating product effectiveness in reducing the risk of infection, but **no products are infallible**.

There are two other forms of prevention: **vaccination** and administration of **domperidone** as a stimulator of the Th1 cell response. However, these should **not be considered as substitutes for repellents**. If they are used, it should be to reinforce the effect of collars or pipettes. This complementary action reduces the number of mosquitoes and parasitic presence in the environment, which potentially reduces the prevalence of infection for other species, including humans.

#### Vaccines

There are some vaccines available against leishmaniasis, one of which has been available in Europe for several years (CaniLeish). Observational studies demonstrated a **reduction in the risk of active infection and the appearance of clinical signs in 70% of cases** (preventive efficacy). In these studies, using Beagles, there were few adverse effects. However, adverse effects appear more frequent when the vaccine is used routinely, especially in small-breed dogs. Vaccination is considered a useful tool, but its use should probably be **limited to larger dogs with high risk factors** (breed, lifestyle).

#### Domperidone

Domperidone causes **stimulation of the cellular immune response** as a side effect. Studies on its use as a treatment for leishmaniosis have not shown good results. On the contrary, observational studies for **domperidone (Leishguard)** as a preventive measure showed a **sevenfold reduction in the infection rate** in dogs when administered according to the prospectus guideline (1 month of treatment every 4 months at the time of greatest sandfly activity).

## Ehrlichiosis/anaplasmosis

### Aetiopathogenesis

Ehrlichiosis (or canine monocytic ehrlichiosis) is a **disease caused by the rickettsia *Ehrlichia canis* and transmitted by the tick *Ripicephalus sanguineus*.**

Anaplasmosis is a disease caused by a bacterium now classified within the genus ***Anaplasma***:

- *A. phagocytophilum* produces infection in granulocytes and eosinophils (formerly canine granulocytic ehrlichiosis) and is transmitted by the tick *Ixodes ricinus*.
- *A. platys* causes platelet infection (canine infectious thrombocytopenia) and is transmitted by *R. sanguineus*.

After **inoculation by the tick**, all of these produce **intracellular infections** in their target cells and signs of **multi-systemic disease** accompanied by cytopenias and arthritis.

In **ehrlichiosis there is an acute phase in the first 10 days** of the infection, which may be subclinical or asymptomatic or cause the characteristic signs of the disease. Amongst dogs subclinically infected, a small proportion may progress to develop the chronic form of the disease with significant involvement of bone marrow.

The pathogenesis of granulocytic anaplasmosis is not well understood, with only the acute phase with fever and arthritis described.

In *A. platys* infections, **thrombocytopenia** occurs and can be cyclic.

### Epidemiology

These are infections transmitted by ticks, which in general must be **attached for a minimum of 24 h to transmit** or inoculate the bacteria. However, a recent study has shown that in the case of E. canis **just 3 h could be enough**.

**Disease prevalence is linked to the distribution of the tick vector**. In areas where *Ripicephalus* predominates, the prevalence of ehrlichiosis and anaplasmosis due to *A. platys* is higher, and in areas where *I. ricinus* predominates, granulocytic anaplasmosis predominates. Concomitant infections with other pathogens transmitted by the same ticks are frequent, and can be significant with regard to clinical signs.

### Clinical signs

#### Ehrlichiosis

The most frequent clinical signs of ehrlichiosis include:

- fever
- anorexia
- depression
- lameness or generalised pain (polyarthritis)
- signs of bleeding due to thrombocytopenia or thrombocytopathy (petechiae, ecchymosis, epistaxis).

The symptoms are generally not severe; however, **serious cases** are documented in which there is:

- ocular disease (uveitis)
- muscle pain (polymyositis)
- neurological signs (multifocal, cerebellar or vestibular involvement)
- kidney disease
- liver disease.

In the **chronic forms of ehrlichiosis**, the presence of pancytopenia (bone marrow hypoplasia) and polyclonal (or monoclonal) gammopathy, accompanied by ocular and/or renal disease, predominates.

The most frequent clinico-pathological abnormalities are:

- thrombocytopenia
- regenerative anaemia
- occasionally, proteinuria due to a glomerular lesion.

In chronic ehrlichiosis the following may be seen:

- pancytopenia (non-regenerative)
- granular lymphocytes
- hypo-albuminaemia
- polyclonal elevations of gamma globulins (even monoclonal).

#### Anaplasmosis

The clinical signs of granulocytic anaplasmosis are:

- fever
- acute muscle and/or joint pain.

A chronic form of the disease has not been described.

The **clinical signs of anaplasmosis** due to *A. platys* are related to **thrombocytopenia**:

Signs of bleeding in mucous membranes, petechiae, ecchymosis and epistaxis.

The most common **clinico-pathological abnormalities** are:

- thrombocytopenia
- regenerative anaemia.

### Diagnosis

Diagnosis is based on the characteristic clinical signs, especially the presence of **thrombocytopenia even in**

**asymptomatic dogs**. In these cases, an attempt should be made to either confirm or rule out the diagnosis, which can be done by:

- antibody detection
- visualisation of bacteria in blood samples
- genome detection using PCR techniques.

### Antibody detection

The detection of antibodies (using IFA and ELISA techniques) is moderately sensitive but not very specific for the diagnosis of disease, since the presence of antibodies does not discriminate between exposure and active infection. In general, in a dog with characteristic clinical signs and an antibody titre >1/80, the diagnosis is reliable. Antibody titre is not indicative of the duration or severity of disease. Problems with sensitivity are due to the fact that, in dogs with acute infection, seroconversion has not yet occurred.

### Visualisation of bacteria in blood samples

The detection of *E. canis* or *Anaplasma* morulae in monocytes or granulocytes and platelets in blood smears, respectively, is **highly specific but very insensitive** (although the latter is improved when the blood smear is harvested from the buffy coat fraction), since these are observed in <10% of cases (Figure 7.43).

### PCR techniques

PCR techniques increase the sensitivity of the diagnosis and confirm it in seronegative dogs in the acute phase of the disease. In general, a **positive PCR on blood confirms that the infection is active**. PCR can also be performed on samples of bone marrow and/or spleen.

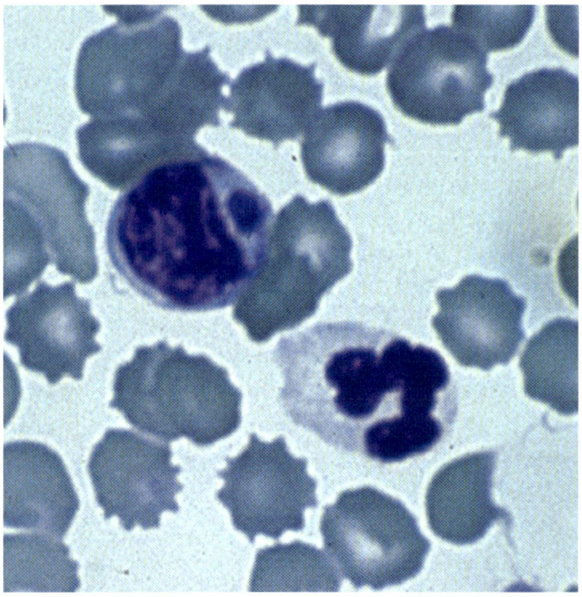

Figure 7.43. *E. canis* morula in the cytoplasm of a monocyte on a blood smear. This is a very insensitive finding, since the number of morulae is very low, but it is very specific and confirms the infection.

### *Treatment*

The treatment of choice is **doxycycline (5 mg/kg/12 h or 10 mg/kg/24 h) for 4 weeks**. Generally, there is a clinical improvement within a few days. Alternatively, it can be combined with imidocarb although in some cases this is not effective. Quinolones are less effective than doxycycline according to some published studies, and are not considered a first choice.

In **severe cases**, especially with neurological involvement and/or an immune-mediated component that does not respond quickly to doxycycline, **short treatments with corticosteroids such as prednisone (1–2 mg/kg/24 h) may be useful**.

In more severe cases, intensive hospital treatment and blood transfusions may be required, although this is unusual.

### *Prognosis*

The prognosis is:

- **Good in acute infections**, especially if there are no renal or neurological complications.
- **Poor in the chronic form** of *E. canis*: most dogs do not fully recover and even die or need to be euthanised as a result of the disease.

### *Prevention*

Prevention is based on the application of effective preventive products against ticks. There are a great variety of products (collars, pipettes, sprays, tablets) available appropriate for different circumstance or type of dog. Vaccines against *E. canis* are being researched, but none are currently commercially available.

## *Borreliosis or Lyme disease*

### *Aetiopathogenesis*

**Lyme disease is an infection caused by the spirochaete *Borrelia burgdorferi* sensu lato** complex (which includes several species, among which *Bb.* sensu estricto has been experimentally shown to cause disease in dogs), **transmitted by ticks of the genus *Ixodes*** (*I. ricinus*, *I. scapularis*).

Most infected dogs suffer a **subclinical infection**, with only a **small percentage showing acute signs of acute neutrophilic mono-arthritis**. **Atypical manifestations** associated with chronic infection (renal, cardiac or neurological) are probably due to **immune-mediated manifestations of disease**, although the details of their pathogenesis are not yet fully understood.

## Epidemiology

Prevalence varies widely according to geographical area and availability of the tick vector. Other forms of transmission, although proven, are not effective or significant. Effective transmission of the bacteria occurs when the **tick ingests the dog's blood for more than 48 hours**. In endemic areas seroprevalence is very high, which makes diagnosis of the real disease difficult. The disease is much more frequent in the USA than in Europe.

## Clinical signs

Borreliosis in dogs is primarily an **acute disease** characterised by:

- fever
- arthritis
- acute lymphadenopathy in joints near the area of tick attachment.

However, **chronic atypical cardiac, neurological, renal and articular** conditions have been described. For example, nephropathy associated with borreliosis does not meet Koch's postulates and has not been proven experimentally.

**Lyme-associated nephropathy** consists of a set of specific lesions (membrano-proliferative **immune-mediated glomerulonephritis** with diffuse tubular necrosis and lymphoplasmacytic interstitial nephritis) in dogs seropositive to borrelia and with a previous episode of arthritis. Symptoms have been seen more frequently in **Labradors, Golden Retrievers and the Shetland Sheepdog**, suggesting a particular interaction between breed, infection and immune response. In these cases, signs of vasculitis, neurological disease and thromboembolism have also been identified.

Any dog diagnosed with borreliosis should be **assessed for the presence of proteinuria** as an indication that renal damage has occurred.

Co-infections with other pathogens transmitted by ticks and other vectors are frequent, and can occasionally be the cause of the disease in dogs that are seropositive for *Borrelia*.

## Diagnosis

There is no simple diagnostic test for borreliosis. Diagnosis is based on:

- The presence of a compatible clinical picture.
- Previous exposure to ticks.
- Ruling out other diseases.
- The presence of anti-*Borrelia* antibodies.
- The appropriate response to treatment.

The **detection of the pathogen by PCR, culture or cytology is extremely difficult**. Bacteria are not easily found in blood, urine, synovial fluid or CSF, but may be found in connective tissue, the synovial capsule and skin (also in lymph nodes and muscles).

Diagnosis generally relies on the **detection of antibodies**. Serological techniques that detect the **specific antibodies against the C6 peptide (surface lipoprotein)** are preferred and do not exhibit interference with vaccine antibodies. There are rapid quantitative and semi-quantitative tests available for clinical use that have **good sensitivity, but the detection of antibodies does not confirm the disease**. However, after effective treatment, **antibody titres against C6 decrease over the following 6 months**, unlike general antibodies.

Recently a **new serological test (Accuplex 4**, Antech Diagnostics) has been developed that detects antibodies **against different *Bb.* proteins** and could **allow better differentiation** between infected and vaccinated dogs, and between acute and chronic infection.

## Treatment

The antibiotics of choice are **doxycycline or amoxicillin for 1 month**. The use of doxycycline is generally preferred as the first choice of treatment, since it also acts on other pathogens that may exist as a co-infection. The **clinical response should be seen within a few days**, and reduces the risk of developing chronic conditions associated with the disease.

Other antibiotics used include third-generation cephalosporins (ceftriaxone) in severe neurological cases; a recent study shows that cefovecin (two doses) can also be effective.

## Prognosis

The **prognosis is good in acute or typical** cases in which the response to doxycycline is rapid and positive. However, it can be reserved or poor in cases where there is renal, cardiac or neurological involvement.

## Prevention

Prevention is based primarily on **good protection against ticks.**

**Vaccination against *Bb.* is controversial** and is not considered an essential or core vaccine. In endemic areas, some veterinarians promote vaccination while others do not. In non-endemic areas, its administration does not make much sense. The efficacy is not 100% and there is a difference of opinion over its protective effects on infection and the appearance of clinical signs. It is considered a safe vaccine and the duration of immunity is 12 months.

## Babesiosis

### Aetiopathogenesis

Information on protozoal infections from the *Babesia* genus in dogs has been available for many years. Thanks to molecular biology techniques, a multitude of species have now been identified, and classified according to morphological appearance into **large species** (*B. canis*) and **small species** (*B. gibsoni*).

**Large species** that infect the dog have certain differences in vector, geographical distribution and clinical signs. These include:

- *B. canis*. Vector: *Dermacentor reticularis*
- *B. rossi*
- *B. vogeli*. Vector: *R. sanguineus*
- *B. bigemina*.

**Small species**, with differences in their epidemiology:

- *B. gibsoni*. Vector: *R. sanguineus*
- *B. conradae*
- *B. microti*-like. Vector: *Ixodes hexagonus*.

The pathogenesis of *Babesia* infections is simple: **an intra- and extravascular haemolysis is caused by an acute immune-mediated reaction against parasitised erythrocytes**. Depending on the severity of the haemolysis and the systemic inflammatory response, **complications associated with haemolysis** can be triggered (acute renal failure, hepatic necrosis, disseminated intravascular coagulation, acute respiratory distress, SIRS and multi-organ failure).

### Epidemiology

There are differences in the prevalence of different forms of babesiosis depending on the **geographical distribution of the various tick vectors**. For example, classical babesiosis (*B. canis*) is common in the north and northeast of Spain and much less frequent in the south, since *Dermacentor* is typically found in fresh, humid climates. On the other hand, babesiosis transmitted by *Rhipicephalus* can have a wider distribution since the tick does not need such specific environmental conditions and is very common in the Mediterranean area. In addition to vector transmission, **vertical transmission has been confirmed by blood transfusions** and by direct contact in fights through wounds, saliva and blood (*B. gibsoni*).

The prevalence of *Babesia* in dogs is variable depending on the geographical area, the group studied and diagnostic technique. There are currently many epidemiological studies available that have used PCR techniques in healthy dogs and in different locations. At the moment, none of the species that affect the dog have been shown to affect humans. There is no clear breed or sex predisposition, except:

- *B. gibsoni* infections in **fighting breeds** (Pit Bull Terrier) due to the route of infection.
- It has been suggested that the following may be more frequent:
  - *B. rossi* in small-breed dogs.
  - *B. canis* in the German Shepherd and Komondor.

**Splenectomised dogs** are at greater risk of suffering from babesiosis.

### Clinical signs

The clinical signs depend on the *Babesia* species. There are a **wide range of clinical signs**, from subclinical infections (there are chronic carriers) to deadly, multisystemic conditions.

The typical and classic clinical sign of babesiosis is **haemolytic anaemia** (intra- and extravascular) with all its clinico-pathological consequences:

- weakness
- anorexia
- fever
- pale mucous membranes
- lymphadenopathy
- splenomegaly
- anaemia
- thrombocytopenia
- jaundice (Figure 7.44)
- haemoglobinuria.

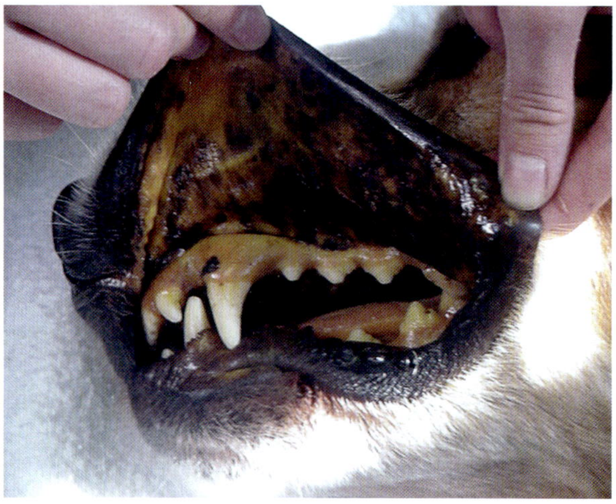

**Figure 7.44.** Oral mucosa of a Labrador Retriever presenting with severe icterus caused by infection with *B. microti*-like. It also presented with a severe acute renal insufficiency that did not improve with treatment, and the patient died.

The symptoms can be more or less serious depending on:

- Age.
- Immune status.
- Other co-infections present.
- The species of *Babesia*:
  - *B. rossi* (present in Africa) is much more serious.
  - *B. microti*-like frequently causes acute kidney disease that worsens the prognosis.
  - *B. gibsoni* and *B. microti*-like present a greater number of more serious systemic complications than those caused by *B. canis* or *B. vogeli*.

## *Diagnosis*

### Direct observation

Clinical diagnosis is based on the observation of ***Babesia* within erythrocytes** in dogs with signs of haemolytic anaemia. The sensitivity of blood smears (especially **capillary blood**, ears for example) is considered good, since dogs in haemolytic crisis usually have a large number of erythrocyte pyroplasmas. However, there may be some **false negatives**.

### PCR

The use of **PCR techniques is recommended** for the confirmation or exclusion of babesiosis in dogs with haemolytic anaemia, especially if infection by any of the small species is suspected. In addition, PCR allows effective **identification of the *Babesia* species**. Samples considered ideal for PCR are **peripheral blood** and spleen aspirations.

### Serological techniques

Serological techniques that **detect antibodies** are useful for epidemiological studies, but not for the diagnosis of the pathology in sick dogs since **a single antibody titre does not discriminate between infection and disease** and, in acute cases, they can be seronegative because antibodies have not yet been produced.

## *Treatment*

The classic treatment of choice for **large species of *Babesia* is imidocarb dipropionate (6.6 mg/kg IM or SC two doses 2 weeks apart)**. The response is usually very good, so much so that if there is not a good clinical response, rethinking the diagnosis is advised since there could be another concurrent infection.

**Babesiosis caused by small species (*B. gibsoni* and *B. microti*-like) should be treated with atovaquone (13.5 mg/kg/8 h PO) and azithromycin (10 mg/kg/24 h PO) for 10 days**.

Other drugs that have been used include:

- **Diminacene (3.5 mg/kg IM as a single dose) and pentamidine** for *B. canis*.
- **Doxycycline** for *B. canis* (improvement in clinical signs).
- **Clindamycin (25 mg/kg/12 h for 2 weeks)** for *B. gibsoni* (improvement in clinical signs).

Results for antibiotic combinations in *B. gibsoni* are not excellent, so these are not considered first-choice treatments but include:

- Clindamycin plus metronidazole and doxycycline.
- Enrofloxacin plus metronidazole and doxycycline.

Many dogs improve rapidly in a few days following commencement of the treatment of choice, especially in *B. canis* infections.

However, in some dogs the symptoms can be serious and may be **accompanied by multiple complications** (hypovolaemia, acute kidney disease, coagulopathies) and require **intensive supportive treatment** (oxygen therapy, blood transfusions, heparin). In some cases there may be a need to consider **administering steroids to curb the immune-mediated response**, which destroys erythrocytes. This is a **controversial decision**, and each case should be assessed individually taking into account the clinical situation and the pros and cons. As a general rule, it is important to consider that it is **not ideal to immunosuppress dogs with babesiosis**.

Use of PCR on peripheral blood or spleen aspirations 1–2 months after treatment, to assess whether there has been parasitological control in addition to improvement of clinical signs, can be useful. This technique allows chronic carriers to be detected. **Small species** (*B. gibsoni*, *B. microti*-like) are more likely to **persist after treatment** and produce chronic infections.

## *Prognosis*

The prognosis is **good in classical babesiosis caused by large species**, although some dogs may arrive in a critical condition and die from the complications of severe haemolytic anaemia. The **prognosis is reserved to poor in babesiosis caused by small species**, frequently associated with renal complications.

## *Prevention*

Babesiosis prevention is based on the **effective control of ticks**. Numerous products are available in different formats that adapt to each individual situation and form of application. Treatments should be applied mainly from April to September in areas where the presence of ticks is more seasonal and, in some cases (*Dermacentor* in northern Spain), during autumn and winter.

There is also a vaccine against *B. canis* which reduces the severity and length of illness in dogs that become infected. The duration of protection is 12 months. It is **not considered an essential or core vaccine**, but it can be useful in highly endemic areas and where the control of ticks with preventive treatments is not sufficient.

## Leptospirosis

### General considerations

Leptospirosis is a disease with a **worldwide distribution**, although prevalence may vary from one country to another. It has recently been considered an **emerging infection** since it is diagnosed more frequently in areas where previously it did not seem so common, although the reason for this is unknown and could simply be due to a greater knowledge of the disease and how to diagnose it.

It is an infection from which many mammalian species can suffer, and where rodents and wild carnivores act as reservoirs and subclinical carriers. Dogs are sensitive to infection and can manifest the disease, unlike cats that are more resistant (they can become infected, but rarely develop the disease). Sick or infected dogs (and cats) can be a source of infection to people by excretion of *Leptospira* in urine.

### Aetiopathogenesis

This infection is caused by a highly mobile **helical Gram-negative spirochaete** from the genus *Leptospira*. The morphology is different from that of other spirochaete genera. There are **numerous species and serovars of *Leptospira*** that can cause disease in the dog. Classification by serovars is based on antigenic characteristics, and is still maintained due to its epidemiological importance and by its tendency to infect certain species.

Leptospirosis is a **blood-borne, multi-systemic disease** with a special **tropism for the kidneys and liver**, but also for other organs such as the eyes (uvea and retina), lungs, pancreas, muscles, meninges, spleen and genitals.

Unlike other Gram-negative bacteria, *Leptospira* does not cause a rapid fulminant disease, probably because of the low endotoxic capacity of its liposaccharides. The **dog's immune response is slow**, since the bacteria evade it, but ultimately the **immune system is able to eliminate the bacteria except from the renal tubules and eyes**, where it can persist for longer.

**Renal injury** consists mainly of **tubular necrosis and acute interstitial nephritis**, caused directly by *Leptospira*. Depending on the severity of the damage, the degree of renal dysfunction can be greater or lesser. **Liver damage consists of hepatocellular necrosis, cholestasis and inflammatory infiltration in hepatic sinusoids**. The severity of hyperbilirubinaemia is associated with a worsening prognosis.

Recently, **pulmonary haemorrhagic syndrome** has been more frequently diagnosed in the dog. The pathogenesis, which is not fully understood in detail, consists of intra-alveolar haemorrhages in the absence of major inflammatory infiltrates, vasculitis or *Leptospira* in large numbers in the lung parenchyma. It is probably a multifactorial lesion with **immune-mediated components and systemic inflammation** due to the direct effects of *Leptospira*, more so in endothelial cells than in the lung parenchyma.

### Epidemiology

*Leptospira* transmission is linked to the skin (via wounds) or mucous membrane contact with urine or water, food or environments contaminated with the organism. In a warm and humid environment, infection can persist for long periods of time, from months to years. After exposure, animals susceptible to infection may develop acute disease.

When **animals that act as a reservoir (rodents) are infected**, they do not develop the disease but **harbour large numbers of Leptospira in their renal tubules**. The dog and the cat can also act as a reservoir if they become infected and do not become ill, eliminating Leptospira via the urine. It is currently understood that dogs are susceptible to infection by multiple serovars and not only by those known as *L. canicola* and *icterohaemorrhagiae*. They can also be infected by serovars of *L. grippotyphosa, australis and sejroe*. There may be geographical differences depending on the animals acting as reservoirs in each area (*L. pomona*, *L. bratislava*, *L. autumnalis*, *L. copenagheni*).

It is possible that clinical cases occur with **seasonality**, linked to rainfall and average temperature. Epidemiological risk factors that have been demonstrated in some studies include:

- Rural environment and countryside.
- Outdoor life.
- Contact with water and wet areas.
- Exposure to rodents and wild animals.
- Living in rescue centres.

Some breeds, such as the German Shepherd, appear more susceptible, but the association has not been clearly demonstrated.

### Clinical signs

Leptospirosis can be **mild or severe** depending on the immune response and serovar involved, and may even present as a **subclinical infection** without the dog showing clinical signs.

The classic clinical sign is the presence of **acute renal failure (AKI)** in conjunction with **hepatitis and acute liver failure** (elevation of liver enzymes and bilirubin). There may be other signs associated with the infection, such as **fever, joint and muscle pain, uveitis, respiratory distress and signs of haemolysis**. Traditionally a suspicion of leptospirosis has been based on the co-existence of acute kidney and liver disease, but it has been shown that both can present as the sole problem and, therefore, leptospirosis should be suspected in dogs with AKI or acute liver disease.

In recent years, **pulmonary haemorrhagic syndrome** has occasionally been identified in dogs with leptospirosis. The presence of severe respiratory distress in animals with a pulmonary radiological pattern from interstitial to reticulo-interstitial-nodular with alveolar foci, particularly in **caudal and dorsal areas**, is characteristic of this condition. Radiological abnormalities can be observed in dogs without respiratory signs. The mortality of this syndrome is high.

Many dogs have clinicopathological signs of involvement in more than one organ, but one-quarter show signs of involvement in a single organ.

Another clinical sign described is **polyuria and intense polydipsia**, with a hyposthenuric urine density (<1.008, in non-azotaemic dogs not showing serious signs of the disease) due to tubular dysfunction and nephrogenic diabetes insipidus. Normally signs of a previous fever are identified.

Other symptoms associated with leptospirosis include:

- coagulopathy and DIC
- serosal effusions
- abortions
- pancreatitis
- intussusception
- myocarditis
- myositis
- meningitis or myelitis.

There is currently no evidence that associates the different clinical signs with infections by specific serovars.

## *Diagnosis*

The clinical diagnosis is based on a combination of serological tests and detection of the pathogen in dogs presenting with compatible clinical signs.

### Laboratory tests

Laboratory abnormalities that can be seen include:

- leucocytosis
- neutrophilia with a leftward shift
- toxic neutropenia
- thrombocytopenia
- anaemia
- azotaemia
- elevated liver enzymes
- hyperbilirubinaemia
- hyper- or hypokalaemia
- hyper- or hypophosphataemia
- hyponatraemia
- hypochloraemia
- elevations of creatine kinase, AST and cardiac troponins
- elevation of coagulation times
- elevated fibrinogen levels
- isosthenuria
- hyposthenuria
- haematuria
- pyuria
- granular cylinders
- glucosuria
- proteinuria.

### Macroscopic agglutination

The detection of **high antibody titres (>1/800)** using the **macroscopic agglutination technique (MAT)** is compatible with leptospirosis. In some cases, titres may not yet be high and must be confirmed by showing **increasing titres (×4) around 1–2 weeks later**. MAT distinguishes between different serovars, although there is cross-reactivity and sometimes the serovar cannot be identified.

Recently vaccinated dogs (3-4 months previously) may have high antibody titres that make diagnosis difficult and, in the initial days of infection, antibody titres may be negative or low until seroconversion occurs.

The sensitivity and specificity of serology in the diagnosis of leptospirosis are variable, there being false negatives and positives, respectively. It is important that the laboratory performing MAT includes the different serogroups and serovars that may exist in the area, to avoid false negatives.

### ELISA

Recently ELISA tests have been developed for the detection of IgM and IgG against *Leptospira*. Some of these exist in the form of a rapid diagnostic kit. The problems and limitations are similar to those of MAT.

### PCR

There are currently PCR tests that can be **performed on urine or blood** for the detection of **leptospiral DNA**. In general, the **sensitivity is high** and allows diagnosis in dogs that are still seronegative. The main problems with lack of sensitivity are when the dog has already received antibiotics and the stage of infection. Performing PCR on blood and urine simultaneously to increase sensitivity is preferable. PCRs offered by commercial laboratories do not allow differentiation between serovars. Urine PCR can be positive in carrier dogs that are not ill. Vaccines do not cause interference with PCR results.

**Simultaneous use of MAT and PCR on blood and urine** is recommended to confirm the diagnosis of leptospirosis in suspected dogs.

#### Other, less useful, tests

Less useful tests include dark-field and fluorescence microscopy. *Leptospira* can also be identified in biopsies of affected organs using specific stains (Levaditi silver). Culture of *Leptospira* is difficult and is not a commonly available technique.

### Treatment

The antibiotics of choice are ampicillin or doxycycline. Generally, **ampicillin (22–30 mg/kg/6–8 h IV)** is used in the dog in a severe or critical state that cannot tolerate the oral route when hospitalised – for example, with AKI that can be oliguric or anuric.

**Doxycycline (5 mg/kg/12 h or 10 mg/kg/24 h PO for 2 weeks)** is used when the oral route is tolerated and in non-critical dogs, being the only antibiotic that has been shown to be capable of eliminating the condition from carriers and *Leptospira* organisms from renal tubules.

Treatment of **AKI should follow the usual recommendations and practices for AKI** due to other causes. The use of closed urine collection systems is essential to monitor production and avoid contact with it. Amounts of fluids should be adapted to the stage of kidney disease, which can be oliguric or polyuric. In some very serious cases, haemodialysis can be useful in keeping the dog alive until renal function is recovered, avoiding overhydration and electrolyte imbalances. Long-term control of renal function is important, as some animals may have chronic kidney disease as a consequence of an acute leptospirosis injury.

Other treatments, which are dependent on the symptoms in each case, include anti-emetics, antacids, analgesics, heparin, oxygen therapy and plasma transfusions. Immunosuppression (steroids and cyclophosphamide in humans) may be indicated in dogs affected by pulmonary haemorrhagic syndrome, but at the time of writing there is insufficient evidence to recommend this treatment.

### Prognosis

The prognosis for leptospirosis is reserved, although it can be very good in mild or moderate cases. Mortality in cases of oliguric or anuric AKI is variable, and depends on the level of intensive medicine that can be practised (for example, haemodialysis).

Doxycycline is advised for the treatment of dogs that live or have been in contact with others diagnosed with leptospirosis.

### Prevention

**Vaccination against leptospirosis is important in dogs at risk** of exposure. Classic vaccines cover the serogroups *L. canicola* and *L. icterohemorrhage*, but not others, and leptospirosis has been diagnosed in vaccinated dogs in Europe. Therefore, administration of tetravalent vaccines is preferable, which also protect against the serogroups *L. bratislava* and *L. gryppotyphosa*. The duration of immunity of vaccines is usually no more than 1 year.

Measures to avoid infection in humans when treating dogs with leptospirosis should be extreme, although the risk of infection is probably low, since there are no documented cases of infected dogs, and seroprevalence in people in contact with sick dogs is low according to studies.

## Main zoonoses of dogs and cats

### General considerations

**Zoonoses are infectious or parasitic diseases transmitted from animals to humans or vice versa**, either **directly** (true zoonoses) or **indirectly** (through contaminated environments). There are numerous zoonotic diseases, some serious and others mild.

This section is not intended to be an exhaustive compilation of all infectious and parasitic diseases that dogs and cats can transmit to humans, but a guide to the most important and the advice that should be given to pet owners to avoid infection.

### Rabies

### Aetiopathogenesis

**Rabies is a viral disease** that has been known about for a long time, caused by infection with a Lyssavirus, one of the few viruses that is **not species-specific**. The definitive host, which can be an **asymptomatic carrier, is the bat**. All other animals, including humans, if infected, suffer from **progressive viral encephalitis** which is fatal once the clinical signs have started. **Humans are infected through animal bites**, including those from dogs and cats suffering from signs of the disease, one of which is aggression. The infection can also be spread by **open wounds coming into contact with saliva** or nerve tissue from affected animals. People bitten by a dog or cat suspected of having rabies should be treated quickly with prophylactic fluids that prevent the infection from progressing to disease.

### Prevention

The prevention of rabies in humans where it is endemic is based on the **vaccination of wild animals** (using bait) and the **mandatory vaccination of domestic pets** such as dogs, cats and ferrets. In rabies-free countries, guidelines from health authorities must be followed because, in some cases vaccination is obligatory. Travelling pets must be vaccinated to cross borders and authorities, especially in rabies-free countries, should avoid allowing entry of unvaccinated animals or during the period in which they could be incubating the disease. For several years, measurement of antibody levels (>0.5 UI/ml) was mandatory for travel to the UK and Scandinavian countries, using official laboratories, within the Pet Travel Scheme, but it is currently no longer necessary. **Veterinarians who suspect that an animal may have rabies should notify official health authorities**.

## Hydatid cyst

### Aetiopathogenesis

The adult cestode parasites (tapeworms) *Echinococcus granulosus* and *E. multilocularis* may be present in the gastrointestinal tract of dogs that do not have any clinical signs. The eggs of these tapeworms are excreted in faeces and can **spread directly or indirectly to people by contact with faeces or with food contaminated with the eggs**. Humans and other animals can develop **large cystic lesions in organs such as the lungs, liver or brain**, a disease that is known as a hydatid cyst and is very serious. Dogs may be at risk of infection due to coprophagy.

### Epidemiology

Currently, the incidence of this zoonosis is low in Western societies where dogs do not feed on offal or raw meat (therefore, they do not become infected), and are also periodically (every 2–6 months, as the case may be) de-wormed for internal parasites with **praziquantel**, which is the drug of choice to treat these parasites.

### Prevention

The small animal veterinarian has an important role in **maintaining routine de-worming in dogs** to avoid this and other diseases. In addition, it is essential to educate owners to collect faeces that their dogs deposit in the environment to avoid environmental contamination with eggs.

## Toxocariasis/larva migrans

### Aetiopathogenesis

Nematode parasites, or roundworms, *Toxocara canis* (dog) and *T. cati* (cat) are commonly present in the gastrointestinal tract, especially of puppies. Humans can be accidentally infected by contact with **environments contaminated with faeces containing eggs of these parasites**, which can persist for weeks to months. Most people who become infected do not develop disease but, in some cases, they can suffer serious consequences due to erratic migration of larvae in viscera, the eyes or central nervous system.

## Toxoplasmosis

### Aetiopathogenesis

Toxoplasmosis is an infection caused by the protozoan *Toxoplasma gondii*, and **cats are the only animals that act as definitive hosts**. This means that they are the only species in which the parasite can infect the intestine, undergo sexual reproduction and, after a series of changes and transformations, be excreted in the faeces in the form of non-sporulated oocysts. The latter **sporulate 1–5 days** later into environmentally resistant forms with infective capacity that can last months to years. These **sporulated oocysts are the forms that indirectly infect the intermediate host** (humans or production animals) and, once the infection and asexual cycle (tachyzoites) of the parasite have been formed (Figure 7.45), they may become **dormant in muscles or CNS** as tissue cysts with bradyzoites (forms of low pathogenicity), which are completely subclinical.

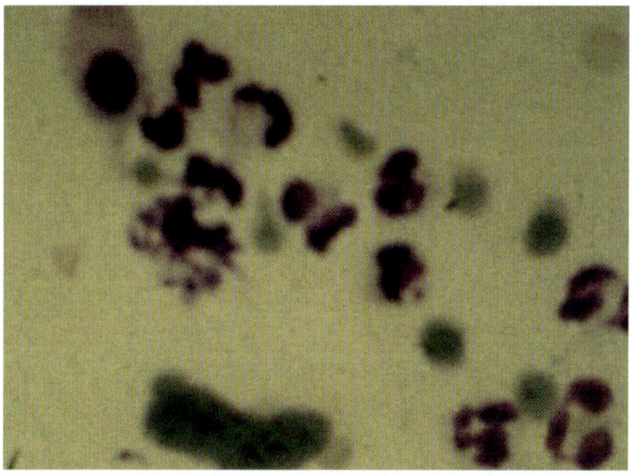

**Figure 7.45.** *Toxoplasma gondii* tachyzoites in a sample of respiratory secretion obtained by broncho-alveolar lavage. The cat was seropositive to FIV and presented with a diffuse pneumonia due to *Toxoplasma*, which suggests an advanced state of immunodeficiency. A cat that is ill with toxoplasmosis does not pose a risk of infection to people unless it is excreting oocysts in faeces at the same time, which is very unlikely.

The most frequent routes of infection in humans are:

- **Ingestion of raw meat** carrying tissue cysts.
- Consumption of **water or food contaminated** with sporulated oocysts.
- **Contact with soil** and earth contaminated with sporulated oocysts (horticulture, agriculture).

Although infection in humans is generally subclinical and of low pathogenicity, it can have **serious consequences if it occurs in the first third of pregnancy** (abortions or malformations) **or in immunosuppressed people** (systemic infections with risk of death).

Direct infection from the cat's own faeces is unusual, since faeces is not normally handled with bare hands and this is even less likely after 24 hours or longer. On the other hand, intestinal infection in cats usually occurs once in a lifetime, during which they excrete oocysts for a period of 7–15 days and do not do so again even if they become re-infected. The percentage of people seropositive to antibodies against *T. gondii* is not significantly different between those who have direct contact with cats and those who do not. This fact reinforces the concept that direct contact with cats is not a frequent or important form of transmission.

#### Prevention

The most effective measures to prevent toxoplasmosis in people are:

- Avoid eating raw or undercooked meat.
- Wearing gloves for horticulture and agriculture.
- Washing vegetables thoroughly.
- Removing faeces from litter boxes daily to avoid contact.
- Always washing hands after being in contact with earth or meat, or having removed faeces from litter boxes.

The most effective measures for prevention of toxoplasmosis in cats are:

- Keeping them indoors.
- Not giving them the chance to hunt and ingest prey.
- Not feeding them raw meat.

### Bartonellosis

#### Aetiopathogenesis

Infection by the bacterium *Bartonella henselae* is the main cause of bartonellosis, or **cat scratch disease**, in humans. Cats can be carriers of this intra-erythrocytic organism in the blood (bacteraemia) subclinically, but rarely show signs of disease or bartonellosis. The route of **transmission between cats is by ingestion of fleas and/or their faeces**. The spread from cats to people occurs through close or very direct contact, playing or sleeping with the cat in bed, by scratches or licking. The transmission of the bacteria to humans is associated with contact with faeces from bacteria-carrying fleas on erosions or wounds on the skin or mucous membranes. There is not a history of being scratched by cats in all cases of bartonellosis in humans.

Bartonellosis **in humans is generally a subclinical infection**, but sometimes it can cause fever and lymphadenitis in immunocompetent people (cat scratch disease) that resolve spontaneously or with antibiotics. However, in **immunosuppressed people** those with AIDS, chronic disease or undergoing immunosuppressive treatments) it can produce **a severe form with fever, endocarditis, sepsis, neuroretinitis, peliosis and bacillary angiomatosis**, which can even be fatal in patients with AIDS.

#### Epidemiology

The prevalence of antibodies in domestic cats is relatively high, especially in young animals.

The prevalence of DNA in feline blood samples is generally low, although PCR techniques incur problems with sensitivity.

#### Prevention

The prevention of bartonellosis in cats is based on the use of effective ectoparasitic measures against fleas.

Prevention in people is based on:

- Washing hands after contact with cats.
- Avoiding aggressive play with cats.
- Avoiding very close contact (licking, sleeping) with cats, especially in the case of older people or those with immunodeficiency.

### Less frequently encountered zoonoses

Table 7.12 lists those zoonoses involving contact with the dog or cat.

## Vaccines and vaccination programmes

### General considerations

The use of vaccines in humans and animals has reduced the prevalence of numerous infectious diseases and some important zoonoses, and should be considered **a success story in medicine**. However, there are people and movements against vaccination, which results in

Table 7.12. Other less frequent zoonoses due to direct contact with cats or dogs.

| Disease | Transmission | Prevention |
|---|---|---|
| *Pasteurella* | Dog and cat bites, aerosolisation, oral or respiratory secretions | Immunosuppressed people: avoid bites and very intimate contact |
| *Capnocytophaga* | Dog and cat bites | Immunosuppressed people: avoid bites |
| Tularaemia (*Francisella tularensis*) | Cat and rodent bites, also mosquito and tick bites | Endemic areas of northern Europe<br>Avoid ectoparasites and contact with at-risk animals |
| Dermatophytosis | Contact with diseased or carrier cats | Mild disease<br>Treat infected cats and the environment |
| Sporotrichosis | Contact with diseased or carrier cats | Serious disease<br>Endemic areas in Brazil and outbreaks in Italy<br>Avoid contact with cats suspected of having or suffering from the disease |
| Bordetellosis (*B. bronchiseptica*) | Contact with carriers and sick dogs and cats | Few cases described in humans, but special attention should be paid in immunosuppressed people |
| Coxielosis (*C. burnetti*) or Q fever | Contact with placentas or foetuses of infected animals, including cats | Few cases described by contact with cats<br>Avoid contact with aborted tissues and foetuses |
| Yersinosis (*Y. pestis*) or plague | Contact with rodent fleas or with diseased cats | Some endemic areas<br>Prevent fleas on cats and avoid contact with rats and rodents |
| Intestinal bacteria (*Campylobacter, Salmonella*) | Contact with dog and cat faeces, carriers and diseased animals | Infrequent<br>Avoid contact with faeces<br>Wash hands |
| Giardiasis (*G. lamblia, G. intestinalis*) | Contact with faeces of infected cats and dogs | Poorly documented<br>*Giardia* variants that infect dogs and cats are not those that affect humans<br>Avoid contact with faeces and wash hands |
| Cryptosporidiosis (*C. parvum, C. felis*) | Contact with faeces of infected cats and dogs | Poorly documented<br>Variants in cats are not so specific as in humans<br>Avoid contact with faeces and wash hands |
| Leptospirosis (*Leptospira* spp. serovars) | Contact with urine from rodents (carriers) and infected dogs or cats | Uncommon via contact with dogs and cats<br>Avoid contact with urine from diseased dogs |
| Brucellosis (*Brucella canis*) | Contact with secretions and reproductive tissues from infected or diseased dogs | Uncommon, but extreme caution when handling secretions and tissues from suspected or infected dogs |
| Mycobacteriosis (mycobacteria from the tuberculosis group [*M. tuberculosis, M. bovis, M. microti*] and from *M. avium* complex) | Contact with respiratory or cutaneous secretions from diseased dogs or cats | The dog and cat are accidental hosts and, in general, transmission is from humans to them<br>However, when diagnosing a mycobacteriosis by zoonotic species, urgent measures must be taken and the separation or euthanasia of the dog or cat should even be assessed, especially if they live with immunosuppressed people |
| Vector-borne diseases (leishmaniosis, borreliosis, babesiosis, dirofilariasis, ehrlichiosis, rickettsiosis) | Indirect transmission through the specific vectors of each disease | Direct contact with infected or diseased dogs or cats is not a risk to humans, but the presence of their vectors is. Prevent vectors (fleas, ticks, mosquitoes, sandflies) with suitable products |

the use of vaccines to decrease in some environments. There are many factors that can cause opposition to vaccination, one of the main ones being the risk of adverse effects.

In the last two decades, and for the first time, groups of experts have been established in the USA and Europe that have developed recommendations and guidelines for vaccination guidelines in dogs and cats. These guidelines are scientific documents based on the best available scientific evidence, without economic criteria or pressure from companies that manufacture and sell vaccines, so that veterinarians can **advise on the best vaccination plans for their patients adapted to the needs of each environment and each animal**. It is possible to find small differences in criteria in the different guides, but this should not be seen as a weak point. In many aspects of vaccination, and in the general prevention of infectious diseases in dogs and cats, there are deficiencies in knowledge and conclusions are drawn from the consensus among experts, so there may be discrepancies.

The general objective of vaccination (and recommendations) is to vaccinate as many dogs and cats as possible against diseases that are considered key.

One of the most important concepts in the subject of vaccination is that of **population or herd immunity**. Epidemiological studies and experiences in human medicine show that, if in a population at risk of an infectious disease >70% of the population is vaccinated and has a good immunity, the prevalence decreases and, over the years, vaccination can even eradicate the illness.

When **population immunity is robust**, pathogens encounter immunised individuals that block the infection from the beginning and there are fewer subclinical infections, and therefore less excretion of the pathogen and a reduced possibility of infecting other individuals. Consequently the **prevalence of pathogen circulation is reduced** and even the percentage of the unvaccinated population is protected. With regard to the vaccination of dogs and cats, this 70 or 80% of the vaccinated population is a long way from being achieved and, even in the best case scenario, there are regions or areas where 50% of dogs or cats have received a correct and adequate vaccination schedule but, as a general rule, the percentage of vaccinated animals ranges from 30 to 50%. This is one of the main reasons why the prevalence of certain infectious diseases, such as parvovirus or distemper, remains high despite the fact that vaccination immunity is effective. **As the percentage of vaccinated individuals decreases (vaccine antagonism), the burden of circulating pathogens is potentially higher and the prevalence of infection and disease increases**.

One of the most important aspects defined in recent years is **which vaccines are essential (core) and which are not (non-core)**, or even not recommended in dogs and cats. From the point of view of companies that manufacture vaccines, all of these are necessary but, from the clinician's, owner's and patient's point of view, this is debatable. For example, there are pathogens to which, due either to their form of transmission or their prevalence in certain areas, it is impossible for a dog or cat to be exposed. In that case the vaccine is considered non-essential and advice is given as to which situations it should be applied or is not essential. On the other hand, there are vaccines whose usefulness or efficacy is debatable in the general population and may not be recommended, or are recommended only in very specific situations.

**Essential vaccines** are those whose application is **recommended in all dogs or cats whatever their lifestyle and living conditions**. These are mainly vaccines against viral diseases in which immunisation is good, even sterilising in some cases, and against viruses that may have a high prevalence and/or environmental resistance, so the prevalence of infection is very high. The zoonotic potential of a pathogen is also important in determining whether a vaccine should be essential or even mandatory.

The only **vaccine that may be mandatory** if considered by the authorities of a country or an area is the **rabies vaccine**. In rabies-endemic areas it is essential that dogs, cats and ferrets are well immunised, since in most cases it is these that spread rabies to the people they live with.

**Non-essential vaccines** are those that are recommended depending on the style or living conditions of the dog or cat, mainly vaccines against bacterial diseases.

## *Types of vaccine*

Different types of vaccines are available, depending on how the pathogen or antigen is formulated in the product.

The most frequently used vaccines are **attenuated vaccines**. In these the pathogen is alive and produces a **subclinical infection in the animal**, so that it develops an immune and memory response. The pathogens have been attenuated in their virulence or pathogenicity in the laboratory by different techniques. They are safe vaccines if used correctly and, in general, these are preferred since they produce **rapid immunity that simulates natural infection**.

**Inactivated vaccines** use antigens or parts of the pathogen that are not capable of producing subclinical infection, and therefore they are **less immunogenic**.

Hence, they must be accompanied by immunogenic substances and cause inflammation so that the cells reach the injection site and then recognise the antigen. They are safe vaccines that produce good immunity, although the duration of immunity may be shorter and adjuvants can produce **local inflammatory reactions** that, in very rare cases, evolve into sarcomas, especially in cats.

In recent years, **recombinant vaccines** have appeared in which viral vectors (non-pathogenic viruses in the vaccinated species) to which a pathogen antigen against which an immune response is desired has been added. They are safe vaccines and do not require the use of adjuvants.

### *Vaccination programmes*

The vaccination guidelines that are recommended are usually **based on a primary vaccination with two doses (2 and 3 months of age)**, revaccination after a year and **annual booster** doses throughout life.

The current recommendations propose the following changes to this classic programme:

- **Primary vaccination**. Administer three (or up to four) doses of essential vaccines in dogs and cats (2, 3 and 4 months, even a first at 6 weeks). This recommendation is based on the results of studies demonstrating that the presence of high levels of maternal immunity for up to 12 or more weeks may interfere with the immune response to the vaccine. Consequently, some dogs or cats are not properly immunised after the traditional last dose at 12 weeks.
- **Revaccination**. Administer at 1 year old or the last dose as a puppy. This recommendation is even being modified to revaccination at 6 months of age rather than waiting until 12 months. There are no scientific studies on this, but it is thought that it might be better to advance revaccination to give greater immunity to dogs or cats at an age at which they are still susceptible to being infected.
- **Adult vaccinations**. Administer booster doses of essential vaccines every 3 years. This recommendation is based on studies of immunity duration demonstrating that, for essential vaccines, if the primary vaccination of dogs and cats is correct, it lasts many years (up to 7) but it is preferable to establish a safety margin (3 years). This does not include non-essential vaccines for which it is not known whether the duration of immunity lasts more than 1 year. This recommendation is also subject to variation depending on the living conditions and the prevalence or environmental burden of infections, or in the case of viruses with frequent genetic modifications (for example, feline calicivirus). In these cases, it is preferable to maintain annual revaccination.

Therefore, the number of vaccinations is increased at the age or stage in which dogs and cats are most susceptible to infections, and decreases at the stage in which it has been shown that there is already good memory immunity if primary vaccination has been performed correctly (essential vaccines). These changes do not affect the immunity of the population as a whole, since these animals are correctly immunised. The real problem is that the percentage of dogs or cats that receives a correct vaccination schedule is not higher.

Recommended vaccination programmes for dogs and cats are listed in Tables 7.13 and 7.14, respectively.

### *Adverse effects*

In general, vaccines have few adverse effects. The most frequent are the following:

- **Immediate type I hypersensitivity** reactions with angioedema, hives, vomiting and, very rarely, systemic signs of anaphylaxis or shock.

Association with **immune-mediated or autoimmune diseases** (anaemia or thrombocytopenia), although their cause–effect relationship has never been demonstrated.

- **Local reactions** with inflammation and pain at the area of application, and also vasculitis or ischaemia that produces focal or multifocal alopecia.
- **Systemic signs of the disease** that has been vaccinated against (rare, although it may occur by accidental inhalation of the attenuated vaccine during preparation).
- **Vaccine failures** due to poor vaccine preservation, insufficient immunisation or an inadequate vaccination programme.

A well-known adverse effect in cats is the development of **sarcoma at the injection site**, whose first denomination was sarcomas associated with vaccines or post-vaccination. They appear in a small number of cats, **associated with chronic or persistent inflammation** at sites where vaccines have been applied, but also with other drugs or exogenous materials such as subcutaneous microchips. Therefore, although vaccines are the major risk factor, it is not an adverse effect directly linked to the vaccine product but, rather, to a malignant transformation of an inflammatory reaction in some predisposed cats. The type of vaccine most associated with this problem is **inactivated vaccines**

Table 7.13. Vaccine recommendations in dogs. Summary of those published in the WSAVA, European ABCD and US AAFP and AAHA guidelines.

| Vaccine | Timeline | Comments |
|---|---|---|
| Parvovirus | (6), 8, 12, 16 weeks | Essential vaccine |
| | Revaccination at 26 or 52 weeks | In some breeds (Rottweiler), additional doses during the first year |
| | Revaccination every 3 years | |
| Distemper | (6), 8, 12, 16 weeks | Essential vaccine |
| | Revaccination at 26 or 52 weeks | |
| | Revaccination every 3 years | |
| Canine infectious hepatitis (adenovirus 2) | (6), 8, 12, 16 weeks | Essential vaccine |
| | Revaccination at 26 or 52 weeks | |
| | Revaccination every 3 years | |
| Rabies | >12 weeks | Vaccine mandatory by law, essential or non-essential depending on the legislation in force in each country or area |
| | Annual revaccination or every 3 years, depending on the type of vaccine | Mandatory vaccination in animals that travel |
| Leptospirosis | 8 and 12 weeks. | Non-essential vaccine, but important in rural and outdoor dogs |
| | Annual revaccination | There are currently new vaccines that extend protection to 4 serovars |
| | | Associated with frequent allergic reactions in small breeds, but there is no scientific evidence to prove it |
| Canine respiratory complex (*Bordetella*, parainfluenza, adenovirus 2) | 8 and 12 weeks. | Non-essential vaccine |
| | Annual revaccination or before going to boarding kennels | Consider in at-risk dogs or in groups and rehoming centres |
| Borreliosis | 12 and 16 weeks. | Essential vaccine |
| | Annual revaccination | Consider only in endemic areas or in dogs that travel to these areas |
| Canine coronavirus | | Vaccine not currently recommended |
| Leishmaniosis | From 6 months of age in seronegative dogs, three separate doses 4 weeks apart | Non-essential vaccine |
| | Annual revaccination | Consider in high-risk dogs or those travelling to endemic areas |
| | | Ensure repellent treatments against sandflies |
| Babesiosis | One dose and annual revaccination | Non-essential vaccine |
| | | Consider in endemic areas and in high-risk dogs |
| | | Maintain preventive tick treatments |

Table 7.14. Vaccine recommendations in cats. Summary of those published in the WSAVA, European ABCD and US AAFP and AAHA guidelines.

| Vaccine | Timeline | Comments |
|---|---|---|
| Herpesvirus | (6), 8, 12, 16 weeks | Essential vaccine |
| | Revaccination at 26 or 52 weeks | Consider annual revaccination in some high-risk situations |
| | Revaccination every 3 years | |
| Calicivirus | (6), 8, 12, 16 weeks | Essential vaccine |
| | Revaccination at 26 or 52 weeks | Consider annual revaccination in some high-risk situations |
| | Revaccination every 3 years | Consider change or rotation of vaccine type if clinical cases appear despite vaccination |
| | | Consider vaccines that protect against more variants |
| Panleukopenia | (6), 8, 12, 16 weeks | Essential vaccine |
| | Revaccination at 26 or 52 weeks | It is one of the vaccines that confers a stronger immunity in properly vaccinated cats |
| | Revaccination every 3 years | |

Table 7.14. Continued

| Vaccine | Timeline | Comments |
|---|---|---|
| Feline leukaemia virus | 9 and 12 weeks. | Vaccine not essential, but highly recommended in outdoor and indoor cats that may have sporadic contact with other cats |
| | Annual revaccination or every 2 or 3 years (different criteria exist) | Perform the antigen test beforehand, and only vaccinate non-viral cats<br>There are recombinant vaccines available without adjuvant |
| Rabies | >12 weeks | Vaccine mandatory by law, essential or non-essential depending on the legislation in force in each country or area |
| | Annual revaccination or every 3 years depending on the type of vaccine | Mandatory vaccination in animals that travel |
| Chlamydiosis | 9 and 12 weeks.<br>Annual revaccination | Non-essential vaccine<br>Consider at-risk cats in endemic groups or communities with high prevalence |
| Feline immunodeficiency | Three separate doses at 2–3 weeks | Non-essential vaccine |
| | Annual revaccination | Marketed in the USA, Japan and Australia |
| Coronavirus/FIP | 16 and 18 weeks.<br>Annual revaccination | Vaccination not recommended<br>Protects against coronavirus infections, not feline infectious peritonitis, in cats and carriers<br>Consider only in at-risk cats that are seronegative, which is unlikely given the high prevalence of coronavirus infections in at-risk cats. |

**with adjuvants**, which are those that produce a greater inflammatory reaction. Changes in the guidelines (revaccinate every 3 years) and in vaccine application sites in cats (avoid the interscapular area, apply in distal areas of the extremities, lateral wall of the abdomen or tail) were implemented with the objective of reducing prevalence of these sarcomas (Figure 7.46).

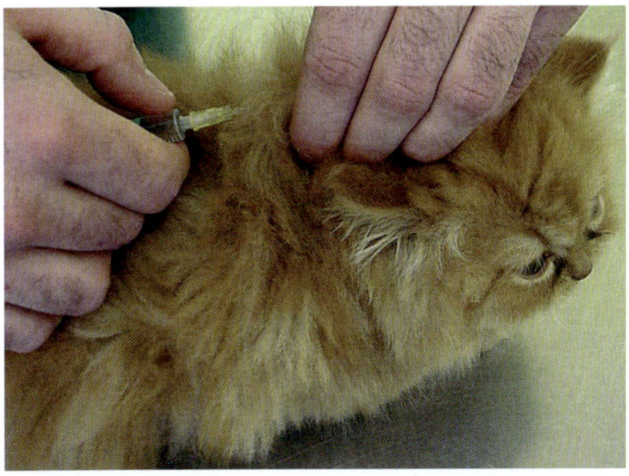

Figure 7.46. Ideally cats should not be vaccinated in the interscapular area (as shown in the photo) given the small risk of inflammation associated with vaccines (and other medications or materials) which can lead to formation of a sarcoma. It is difficult to completely remove sarcomas from this area. Currently subcutaneous vaccination is mainly recommended in the distal areas of the limbs.

## Bibliography

### Feline infectious diseases

#### Respiratory infections


Ballin, A.C., Schulz, B., Helps, C., Sauter-Louis, C., Mueller, R.S. and Hartmann K. (2014) Limited efficacy of topical recombinant feline interferon-omega for treatment of cats with acute upper respiratory viral disease. *Veterinary Journal* 202(3), 466–470.

Bol, S. and Bunnik, E.M. (2015) Lysine supplementation is not effective for the prevention or treatment of feline herpesvirus 1 infection in cats: a systematic review. *BMC Veterinary Research* 11, 284.

Fernandez, M., Manzanilla, E.G., Lloret, A., León, M. and Thibault, J.C. (2016) Prevalence of feline herpesvirus-1, feline calicivirus, *Chlamydophila felis* and *Mycoplasma felis* DNA and associated risk factors in cats in Spain with upper respiratory tract disease, conjunctivitis and/or gingivostomatitis. *Journal of Feline Medicine and Surgery* https://doi.org/10.1177/1098612X16634387.

Gruffydd-Jones, T., Addie, D., Belák, S., Boucraut-Baralon, C., Egberink, H., Frymus, T. et al. (2009) *Chlamydophila felis* infection. ABCD guidelines on prevention and management. *Journal of Feline Medicine and Surgery* 11(7), 605–609.

Gutzwiller, M.E., Brachelente, C., Taglinger, K., Suter, M.M., Weissenböck, H. and Roosje, P.J. (2007) Feline herpes dermatitis treated with interferon omega. *Veterinary Dermatology* 18, 50–54.

Hartmann, A.D., Helps, C.R., Lappin, M.R., Werckenthin, C. and Hartmann, K. (2008) Efficacy of pradofloxacin in cats with feline upper respiratory tract disease due to *Chlamydophila felis* or *Mycoplasma* infections. *Journal of Veterinary Internal Medicine* 22(1), 44–52.

Hora, A.S., Tonietti, P.O., Guerra, J.M., Leme, M.C., Pena, H.F., Maiorka, P.C. et al. (2013) Felid herpesvirus 1 as a causative agent of severe nonsuppurative meningoencephalitis in a domestic cat. *Journal of Clinical Microbiology* 51(2), 676–679.

Jas, D., Frances-Duvert, V., Vernes, D., Guigal, P.M. and Poulet, H. (2015) Three-year duration of immunity for feline herpesvirus and calicivirus evaluated in a controlled vaccination-challenge laboratory trial. *Veterinary Microbiology* 177(1–2), 123–131.

Lee, M., Bosward, K.L. and Norris, J.M. (2010) Immunohistological evaluation of feline herpesvirus-1 infection in feline eosinophilic dermatoses or stomatitis. *Journal of Feline Medicine and Surgery* 12, 72–79.

Malik, R., Lessels, N.S., Webb, S., Meek, M., Graham, P.G., Vitale, C. et al. (2009) Treatment of feline herpesvirus-1 associated disease in cats with famciclovir and related drugs. *Journal of Feline Medicine and Surgery* 11, 40–48.

Möstl, K., Addie, D.D., Boucraut-Baralon, C., Egberink, H., Frymus, T., Gruffydd-Jones, T. et al. (2015) Something old, something new: Update of the 2009 and 2013 ABCD guidelines on prevention and management of feline infectious diseases. *Journal of Feline Medicine and Surgery* 17(7), 570–582.

Radford, A.D., Addie, D., Belák, S., Boucraut-Baralon, C., Egberink, H., Frymus, T. et al. (2009) Feline calicivirus infection: ABCD guidelines on prevention and management. *Journal of Feline Medicine and Surgery* 11, 556–564.

Schulz, C., Hartmann, K., Mueller, R.S., Helps, C. and Schulz, B.S. (2015) Sampling sites for detection of feline herpesvirus-1, feline calicivirus and *Chlamydia felis* in cats with feline upper respiratory tract disease. *Journal of Feline Medicine and Surgery* 17(12), 1012–1019.

Stiles, J. (2014) Ocular manifestations of feline viral diseases. *Veterinary Journal* 201(2), 166–173.

Thiry, E., Addie, D., Belák, S., Boucraut-Baralon, C., Egberink, H., Frymus, T. et al. (2009) Feline herpesvirus infection: ABCD guidelines on prevention and management. *Journal of Feline Medicine and Surgery* 11, 547–555.

Thomasy, S.M., Lim, C.C., Reilly, C.M., Kass, P.H., Lappin, M.R. and Maggs, D.J. (2011) Evaluation of orally administered famciclovir in cats experimentally infected with feline herpesvirus type-1. *American Journal of Veterinary Research* 72(1), 85–95.

## Chronic feline gingivostomatitis (CFGS)

Arzi, B., Mills-Ko, E., Verstraete, F.J., Kol, A,. Walker, N.J., Badgley, M.R. et al. (2016) Therapeutic efficacy of fresh, autologous mesenchymal stem cells for severe refractory gingivostomatitis in cats. *Stem Cells Translational Medicine* 5(1), 75–86.

Belgard, S., Truyen, U., Thibault, J.C. et al. (2010) Relevance of feline calicivirus, feline immunodeficiency virus, feline leukemia virus, feline herpesvirus and *Bartonella henselae* in cats with chronic gingivostomatitis. *Berliner und Münchener tierärztliche Wochenschrift* 123(9–10), 369–376.

Bellei, E., Dalla, F., Masetti, L., Pisoni, L. and Joechler, M. (2008) Surgical therapy in chronic feline gingivostomatitis (FCGS). *Veterinary Research Communications 32 (Suppl. 1)*, S231–S234.

Dolieslager, S.M., Bennett, D., Johnston, N. and Riggio, M.P. (2013) Novel bacterial phylotypes associated with the healthy feline oral cavity and feline chronic gingivostomatitis. *Research in Veterinary Science* 94(3), 428–432.

Dolieslager, S.M., Lappin, D.F., Bennett, D., Graham, L., Johnston, N. and Riggio, M.P. (2013) The influence of oral bacteria on tissue levels of Toll-like receptor and cytokine mRNAs in feline chronic gingivostomatitis and oral health. *Veterinary Immunology and Immunopathology* 151(3–4), 263–274.

Dolieslager, S.M., Riggio, M.P., Lennon, A., Lappin, D.F., Johnston, N., Taylor, D. et al. (2011) Identification of bacteria associated with feline chronic gingivostomatitis using culture-dependent and culture-independent methods. *Veterinary Microbiology* 148(1), 93–98.

Dowers, K.L., Hawley, J.R., Brewer, M.M., Morris, A.K., Radecki, S.V. and Lappin, M.R. (2010) Association of *Bartonella* species, feline calicivirus, and feline herpesvirus 1 infection with gingivostomatitis in cats. *Journal of Feline Medicine and Surgery* 12(4), 314–321.

Harley, R., Gruffydd-Jones, T.J. and Day, M.J. (2011) Immunohistochemical characterization of oral mucosal lesions in cats with chronic gingivostomatitis. *Journal of Comparative Pathology* 144(4), 239–250.

Hennet, P.R., Camy, G.A., McGahie, D.M. and Albouy, M.V. (2011) Comparative efficacy of a recombinant feline interferon omega in refractory cases of calicivirus-positive cats with caudal stomatitis: a randomised, multi-centre, controlled, double-blind study in 39 cats. *Journal of Feline Medicine and Surgery* 13(8), 577–587.

Quimby, J.M., Elston, T., Hawley, J., Brewer, M., Miller, A. and Lappin, M.R. (2008) Evaluation of the association of *Bartonella species*, feline herpesvirus 1, feline calicivirus, feline leukemia virus and feline immunodeficiency virus with chronic feline gingivostomatitis. *Journal of Feline Medicine and Surgery* 10(1), 66–72.

Rolim, V.M., Pavarini, S.P., Campos, F.S., Pignone, V., Faraco, C., Muccillo, M.S. et al. (2016) Clinical, pathological, immunohistochemical and molecular characterization of feline chronic gingivostomatitis. *Journal of Feline Medicine and Surgery* https://doi.org/10.1177/1098612X16628578.

## Gastrointestinal infections

Ballweber, L.R., Xiao, L., Bowman, D.D., Kahn, G. and Cama, V.A. (2010) Giardiasis in dogs and cats: update on epidemiology and public health significance. *Trends in Parasitology* 26, 180–189.

De Santis-Kerr, A.C., Raghavan, M., Glickman, N.W., Caldanaro, R.J., Moore, G.E., Lewis, H.B., Schantz, P.M. et al. (2006) Prevalence and risk factors for *Giardia* and *coccidia* species of pet cats in 2003–2004. *Journal of Feline Medicine and Surgery* 8, 292–301.

Gruffydd-Jones, T., Addie, D., Belák, S., Boucraut-Baralon, C., Egberink, H., Frymus, T. et al. (2013) Tritrichomoniasis in cats: ABCD guidelines on prevention and management. *Journal of Feline Medicine and Surgery* 15(7), 647–649.

Gruffydd-Jones, T., Addie, D., Belák, S., Boucraut-Baralon, C., Egberink, H., Frymus, T. et al. (2013) Giardiasis in cats: ABCD guidelines on prevention and management. *Journal of Feline Medicine and Surgery* 15(7), 650–652.

Jakel, V., Cussler, K., Hanschmann, K.M., Truyen, U., König, M., Kamphuis, E. et al. (2012) Vaccination against feline panleukopenia: implications from a field study in kittens. *BMC Veterinary Research* 8, 62.

Keith, C.L., Radecki, S.V. and Lappin, M.R. (2003) Evaluation of fenbendazole for treatment of *Giardia* infection in cats concurrently infected with *Cryptosporidium parvum*. *American Journal of Veterinary Research* 64, 1027–1029.

McGlade, T.R., Robertson, I.D., Elliot, A.D. and Thompson, R.C. (2003) High prevalence of *Giardia* detected in cats by PCR. *Veterinary Parasitology* 110, 197–205.

Miró, G., Hernández, L., Montoya, A., Arranz-Solís, D., Dado, D., Rojo-Montejo, S. et al. (2011) First description of naturally acquired *Tritrichomonas foetus* infection in a Persian cattery in Spain. *Parasitology Research* 109(4), 1151–1154.

Olson, M.E., Leonard, N.J. and Srout, J. (2010) Prevalence and diagnosis of *Giardia* infection in dogs and cats using a fecal antigen test and fecal smear. *Canadian Veterinary Journal* 51, 640–642.

Paris, J.K., Wills, S., Balzer, H.J., Shaw, D.J. and Gunn-Moore, D.A. (2014) Enteropathogen co-infection in UK cats with diarrhea. *BMC Veterinary Research* 10, 13.

Sotiriadou, I., Pantchev, N., Gassmann, D. and Karanis, P. (2013) Molecular identification of *Giardia* and *Cryptosporidium* from dogs and cats. *Parasite* 20, 8.

Spada, E., Proverbio, D., Della Pepa, A., Domenichini, G., Bagnagatti De Giorgi, G., Traldi, G. et al. (2013) Prevalence of faecal-borne parasites in colony stray cats in northern Italy. *Journal of Feline Medicine and Surgery* 15(8), 672–677.

Stuetzer, B. and Hartmann, K. (2014) Feline parvovirus infection and associated diseases. *Veterinary Journal* 201(2), 150–155.

Truyen, U., Addie, D., Belák, S., Boucraut-Baralon, C., Egberink, H., Frymus, T., Gruffydd-Jones, T. et al. (2009) Feline panleukopenia. ABCD guidelines on prevention and management. *Journal of Feline Medicine and Surgery* 11(7), 538–546.

Truyen, U. and Parrish, C.R. (2013) Feline panleukopenia virus: its interesting evolution and current problems in immunoprophylaxis against a serious pathogen. *Veterinary Microbiology* 165(1–2), 29–32.

Xenoulis, P.G., Lopinski, D.J., Read, S.A., Suchodolski, J.S. and Steiner, J.M. (2013) Intestinal *Tritrichomonas foetus* infection in cats: a retrospective study of 104 cases. *Journal of Feline Medicine and Surgery* 15(12), 1098–1103.

Yao, C. and Köster, L.S. (2015) *Tritrichomonas foetus* infection, a cause of chronic diarrhea in the domestic cat. *Veterinary Research* 46, 35.

## *Coronavirus infections*

Addie, D., Belák, S., Boucraut-Baralon, C., Egberink, H., Frymus, T., Gruffydd-Jones, T. et al. (2009) Feline infectious peritonitis: ABCD guidelines on prevention and management. *Journal of Feline Medicine and Surgery* 11, 594–604.

Chang, H.W., Egberink, H.F., Halpin, R., Spiro, D.J. and Rottier, P.J. (2012) Spike protein fusion peptide and feline coronavirus virulence. *Emerging Infectious Diseases* 18(7), 1089–1095.

Doenges, S.J., Weber, K., Dorsch, R., Fux, R., Fischer, A., Matiasek, L.A. et al. (2016) Detection of feline coronavirus in cerebrospinal fluid for diagnosis of feline infectious peritonitis in cats with and without neurological signs. *Journal of Feline Medicine and Surgery* 18(2), 104–109.

Felten, S., Weider, K., Doenges, S., Gruendl, S., Matiasek, K., Hermanns, W. et al. (2017) Detection of feline coronavirus spike gene mutations as a tool to diagnose feline infectious peritonitis. *Journal of Feline Medicine and Surgery* 19(4), 321–335.

Gunn-Moore, D.A., Gruffydd-Jones, T.J. and Harbour, D.A. (1998) Detection of feline coronaviruses by culture and RT-PCR of blood samples from healthy cats and cats with clinical feline infectious peritonitis. *Veterinary Microbiology* 8, 69–72.

Ishida, T., Shibanai, A., Tanaka, S., Uchida, K. and Mochizuki, M.C. (2004) Use of recombinant feline interferon and glucocorticoid in the treatment of feline infectious peritonitis. *Journal of Feline Medicine and Surgery* 6, 107–109.

Legendre, A.M. and Bartges, J.W. (2009) Effect of Polyprenyl Immunostimulant on the survival times of three cats with the dry form of feline infectious peritonitis. *Journal of Feline Medicine and Surgery* 11(8), 624–626.

Longstaff, L., Porter, E., Crossley, V.J., Hayhow, S.E., Helps, C.R. and Tasker, S. (2017) Feline coronavirus quantitative reverse transcriptase polymerase chain reaction on effusion samples in cats with and without feline infectious peritonitis. *Journal of Feline Medicine and Surgery* 19(20), 240–245.

Pedersen, N.C. (2014) An update on feline infectious peritonitis: virology and immunopathogenesis. *Veterinary Journal* 201(2), 123–132.

Pedersen, N.C. (2014) An update on feline infectious peritonitis: diagnostics and therapeutics. *Veterinary Journal* 201(2), 133–141.

Porter, E., Tasker, S., Day, M.J., Harley, R., Kipar, A., Siddell, S.G. et al. (2014) Amino acid changes in the spike protein of feline coronavirus correlate with systemic spread of virus from the intestine and not with feline infectious peritonitis. *Veterinary Research* 45, 49.

Riemer, F., Kuehner, K.A., Ritz, S., Sauter-Louis, C. and Hartmann, K. (2016) Clinical and laboratory features of cats with feline infectious peritonitis – a retrospective study of 231 confirmed cases (200–2010). *Journal of Feline Medicine and Surgery* 18(4), 348–356.

Ritz, S., Egberink, H. and Hartmann, K. (2007) Effect of feline interferon-omega on the survival time and quality of life of cats with feline infectious peritonitis. *Journal of Veterinary Internal Medicine* 21(6), 1193–1197.

Vennema, H., Poland, A., Foley, J. and Pedersen, N.C. (1008) Feline infectious peritonitis arise by mutation from endemic feline enteric coronaviruses. *Virology* 243, 150–157.

## *Retrovirus infections*

Bęczkowski, P.M., Litster, A., Lin, T.L., Mellor, D.J., Willett, B.J. and Hosie, M.J. (2015) Contrasting clinical outcomes in two cohorts of cats naturally infected with feline immunodeficiency virus (FIV). *Veterinary Microbiology* 176(1–2), 50–60.

Boesch, A., Cattori, V., Riond, B., Willi, B., Meli, M.L., Rentsch, K.M. et al. (2015) Evaluation of the effect of short-term treatment with the integrase inhibitor raltegravir (Isentress) on the course of progressive feline leukemia virus infection. *Veterinary Microbiology* 175(2–4), 167–178.

Crawford, P.C., Slater, M.R. and Levy, J.K. (2005) Accuracy of PCR assays for the diagnosis of feline immunodeficiency infection in cats. *Journal of the American Veterinary Medical Association* 226(9), 1503–1507.

De Mari, K., Maynard, L., Sanquer, A., Lebreux, B. and Eun, H.M. (2004) Therapeutic effects of recombinant feline interferon omega on feline leukemia virus infected cats and felv / fiv coinfected symptomatic cats. *Journal of Veterinary Internal Medicine* 18, 477–482.

De Oliveira Medeiros, S., Abreu, C.M., Delvecchio, R., Ribeiro, A.P., Vasconcelos, Z., de Moraes Brindeiro, R. et al. (2016) Follow-up on long-term antiretroviral therapy for cats infected with feline immunodeficiency virus. *Journal of Feline Medicine and Surgery* 18(4), 264–272.

Gil, S., Leal, R.O., McGahie, D., Sepúlveda, N., Duarte, A., Niza, M.M. et al. (2014) Oral recombinant feline interferon-omega as an alternative immune modulation therapy in FIV positive cats: clinical and laboratory evaluation. *Research in Veterinary Science* 96(1), 79–85.

Hartmann, K. (2015) Efficacy of antiviral chemotherapy for retrovirus-infected cats: What does the current literature tell us? *Journal of Feline Medicine and Surgery* 17(11), 925–939.

Helfer-Hungerbuehler, A.K., Spiri, A.M., Riond, B., Grest, P,. Boretti, F.S. and Hofmann-Lehmann, R. (2015) No benefit of therapeutic vaccination in clinically healthy cats persistently infected with feline leukemia virus. *Vaccine* 33(13), 1578–1585.

Hosie, M.J., Addie, D., Belák, S., Boucraut-Baralon, C., Egberink, H., Frymus, T. et al. (2009) Feline inmunodeficiecy: ABCD guidelines on prevention and management. *Journal of Feline Medicine and Surgery* 11, 575–584.

Lutz, H., Addie, D., Belák, S., Boucraut-Baralon, C., Egberink, H., Frymus, T. et al. (2009) Feline leukemia: ABCD guidelines on prevention and management. *Journal of Feline Medicine and Surgery* 11, 565–574.

Nesina, S., Katrin Helfer-Hungerbuehler, A., Riond, B., Boretti, F.S., Willi, B., Meli, M.L. et al. (2015) Retroviral DNA – the silent winner: blood transfusion containing latent feline leukemia provirus causes infection and disease in naïve recipient cats. *Retrovirology* 12, 105.

Pedretti, E., Passeri, B., Amadori, M., Isola, P., Di Pede, P., Telera, A. et al. (2006) Low dose interferon alpha treatment for feline immunodeficiency virus infection. *Veterinary Immunology and Immunopathology* 109, 245–254.

Stuetzer, B., Brunner, K., Lutz, H. and Hartmannm K. (2013) A trial with 3'-azido-2',3'-dideoxythymidine and human interferon-$\alpha$ in cats naturally infected with feline leukaemia virus. *Journal of Feline Medicine and Surgery* 15(8), 667–671.

Torres, A.N., Mathiason, C.K. and Hoover, E.A. (2005) Re-examination of feline leukemia virus: host relationships using RT-PCR. *Virology* 332, 272–283.

### *Haemoplasmosis*

Reynolds, C.A. and Lappin, M.R. (2007) *"Candidatus Mycoplasma haemominutum"* infections in 21 client-owned cats. *Journal of the American Animal Hospital Association* 43, 249–257.

Sykes, J.E. (2010) Feline hemotropic mycoplasmas. *Veterinary Clinics of North America Small Animal Practice* 40(6), 1157–1170.

Tasker, S. (2010) Haemotropic mycoplasmas: what's the real significance in cats? *Journal of Feline Medicine and Surgery* 12, 369–381.

Tasker, S., Peters, I.R., Papasouliotis, K., Cue, S.M., Willi, B., Hofmann-Lehmann, R. et al. (2009) Description of outcomes of experimental infection with feline hemoplasmas: copy numbers, haematology, Coombs' testing and blood glucose concentrations. *Veterinary Microbiology* 139, 323–332.

## *Canine infectious diseases*

### *Viral infections in puppies*

#### Canine parvovirus

de Mari, K., Maynard, L., Eun, H.M. and Lebreux, B. (2003) Treatment of canine parvoviral enteritis with interferon omega in a placebo-controlled field trial. *Veterinary Record* 152, 105–108.

Hernández-Blanco, B. and Catala-López, F. (2015) Are licensed canine parvovirus (CPV2 and CPV2b) vaccines able to elicit protection against CPV2c subtype in puppies? A systematic review of controlled clinical trials. *Veterinary Microbiology* 180(1–2), 1–9.

Mohr, A.J., Leisewitz, A.L., Jacobson, L.S., Steiner, J.M., Ruaux, C.G. and Williams, D.A. (2003) Effect of early enteral nutrition on intestinal permeability, intestinal protein loss, and outcome in dogs with severe parvoviral enteritis. *Journal of Veterinary Internal Medicine* 17, 791–798.

Proksch, A.L., Unterer, S., Speck, S., Truyen, U. and Hartmann, K. (2015) Influence of clinical and laboratory variables on faecal antigen ELISA results in dogs with canine parvovirus infection. *Veterinary Journal* 204(3), 304–308.

#### Distemper

Elia, G., Camero, M., Losurdo, M., Lucente, M.S., Larocca, V., Martella, V. et al. (2015) Virological and serological findings in dogs with naturally occurring distemper. *Journal of Virological Methods* 213, 127–130.

Martella, V., Elia, G. and Buonavoglia, C. (2008) Canine distemper virus. *Veterinary Clinics of North America Small Animal Practice* 38(4), 787–797.

Pesavento, P.A. and Murphy, B.G. (2014) Common and emerging infectious diseases in the animal shelter. *Veterinary Pathology* 51(2), 478–491.

Viitanen, S.J., Lappalainen, A. and Rajamäki, M.M. (2005) Co-infections with respiratory viruses in dogs with bacterial pneumonia. *Journal of Veterinary Internal Medicine* 29(2), 544–551.

#### Coronavirus

Godsall, S.A., Clegg, S.R., Stavisky, J.H., Radford, A.D. and Pinchbeck, G. (2010) Epidemiology of canine parvovirus and coronavirus in dogs presented with severe diarrhoea to PDSA PetAid hospitals. *Veterinary Record* 167(6), 196–201.

Priestnall, S.L., Mitchell, J.A., Walker, C.A., Erles, K. and Brownlie, J. (2014) New and emerging pathogens in canine infectious respiratory disease. *Veterinary Pathology* 51(2), 492–504.

Schulz, B.S., Kurz, S., Weber, K., Balzer, H.J. and Hartmann, K. (2014) Detection of respiratory viruses and *Bordetella bronchiseptica* in dogs with acute respiratory tract infections. *Veterinary Journal* 201(3), 365–369.

Zicola, A., Jolly, S., Mathijs, E., Ziant, D., Decaro, N., Mari, V. and Thiry, E. (2012) Fatal outbreaks in dogs associated with pantropic canine coronavirus in France and Belgium. *Journal of Small Animal Practice* 53(5), 297–300.

#### Canine infectious tracheobronchitis

Kawakami, K., Ogawa, H., Maeda, K., Imai, A., Ohashi, E., Matsunaga, S. et al. (2010) Nosocomial outbreak of serious canine infectious tracheobronchitis (kennel cough) caused by canine herpesvirus infection. *Journal of Clinical Microbiology* 48(4), 1176–1181.

Radhakrishnan, A., Drobatz, K.J., Culp, W.T. and King, L.G. (2007) Community-acquired infectious pneumonia in puppies: 65 cases (1993–2002). *Journal of the American Veterinary Medical Association* 230, 1493–1497.

Schulz, B.S., Kurz, S., Weber, K., Balzer, H.J. and Hartmann, K. (2014) Detection of respiratory viruses and *Bordetella bronchiseptica* in dogs with acute respiratory tract infections. *Veterinary Journal* 201(3), 365–369.

Viitanen, S.J., Lappalainen, A. and Rajamäki, M.M. (2015) Co-infections with respiratory viruses in dogs with bacterial pneumonia. *Journal of Veterinary Internal Medicine* 29(2), 544–551.

## Vector-borne diseases

### Leishmaniosis

Maroli, M., Gradoni, L., Oliva, G., Castagnaro, M., Crotti, A., Lubas, G. et al. (2010) Guidelines for prevention of leishmaniasis in dogs. *Journal of the American Veterinary Medical Association* 236(11), 1200–1206.

Paltrinieri, S., Solano-Gallego, L., Fondati, A., Lubas, G., Gradoni, L., Castagnaro, M. et al. (2010) Guidelines for diagnosis and clinical classification of leishmaniasis in dogs. *Journal of the American Veterinary Medical Association* 236(11), 1184–1191.

Solano-Gallego, L., Miró, G., Koutinas, A., Cardoso, L., Pennisi, M.G., Ferrer, L. et al. (2011) LeishVet guidelines for the practical management of canine leishmaniosis. *Parasites & Vectors* 4, 86.

### Ehrlichiosis/anaplasmosis

Sainz, Á., Roura, X., Miró, G., Estrada-Peña, A., Kohn, B., Harrus, S. et al. (2015) Guidelines for veterinary practitioners on canine ehrlichiosis and anaplasmosis in Europe. *Parasites & Vectors* 8, 75.

Villaescusa, A., García-Sancho, M., Rodríguez-Franco, F., Tesouro, M.Á. and Sainz, Á. (2015) Effects of doxycycline on haematology, blood chemistry and peripheral blood lymphocyte subsets of healthy dogs and dogs naturally infected with *Ehrlichia canis*. *Veterinary Journal* 204(3), 263–268.

### Borreliosis or Lyme disease

Cardoso, L., Mendão, C. and Madeira de Carvalho, L. (2012) Prevalence of *Dirofilaria immitis*, *Ehrlichia canis*, *Borrelia burgdorferi* sensu lato, *Anaplasma* spp. and *Leishmania infantum* in apparently healthy and CVBD-suspect dogs in Portugal – a national serological study. *Parasites & Vectors* 5, 62.

Chomel, B. (2015) Lyme disease. *Revue Scientifique et Technique* 34(2), 569–576.

Littman, M.P. (2013) Lyme nephritis. *Journal of Veterinary Emergency and Critical Care (San Antonio)* 23(2), 163–173.

Moroff, S., Woodruff, C., Woodring, T., Sokolchik, I. and Lappin, M.R. (2015) Multiple antigen target approach using the Accuplex4 BioCD system to detect *Borrelia burgdorferi* antibodies in experimentally infected and vaccinated dogs. *Journal of Veterinary Diagnostic Investigation* 27(5), 581–588.

Pantchev, N., Pluta, S., Huisinga, E., Nather, S., Scheufelen, M., Vrhovec, M.G. et al. (2015) Tick-borne diseases (Borreliosis, Anaplasmosis, Babesiosis) in German and Austrian dogs: status quo and review of distribution, transmission, clinical findings, diagnostics and prophylaxis. *Parasitology Research* 114 (Suppl. 1), S19–S54.

Wagner, B., Johnson, J., Garcia-Tapia, D., Honsberger, N., King, V., Strietzel, C. et al. (2015) Comparison of effectiveness of cefovecin, doxycycline, and amoxicillin for the treatment of experimentally induced early Lyme borreliosis in dogs. *BMC Veterinary Research* 11, 163.

### Babesiosis

Ayoob, A.L., Hackner, S.G. and Prittie, J. (2010) Clinical management of canine babesiosis. *Journal of Veterinary Emergency and Critical Care* 20, 77–89.

Camacho-Garcia, A.T. (2006) *Piroplasma* infection in dogs in northern Spain. Veterinary Parasitology 138, 97–102.

Solano-Gallego, L. and Baneth, G. (2011) Babesiosis in dogs and cats – expanding parasitological and clinical spectra. *Veterinary Parasitology* 181, 48–60.

### Leptospirosis

Klaasen, H.L., Van der Veen, M., Sutton, D. and Molkenboer, M.J. (2014) A new tetravalent canine leptospirosis vaccine provides at least 12 months immunity against infection. *Veterinary Immunology and Immunopathology* 158(1–2), 26–29.

Schuller, S., Francey, T., Hartmann, K., Hugonnard, M., Kohn, B., Nally, J.E. et al. (2015) European consensus statement on leptospirosis in dogs and cats. *Journal of Small Animal Practice* 56(3), 159–179.

## Main zoonoses of dogs and cats

Baneth, G., Thamsborg, S.M., Otranto, D., Guillot, J., Blaga, R., Deplazes, P. et al. (2016) Major parasitic zoonoses associated with dogs and cats in Europe. *Journal of Comparative Pathology* 155(Suppl. 1), S54–S74.

European Scientific Council Companion Animal Parasites Guidelines http://www.esccap.org/guidelines/#.VzbX7lTyhdg.

Hartmann, K., Addie, D., Belák, S., Boucraut-Baralon, C., Egberink, H., Frymus, T. et al. (2013) *Toxoplasma gondii* infection in cats: ABCD guidelines on prevention and management. *Journal of Feline Medicine and Surgery* 15(7), 631–637.

Pennisi, M.G., Marsilio, F., Hartmann, K., Lloret, A., Addie, D., Belák, S. et al. (2013) *Bartonella* species infection in cats: ABCD guidelines on prevention and management. *Journal of Feline Medicine and Surgery* 15(7), 563–569.

Wang, A. and Greene, C.E. (2014) Pet-associated Illness. In: Bonagura, R. and Twedt, S. (eds) *Kirk's Current Veterinary Therapy XV*. Elsevier Saunders, St Louis, MO, pp. 1244–1249.

## Vaccines and vaccination programmes

Day, M.J., Horzinek, M.C., Schultz, R.D. and Squires, R.A. (2016) WSAVA Guidelines for the vaccination of dogs and cats. *Journal of Small Animal Practice* 57(1), E1–E45.

Hartmann, K., Day, M.J., Thiry, E., Lloret, A., Frymus, T., Addie, D. et al. (2015) Feline injection-site sarcoma: ABCD guidelines on prevention and management. *Journal of Feline Medicine and Surgery* 17(7), 606–613.

Horzinek, M.C. (2010) Vaccination protocols for companion animals: the veterinarian's perspective. *Journal of Comparative Pathology* 42(Suppl. 1), S129–S132.

Horzinek, M.C. and Thiry, E. (2009) Vaccines and vaccination: the principles and the polemics. *Journal of Feline Medicine and Surgery* 11(7), 530–537.

Hosie, M.J., Addie, D.D., Boucraut-Baralon, C., Egberink, H., Frymus, T., Gruffydd-Jones, T. et al. (2015) Matrix vaccination guidelines: 2015 ABCD recommendations for indoor/outdoor cats, rescue shelter cats and breeding catteries. *Journal of Feline Medicine and Surgery* 17(7), 583–587.

## Tests

### Infectious diseases in cats

1. **Regarding FIP, which of the following statements is correct?**
   A) In a healthy cat, the higher the titre of anti-coronavirus antibodies, the greater the probability of suffering from FIP.
   B) Corticosteroids improve the clinical signs but decrease survival in cats with FIP.
   C) The titre of anti-coronavirus antibodies has some correlation with the load of excreted coronavirus in a transient or permanent infection.
   D) Coronavirus PCR on blood is the confirmatory test for FIP because, if virus is found in blood, it must mean the cat is sick with FIP.
2. **An unvaccinated, 10-month-old cat has fever, sneezing, purulent nasal discharge and conjunctivitis that have developed over 2 days. Of the following statements, which one is correct?**
   A) PCR tests for herpes and calicivirus should be done to determine the exact aetiology and to be able to choose the best treatment.
   B) If the condition is caused by herpes or calicivirus, once overcome, vaccination is not necessary since it will be immunised for a lifetime.
   C) It is probably a viral condition with secondary bacterial infection, and the bacterium that is most likely to be producing the respiratory signs is *Chlamydophila felis*.
   D) One should start treatment with oral doxycycline (in a suspension) and an ophthalmic ointment of tetracyclines combined with an anti-herpetic ophthalmic ointment, and administer the treatment for 7–10 days.
3. **Regarding the rapid diagnosis tests for retroviruses, FeLV and FIV, there is only one correct answer:**
   A) They are tests that detect antibodies, and therefore the results must be confirmed with tests that detect antigens.
   B) A 3-month-old kitten testing positive for FIV may not be infected by the virus.
   C) A 3-month-old kitten testing positive for FeLV is not considered a reliable result and should be confirmed with a PCR.
   D) A cat recently vaccinated for FeLV may give a false positive in the detection of p27 by ELISA.
4. **A clinically healthy, 1-year-old cat has tested positive for a feline leukaemia on ELISA; how is the result interpreted?**
   A) A positive result indicates viraemia; if it is not a false positive, this cat will become ill and die before it is 3 years old.
   B) A positive result may indicate a previous exposure to the virus without actually having an infection at this time, so the test should be repeated in 6 weeks.
   C) The positive result indicates viraemia, but not necessarily that it is a persistent viraemia and a progressive infection, and therefore it would be better to do other tests.
   D) Only if the cat is positive on a provirus PCR can it be ensured that the infection is progressive.
5. **A radiograph of a 1-year-old cat with dyspnoea and fever shows pleural effusion; what is the diagnosis?**
   A) If the serum anti-coronavirus antibody titre is high, the diagnosis is certain to be FIP.
   B) If the total pleural fluid proteins are high and cytology shows a predominance of neutrophils and lymphocytes, the diagnosis of FIP is confirmed.
   C) If the coronavirus PCR on the pleural fluid is negative, it is not FIP.
   D) None of the above is correct.
6. **Regarding vaccines in cats, which of the following statements is correct?**
   A) In a cat that lives indoors 100% of the time, the trivalent vaccine is not necessary; if it is advised, it is for economic criteria and to force owners to take their cats to the practice and examine them.
   B) The immunity gap consists of a period of time in which the values of maternal antibodies are very low and, therefore, the animal is totally unprotected against infections.
   C) The feline panleukopenia vaccine protects against the signs of the disease, but not the infection, unlike what happens in the case of herpes and caliciviruses.
   D) None of the above is correct.

**7. A 14-year-old cat has been diagnosed with diffuse intestinal lymphoma by biopsy.**
A) The majority of such cases involve persistent viraemia due to FeLV.
B) Chemotherapy should not be used as a treatment, given the risk of immunosuppression and reactivation of a latent FeLV infection.
C) Although ELISA and provirus PCR on blood and bone marrow are negative, this lymphoma originated from a previous infection with FeLV virus.
D) None of the above is correct.

**8. Which of the following statements about upper respiratory tract infections is correct?**
A) *Chlamydophila* infections typically cause conjunctivitis, rhinotracheitis and pneumonia in the most severe cases.
B) Cats permanently infected by FHV-1 release the virus constantly and are a source of virus in the environment.
C) FHV-1 (herpesvirus) has an ocular tropism, especially in the uvea and retina.
D) In an affected cat with a deep stromal corneal ulcer, FVH-1 PCR may be negative.

**9. A 6-year-old stray cat picked up from the street and appears to be clinically healthy, with a normal blood count, serum biochemistry and urine tests, but tested positive on FIV ELISA. What conclusion can be drawn from this?**
A) It will die within 3 years.
B) It is advisable to repeat the test in 6–8 weeks to rule out a false positive on the first test.
C) It is essential to do an FIV PCR, since ELISAs are unreliable. This can also detect antibodies, and it could be that the cat was not actually infected.
D) It is a very serious mistake to allow it to live with another cat, since this is a highly contagious infection.

**10. On abdominal ultrasound of a 2-year-old cat with recurrent fever, apathy, weight loss and bilateral uveitis, mesenteric lymphadenopathy is observed. Which of the following is correct?**
A) FIP is highly unlikely since the presence of effusions is not observed.
B) If the anti-coronavirus antibody titre is high positive, a diagnosis of FIP is confirmed.
C) If there is no increase in gamma globulins in the serum proteinogram, it is certain that it is not FIP.
D) Cytology of ultrasound-guided lymph node aspiration with an inflammatory pyogranulomatous pattern indicates that FIP is likely.

**11. Regarding a cat suffering from confirmed feline chronic gingivostomatitis, which of the following is true?**
A) It is not worth performing FCV PCR on an oral swab since 100% of cats are positive. This disease is caused by a chronic FCV infection.
B) If the FCV PCR of an oral swab is positive, complete exodontics is contraindicated.
C) It is a multifactorial disease with a considerable immune-mediated component, as suggested by the histological and cytokine patterns and the clinical response to immunosuppressants.
D) Total exodontics produce good results, with a 40–50% chance of complete cure or significant improvement.

**12. In a 6-month-old cat with pleural and abdominal effusion, a diagnosis of FIP has been confirmed. Which of the following is true?**
A) Corticosteroids are contraindicated as they worsen immunosuppression.
B) A treatment with high-dose feline interferon omega, 106 MUI/kg/24 h SC for 7 days, guarantees higher survival and improvement of clinical signs.
C) There is a high chance it will die within 1 month.
D) Because corticosteroids plus Polyprenil Immunostimulant have shown good survival results in cats with the wet form of FIP, this would be the best treatment.

**13. Regarding the diagnosis of retroviruses (FeLV and FIV), which of the following is true?**
A) Provirus PCR on FeLV DNA positive in blood means that the cat is infected, is viral and is eliminating the virus through saliva.
B) The subclinical or asymptomatic phase of FIV infection can last at least 3 years, following which immunodeficiency syndrome develops.
C) Proviral DNA from FIV DNA is unreliable because the virus does not integrate in the genome of feline cells in the same way that FeLV does.
D) IFA on blood smears can be used to discriminate a transient from a permanent viraemia in cats with FeLV-positive ELISA.

**14. Adult and aged cats with signs of systemic vasculitis, limb oedema, oral ulcers, jaundice and high fever are dying in a colony of street cats that is being monitored. An outbreak of virulent systemic calicivirus is still pending confirmation. Indicate which of the following is correct.**

A) The youngest kittens will soon begin to die in the same way, especially those that are not vaccinated.
B) Ideally, sick cats should be hospitalised so that they can receive intensive treatment.
C) If it is not a systemic calicivirosis, it is most likely an outbreak of feline infectious peritonitis.
D) Great care should be taken, due to the risks of infection by fomites, with your own cats and other patients at the practice. In addition, it is also possible that not many young kittens will become ill and die.

**15. An 8-month-old cat with obstructive upper respiratory signs (rales, noisy breathing) does not respond to antibiotics, nonsteroidal anti-inflammatory drugs or lysine. In recent weeks, famciclovir has been given at 80 mg/kg/8 h because a herpesvirus PCR was positive, but it does not improve with this either. Which of the following options is correct?**

A) It is most likely to be a chronic herpesvirus that will never be cured.
B) Herpesvirus PCR has shown a false-positive result and it is possibly suffering from another disease, for example a nasopharyngeal polyp.
C) The cat probably has a nasopharyngeal polyp; studies have shown that polyps are caused by chronic herpesvirus infection.
D) None of the above is correct.

**16. Which of the following could be the treatment of the future for chronic gingivostomatitis that does not respond to exodontics or the usual medical treatments?**

A) $CO_2$ laser surgery.
B) New, more specific, immunosuppressants.
C) Specific antivirals effective against calicivirus.
D) Stem cells.

### Infectious diseases in dogs, zoonoses and vaccines

**1. Regarding leptospirosis, which of the following statements is correct?**

A) Unvaccinated dogs exposed to *Leptospira* become ill or are not infected; there are no subclinical infections.
B) Infections in which signs of disease are evident are those produced caused the serovars canicola and icterohemorragie.
C) There are environmental and lifestyle factors in the dog that influence a greater or lesser risk of exposure to the bacterium.
D) Cats do not suffer from this infection.

**2. Regarding borreliosis, which of these statements is correct?**

A) The *Borrelia* transmitter vector is the *Dermacentor* tick.
B) Diagnosis is simple, using PCR techniques on blood or urine.
C) A positive result for the detection of C6 antipeptide antibodies confirms a diagnosis of borreliosis.
D) None of the above is correct.

**3. Regarding babesiosis, which of the following statements is correct?**

A) The tick that transmits *Babesia canis* is from the genus *Rhipicephalus*, and *B. gibsoni* is from the genus *Dermacentor*.
B) Babesia infections have significant zoonotic potential.
C) With proper treatment, babesiosis always has a good prognosis.
D) *B. microti*-like infections have been associated with the development of severe kidney disease.

**4. Regarding a clinically healthy dog being tested for leishmaniasis, which of the following statements is true?**

A) If it is seropositive, it should be treated to prevent the disease from progressing further.
B) The test of choice is a quantitative PCR on blood: if it is positive, it has leishmaniasis.
C) The test of choice is a rapid snap test: if it is positive, it must be confirmed with a quantitative PCR on blood.
D) It should be based on the range of antibody titres and the presence or absence of analytical abnormalities (blood count, biochemistry, electrophoresis) frequently found with the disease.

5. **In a sick dog in which leptospirosis is suspected, which of the following statements is true?**
   A) The presence of thrombocytopenia is not typical.
   B) Respiratory distress and a diffuse interstitial pulmonary radiological pattern with alveolar opacities may be seen.
   C) If PCR is requested it is better to perform it on urine, since on blood it does not have good sensitivity.
   D) Quinolones are the most effective antibiotics.
6. **A 5-year-old dog has been referred to the hospital for treatment of acute polyuric kidney disease with suspected leptospirosis. It has been treated for 2 days with ampicillin and fluids and the serology result (MAT) is awaited; 24 hours after admission, signs of tachypnoea and respiratory distress begin. Which of the following options is the most logical?**
   A) Send urine samples for *Leptospira* PCR, in order to interpret the results together with those of MAT.
   B) If a diffuse interstitial pattern with alveolar consolidation is observed on radiography, leptospirosis should be ruled out and other aetiologies considered.
   C) If a diffuse reticulonodular interstitial pattern is observed on radiography, treatment with high-dose glucocorticoids should be started.
   D) Chest radiography is indicated and, if there is no vomiting and oral administration of medications is tolerated, start the administration of doxycycline at 5 mg/kg/12 h.
7. **A dog diagnosed with haemolytic anaemia has a haematocrit of 15% in which *Babesia* (large species) has been detected in erythrocytes on a blood smear. Which of the following statements is true?**
   A) If there is thrombocytopenia, there is certain to be co-infection with another pathogen since babesiosis does not cause a decrease in platelets.
   B) If the dog is cured, following treatment it will be immunised for life.
   C) The risk of severe acute kidney disease is very high.
   D) None of the above is correct.
8. **In which of the following should clinical suspicions of borreliosis be highest?**
   A) A young dog with fever and widespread pain (especially in the carpus, tarsus and neck area) that have developed over 2 months.
   B) A dog with polyarthritis and proteinuria.
   C) A dog with acute lameness of one limb, presenting with pain and inflammation in the knee joint and on which ticks have been seen.
   D) A dog with intermittent lameness and on which ticks of the genus *Dermacentor* have been observed.
9. **In a 4-year-old Belgian Shepherd dog presenting generalised lymphadenopathy and subcutaneous inflammation in one of its carpi, without other clinical signs, which of the following tests should be performed?**
   A) Serology for *Leishmania* and, if positive, start treatment.
   B) Obtain bone marrow by puncturing the costochondral junction. If *Leishmania* is not observed on cytology, leishmaniasis can be ruled out.
   C) Request a *Leishmania* PCR on blood, which is much more reliable than serology since the pathogen is detected.
   D) If there is non-regenerative anaemia, polyclonal gammopathy, proteinuria and the anti-leishmanial antibody titre is highly positive, this is a reliable diagnosis of leishmaniasis, so start treatment.
10. **In a healthy blood donor dog, a positive *Leishmania* PCR has been obtained from blood. What procedure should be followed?**
    A) Ignore it because it is a false positive, since with a positive PCR on blood it should be showing clinical signs.
    B) Perform tests that include a complete blood count, proteinogram, renal function, proteinuria and anti-leishmanial antibody titre. If all results are normal, the PCR was a false positive.
    C) Start treatment immediately.
    D) None of the above is completely correct.
11. **A 4-month-old puppy from a pet shop presents with signs of acute diarrhoea, some vomiting, loss of appetite and fever. Which of the following statements is correct?**
    A) The most likely diagnosis is coronavirus infection.
    B) If there is marked neutropenia on the blood count, the first differential diagnosis should be distemper.
    C) If a parvovirus antigen ELISA test on stools is negative, parvovirus can be ruled out.
    D) Answers A–C are incorrect.

**12. Regarding bartonellosis or cat scratch disease, which of the following statements is correct?**

A) The virus that causes it is transmitted through fleas.
B) It is spread by cat bites and scratches to susceptible people.
C) It can manifest itself in immunocompetent and immunosuppressed people.
D) Answers A–C are incorrect.

**13. Regarding vaccination in dogs and cats, which of the following statements is correct?**

A) In general, inactivated vaccines are much less effective than attenuated.
B) Recombinant vaccines carry adjuvants to provide immunogenicity.
C) Vaccines against feline leukaemia virus are all inactivated.
D) Answers A–C are incorrect.

**14. Primary vaccination consists of a series of repeated doses during the puppy stage; which of the following statements is correct?**

A) This ensures good immunity at a time when the immune system is immature and responds poorly to vaccines.
B) This ensures good immunity at a time when maternal antibody levels could interfere with response to the vaccine.
C) There is no scientific evidence of the usefulness of multiple doses in primary vaccination.
D) None of the above is true.

**15. Regarding distemper virus, which of the following statements is true?**

A) It is a DNA virus with a systemic tropism.
B) It produces acute infections: if in 2 weeks the disease has not progressed, the dog will recover.
C) Occasionally, blood PCR is negative in infected dogs.
D) Answers A–C are all true.

**16. A gynaecologist has advised a pregnant owner to get rid of the cat she has at home (an indoor cat that goes out onto a balcony without access to the outside), because it has shown to be positive for toxoplasmosis by antibody testing. Which of the following should the veterinarian advise?**

A) Although the risk of infection is very low, follow the doctor's advice to cover your back.
B) Perform diagnostic tests on the cat – for example, antibody titres in blood: if the cat is positive, the risk is much higher so you should follow the doctor's instructions.
C) Advise that there is no risk whatsoever because she is already seropositive, and that it is precisely because she has a cat at home and has already been exposed to the parasite.
D) None of the above.

## Clinical case 1

**Signalment**: 8-year-old common European cat, 2.5 kg.
**Reason for consultation**: Referred for corneal ulcers that have not healed and chronic gingivostomatitis (proliferative caudal stomatis). Undergoing treatment with high-dose corticosteroids >1 year; has also been treated with antibiotics, dental hygiene procedures and NSAIDs.
**Clinical history**: The eye disease appeared 1 month ago with bilateral uveitis, fever, weight loss and IgG toxoplasma titre 1/50; was treated with clindamycin 25 mg/kg/12 h plus dexamethasone and chloramphenicol eye drops. Worsening after 1 week, a deep OS ulcer appeared, dexamethasone administration was stopped, topical atropine was added and the case was referred.
**Physical examination**: BCS (body condition score) 2/5, poor-quality hair appearance, apathy, mild dehydration (5%), fever (40°C), moderate hepatomegaly, proliferative gingivostomatitis and severe caudal stomatitis. The remainder of the physical exam was without notable abnormalities.
**Eye examination**: Blepharospasm, mucosal secretion, lack of response to threat and dazzle reflexes, pupillary reflexes not present, normal Schirmer tear test, deep stromal corneal ulcers, diffuse endothelial corneal oedema, Tindal 4+ OU, tonometry 35 mmHg RE and 32 mmHg OS, not possible to evaluate lens and fundus.
**Haematology, blood biochemistry and urinalysis**: Mild mature neutrophilia, monocytosis, hyperglycaemia >350 mg/dl, mild azotaemia, polyclonal gammopathy, fructosamine 600 mg/dl, urine density 1.035, proteinuria 2+, glycosuria 4+, ketonuria 2+.
**Thoracic radiography**: No abnormalities.

**Abdominal ultrasound**: Hepatomegaly, diffuse hyper-echogenicity, remainder of the abdomen normal, liver cytology shows normal hepatocytes and neutrophils.
**Serologies**: Coronavirus antibodies (+) 1/320, cryptococcal antigen latex (–), *Ehrlichia* antibodies (–) 1/20, *Leishmania* antibodies (+ maximum) 300%, *Toxoplasma* IgG (+ low) 1/50.

1. **Based on this information, what is the most likely cause of the eye disease in this cat?**
   A) Herpesvirus.
   B) Toxoplasmosis.
   C) Leishmaniosis and FIP.
   D) Leishmaniosis.
2. **What is the most likely cause of the diabetes mellitus?**
   A) It is not diabetes, it is a stress hyperglycaemia.
   B) An immune-mediated type I diabetes.
   C) A secondary diabetes associated with corticosteroid depot treatment.
   D) None of the above.
3. **What should be the initial approach to the management of diabetes mellitus?**
   A) Intermediate-acting insulin and fibre-rich diet.
   B) Oral hypoglycaemic agents such as glipizide.
   C) Glargine-type long-acting insulin every 24 h and a low-carbohydrate diet.
   D) Glargine-type long-acting insulin every 12 h and a low-carbohydrate diet.
4. **How could the diagnosis of eye disease be confirmed?**
   A) Cytology and/or PCR for *Leishmania* on bone marrow.
   B) In the event that one of the eyes has to be enucleated, performing a histological study and immunohistochemical tests for *Leishmania* and coronavirus.
   C) By coronavirus and *Leishmania* PCR on blood.
   D) Both A and B are correct.
5. **If the final diagnosis of the eye disease is leishmaniosis, what would be the most appropriate treatment?**
   A) Euthanasia, because leishmaniasis in cats has a very poor prognosis.
   B) High-dose glucantime (100 mg/kg/day) and allopurinol (10 mg/kg/12 h).
   C) Stop cortisone treatment and start allopurinol at 10 mg/kg/12 h, treat diabetes correctly and note progression in a few weeks.
   D) It is impossible because cats do not suffer from leishmaniosis.
6. **What is the most appropriate treatment for chronic gingivostomatitis in this cat?**
   A) Swap cortisone for cyclosporine and interferon omega at low doses.
   B) Stop cortisone treatment and consider complete exodontics when the signs of leishmaniosis and diabetes have improved.
   C) It is impossible to manage chronic gingivostomatitis without high doses of cortisone.
   D) This cat must be euthanised because she has no chance of improving.

## Clinical case 2

**Signalment**: 9-year-old, uncastrated male Schnauzer dog.
**Reason for consultation**: Referral from another veterinarian for weakness and apathy, which has been developing over 1 month.
**History and clinical history**: Vaccines and de-worming up to date, urban life and goes outside when on holiday; no history of fleas or ticks. The dog was taken to its usual veterinarian, who performed tests: non-regenerative anaemia, 21% haematocrit, 2,990,000/mcl RBC, haemoglobin 8.7 g/dl, reticulocytes 42,159/mcl, neutrophilic leucocytosis 20,200/mcl, thrombocytopaenia 58/mcl, anisocytosis, 7% erythroblasts, hypo-albuminaemia 0.8 g/dl, hyperglobulinaemia 5 g/dl, *Leishmania* snap test (–), hepatosplenomegaly, suspected possible haematopoietic neoplasia.
**Physical examination**: BC 2/5, 13 kg, 38.7°C, mild depression, outpatient, HR 120 ppm, RR 32 rpm, cardiopulmonary auscultation without abnormalities, hepatosplenomegaly, absence of pain, SAP 140 mmHg.

**Tests include**: Blood count, serum biochemistry, proteinogram and urinalysis. Results similar to the referring veterinarian's blood count, blood parasites are not observed on the smear, mild elevation of liver enzymes, severe hypoalbuminaemia, polyclonal gammopathy, urine density 1,020, inactive sediment, UPC ratio 7.60, other values normal (including creatinine).
**Snap 4Dx test**: *Ehrlichia* (+); *Anaplasma*, *Borrelia* and *Filaria* (–).
**Abdominal ultrasound**: Hepatomegaly with homogeneous parenchyma and moderate splenomegaly, abnormalities compatible with inflammation, extramedullary haematopoiesis or infiltrative neoplasia in spleen and liver cytology, absence of neoplastic cells compatible with extramedullary haematopoiesis.
**Serologies**: In commercial laboratory, IFI *Ehrlichia* (+) 1/640, ELISA *Leishmania* (+ low) 20%.

1. **Based on the clinical signs and results obtained, indicate which of the following is the most likely diagnosis.**
   A) Autoimmune disease in a non-diseased *Ehrlichia*-seropositive dog.
   B) Acute ehrlichiosis with renal involvement.
   C) Chronic ehrlichiosis with secondary glomerulopathy.
   D) More tests are needed to reach a diagnosis.
2. **What treatment would be most appropriate based on the information available?**
   A) Enrofloxacin, high-protein diet, enalapril and aspirin at low doses.
   B) Enrofloxacin, restricted-protein diet (renal), enalapril and aspirin at low doses.
   C) Doxycycline, high protein diet, enalapril and low-dose aspirin.
   D) Doxycycline, protein-restricted diet (renal), enalapril and aspirin at low doses.
3. **How would you classify this patient's kidney disease if the kidney damage had been established >2 months?**
   A) Borderline normotensive proteinuric IRIS I chronic kidney disease.
   B) Normotensive proteinuric IRIS II chronic kidney disease.
   C) Normotensive proteinuric IRIS I chronic kidney disease.
   D) If there is no azotaemia, it cannot be diagnosed as chronic kidney disease.
4. **After 4 weeks of treatment there has been a significant improvement in clinical status, weight and blood count; cytopenias have been corrected but gammopathy persists and the UPC ratio is 3.4 with albumin levels 1.90 g/dl. Which of the following should be recommended?**
   A) Continue with the same treatment.
   B) Continue the same treatment except for enalapril, which is increased every 12 h (0.5 mg/kg) instead of every 24 h as it was at the start.
   C) Same as B and but stop giving aspirin.
   D) Same as B and but stop giving aspirin and the renal diet.
5. **At 6 months the general condition is good, albumin is 2.24 g/dl, and the UPC ratio is 1.4, the Ehrlichia IFI is positive at 1/640, the animal has been receiving doxycycline for 2 months and continues with renal treatment. Which of the following statements is correct?**
   A) The high titre indicates that the infection is persisting.
   B) An *Ehrlichia* PCR could be done on blood or on a spleen or bone marrow aspiration to check whether pathogens are detected.
   C) The high titre indicates that the problem was not ehrlichiosis, otherwise it would have diminished as the patient improved.
   D) None of the above.
6. **Indicate which option is correct regarding chronic ehrlichiosis.**
   A) The diagnosis is based on high antibody titres in dogs with pancytopenia and polyclonal – and even monoclonal – gammopathy in some cases, and rules out the presence of other concurrent infections.
   B) Ideally the diagnosis should be confirmed with the observation of morulae in monocytes and/or positive PCR on blood or bone marrow.
   C) Antibodies may remain persistently high.
   D) All of the above are correct.

## Correct answers

### Test

Infectious diseases in cats

| | | |
|---|---|---|
| 1. C | 7. D | 13. D |
| 2. D | 8. D | 14. D |
| 3. B | 9. B | 15. D |
| 4. C | 10. D | 16. D |
| 5. D | 11. C | |
| 6. D | 12. C | |

Infectious diseases in dogs, zoonoses and vaccines

| | | |
|---|---|---|
| 1. C | 7. D | 13. D |
| 2. D | 8. C | 14. B |
| 3. D | 9. D | 15. C |
| 4. D | 10. D | 16. D |
| 5. B | 11. D | |
| 6. D | 12. D | |

### Clinical case 1

1. D
2. C
3. D
4. D
5. C
6. B

### Clinical case 2

1. C
2. D
3. C
4. B
5. B
6. D

# 8

# Ophthalmology

Alejandro Bayón

## Chapter summary

## Introduction

Do you observe the patient from the moment they enter the consult room? Simply watching how an animal interacts with an unfamiliar environment gives the clinician precious clues as to that animal's ability to see.

Unfortunately, in many cases, by the time blindness has occurred there is little hope of recovering vision. Treating the patient becomes a matter of controlling pain and looking for the underlying problems that could have caused their sight loss. This serves to emphasize how important a thorough ocular examination is because a condition caught early has a much better chance of successful resolution or control.

This chapter takes an overview of all the skills and procedures necessary for a clinician to feel confident about conducting a meaningful eye examination. In addition, it reviews systemic conditions that have an ocular manifestation, so that the clinician does not get 'tunnel vision' when they encounter a patient with eye problems.

### Key learning points

- How to perform an eye examination and test ocular reflexes.
- Gain an understanding of the pathological conditions that can affect each part of the eye.
- Appreciate systemic conditions that have ophthalmological sequelae.

## Ophthalmological examination

The assessment of a patient with ophthalmic concerns is based on a **detailed clinical history**, a thorough examination of both **ocular and periocular structures**, plus **specific diagnostic tests** as suggested by the former.

### *Evaluation of sight*

From the moment the animal enters the consult room, **observe how it** interacts with this unfamiliar environment. Their behaviour while taking a clinical history can also be illuminating.

For example:

- Do they collide with objects?
- Do they have a fixed gaze?
- Do they refuse to move?

The **animal's vision** is tested first in **normal light** and then in **low light**.

Vision is assessed by response to:

- hand movements
- bright lights
- throwing balls of cotton wool in the animal's field of vision.

Other tests used to assess vision are:

- threat or menace test
- maze test
- following a laser beam.

The threat or **menace response is more useful in dogs** than cats, with the latter often showing little response. Care must be taken when performing the menace test not to move air or touch a whisker, which may make it appear the animal can see.

### *Clinical history*

A **complete and detailed clinical history** is an important part of the diagnostic process.

Questions to ask include the following:

- How is the animal housed and what is their **diet**?
- Have they suffered from any other eye conditions in the past?
- When did the problem first occur?
- Do they have problems seeing during the **day or night**?
- Do they **stumble**?
- Is there an ocular discharge, and if so, what does it look like?
- Have the eye(s) **changed colour**?
- Have there been **behavioural changes**?

- Has the animal suffered from any **systemic conditions**?
- Is there any **family history** of disease?

## Basic eye exam

It is advisable to follow an **orderly sequence** when performing an eye examination since certain tests may interfere with others, for example:

- Perform a **Schirmer's test and collect samples for culture first** before applying drops or manipulating the eye.
- **Measure** (indentation or applanation tonometry) intraocular pressure; this requires topical anaesthesia and must be performed before the patient is handled excessively.
- **Mydriatics** to facilitate the examination of the lens, vitreous chamber and retina should only be used once intraocular pressure has been measured.

### Schirmer's test

The **Schirmer's test is a semi-quantitative** method for measuring the aqueous fraction of tear fluid.

This test is performed with individually packaged **sterile strips of absorbent paper**, with a cut-out notch at 5 mm from the end. Fold the strip at the level of the notch and insert at the bottom of the **lower conjunctival sac for one minute** (Figure 8.1). Normally, the animal closes the eyelids during the test. The measurement should be taken from the notch to the end of the moistened part immediately after removing the strip.

The **result is not linear**; therefore, obtaining a value in 30 seconds does not imply that it will be doubled in one minute.

There are two types of Schirmer's test.

- **Test 1** is used to measure basal and reflex tear production (most common).
- In **Test 2**, corneal sensitivity is eliminated with topical anaesthesia.

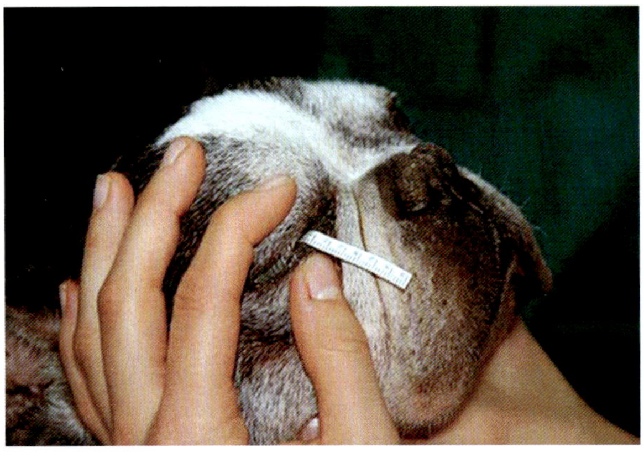

Figure 8.1. Performing the Schirmer's test.

**Normal values** from the Schirmer's test are:

- dogs: 21.9 ± 14 mm/minute
- cats: 20 ± 4.5 mm/minute.

### Photomotor reflexes

First assess the **size, shape and symmetry of the pupils** in a resting state (backlighting technique) (Figure 8.2). **Pupillary reactivity is examined in low light with a bright light source.**

The reflex by which the pupil contracts in response to light arriving at the retina is called the **pupillary light reflex (PLR)**. In most mammals, **pupillary miosis of the illuminated eye (direct) is slightly higher** than that of the non-illuminated contralateral eye (indirect or consensual) because only 30% decussation occurs in the optic chiasma. Assess both the direct (in the examined eye) and indirect (the response of the other eye) PLR.

Remember that the **PLR is a subcortical reflex** that requires relatively little retinal function. Therefore, **a positive direct reflex is not an indicator of vision.**

Pupillary reflexes are affected by:

- the animal's mental state
- ambient lighting
- the animal's age
- the administration of topical and/or systemic drugs
- stimulus intensity.

### Cultures and cytology

**Obtain culture samples before administering eye drops** since many contain bacteriostatic agents. This is done with sterile wet swabs, taking special care not to touch the skin and hair. The goal is to **perform antibiograms.**

For **cytology, first apply a topical anaesthetic, then scrape the conjunctiva vigorously** but without causing bleeding using a Kimura spatula, the back of

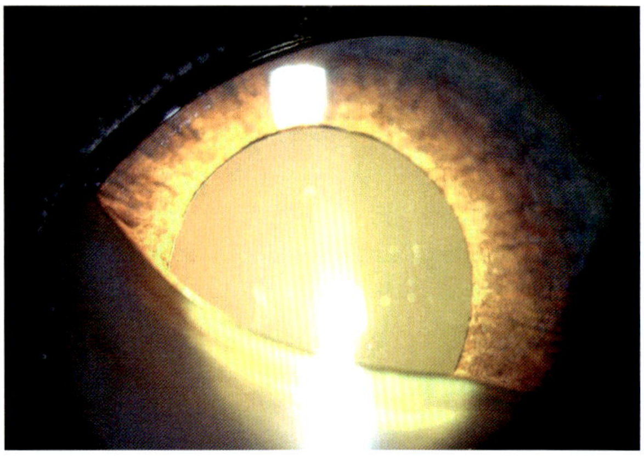

Figure 8.2. Backlighting technique to assess pupil size and shape.

a scalpel blade or brushes. Place the samples on slides, which are then stained using different stains as appropriate (Gram, Giemsa, Diff-Quik, etc.).

### *Tonometry*

**Tonometry measures intraocular pressure (IOP).** It is used to diagnose uveitis and glaucoma, and to measure the response to treatment.

**Normal values are 10–20 mmHg**, with variations due to:

- the individual
- the technique used
- the time of day when the measurement is taken.

Patient collaboration is an important factor. Care should be taken to **minimize the pressure applied around the neck or orbital area** and when separating the eyelids.

#### IOP measurement methods

The Schiötz tonometer (Figure 8.3) consists of three parts: the piston; the mounting platform; and the handle. It also has **different weights (5.5 g, 7.5 g, 10.0 g and 15.0 g)**. The greater the weight applied to the eye, the greater the indentation. Apply a single drop of **topical anaesthetic** onto the ocular surface before placing the tonometer. Hold the patient to position the vertical ocular surface and carefully open the eyelids. The figure obtained is interpreted in the tables corresponding to the weight used. **Normal values are 20–30 ± 5 mmHg.**

Applanation tonometry is based on the principle that **the force required to flatten a given area of a sphere is equal to the pressure inside the sphere**. Apply anaesthetic eye drops before tonometry. The eyelids are carefully opened; then, perform multiple delicate touches parallel to the cornea. Accuracy is determined by the instrument and must always be around 5%. Normal values are 16–18 ± 5 mmHg.

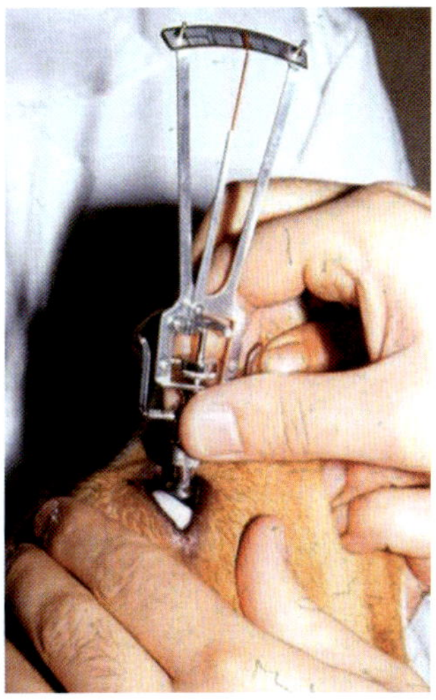

Figure 8.3. Indentation tonometry using the Schiötz tonometer.

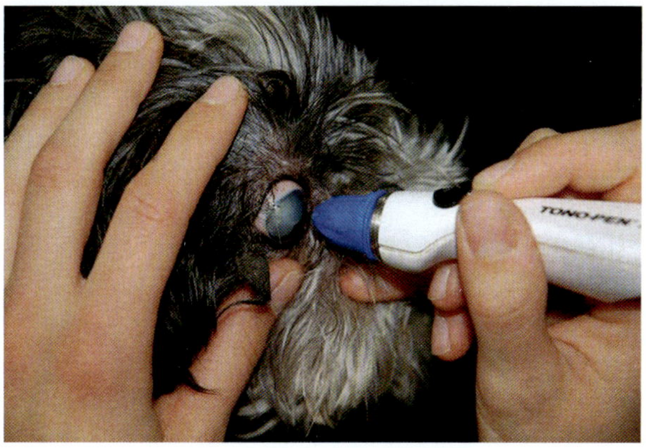


Figure 8.4. Applanation tonometry using a Tono-Pen®.

Advantages of the Tono-Pen® (Figure 8.4) to carry out applanation tonometry include the following.

- It is not necessary to keep the patient's head upright.
- It can be applied on irregular corneas due to the small probe size.
- It shows the pressure directly in mmHg.

The Tonovet® (Figure 8.5) works by launching a small probe with the rounded end at a fixed distance from the cornea and assessing the movement of the tonometer head as it contacts the cornea and returns (rebounds) towards the instrument. This method is affected by the tension on the ocular surface, so it must be performed before administering any eye drops. **Normal values are 1–2 mmHg lower than with the Tono-Pen®.**

## *Ophthalmic examination*

### *Orbit and annexes*

With regard to the orbit, pay attention to the following:

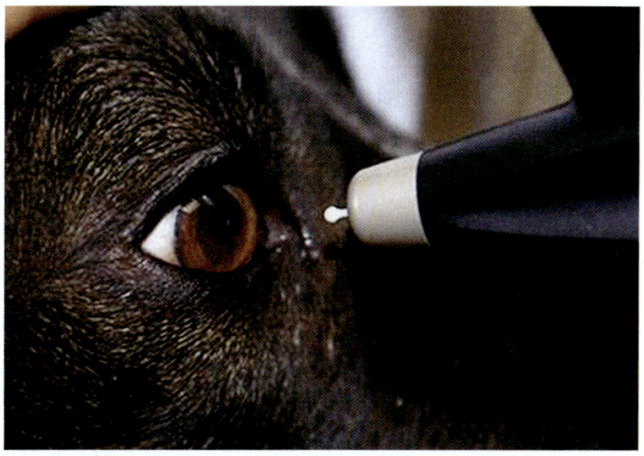

Figure 8.5. Rebound tonometry, using the Tonovet®.

- **symmetry**, comparing one eye with the other
- the relationship between **the eye and the orbit**
- whether there are **deformities or changes in size**
- the presence or absence of **strabismus and nystagmus**
- the position of the eyelid (Figure 8.6), to assess the **relative size of the eyeball**.

Likewise, the following should also be assessed:

- **Examine the mouth and palate** around the area of the orbital floor (after the last molar) (Figure 8.7).
- **Palpate the orbital margin**.
- Perform **retropulsion of the eyeball** (Figure 8.8).

## Eyelids

**Magnification and good illumination** are important when examining the eyelids to detect conditions such as **distichiasis and ectopic cilia**, which can otherwise go unnoticed.

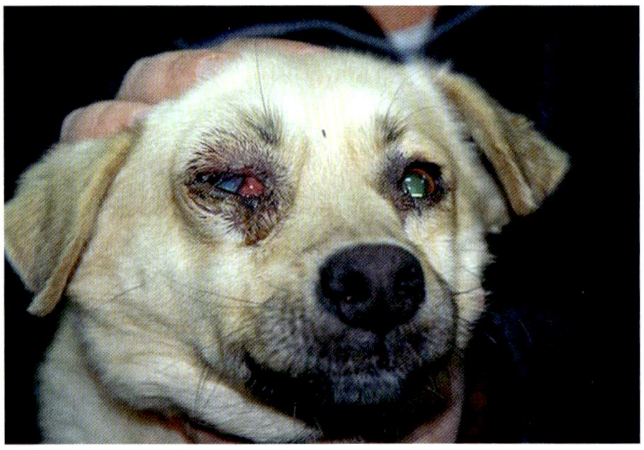

**Figure 8.6.** Examination of the orbit. Proptosis and signs of pain in the right eye (blepharospasm, epiphora and protrusion of the nictitating membrane (third eyelid)).

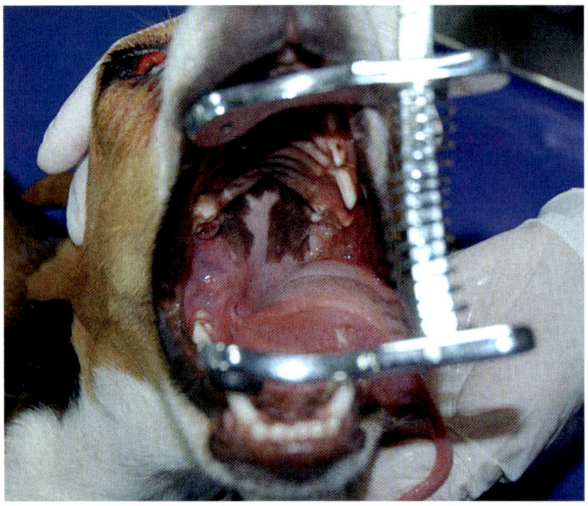

**Figure 8.7.** Examination of the orbit. Presence of a lumpy area behind the last molar on the right-hand side in a dog diagnosed with an orbital abscess.

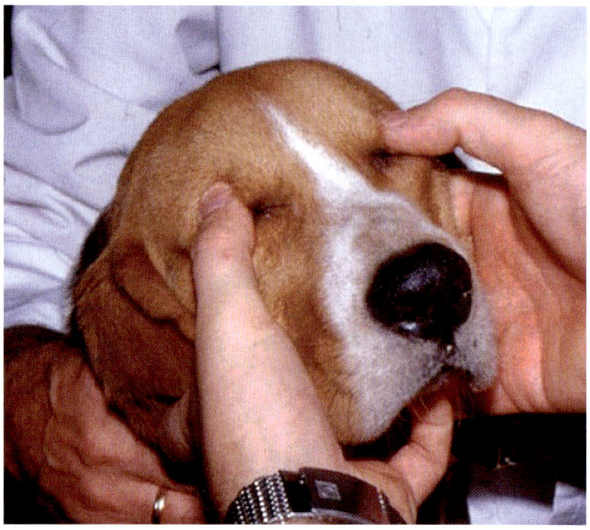

**Figure 8.8.** Examination of the orbit. Retropulsion of the eyeball.

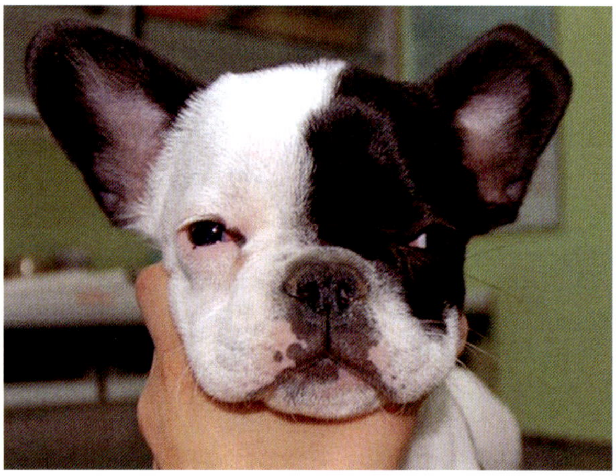

**Figure 8.9.** Examination of the eyelids. Position, function and structure.

- The tarsal borders are regular and slightly arched, allowing for easy visualization of the opening of the Meibomian glands.
- In **dogs, eyelashes or cilia** in the upper eyelid are in three irregular rows. **Cats do not have cilia**.

Assess **abnormalities in position, function and structure of the eyelids** (Figure 8.9), checking they are in contact with the ocular surface. Also observe the integrity and speed of blinking.

## Conjunctiva

Evert the eyelids to examine the eyelid conjunctiva and observe the following:

- colour and vascularization
- if there is an excess of lymphoid follicles
- the presence of lacerations, masses, abnormal growths, haemorrhage or oedema.

Also assess the **palpebral and bulbar conjunctiva of the nictitating membrane** and conjunctival sac since they can be affected by different conditions (for example, presence of foreign bodies or follicular conjunctivitis).

### *Nictitating membrane (third eyelid)*

Evaluate the nictitating membrane with respect to:

- the **conformation of the free edge** (related to the horizontal and vertical branches of its cartilage)
- the **gland located at its base**, which can suffer from prolapses, causing the so-called 'cherry eye'.

### *Sclera*

The objective of examining the sclera is to detect changes in colour, abnormal masses and lacerations.

Regarding vascularization, it is important to remember that:

- The perilimbal scleral vessels are straight, small and immobile.
- The conjunctival vessels are branched, large and mobile.

These vascularization characteristics can be used to:

- **Differentiate conjunctivitis from iridocyclitis** by using **phenylephrine eye drops**: the former results in blanching of the vascularization.
- **Identify glaucoma**, which causes enlargement and congestion of the episcleral veins; this persists even after glaucoma has been controlled.

### *Cornea*

**The cornea is smooth, transparent**, bright, avascular and non-pigmented. Examine the cornea carefully to assess loss of transparency, opacities, vascularization, pigmentation, dryness, growths, foreign bodies, lacerations, contour changes and ulcers.

As a result of different conditions in the cornea, two types of vascularization can appear:

- **Superficial**. This is formed from the vessels present in the first third of the stroma. It is continuous and arborized and is associated with superficial conditions (Figure 8.10).
- **Deep**. This consists of small, deep vessels that travel little distance in the cornea and form a kind of brush in the limber area. It is associated with intraocular inflammation (Figure 8.11).

To complete the corneal examination, vital **topical stains** should be used. (It is important to perform an intensive wash with Ringer Lactate solution after application.)

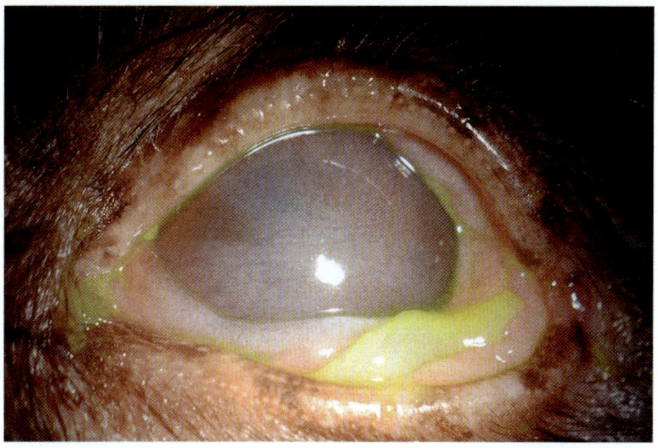

**Figure 8.10.** Superficial corneal vascularization. Note the presence of long, branching vessels.

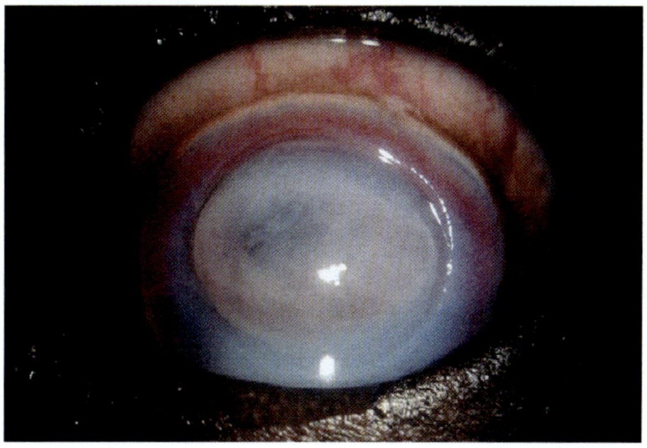

**Figure 8.11.** Deep corneal vascularization. Note the presence of short vessels in the limbal area.

- **Fluorescein**. Available as paper strips and eye drops. When there is an epithelial lesion in the cornea, fluorescein is retained in the stroma. This test is also useful to assess the patency of the nasolacrimal duct (Jones test).
- **Rose Bengal**. Available as paper strips. It can be used to evaluate the integrity of the corneal and conjunctival epithelium. It produces an intense red in the case of cell death and degeneration, indicating mucin defects in the tear film. It is used in the diagnosis of keratoconjunctivitis sicca (KCS) and keratitis of different origins. This test causes corneal pain due to irritation of the nerve endings.

### *Anterior chamber*

Assess **the transparency and depth** of the anterior chamber.

An **increase in protein and cellularity causes the Tyndall effect**, which can be seen with intense light and magnification (Figure 8.12). The Tyndall effect gives the impression of particles moving through the light beam or hazy smoke in the anterior chamber.

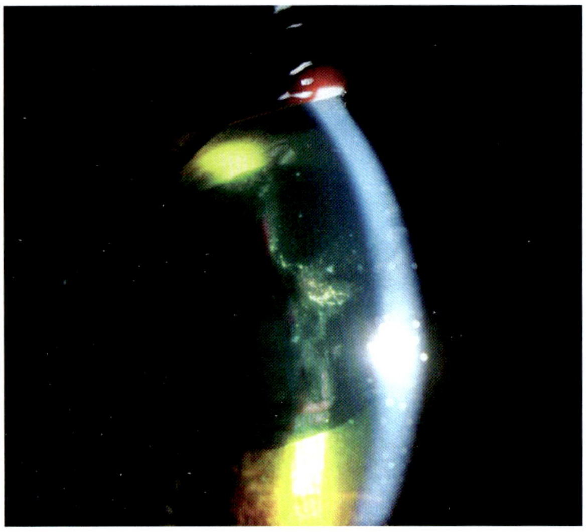

**Figure 8.12.** Image showing the Tyndall effect in the anterior chamber.

### *Iris*

Assess the following:

- iris **colour**, in three distinct areas:
  - the pupillary margin
  - the collarette
  - the base.
- **pupillary shape and size**
- the **surface** of the iris
- **movement**.

On examination, adhesions may be observed between the iris and anterior lens capsule or the corneal endothelium (Figure 8.13). They may be congenital or secondary to conditions causing intraocular inflammation.

### *Lens*

The **lens is a transparent, avascular structure**. Before assessing the lens and posterior structures, the **pupil**

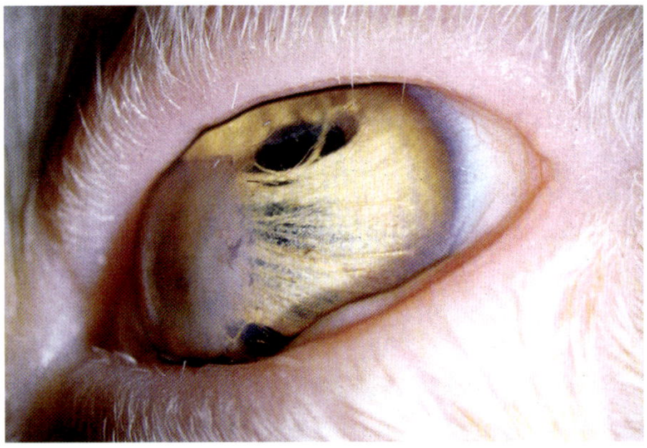

**Figure 8.13.** Persistent membranous pupils in a cat. Note the adhesions of the iris with the corneal endothelium.

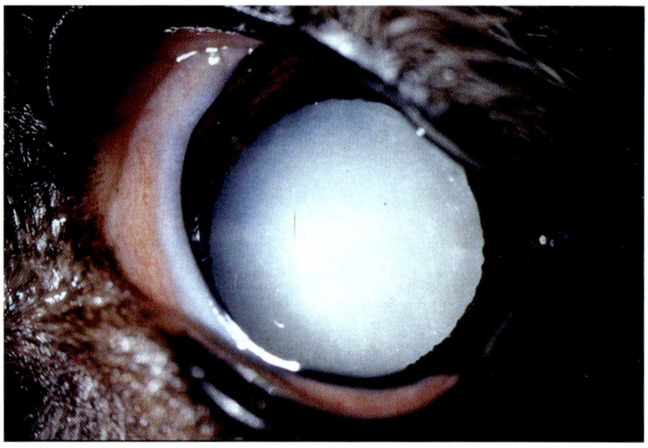

**Figure 8.14.** Presence of mature opacity of the lens after dilation with tropicamide.

**must be dilated by applying 1% topical** tropicamide (1 drop every 10 minutes for 20 minutes).

The purpose of the examination is to rule out:

- **opacities** (Figure 8.14). Assess opacities via a spotlight or slit-lamp biomicroscopy looking for Purkinje images. (The latter are reflections of light from the internal structures of the eye.) Do not confuse sclerosis of the lens with cataracts: sclerosis does not impede vision or ophthalmoscopic visualization of the fundus, whereas cataracts do.
- lens **displacement**.
- alterations in size.

### *Vitreous humour*

The vitreous humour is a **clear gel** located between the posterior capsule of the lens and the retina.

Vitreous examination consists of:

- anterior vitreous humour: focal illumination and magnification
- posterior vitreous humour: ophthalmoscopy or biomicroscopy associated with the lens.

Vitreous anomalies that can be observed are:

- vitreous meshes
- asteroid hyalosis
- synchysis scintillans
- vascularization (hyaloid vessel remnants)
- haemorrhage
- inflammatory cell infiltrates (vitreous Tyndall).

### *Fundus of the eye*

Examination of the fundus requires the following.

#### Direct ophthalmoscopy

A direct ophthalmoscope **examines the eye directly** (Figure 8.15), without the interposition of a condensing

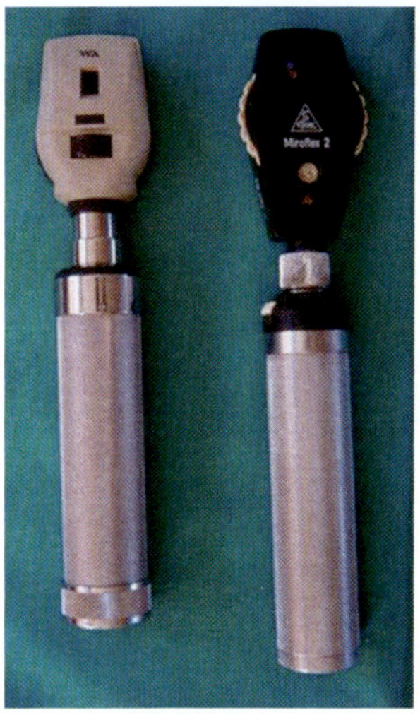

**Figure 8.15.** Direct ophthalmoscopes.

lens between the instrument and the patient. The area visualized is approximately two discs in diameter. **The image is direct, real and upright, and is magnified 17–19 times**.

At the beginning of the examination, the **ophthalmoscope (dioptre) numbering should be placed at 0** and then moved to positive (black) and negative (red) numbers. The **optimal retinal focus is usually around +3**, with +8 and +12 to assess the lens and set at **+20 to assess the cornea**.

## Indirect ophthalmoscopy

Indirect ophthalmoscopy complements direct ophthalmoscopy (Figure 8.16). The technique involves directing a very bright light source along a 0-degree axis with the visual axis, with the interposition of a condensing lens (+20 D). The **image formed is inverted**.

The advantages over direct ophthalmoscopy are the **perception of depth**, greater visual field, greater ease of visualization of the **peripheral fundus**, ease

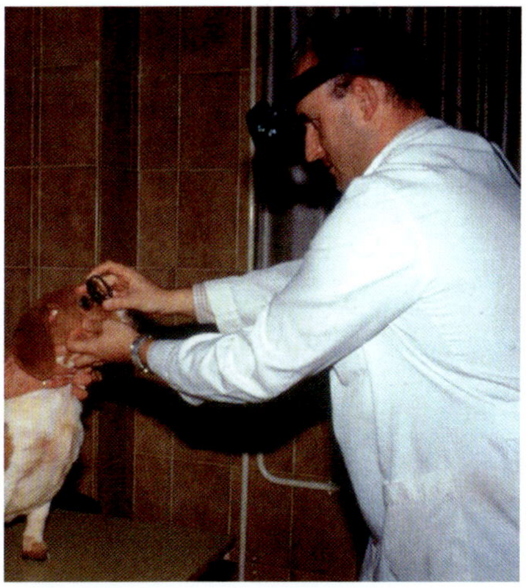

**Figure 8.16.** Indirect ophthalmoscope used with a +20 D condensing lens.

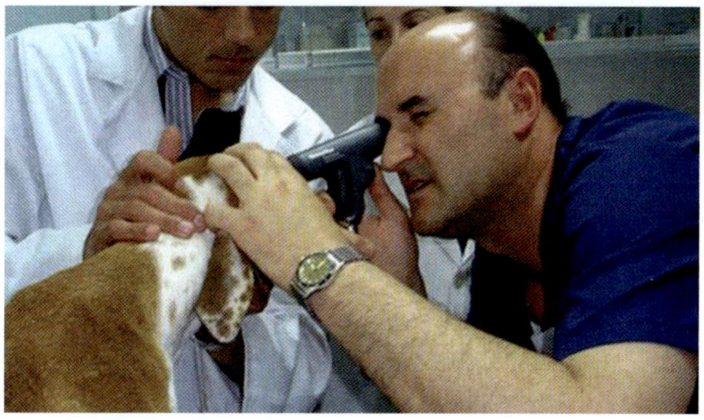

**Figure 8.17.** Ophthalmoscopy using a PanOptic® ophthalmoscope.

of compensation for refractory errors and eye movements, **stereopsis** and greater distance between the observer and the patient. The **disadvantage is lower magnification** of specific areas.

A PanOptic® ophthalmoscope can be used to become familiar with examination of the fundus (Figure 8.17).

When visualizing the fundus, always consider **species and breed specific variations** (Figures 8.18–8.21). The following should be examined:

- the **tapetal area** (shiny)
- the **non-tapetal area**
- retinal **vascularization**
- the **optic nerve**.

The objective of examining the fundus is to identify:

- changes in appearance
- retinal detachments
- hypoplasia or chorioretinal dysplasia
- thinning
- congestion
- haemorrhage
- coloboma

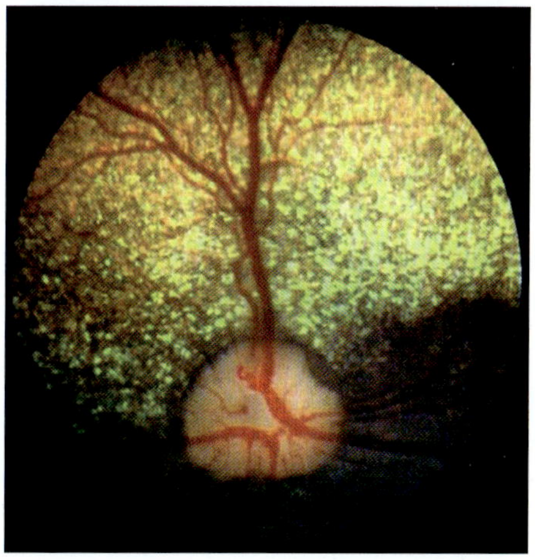

**Figure 8.18.** Fundus of a normal eye in a dog.

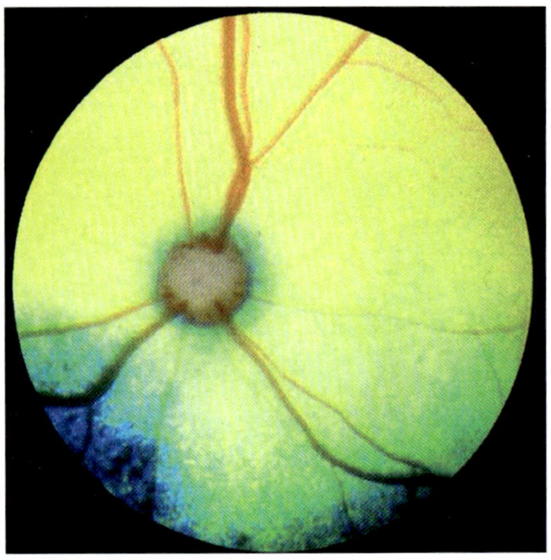

**Figure 8.19.** Fundus of a normal eye in a cat.

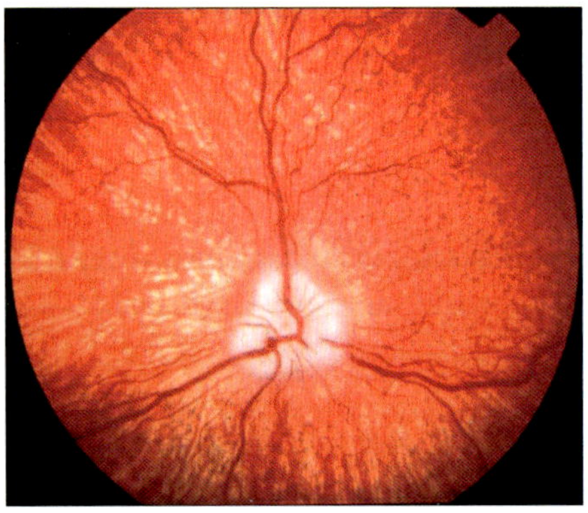

**Figure 8.20.** Fundus of a normal albino eye in a dog.

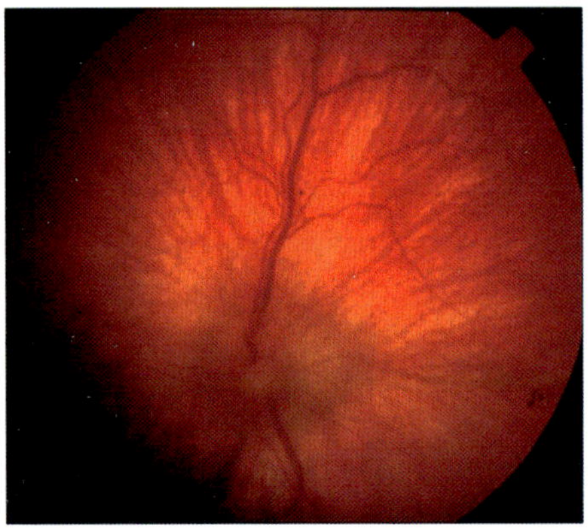

**Figure 8.21.** Fundus of a normal albino eye in a cat.

- scars
- pigmentation changes
- foci of inflammation
- specific abnormalities of the optic nerve (size, shape and colour) plus masses, excavations and colobomas should be examined.

## *Special diagnostic procedures*

It is important to be aware of various special diagnostic procedures so that in specific cases, where appropriate, referral can be advised.

### *Gonioscopy*

Gonioscopy facilitates assessment of the iridocorneal angle and drainage of the aqueous humour.

A special **goniolens is placed directly onto the cornea**, so there is no air between the lens and cornea. With a **refractive index close to that of the cornea** and with internal reflection eliminated, the **drainage angle can be observed directly**. The goniolens can also be combined with magnification instruments, such as the biomicroscope.

#### Types of goniolenses

- **Direct**, for example, the Koeppe goniolens (Figure 8.22)
- **Indirect**, for example, the Goldmann goniolens.

In compliant patients, the application of anaesthetic eye drops is often enough to facilitate examination, but in other cases sedation may be necessary.

Gonioscopy is mainly used to assess the following:

- if the angle is **open, narrow or closed**
- if the angle is **obstructed** by mesodermal remains
- if there are **foreign bodies, tumours or inflammatory exudates**.

### *Ultrasound*

Ultrasound is useful to:

- **Visualize posterior structures** where opacity prevents direct observation.
- Evaluate **orbital structures**.
- **Guide** fine needle aspiration.

Currently, many general ultrasound machines can be used for ophthalmology. The technique consists of administering **topical anaesthetic eye drops** and placing the transducer gel and probe directly on the corneal surface or over the eyelids (Figure 8.23).

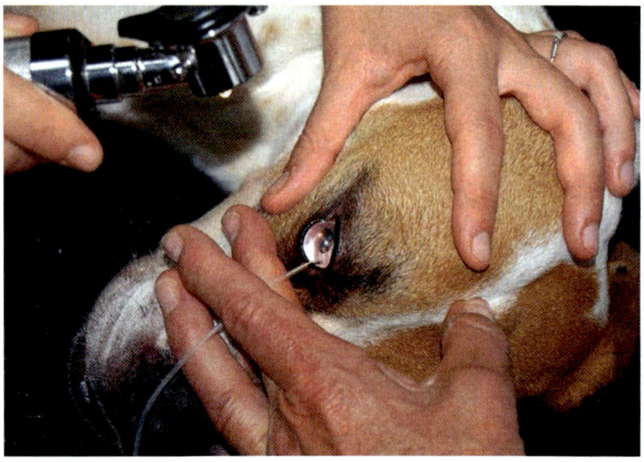

**Figure 8.22.** Gonioscopy using a Koeppe goniolens.

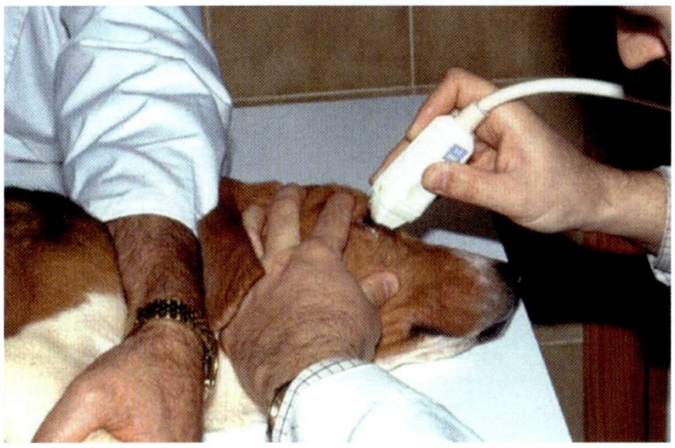

**Figure 8.23.** Ocular ultrasound.

### *Slit-lamp biomicroscopy*

**Slit-lamp biomicroscopy** is commercially available in portable and stationary devices (Figure 8.24). Its big advantage is the integration of the light source and magnification into the same equipment. In addition, the light beam can be shifted to the sides, allowing optical cross sections of the eye and identification of the sites of lesions.

### *Others*

- electroretinography (Figure 8.25)
- fluorescein angiography
- computed tomography (CT) (Figure 8.26)
- magnetic resonance imaging (MRI)
- optical coherence tomography (OCT) (Figure 8.27).

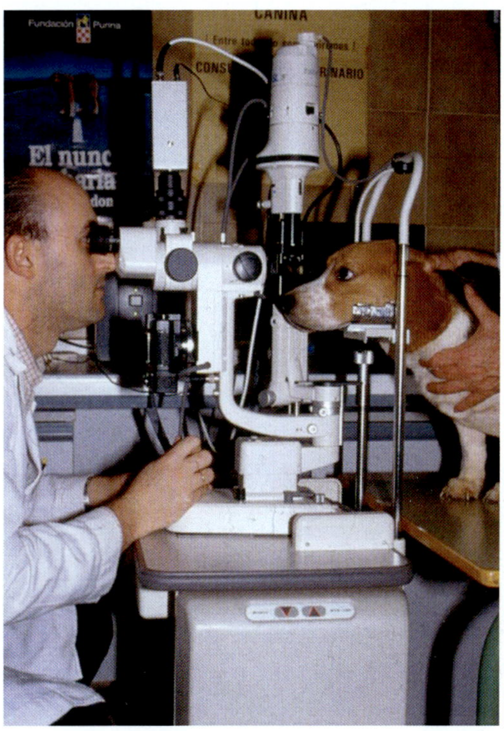

**Figure 8.24.** Slit-lamp biomicroscopy examination.

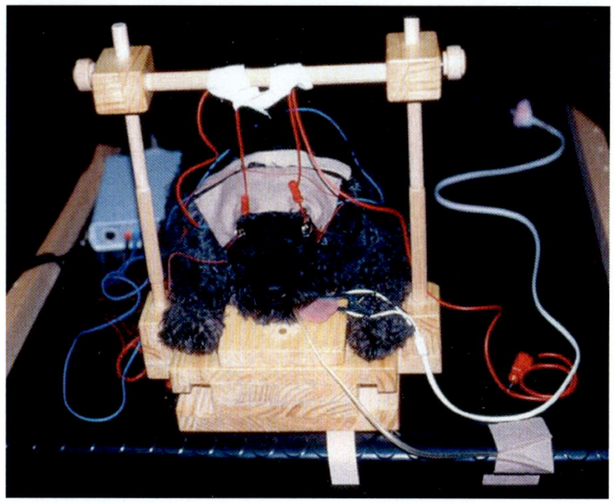

**Figure 8.25.** Electroretinography in a dog.

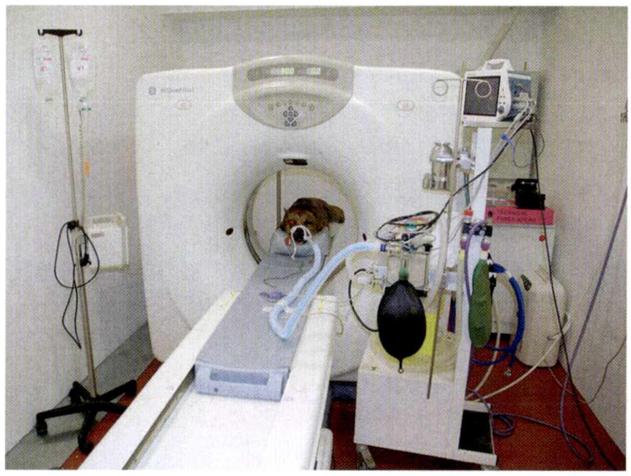

**Figure 8.26.** CT in a dog with an orbital pathology.

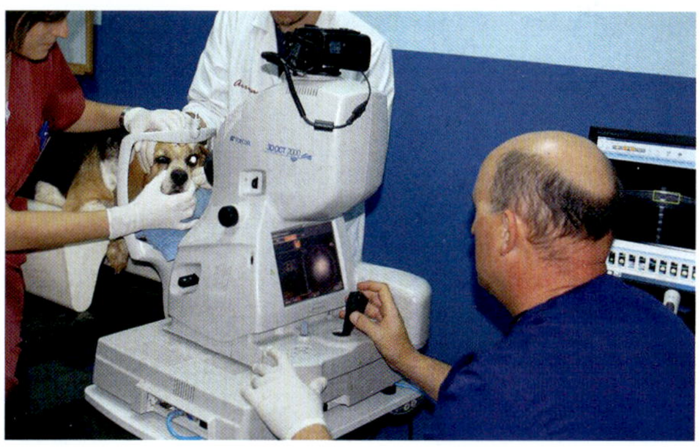

**Figure 8.27.** OCT in a dog.

## Eyelids

### *General aspects*

The eyelids consist of a fibrous tarsal and muscular lamina, lined on the inner side by the conjunctiva and on the outer side by a thin, more mobile and flexible skin than the rest of the skin on the body.

Specialized attached structures include:

- eyelashes:
  - In **dogs**, these are present on the margin of the **upper eyelid**.
  - **Cats do not have eyelashes**, but a line of **modified cilia** with similar functionality to eyelashes.
- glands: (The following are distinguished between.)
  - **glands of Moll (ciliary glands)**. These are modified sweat glands in the margin of the eyelid near the base of the hairs.
  - **glands of Zeis**. These are rudimentary sebaceous glands that open in the hair follicles.
  - **tarsal or Meibomian glands** (Figure 8.28). These are modified sebaceous glands located on the tarsal plate.

Basic functions of the eyelids include:

- **physical protection** against trauma
- distribution of the precorneal tear film
- **reduced tear evaporation**
- drainage of tears towards the puncta and maintenance of a uniform thickness of the tear film without modifying its optical properties.

## Congenital and developmental structural abnormalities

**Puppies and kittens are born with closed eyelids** to protect the cornea and conjunctiva until the tear system has developed completely. **Opening occurs between 10 and 14 days** of age.

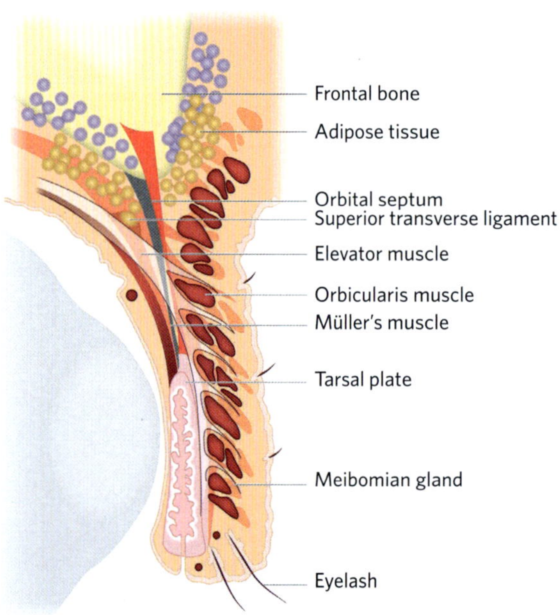


Figure 8.28. Diagram of palpebral structures.

### *Premature opening of the eyelids*

#### Epidemiology

Premature opening of the eyelids is rare.

#### Clinical signs

Premature opening causes:

- corneal desiccation
- keratitis
- corneal ulcers
- conjunctivitis.

If these consequences are not addressed, premature opening can evolve into:

- corneal perforation
- endophthalmitis.

#### Treatment

Regular application of ophthalmic lubricating ointments or **artificial teardrops**.

### *Delayed opening of the eyelids*

#### Aetiopathogenesis

Associated with an accumulation of mucus and, sometimes, infection (*Chlamydophila felis* or herpesvirus in cats and *Staphylococcus* spp. in dogs and cats), in which case it is called **neonatal ophthalmia (ophthalmia neonatorum)** (Figure 8.29).

#### Epidemiology

**Delayed opening of the eyelids** or ankyloblepharon is more common than early opening in both dogs and cats.

#### Treatment

Treatment includes:

- **atraumatic separation** of the eyelids. Once the eyelids have been opened, the eye should

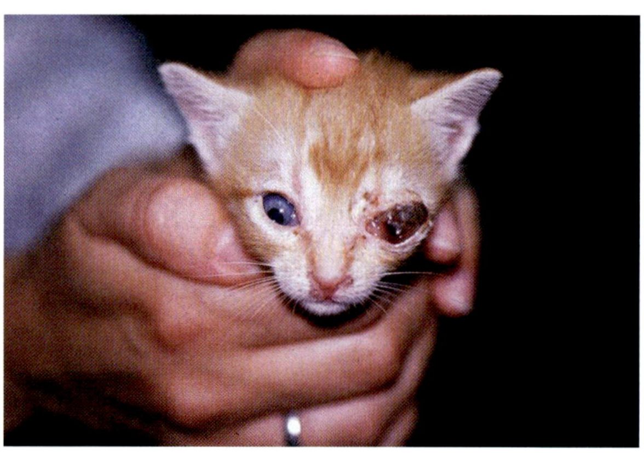

Figure 8.29. Appearance of the eye in a case of neonatal ophthalmia (ophthalmia neonatorum).

be examined for the presence of corneal ulceration.

- **drainage and cleaning of secretions** by irrigation with physiological saline or Ringer's lactate solution
- application of a specific **topical antibiotic**.

### *Agenesis or palpebral coloboma*

#### Definition

**Congenital absence of a portion of the eyelid.**

#### Aetiopathogenesis

Palpebral coloboma is associated with **excessive evaporation and an incorrect dispersion of tear fluid**, as well as with **trichiasis**.

#### Epidemiology

Palpebral coloboma is more common in **cats**, especially affecting the **lateral portion of the upper eyelid**.

#### Clinical signs

Palpebral coloboma may cause:

- keratoconjunctivitis
- pain
- corneal ulcers.

#### Treatment

Treatment is surgical (blepharoplasty).

## *Eyelash abnormalities*

### *Definitions*

- **Distichiasis**. Presence of **eyelashes that emerge through the Meibomian gland openings**. Generally, when these cilia are thin and soft, they do not cause irritation and have no clinical significance (Figure 8.30).
- **Trichiasis**. Presence of eyelashes or **hairs from adjacent skin** in a normal anatomical location **that make contact with the conjunctiva and/or cornea**. This abnormality can be primary or secondary, as occurring in cases of prominent nasal folds (Figure 8.31), palpebral colobomas, palpebral agenesis and entropion.
- **Ectopic cilia**. Presence of **an eyelash that emerges from the Meibomian gland through the palpebral conjunctiva**, especially in the upper eyelid (Figure 8.32), producing significant corneal irritation and often ulcers in the upper temporal area.

### *Epidemiology*

These abnormalities are **more frequent in dogs** than cats.

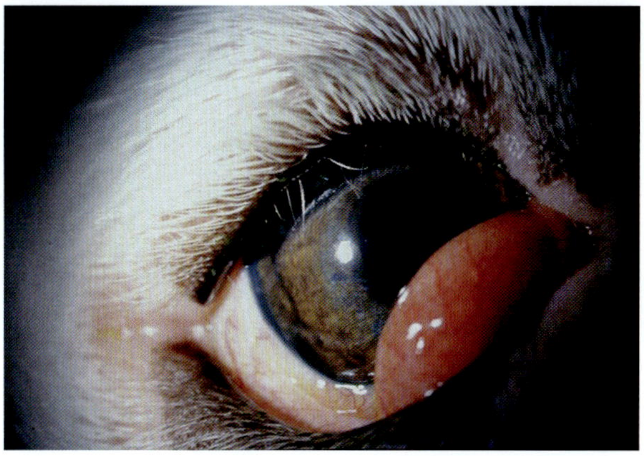

**Figure 8.30.** Distichiasis in an English bulldog. In addition, there is prolapse of the third eyelid.

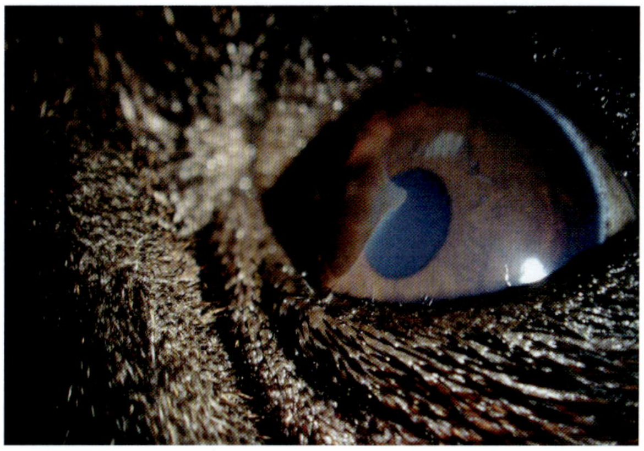

**Figure 8.31.** Trichiasis in a pug dog with prominent nasal folds that cause the appearance of corneal pigment.

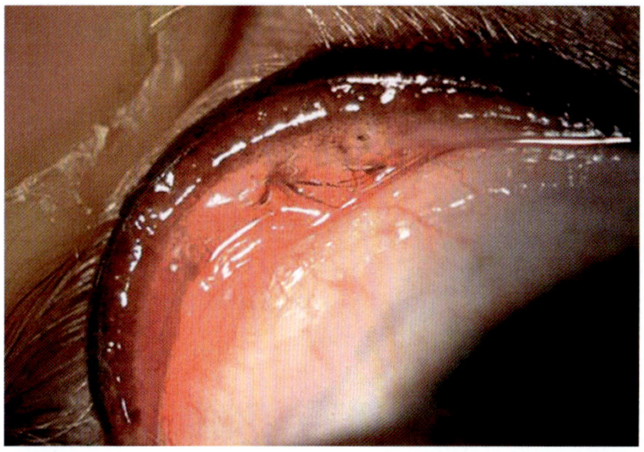

**Figure 8.32.** Presence of ectopic cilia that emerge from the body of the Meibomian gland through the palpebral conjunctiva.

### *Clinical signs*

All eyelash abnormalities produce very similar clinical signs, including:

- epiphora
- blepharospasm
- chronic conjunctival hyperaemia
- corneal ulcers.

### Treatment

In all cases, treatment involves surgical intervention, such as:

- surgical resection
- cryoepilation
- electrodepilation.

## Palpebral fissure or palpebral opening abnormalities

### Definition

Abnormalities of the eyelid (palpebral) fissure include:

- macroblepharon or **macropalpebral fissure** (excessively large palpebral opening)
- microblapharon or **micropalpebral fissure** (reduction in size of the eyelid opening).

### Treatment

Surgical, whenever secondary ocular signs are observed.

## Entropion

### Definition

Inversion of the eyelid margin.

### Aetiopathogenesis

Entropion may be:

- **conformational** or congenital (Figures 8.33 and 8.34)
- **spastic**, caused by painful lesions to the eyeball (Figure 8.35)
- **cicatricial (scar-forming)**
- associated with changes in the position of the eyeball (**enophthalmos**)
- associated with changes to the size of the eyeball (**ptosis or microphthalmos**).

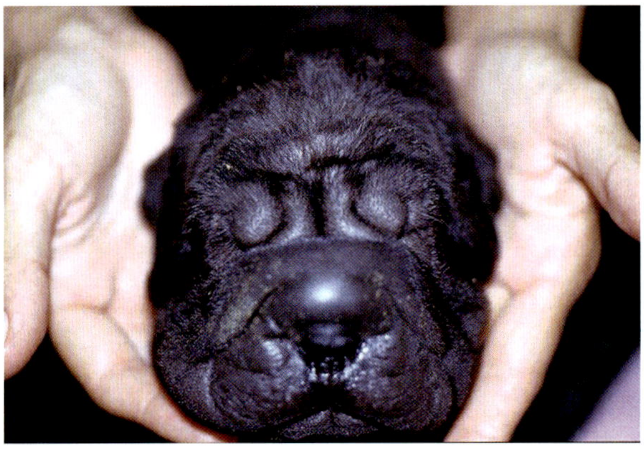

**Figure 8.33.** Congenital entropion in a Shar-Pei.

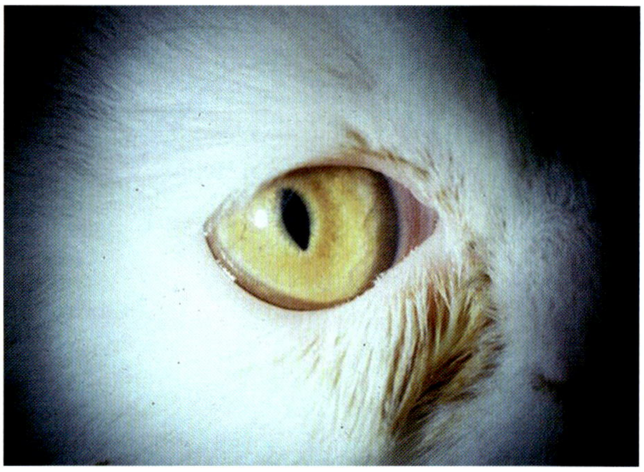

**Figure 8.34.** Medial congenital entropion in a Persian cat.

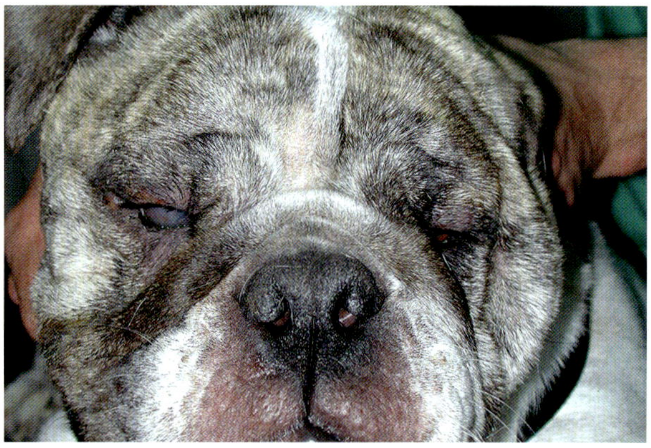

**Figure 8.35.** Acquired entropion due to uveitis in a dog diagnosed with leishmaniasis.

### Epidemiology

**Conformational entropion is hereditary in many dog breeds** including (among others): chow chow; English bulldog; Irish setter; Labrador retriever; golden retriever; St Bernard; Shar-Pei; Rottweiler; and Great Dane.

### Clinical signs

Frequently, clinical evidence of **conformational entropion appears months after birth**, as skull development occurs and facial skin folds grow, although it can also manifest itself at the time of eyelid opening.

In some cases, entropion reduction or even resolution occurs with maturity. Therefore, **surgery should be delayed until facial maturity** is reached.

Clinical signs include:

- eyelid curling
- blepharospasm
- excoriation
- maceration of the palpebral surface due to being in continuous contact with tears
- scratching of the affected area
- epiphora or mucoid discharge

- conjunctival hyperaemia
- corneal ulcers
- corneal melanosis, in chronic cases
- vascularization, in chronic cases.

#### Treatment
An appropriate surgical technique selected according to facial maturity, breed, entropion severity and economic considerations.

### Ectropion

#### Definition
**Eversion of the lower eyelid** (Figure 8.36).

#### Aetiopathogenesis

- Conformational ectropion is most common in breeds that have **excess facial skin folds**.
- Cicatricial ectropion is due to palpebral lacerations or surgery that overcorrected entropion.

#### Epidemiology
Ectropion is less frequent than entropion.

The most common type of ectropion is conformational, in breeds such as the retrievers, St Bernard, bloodhounds and cocker spaniel.

#### Clinical signs
Corneal/conjunctival lesions due to overexposure.

#### Treatment
Surgical treatment is the treatment of choice for animals with:

- conjunctivitis
- keratitis
- exfoliative blepharitis due to epiphora
- secondary keratoconjunctivitis sicca.

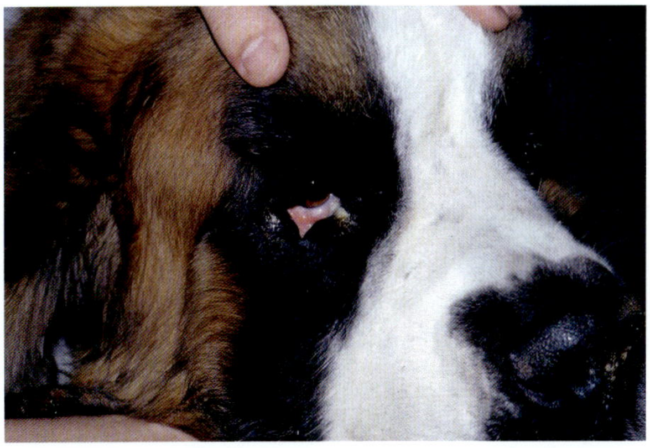

**Figure 8.36.** Conformational ectropion in a St Bernard dog.

## Acquired abnormalities

### Chalazion

#### Aetiopathogenesis
This is a **non-neoplastic enlargement of the Meibomian gland** due to the production of thickened secretions and blockage of the duct (Figure 8.37).

#### Diagnosis
This is not generally a painful condition. Chalazion has a **yellow-white appearance** when observed through the palpebral conjunctiva or skin.

#### Treatment
Surgical drainage of the gland.

### Stye and Meibomian adenitis

#### Aetiopathogenesis
**Purulent bacterial infection** (*Staphylococcus aureus*) of the following:

- gland of Zeis (external stye)
- Meibomian gland (internal stye).

This often affects multiple glands, in which case it is called meibomitis, tarsal or Meibomian adenitis or marginal blepharitis.

#### Clinical signs
Meibomian adenitis causes more **inflammation and pain** than chalazion.

Clinical signs include:

- variable erythema and inflammation of the eyelid margin
- pruritus
- pain
- chemosis
- purulent conjunctivitis.

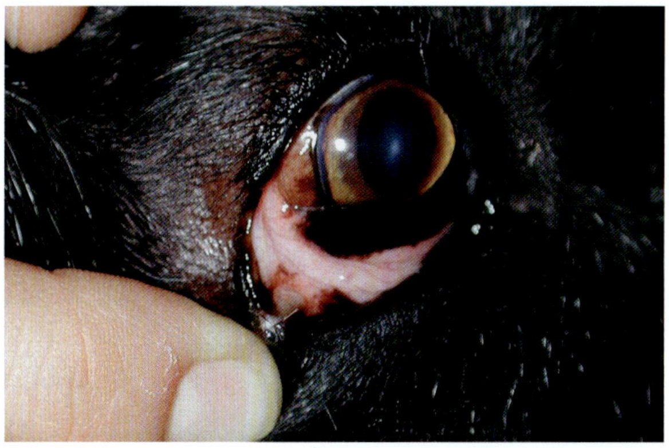

**Figure 8.37.** Chalazion.

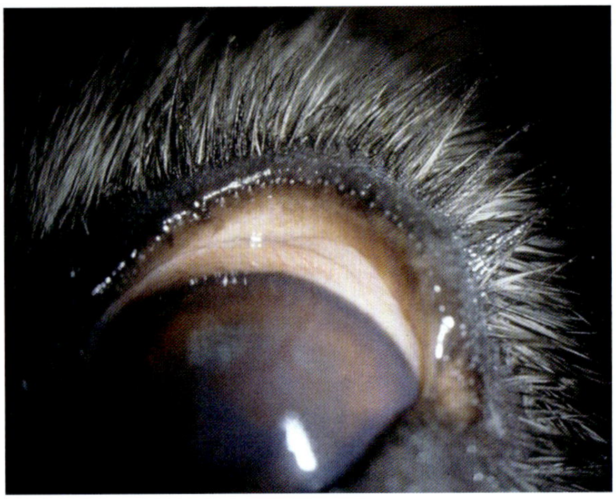

**Figure 8.38.** Meibomitis or tarsal adenitis, which secondarily causes a dry eye.

If lubricating secretions are retained, this may result in **secondary KCS** (Figure 8.38).

### Treatment

Treatment involves the administration of **systemic antibiotics** (amoxicillin + clavulanic acid, doxycycline, cephalosporin) and the use of **topical antibiotics with corticosteroids**.

## Blepharitis

### Aetiopathogenesis

Blepharitis or **palpebral inflammation** is usually **part of a generalized skin condition**, which is more evident in this area because of its greater vascularization. Therefore, patients with blepharitis should undergo a **complete dermatological examination**.

For owners, blepharitis is the most striking aspect of the skin condition because it is most easily visible on the mucocutaneous junction.

### Aetiology

- Parasitic:
  - *Sarcoptes scabiei* (dog)
  - *Demodex* spp. (Figure 8.39)
  - *Notoedres cati* (cat)
  - ticks
  - mosquito bites
  - *Habronema* spp.
  - *Leishmania* spp.
- Infectious:
  - bacterial (Figure 8.40) (*Staphylococcus* spp., *Corynebacterium* spp., *Mycobacterium* spp.)
  - viral (feline herpesvirus type 1)
  - fungal (e.g. *Microsporum canis*, *Microsporum gypseum*, *Tricophyton mentagrophytes*).
- Allergic:
  - atopic dermatitis
  - food allergy
  - contact dermatitis
  - hypersensitivity to medications.
- Autoimmune:
  - pemphigus (Figure 8.41) (foliaceous, vulgar and erythematous)
  - lupus (discoid, erythematous)
  - uveodermatological syndrome
  - alopecia areata
  - nodular panniculitis.
- Neoplastic
  - squamous cell carcinoma
  - melanoma
  - histiocytoma.

### Clinical signs

The **aetiology of blepharitis is multifactorial**, so the appearance of the eyelid lesions varies and can include peeling, alopecia, oedema, papules, pustules, scabs, ulcers, etc.

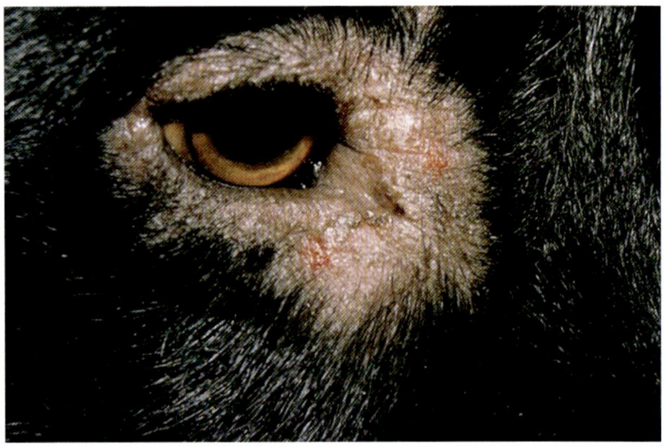

**Figure 8.39.** Parasitic blepharitis (*Demodex* spp.).

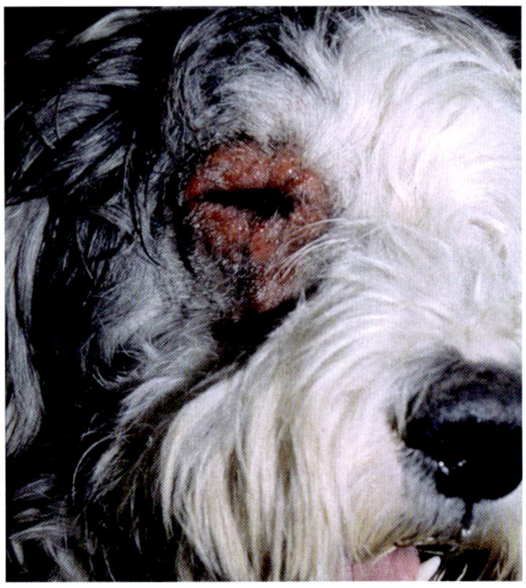

**Figure 8.40.** Bacterial blepharitis (*Staphylococcus* spp.).

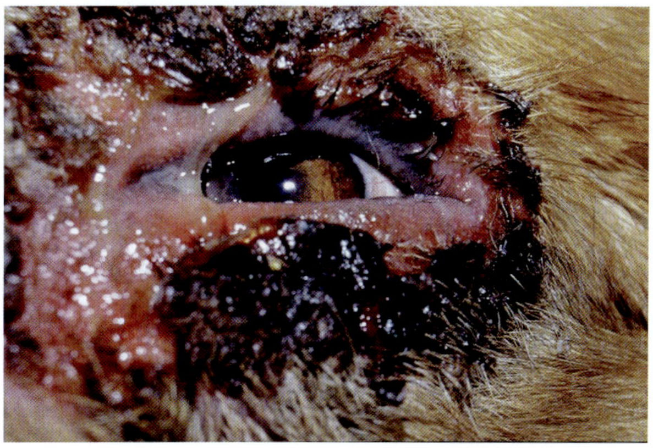

**Figure 8.41.** Autoimmune blepharitis (pemphigus).

### *Treatment*

The treatment of blepharitis should be **based on its aetiology**; most cases requires systemic treatments.

## *Neoplasms*

### *Epidemiology*

**Palpebral tumours are relatively common** in domestic species. Those most frequently encountered in dogs include:

- Meibomian gland adenoma (Figure 8.42)
- papilloma
- carcinoma (Figure 8.43)
- histiocytoma
- melanoma
- in cats, squamous cell carcinoma (Figure 8.44).

### *Treatment*

All **neoplasms require surgery** and histological examination.

In many cases, cryotherapy is particularly useful since tumour cells are differentially affected more than the eyelids.

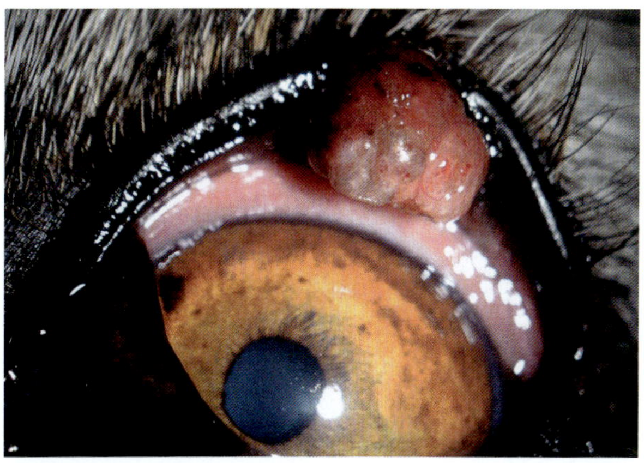

**Figure 8.42.** Adenoma of the Meibomian gland.

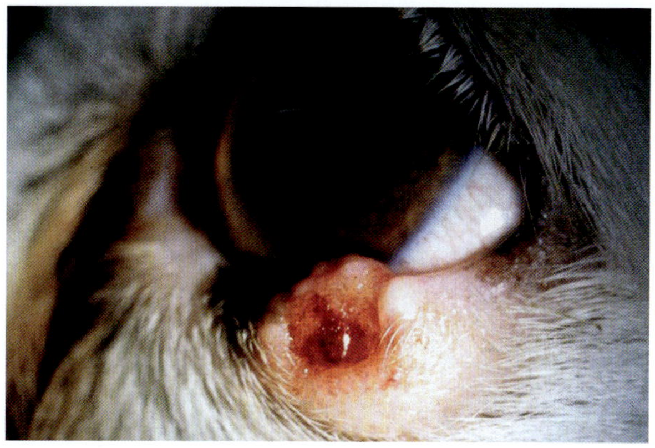

**Figure 8.43.** Palpebral carcinoma in a dog.

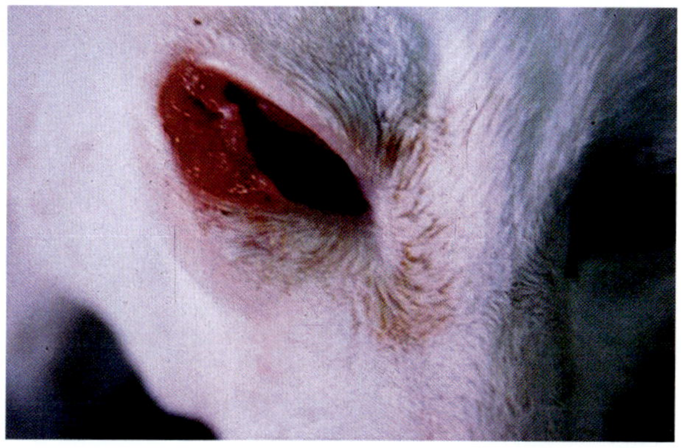

**Figure 8.44.** Squamous cell carcinoma in a cat.

# Conjunctiva

## *General aspects*

The conjunctiva is a mobile mucous membrane that covers the following (Figure 8.45):

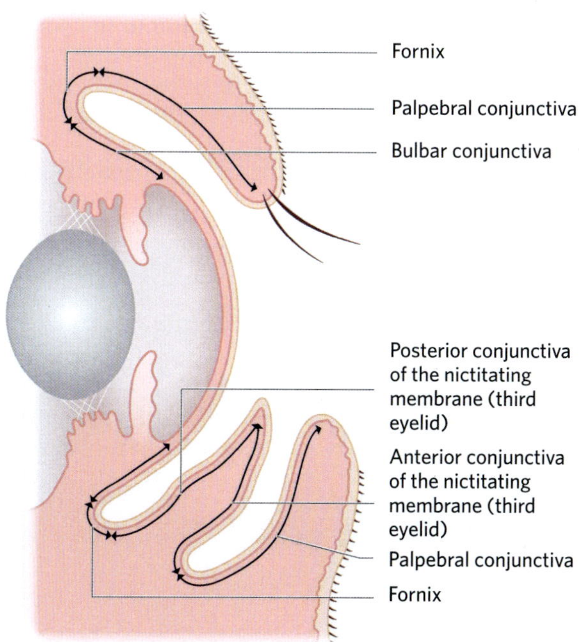


**Figure 8.45.** Distribution of the conjunctiva.

- the **inner surface** of the eyelids (palpebral conjunctiva)
- the **anterior portion** of the eyeball adjacent to the limbus (bulbar conjunctiva)
- the **inner and outer surfaces of the third eyelid**.

The **junction between the bulbar and palpebral conjunctiva is called the sacral fundus** or conjunctival fornix.

The conjunctiva consists of a **non-keratinized columnar epithelium with goblet cells** that contribute to the production of tear film mucin.

This **mucous membrane is the most exposed in the body**. It responds quickly to harmful stimuli due to the presence of lymphoid follicles, which are particularly numerous in the bulbar surface of the third eyelid.

## Congenital abnormalities

### Conjunctival dermoid

#### Definition

Conjunctival dermoids consist of **areas of ectopic skin** complete with associated structures. In the dog, these generally affect the lateral edge of the cornea or the sclerocorneal limbus (Figure 8.46).

#### Treatment

Surgical excision of the conjunctival dermoid.

## Acquired abnormalities

### Conjunctivitis

#### Definition

Conjunctivitis is **swelling and irritation of the ocular conjunctiva**.

#### Classification

Conjunctivitis is variously classified according to:

- duration:
  - acute
  - subacute
  - chronic
  - recurrent
- nature of the ocular **discharge:**
  - mucoid
  - purulent
  - mucopurulent
  - haemorrhagic
- **appearance**:
  - follicular
  - membranous
  - pseudomembranous
  - ligneous
- **aetiology**:
  - aetiology is the most relevant classification since the treatments administered should be specific to the inciting condition.

#### Aetiology

- **irritants** (Figure 8.47):
  - external (foreign bodies, dust, sand, smoke, low humidity, air, allergens, etc.)
  - internal (tear deficiency, entropion, distichiasis, trichiasis, ectropion, etc.).
- **infectious**:
  - bacterial (*Staphylococcus* spp., *Streptococcus* spp.)
  - chlamydia (cat)
  - viral (**herpesvirus type 1** in the cat, distemper and adenovirus 1 and 2 in the dog)
  - fungal (*Candida* spp., *Aspergillus* spp.)
  - parasitic (*Thelazia* spp.).
- immune-mediated:
  - exposure to antigens.
- due to orbital abnormalities:
  - cellulitis
  - abscesses.

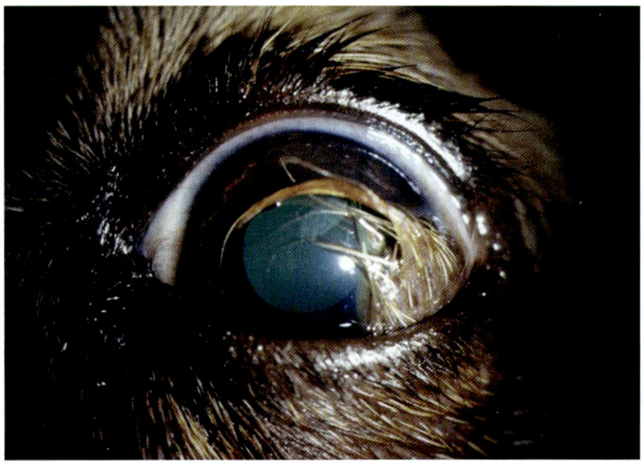

**Figure 8.46.** Corneal/conjunctival dermoid.

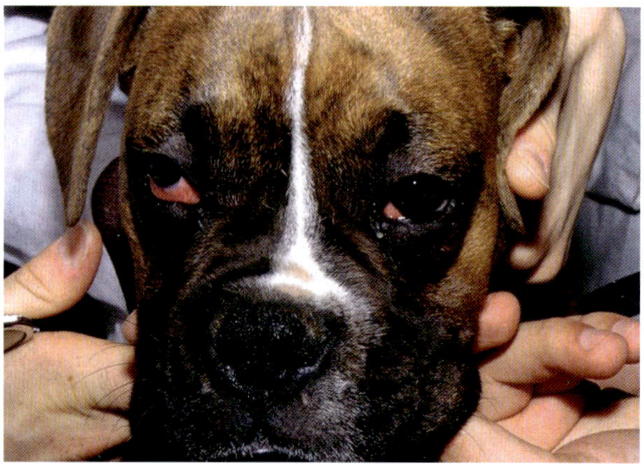

**Figure 8.47.** Conjunctivitis due to irritants after being outside in the countryside.

### Clinical signs

General clinical signs include:

- hyperaemia, due to dilation of the conjunctival vessels
- chemosis (conjunctival oedema) (Figure 8.48)
- subconjunctival haemorrhage
- follicular hyperplasia (Figure 8.49), seen usually in chronic conditions
- ocular discharge, the nature of which depends on the aetiology.

### Diagnosis

Diagnosis is based on the results of:

- complete eye examination
- ocular retropulsion
- Schirmer's test
- bacterial culture
- cytology
- conjunctival biopsy.

### Treatment

Treatment depends on the aetiology, for example:

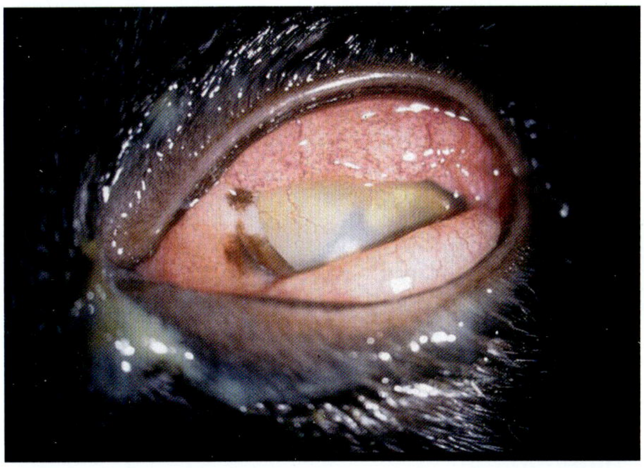

**Figure 8.48.** Presence of chemosis and conjunctival hyperaemia in a cat (herpesvirus type 1).

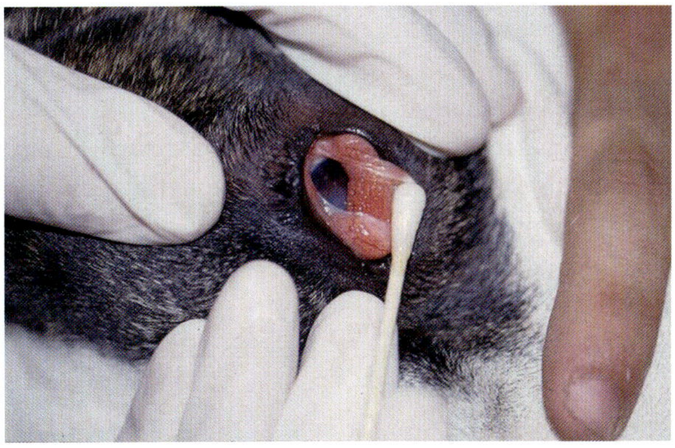

**Figure 8.49.** Presence of follicular hyperplasia in the bulbar conjunctiva of the third eyelid.

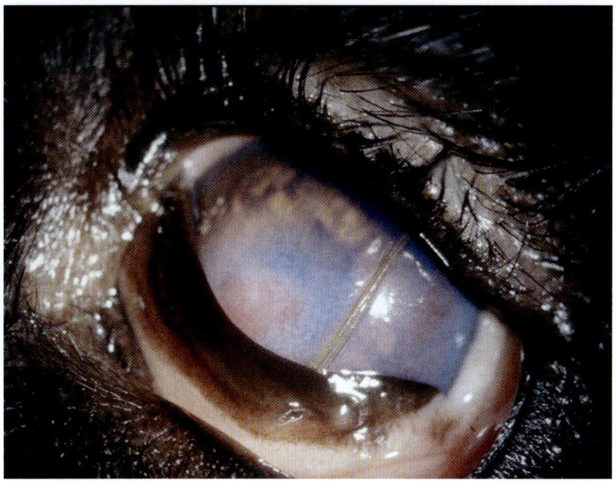

**Figure 8.50.** Presence of a plant-type foreign body in the bulbar conjunctiva of the third eyelid.

- **removal of foreign bodies** (Figure 8.50)
- **surgical techniques** to correct congenital eyelid abnormalities
- **topical antibiotic therapy**. Most animals respond to treatment with broad-spectrum antimicrobial agents administered topically. In cases where there is no response, a culture and an antibiogram are recommended.
- **corticosteroids**. Generally, they should only be used in non-infectious conditions. Therefore, they should not be considered as a routine treatment for conjunctivitis and should not be prescribed without having made a specific diagnosis.
- **cleaning agents**. The elimination of accumulations of eye discharges facilitates the penetration of ophthalmic medication and allows animals to feel more comfortable. Ringer's lactate solution or commercial solutions can be used for irrigation.
- **antiviral agents**. Trifluridine and idoxuridine are the most commonly used. For cats, systemic L-lysine (reduces virus replication) and topical interferon should be added. Systemic antivirals may also be appropriate in some cases.

## *Neoplasms*

### *Aetiopathogenesis*

Conjunctival neoplasms can be primary or metastatic.

Types of conjunctival neoplasia:

- **squamous cell carcinoma** (Figure 8.51) is the most frequent
- haemangioma
- haemangiosarcoma
- melanoma
- papilloma
- mastocytoma.

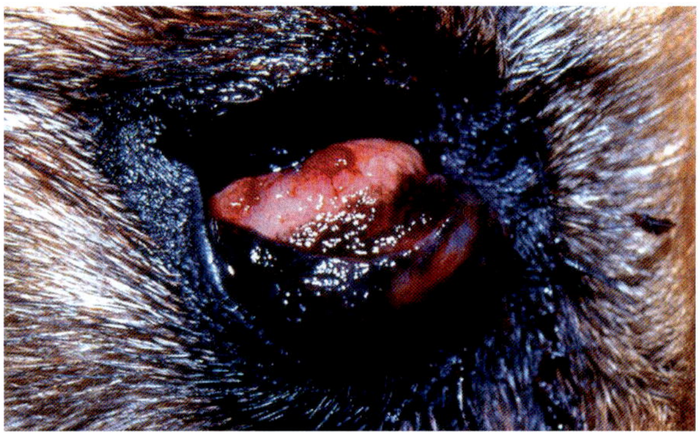

**Figure 8.51.** Squamous cell carcinoma of the conjunctiva.

### Diagnosis

Biopsy or fine needle aspirates can be used to make a diagnosis.

## Nictitating membrane (third eyelid)

### General aspects

The third eyelid or **nictitating membrane is a mobile, protective glandular structure**, located between the cornea and the lower eyelid in the medial portion of the lower conjunctival sac.

It is formed by the following structures:

- **T-shaped cartilage**, which provides stiffness
- **gland** of the nictitating membrane (third eyelid)
- **conjunctiva** that covers the bulbar and palpebral surfaces
- numerous **lymphoid follicles** under the bulbar surface.

The **main functions** of the third eyelid include:

- tear film distribution
- corneal protection
- production of the aqueous fraction of the tear film, as well as immunoglobulins.

### Eversion of nictitating membrane

#### Definition

Eversion of the nictitating membrane (third eyelid) is when the **exterior margin of the nictitating membrane curls outwards** due to an abnormal curvature in the vertical portion of the cartilage (Figure 8.52). This abnormality can be unilateral or bilateral.

#### Aetiopathogenesis

A **hereditary basis** is suspected. Injuries and inappropriate sutures in the nictitating membrane (third eyelid) can also result in eversion.

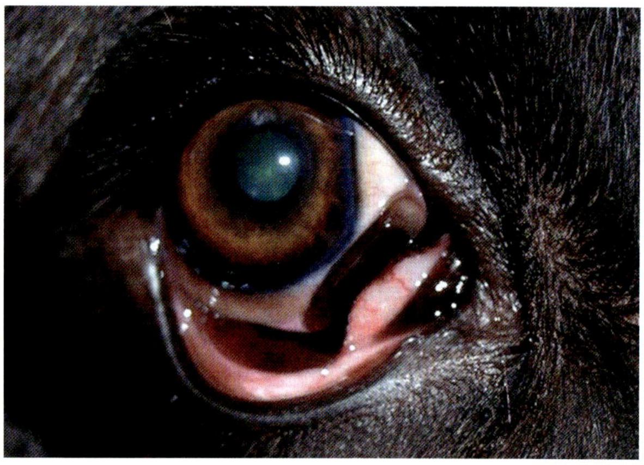

**Figure 8.52.** Eversion of the nictitating membrane (third eyelid) due to an abnormal curvature in the vertical portion of the cartilage.

#### Epidemiology

Although mainly seen in **young dogs**, eversion can occasionally develop in middle-aged dogs.

**Predisposed breeds** include the Weimaraner, St Bernard, Newfoundland, Great Dane and Irish setter, among others.

#### Treatment

**Treatment is surgical**, to correct a cosmetic problem that can cause secondary conjunctivitis and keratitis.

### Prolapse of the gland of the nictitating membrane (third eyelid) (Cherry eye)

#### Aetiopathogenesis

It usually occurs after **lymphoid hyperplasia** (exposure of young animals to environmental antigens), when there is a **laxity in the retinaculum** that should fix the nictitating membrane (third eyelid) to the periorbital one.

#### Epidemiology

There is a **genetic predisposition in brachycephalic animals**, although it can be seen in any breed.

This condition, also called 'cherry eye', is primarily seen in dogs and, occasionally, in cats.

#### Clinical signs

It has a characteristic appearance: a **reddish follicular mass behind the nictitating membrane (third eyelid)**, which normally protrudes from its margin (Figure 8.53).

The condition occurs bilaterally and asynchronously.

#### Clinical signs

Clinical signs include:

- epiphora
- conjunctivitis.

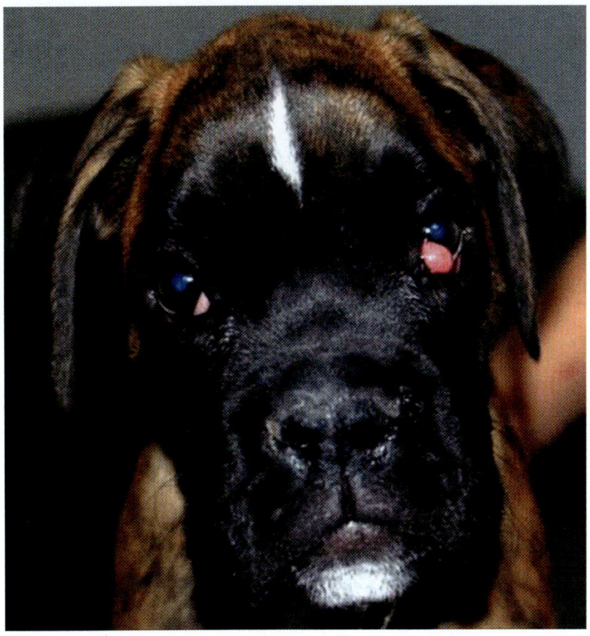

**Figure 8.53.** Prolapse of the gland of the nictitating membrane (third eyelid).

### Treatment
The gland should be **repositioned**, **never removed**, by surgical techniques to allow tear secretion and prevent exposure of the gland and conjunctiva, thus avoiding consequent dryness, inflammation, infection and aesthetic alterations.

## Plasmoma

### Definition
Plasmoma is **plasmacytic infiltration of the nictitating membrane (third eyelid)**.

### Aetiology
Unknown (possibly autoimmune).

### Epidemiology
**German shepherd** dogs have a clear breed predisposition.

### Clinical signs
It involves **thickening and depigmentation of the free edge of the nictitating membrane** (Figure 8.54).

### Treatment
Topical corticosteroids.

## Follicular conjunctivitis

### Aetiopathogenesis
This is an **immune-mediated condition**, usually secondary to chronic antigenic stimulation.

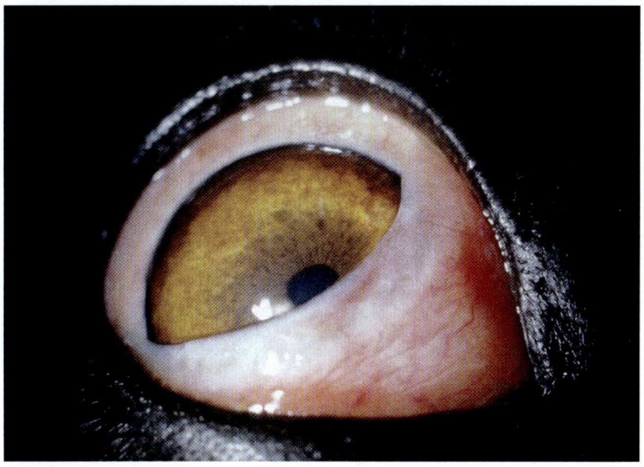

**Figure 8.54.** Plasmoma in a German shepherd dog. Note the depigmentation of the free edge of the third eyelid.

### Clinical signs
Inflammation and hypertrophy of the lymphoid follicles present on the bulbar surface of the nictitating membrane (third eyelid) (Figure 8.49).

### Treatment
Although the use of **topical corticosteroids** can reduce inflammation, treatment is aimed at treating the cause of the condition.

## Neoplasms

### Epidemiology
The most frequent types of neoplasms are:

- lymphoma
- haemangioma or haemangiosarcoma
- adenocarcinoma.

### Diagnosis
Animals that present with these neoplasms should undergo a thorough examination of the orbit, regional lymph nodes and other **distant locations for metastases**.

### Treatment
**Surgical excision of malignant tumours** is recommended except for **lymphoma, which can be treated with systemic chemotherapy**.

# Lacrimal apparatus

## General aspects

The lacrimal apparatus consists of the following structures, which contribute to **tear production** (Figure 8.55) and its **drainage** (Figure 8.56):

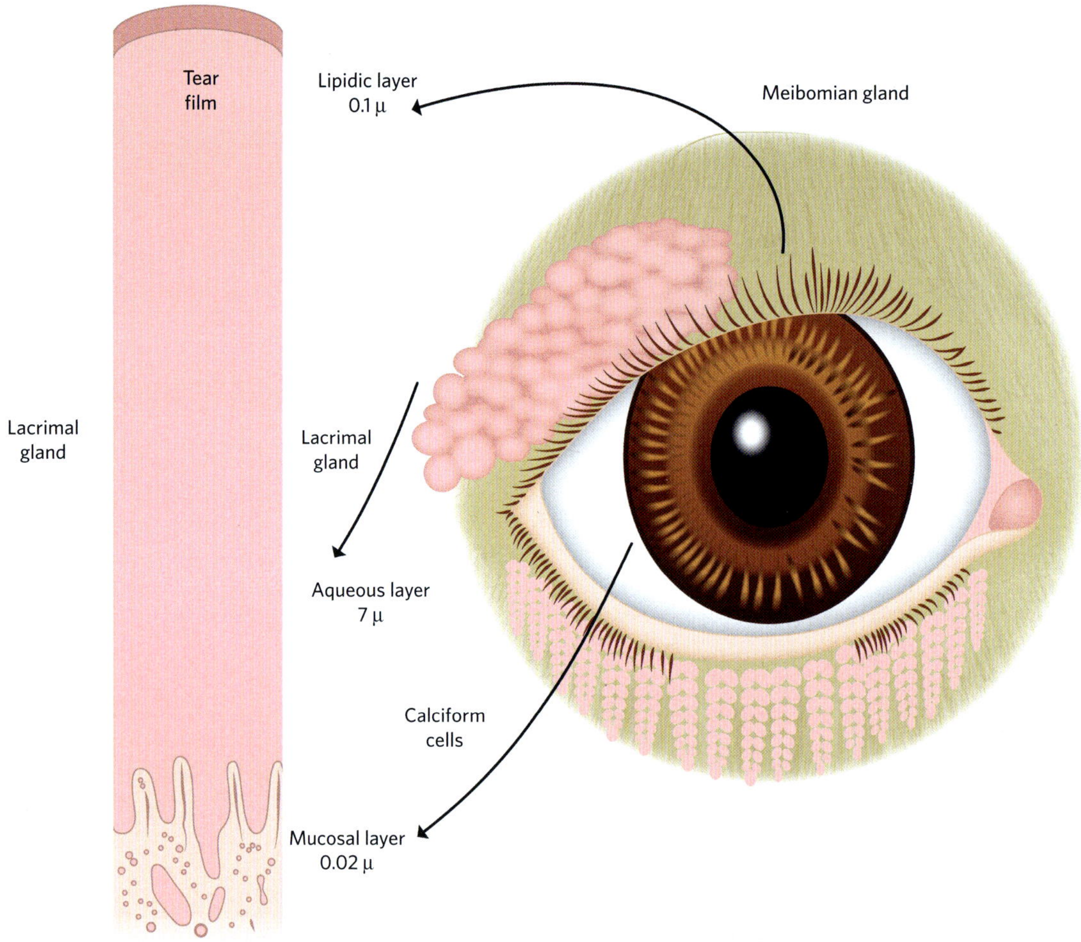


**Figure 8.55.** Diagram showing the structures that give rise to the different tear film layers.

- main lacrimal gland (located under the orbital ligament, with several excretory ducts that open into the temporal area of the conjunctiva of the upper eyelid) and the nictitating membrane (third eyelid)
- accessory lacrimal glands (fundamentally Meibomian glands)
- precorneal tear film
- lacrimal punctum and canaliculi
- lacrimal sac
- nasolacrimal duct
- nasal punctum.

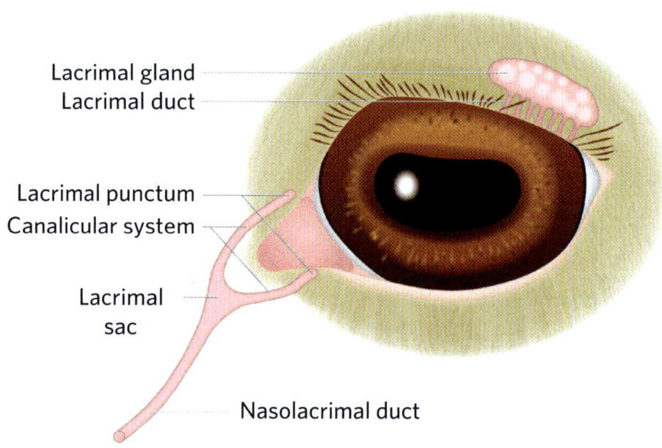


**Figure 8.56.** Diagram of the lacrimal drainage system. Lacrimal punctum, canalicular system, lacrimal sac and nasolacrimal duct, which flow into the inferior nasal meatus.

The **precorneal tear film** covers the cornea and conjunctiva. It consists of **three layers** with different compositions and a thickness of 8–9 μm:

1. **Lipid layer** (outer layer). It has a thickness of 0.1 μm. It is composed of oily substances and phospholipids from the Meibomian and Zeis glands. Its functions are:
   - **avoid evaporation** of the aqueous layer
   - unite the tear film with the cornea at the palpebral edges
   - **avoid overflow** thanks to its high surface tension.
2. **Aqueous layer** (intermediate layer). Mainly consisting of water, it is derived from the main tear gland and nictitating membrane (third eyelid). It is 7 μm thick. Its functions are:
   - **removal of foreign bodies** and bacteria
   - **lubrication** of the eyelids and nictitating membrane (third eyelid)

- **provide the cornea with nutrients** (oxygen, amino acids, vitamin A, growth factors and antibodies)
- provide a **smooth surface** for proper optical efficiency
- act as a source of **antibacterial** substances (immunoglobulins, lactoferrin and lysozyme).

3. **Mucous layer** (inner layer). It is 1–2 μm thick.
   - It consists of mucoproteins from the conjunctival goblet cells. These mucoproteins are bipolar, with a lipophilic part (associated with the corneal epithelium) and a hydrophilic part (associated with the aqueous tear layer).

## Abnormalities in tear function

These can be classified in two categories:

1. **Inability of the drainage system to eliminate the tears produced**. This may be caused by:
   - obstruction of the drainage system
   - overproduction of tears
   - the clinical sign is epiphora
   - precorneal tear film production failure may be:
     - quantitative (insufficient aqueous layer)
     - qualitative (insufficient lipid or mucous layer).

   It causes secondary conjunctivitis and keratitis.

2. **Alterations of tear function** in relation to tear drainage.

## Dacryocystitis

### Definition

**Inflammation of the lacrimal sac and nasolacrimal duct**.

### Aetiology

Although occasionally a foreign body (plant debris, sand, dust and concretions of mucopurulent material) is the inciting cause, in most patients the primary cause cannot be determined (Figure 8.57).

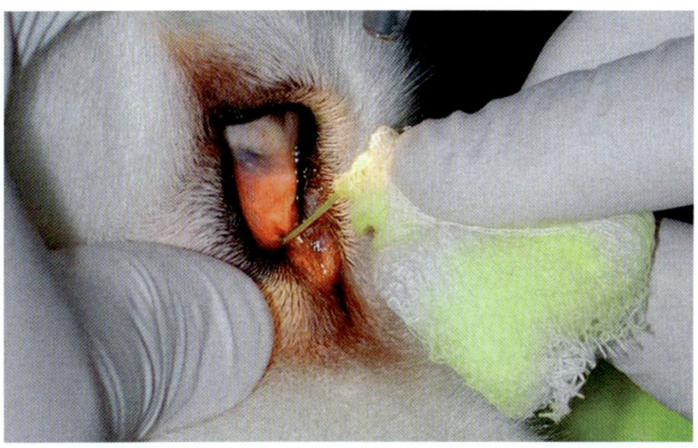

**Figure 8.57.** Dacryocystitis. Extraction of a mucopurulent exudate from the lacrimal orifice.

### Clinical signs

- **Ocular discharge** at the medial canthus. This exudate, either simply tear or mucopurulent exudate, may have layers of purulent and clear material and even gas bubbles.
- **Mild conjunctivitis**, especially in the medial area. In cases of chronic dacryocystitis, chronic unilateral recurrent conjunctivitis may be the only clinical sign, with a temporary response after washing and applying antibiotics.
- Appearance of **mucopurulent material at the tear punctum** after applying pressure in the medial area, with the presence of pain in some cases.
- Erythematous **pain and dermatitis of the medial canthus** on certain occasions.
- In severe cases, **tear sac abscesses** and even formation of large cavities can be seen.

### Diagnosis

Diagnosis is based on clinical signs, especially visualization of the mucopurulent material at the tear punctum.

The exact location of the obstruction can be determined by:

- cannulation
- dacryocystorhinography
- CT
- MRI.

### Treatment

The treatment of choice is **catheterization of the lacrimal system** for 2–3 weeks.

In some cases, daily lavage with antibiotic eye drops and the application of corticosteroids may be effective (Figure 8.58).

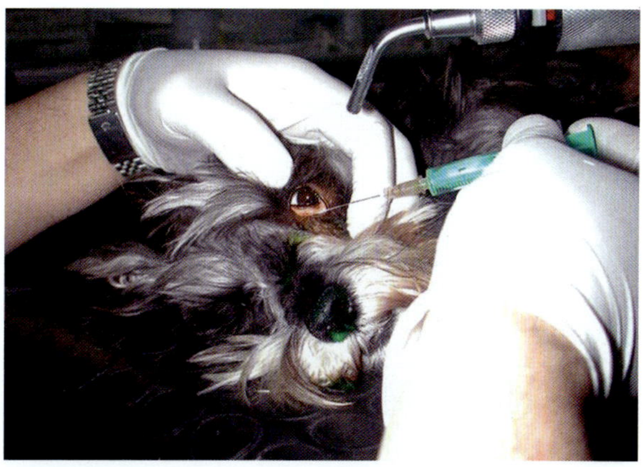

**Figure 8.58.** Catheterization and lavage of the lacrimal duct. The rinsing solution contains a drop of fluorescein so that it can be seen when it exits the nose.

When severe dermatitis or abscesses exist, systemic antibiotic therapy should be administered. In the most severe cases, where there is obstruction, a dacryocystotomy is recommended.

## Tear punctum atresia, ectopia and imperforate lacrimal punctum

### Definition
**Lacrimal duct occlusion**, usually lower.

### Aetiopathogenesis
In dogs, it is considered a **congenital condition**.

In cats, the most common cause is scarring of the tear punctum due to conjunctivitis caused by herpesvirus type 1.

### Epidemiology
**Predisposed dog breeds** include the American cocker spaniel, Bedlington terrier, golden retriever, miniature and toy poodle and Samoyed.

### Clinical signs
The main clinical sign is **epiphora** (Figure 8.59), which causes a reddish-brown coloration of the facial hair around the medial canthus of the eye.

Many animals remain asymptomatic until they reach several weeks of age.

### Diagnosis
Diagnosis is made using magnification, after checking that the tear duct cannot be cannulated. In most cases, a layer of conjunctiva is observed over the tear punctum.

Differential diagnoses can include:

- trichiasis
- distichiasis
- entropion.

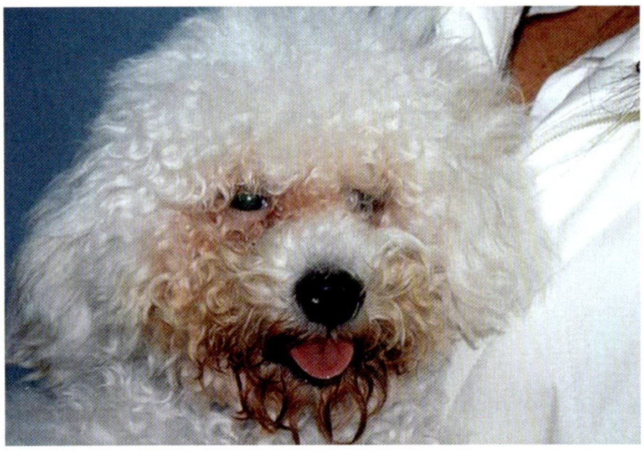

**Figure 8.59.** Atresia of the lacrimal puncta. Note the red/brown-coloured discharge on the face hair due to crying.

### Treatment
Surgical.

## Precorneal tear film deficiency: mucin deficiency

### Aetiology
A **decrease in the number of conjunctival goblet cells**, caused by chronic inflammation, metaplasia, hypoplasia or fibrosis, can cause mucin deficiency in dogs and cats.

### Clinical signs
The clinical signs are the same as for keratoconjunctivitis sicca, except that the Schirmer's test may be normal or slightly reduced.

### Diagnosis
Diagnostic tests include:

- tear break-up time (less than 5 seconds)
- conjunctival biopsy, to confirm the lowest number of caliciform cells.

### Treatment
**Topical 2% cyclosporine** applied together with artificial teardrops containing polyvinylpyrrolidone or methylcellulose derivatives, which simulate natural mucins.

## Precorneal tear film deficiency: lipid deficiency

### Aetiopathogenesis
This type of tear film deficiency is characteristic of inflammation of the eyelid margin and Meibomian glands.

The most frequent causes are:

- staphylococcal infections and *Malassezia* associated with blepharitis
- generalized seborrhoea
- atopy
- demodicosis.

The aberrant lipids generated can be directly toxic to the epithelial cells, resulting in the loss of the epithelial layer and, therefore, a dispersion of the tear film, which causes a dry eye.

### Clinical signs
Clinical signs include:

- blepharitis
- swelling of the opening of the Meibomian glands

- hyperaemia of the mucocutaneous junction
- mucous or mucopurulent discharge
- chalazion
- due to the transparency of the conjunctiva, the glands appear yellowish with a paste-like content
- conjunctival hyperaemia
- keratitis
- areas of corneal oedema
- corneal erosion.

### Treatment

Treatment includes:

- **hot compresses 2–3 times daily** (gel masks heated in the microwave are currently used)
- systemic and topical **antibiotic therapy** specific to culture and antibiogram done on a sample taken from the eyelid edge
- topical application of lipid substitutes, such as **mineral oil or lanolin**.

Systemic and topical corticosteroids can also help when there is a lot of inflammation around the ducts of the Meibomian glands. (Do not apply if there is corneal erosion.)

## Keratoconjunctivitis sicca

### Aetiopathogenesis

KCS consists of **chronic inflammation of the cornea and conjunctiva caused by insufficient tear production** (aqueous fraction).

### Causes

Causes of KCS include the following:

- pharmacological:
  - non-steroidal anti-inflammatory drugs (etodolac)
  - sulfa-containing derivatives (trimethoprim/sulfamethoxazole, sulfadiazine, sulfasalazine)
  - topical and systemic atropine.
- general anaesthesia
- surgical
  - removal of the nictitating membrane (third eyelid) gland (KCS appears after 3–4 years)
  - sectioning of the facial nerve in ear surgeries.
- immunological. This is most frequent in dogs. KCS is caused by the immune-mediated destruction of tissues due to rupture of the blood–lacrimal barrier.
  - systemic autoimmune conditions that can cause this type of KCS:
    - Sjögren syndrome
    - systemic lupus erythematosus
    - pemphigus foliaceus
    - rheumatoid arthritis
    - polymyositis and polyarthritis
    - atopy.
- hypothyroidism
- diabetes mellitus
- glomerulonephritis
- ulcerative colitis
- traumatic, due to orbital and supraorbital traumas that directly affect the glands or their innervation. It may accompany proptosis of the eyeball
- infectious:
  - canine distemper (temporary KCS)
  - leishmaniasis
  - feline herpesvirus.
- congenital:
  - in dogs with congenital acinar hypoplasia, in breeds such as the pug dog, chihuahua and Yorkshire terrier
  - in cats with palpebral agenesis due to the absence of glands or their ducts.
- degenerative: senile atrophy of the tear glands in dogs over 10 years old
- due to radiotherapy
- neurogenic:
  - loss of parasympathetic innervation of the lacrimal glands
  - trigeminal abnormalities
  - feline dysautonomia.

### Epidemiology

The **most commonly affected breeds** are the American cocker spaniel, Boston terrier, Cavalier King Charles spaniel, English bulldog, springer spaniel, Lhasa apso, miniature schnauzer, Pekingese, pug dog, poodle, West Highland white terrier and Yorkshire terrier.

### Clinical signs

Clinical signs depend on whether the condition is unilateral or bilateral, acute or chronic and temporary or permanent:

- **mucous or mucopurulent discharge** (Figure 8.60). The secretion is thick, viscous and adheres to the ocular surface because of an increase in mucin production and a reduction in aqueous tear fraction. The purulent component can be sterile or with secondary bacterial infection.
- thickened **hyperaemic conjunctiva** with chemosis
- **blepharospasm** and protrusion of the nictitating membrane (third eyelid), depending on the degree of irritation caused by blinking
- corneal vascularity (superficial and deep) and **pigmentation** in cases of chronic KCS (Figure 8.61)

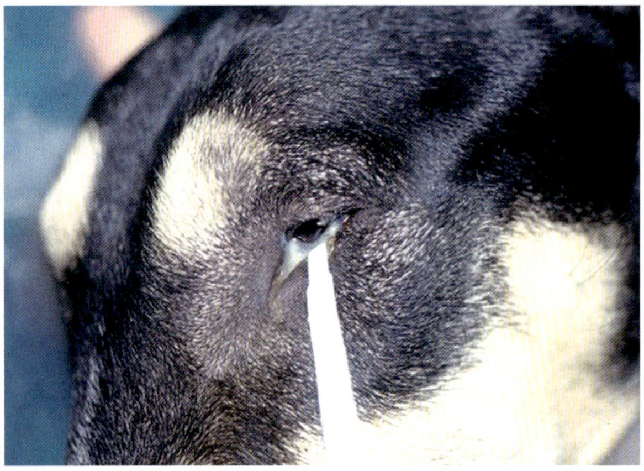

**Figure 8.60.** Mucopurulent discharge in a dog with KCS.

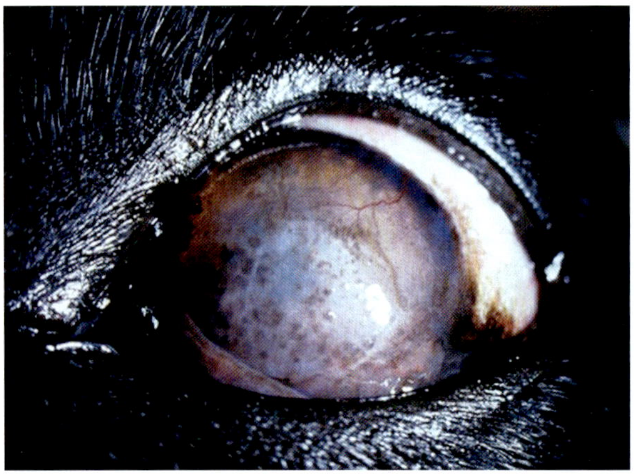

**Figure 8.61.** Chronic KCS. Corneal vascularization and pigmentation.

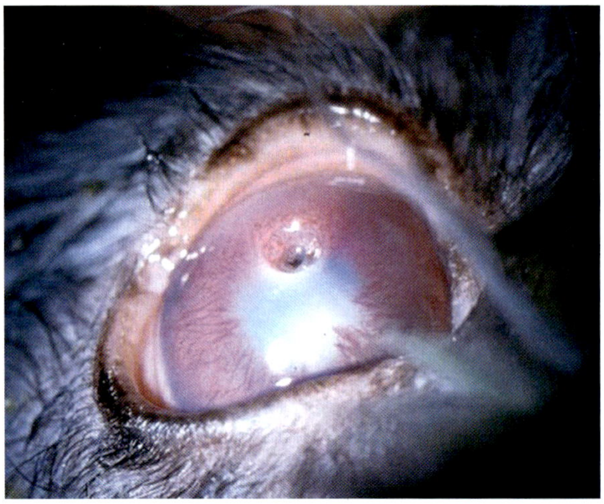

**Figure 8.62.** Chronic KCS. Vascularization and deep central corneal ulcer.

- **corneal ulceration** in severe or acute cases, especially in the central area; perforation and endophthalmitis may occur (Figure 8.62)
- **loss of corneal shine** caused by dryness, which is present in 25% of dogs
- dryness in the nostril of the affected side, especially in neurogenic KCS due to the involvement of the lateral nasal gland
- chronic staphylococcal blepharitis
- loss of vision.

### *Treatment*

Medical therapy that requires periodic check-ups:

- Clean the ocular and periocular tissues with commercial solutions.
- Stimulate natural tear production.
- Use **2% cyclosporine in corn oil**. This produces immunomodulation by inhibiting helper T cells and directly stimulating tear production, blocking the cyclophilin receptor and inhibiting prolactin, which in turn limits tear production. In addition, cyclosporine reduces corneal pigmentation, reduces inflammation and improves mucin secretion. Administration schedule: **every 12 hours**. If there is no response in 1 month, it can be prescribed every 8 hours.
- Use **0.02% tacrolimus**. This is a powerful immunomodulator with a mechanism of action like cyclosporine.
- Use 2% pilocarpine. Pilocarpine can be used in cases of neurogenic KCS secondary to parasympathetic denervation because of cholinergic stimulation (1 drop in food per 10 kg of weight twice daily).
- Apply **artificial tears**:
  - solutions of polyvinyl alcohol (very aqueous), dextran, methylcellulose, viscoelastic agents (chondroitin sulphate, sodium hyaluronate)
  - lanolin ointments, although the response to them is worse than with solutions.
- Reduce inflammation to the eye surface.
  - If the anti-inflammatory action of cyclosporine is not enough, **0.1% dexamethasone or 1% prednisolone** may be administered topically every 6–8 hours to reduce corneal vascularization. It is important to rule out the existence of corneal ulcers since they may evolve into corneal perforation.
  - Use **non-steroidal anti-inflammatory drugs (NSAIDs)** (flurbiprofen), with the same precautions.
- **Control secondary infections**. The presence of a purulent discharge does not imply a bacterial infection. If a corneal ulcer is present, topical antibiotics should be applied.
- Remove excess mucus. If washing is not enough, mucolytics such as topical 5% N-acetyl cysteine should be used temporarily.

In cases where there is no improvement after at least 6 months of medical therapy, **surgical treatment (transposition of the parotid duct)** can be performed, but it has many side effects, such as the appearance of a mineralized whitish substance on the ocular surface.

The use of inoculated stem cells directly into the glands is currently being investigated and has shown encouraging results.

## Cornea

### *General aspects*

The cornea is a **transparent fibrous tissue**. In domestic species, the horizontal diameter is greater than the vertical one. Thickness varies between species and corneal regions, but the range is 0.5–0.8 mm.

It consists of the following layers:

1. **stratified epithelium**, non-keratinized, with basement membrane and hemidesmosomes
2. **stroma**, which is mainly formed of collagen
3. **Descemet's membrane**
4. **endothelial**. It works as an ion pump between the stroma and aqueous humour, keeping the stroma relatively dehydrated. In adults, it has a limited regenerative capacity.

Because of its curvature and transparency, the cornea is **the ocular surface with the highest refractive optical power**.

The transparency of the cornea is due to:

- absence of blood vessels
- relative low cell density
- absence of melanin
- maintenance of a relative state of dehydration
- smooth optical surface (provided by the tear film)
- structure of stromal collagen fibrils
- absence of keratinization.

### *Congenital abnormalities of the cornea*

#### *Microcornea*

##### Diagnosis

This condition is generally **unilateral** and associated with **microphthalmia**.

Diagnosis is made by **comparing the vertical and horizontal diameters of the corneas of both eyes** (Figure 8.63).

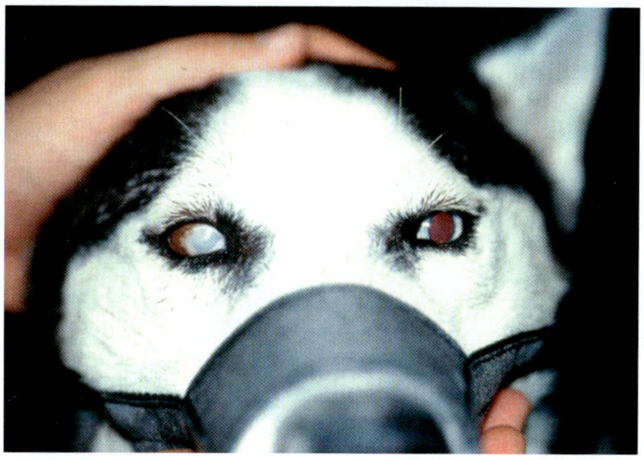

**Figure 8.63.** Microcornea in the right eye associated with microphthalmia.

#### *Dermoid cyst*

##### Definition

**Presence of skin and its associated structures attached to the corneal surface** (Figure 8.64).

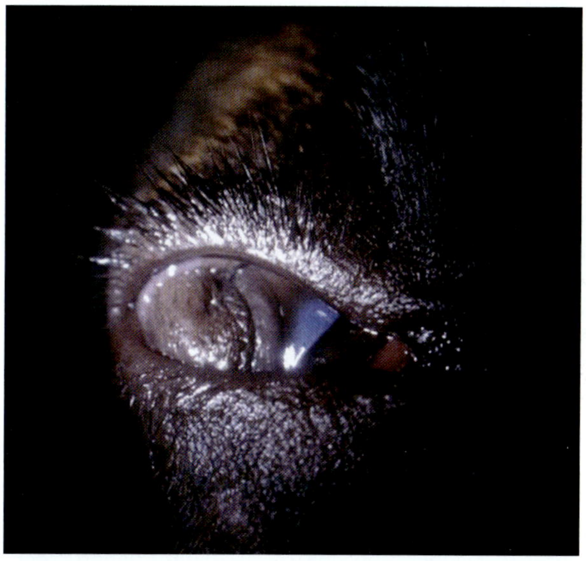

**Figure 8.64.** Corneal dermoid cyst.

Other structures such as the conjunctiva, the third eyelid, eyelid margin and the limbus may also be involved.

##### Epidemiology

It is considered hereditary in:

- Burmese cat
- some dog breeds, including the Dalmatian, St Bernard and dachshund.

##### Clinical signs

It can lead to:

- corneal opacity
- conjunctival hyperaemia
- ocular discharge.

##### Treatment

Surgical excision by keratectomy.

## *Persistent pupillary membranes*

### Aetiopathogenesis

Persistent pupillary membranes are a **hereditary abnormality** that arise as a failure of the uveal tract to regress during embryogenesis and postnatal development.

### Clinical signs

They can cause corneal opacity if they connect the iris collarette with the corneal endothelium, causing corneal oedema, melanosis and/or fibrosis (Figure 8.13).

The **effect on vision** varies according to severity and location.

### Treatment

These **do not require treatment**.

## *Corneal lipid dystrophy*

### Aetiopathogenesis

Deposit of lipids and, occasionally, minerals in the anterior stroma (Figure 8.65). The deposits are generally **central**, **static or very-slow-progressing**, and bilateral, and may be asymmetrical. They can take multiple forms (circular, oval and arch-shaped). **The condition is familial**.

### Epidemiology

It is common in dogs but rare in cats.

### Differential diagnosis

Corneal lipid dystrophy should be distinguished from corneal degeneration due to circulating hyperlipidaemia, taking the following characteristics of dystrophy into account:

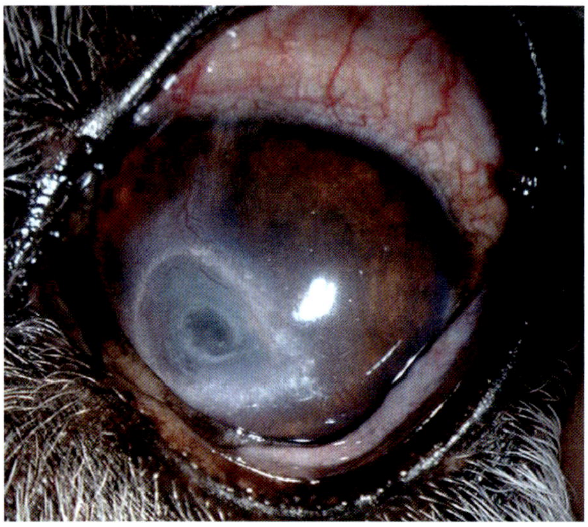

**Figure 8.65.** Lipid dystrophy. Note the lipid and mineral deposits in the anterior stroma.

- It is not inflammatory.
- There is no connection to the limbus.
- Animals have normal cholesterol and triglyceride levels.

# *Acquired abnormalities*

## *Corneal ulcer*

### Definition

Corneal ulcers are considered **a keratopathy where there is loss of epithelium and other corneal layers**.

They may also be called ulcerative keratitis because of the inflammatory phenomena that accompany the ulcer.

### Classification

**Depth-dependent** (Table 8.1):

- superficial
- deep
- descemetocele
- perforated.

According to **development:**

- complicated
- non-complicated. Ulcers resolve without veterinary attention.

Table 8.1. Classification of corneal ulcers.

| Type of ulcer | Affected layers | Development |
|---|---|---|
| Superficial | Epithelial, basal membrane, variable | Non-complicated, progressive |
| Some depth | Epithelial, basal membrane, 1/4–1/3 stroma | Non-complicated, progressive |
| Moderate | Epithelial, basal membrane, 1/2 stroma | Non-complicated, progressive |
| Deep | Epithelial, basal membrane, 2/3–3/4 stroma | Non-complicated, progressive |
| Descemetocele | Epithelial, basal membrane, stroma | Complicated, progressive |
| Prolapsed iris | Epithelial, basal membrane, stroma, Descemet's membrane, endothelial | Complicated, progressive |

## Aetiology

**Excessive abrasion of the cornea** may be caused by:

- endogenous causes:
  - abnormalities in eyelid conformation
  - eyelash abnormalities
  - tear film deficit
  - exophthalmos
  - buphthalmos.
- exogenous causes:
  - trauma
  - chemical substances
  - retention of foreign bodies in the conjunctival fornix
  - infectious agents; mainly viruses since bacteria alone do not primarily cause this abnormality.

## Clinical signs

Clinical signs of superficial ulcers include:

- **pain** because this is where the sensitive nerve endings are (less pain in brachycephalic dogs). The pain is manifested by:
  - **blepharospasm**
  - **photophobia**
  - lacrimation
  - serous or purulent discharge
  - irregular surface with peripheral oedema
  - superficial vascularization may appear quickly and is directed to the damaged area.

Clinical signs of **deep ulcers** include:

- increased surface irregularity
- **reduced pain**
- superficial and deep vascularization (perikeratic circle)
- rounded or oval shape, central location and, frequently, jelly-like appearance (Figure 8.66).

## Diagnosis

It is based on:

- clinical history
- Schirmer's test
- assessment of corneal and palpebral reflexes
- anatomical evaluation of the eyelids, conjunctiva and nictitating membrane (third eyelid)
- biomicroscopy
- culture, if infection is suspected
- fluorescein test (Figure 8.67). It is important to differentiate whether they are superficial ulcers, deep ulcers, descemetoceles or perforations.

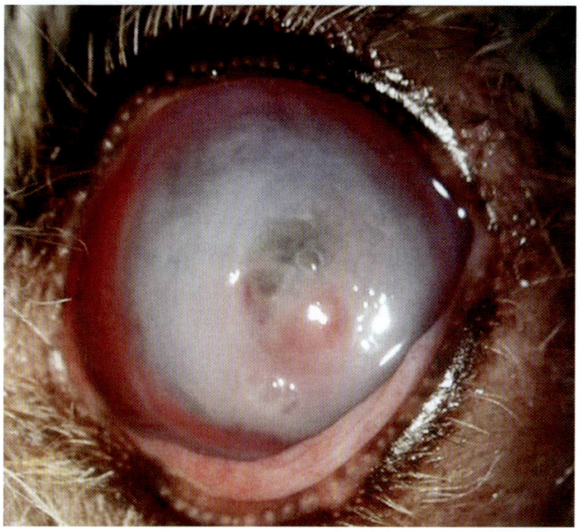

**Figure 8.66.** Deep corneal ulcer with a gelatinous appearance and perikeratic circle (melting ulcer).

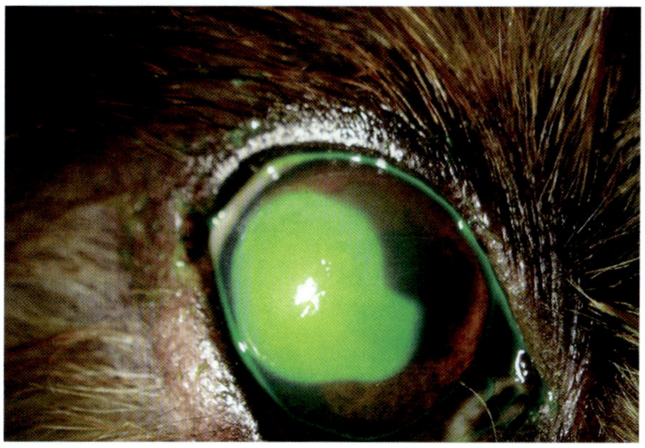

**Figure 8.67.** Corneal ulcer stained with fluorescein. Superficial vascularization and oedema can be seen.

## Treatment

Generally, **corticosteroids and topical NSAIDs are contraindicated** in the treatment of any type of ulcer.

### *Treatment of simple and superficial ulcers*

This consists of:

- eliminating the cause
- eliminating the pain. Topical administration of **1% atropine twice daily for 3 days**. In addition to reducing pain, atropine prevents the formation of synechiae (adhesions) if there is a concomitant uveitis.
- **topical broad-spectrum antibiotic therapy** should be administered three or four times daily.

If within 7 days signs have not resolved or there is no improvement, the aetiological diagnosis should be reconsidered.

### *Treatment of complicated or deep (stromal) ulcers and descemetoceles*

**These ulcers should always be considered infected.** Treatment consists of:

- administration of **specific topical antibiotics every hour for 1–2 days** and then 6 times daily
- control of tissue destruction with **collagenase inhibitors** (e.g. the animal's own serum, acetylcysteine or edetic acid)
- if the ulcer is deeper than half of the corneal thickness, a fibrovascular infiltration is required. This can be achieved quickly with the **placement of conjunctival grafts**.

## *Pigmentary keratitis*

### Aetiopathogenesis

Pigmentary keratitis, also called corneal melanosis, is simply a clinical sign of chronic keratitis due to:

- chronic exposure in brachycephalic breeds (Figure 8.68)
- eyelash abnormalities
- tear film abnormalities
- any combination thereof.

### Treatment

Aetiological treatment to stop further melanin deposits. The existing melanin will slowly disappear. Therefore, rapid detection of the cause and its correction is important.

## *Chronic superficial keratoconjunctivitis*

### Aetiopathogenesis

Also called **Uberreiter's syndrome**, this is an **immune-mediated condition** that causes inflammation of the cornea and conjunctiva. Note the **presence of pannus** (non-specific corneal vascularization). The exact aetiology is unknown, although the existence of cellular immunity against uveal and corneal antigens has been proved.

It occurs especially in **dogs that live at certain altitudes**; **ultraviolet radiation** is proposed as being responsible for altering tissue antigenicity in susceptible corneas.

### Pathophysiological development

1. In early stages, corneal epithelial cells proliferate and the superficial stroma is infiltrated by plasma cells and lymphocytes (Figure 8.69).
2. As the condition progresses, melanocytes, histiocytes and fibrocytes enter the cornea, and oedema and neovascularization are formed (Figure 8.70).
3. In more advanced stages, the corneal epithelium and anterior stroma become strongly melanotic and vascularized, and the epithelium is keratinized. A fibrous granulation tissue that retains fluorescein may also appear, giving the impression of an ulcer.

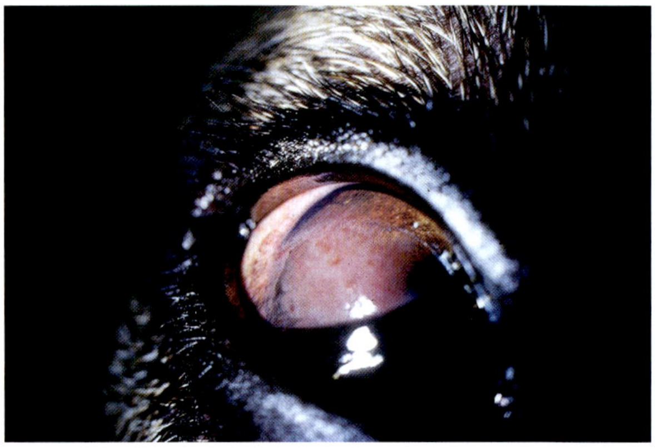

**Figure 8.69.** Superficial chronic keratoconjunctivitis in a German shepherd. Early stage (infiltration of plasma cells and lymphocytes).

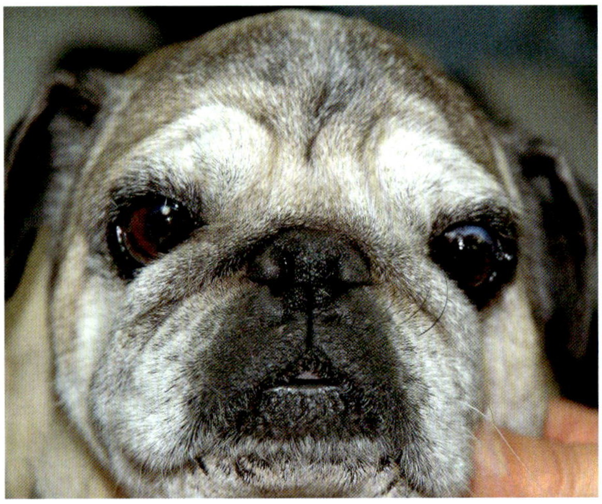

**Figure 8.68.** Pigmentary keratitis in a pug dog.

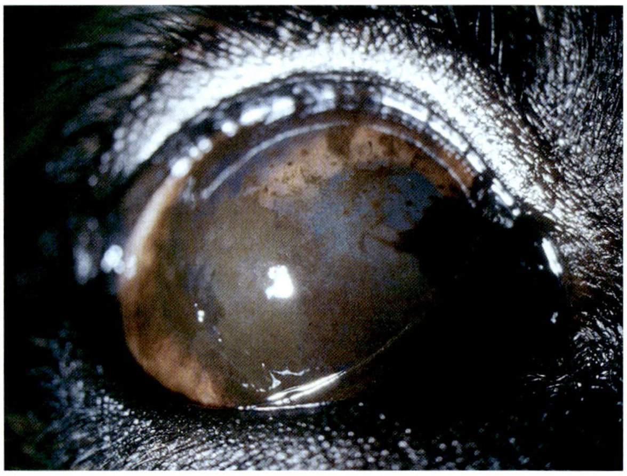

**Figure 8.70.** Superficial chronic keratoconjunctivitis in a German shepherd. Advanced stage (pigmentation and vascularization).

The condition can start, in order of importance, in the following quadrants:

1. temporal
2. nasal
3. lower
4. upper.

### Epidemiology

Although there is a predisposition in the **German shepherd and greyhound breeds**, it can affect any breed.

### Clinical signs

- **Vascularization and corneal melanosis** first appear in the temporal limbus and gradually extend towards the centre and other quadrants. The entire cornea may be affected and cause visual problems.
- **Oedema and corneal degeneration** are located 1–3 mm ahead of the advancing lesion.
- There is also **depigmentation, thickening of the free edge of the nictitating membrane** (**third eyelid**) and eye discharge, which may appear even before corneal lesions.

Lesions are more serious when the condition occurs at an early age.

### Diagnosis

Diagnosis is based on the history, clinical signs and corneoconjunctival cytology.

### Treatment

There is no cure. It is important to institute lifelong treatment, with the minimum medication necessary so that the condition does not progress or recur.

Initial treatment consists of:

- **topical corticosteroids** (0.1% dexamethasone or 1% prednisolone) 4 times daily
- **topical 2% cyclosporine A** twice daily.

At 3–4 weeks, animals generally show improvement and corticosteroids are discontinued, continuing exclusively with 2% cyclosporine A.

## *Corneal sequestration*

### Definition

Also called **feline corneal necrosis**, corneal mummification or keratitis nigrum.

### Aetiology

The cause of the condition is unknown.

It can occur in animals without any ophthalmic history, although it usually happens after the following:

- chronic ulcers
- herpesvirus.

### Epidemiology

It affects all breeds of cat but breeds with a predisposition are **Persian, Burmese, Himalayan and Siamese.**

There are also cases described in the dog.

### Clinical signs

The most typical sign is the appearance in the cornea of **an amber or black focus**, usually centrally, **surrounded by a wider area of superficial ulceration** (Figure 8.71). The black material is pigmented, necrotic cornea, not melanin.

The lesions are painful, causing blepharospasm and epiphora.

Depending on the chronicity, it can be accompanied by:

- vascularization
- oedema
- infiltration of white blood cells into the stroma as a reaction to necrotic tissue.

### Treatment

Surgical removal by keratectomy; if necessary, placement of a conjunctival graft or amniotic membrane is recommended.

## *Neoplasms*

### Aetiopathogenesis

The cornea and sclera are not the origin of tumours, rather they are important barriers that prevent the diffusion of intraocular neoplasms to other parts of the body, and the diffusion of orbital tumours and attached organs.

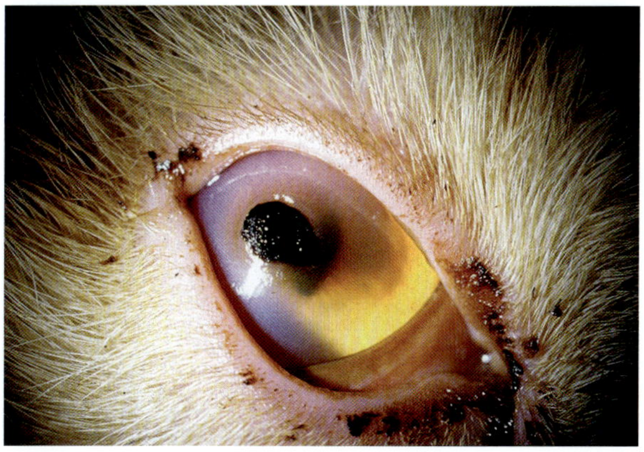

**Figure 8.71.** Corneal sequestration in a cat.

The **only place prone to the formation of neoplasms is the sclerocorneal limbus**.

The tumours seen most frequently are:

- haemangiomas/haemangiosarcomas
- limbal melanoma (Figure 8.72).

### Epidemiology

**Primary corneal tumours are rare**.

## Uvea

### *General aspects*

Anatomically, the uveal tract is divided into two areas:

- **anterior uvea**, consisting of the iris and ciliary body
- **posterior uvea**, formed by the choroid.

The uveal tract plays an important role in maintaining the **blood–eye barrier**. The conditions that affect the uveal tract frequently cause this barrier to break, allowing the **exudation of excessive amounts of proteins or cells in the aqueous and vitreous humours, and the subretinal space**.

The blood–eye barrier is formed by:

- the blood–retinal barrier, which consists of:
  - the vascular endothelium of the retinal capillaries
  - the pigmented epithelium of the retina.
- the **blood–water barrier**, which consists of:
  - the vascular endothelium of the iris
  - the non-pigmented epithelium of the ciliary body.

Most large molecules, especially proteins, cannot pass through or between the cells that make up these barriers.

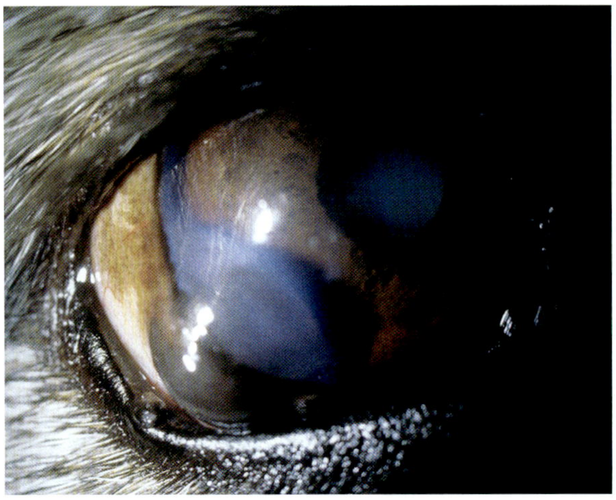

**Figure 8.72.** Limbal melanoma in a dog.

### *Abnormalities*

### *Uveitis*

#### Definition

**Uveitis refers to inflammation of part or all the uveal tract**, consisting of the iris, ciliary body and choroid.

#### Classification

The classification of uveitis depends on the **area affected**:

- **anterior** uveitis (affecting the iris and possibly the ciliary body)
- **posterior** uveitis (affecting the choroid)
- **panuveitis** (uveal tract).

According to the **histological nature**:

- suppurative uveitis
- non-suppurative uveitis
- granulomatous uveitis
- non-granulomatous uveitis.

According to the **starting point** of the condition:

- endogenous uveitis
- exogenous uveitis.

According to **the aetiology**:

- **infectious**:
  - **viral**.
    - canine distemper
    - adenovirus type 1 and 2 (naturally or post-vaccination causing 'blue eye disease')
    - feline infectious peritonitis (most frequent in cats)
    - feline leukaemia virus
    - feline immunodeficiency virus (FIV)
    - canine and feline herpesvirus.
  - **bacterial**.
    - septicaemia/endotoxaemia due to any cause
    - leptospirosis
    - brucellosis
    - borreliosis (Lyme disease).
  - **parasitic**.
    - protozoal (leishmaniasis, toxoplasmosis and babesiosis)
    - rickettsial (ehrlichiosis)
    - helminthic (dirofilariasis, ascariasis)
  - **fungal** (uncommon).
    - aspergillosis
    - blastomycosis
    - histoplasmosis
    - cryptococcosis.

- **immunological**:
  - uveodermatological syndrome
  - phaco-induced uveitis
  - vasculitis
  - thrombocytopenia.
- **metabolic**:
  - diabetes mellitus
  - systemic hypertension
  - hyperlipidaemia.
- **systemic**:
  - pyometra
  - prostatitis.
- **traumatic**:
  - penetrating injuries (including iatrogenic after surgery)
  - blunt trauma.
- **neoplastic**. Almost all primary or secondary eye tumours cause uveitis. Some of the most frequent are:
  - melanoma
  - lymphosarcoma.
- **pharmacological**:
  - prostaglandin-derived medications (latanoprost)
  - pilocarpine and other parasympathomimetics.

Despite all the classifications, there are **many cases of idiopathic uveitis** (possibly immune-mediated) where treatment should be aimed at treating inflammation and avoiding subsequent damage.

## Clinical signs

Clinical signs include:

- **pain** (photophobia, blepharospasm, epiphora and even anorexia and depression)
- conjunctival hyperaemia and **circumcorneal ciliary injection** (deep, perilimbal and parallel vessels)
- **corneal oedema**. Endothelial damage (Figure 8.73)
- reduction or disappearance of pupillary reflexes (mainly posterior)
- **miosis**. Irritation of the pupillary sphincter muscle by prostaglandins. Resistance to pharmacological mydriasis
- **reduced intraocular pressure**. Inflammation of the ciliary processes decreasing aqueous humour production
- **hyperpigmentation of the iris**, oedema, neovessels and irregular surface
- **Tyndall effect**. Disruption of the blood–eye barrier with protein loss. Rated from 0 to +4. There is also an outflow of cells (lymphocytes, neutrophils and erythrocytes), which if present in large quantities form a sediment and cause **hypopyon and hyphaema** (Figure 8.74). In the case of posterior

Table 8.2. Differential diagnoses for a red eye.

| | Conjunctivitis | Keratitis | Ulcerative keratitis | Uveitis | Glaucoma |
|---|---|---|---|---|---|
| IOP | Normal | Normal | Normal | Low | High |
| Pupillary size | Normal | Normal | Normal | Miosis | Mydriasis |
| Fluorescein | Negative | Negative | Positive | Negative | Negative |
| Neovascularization | Absent | Present | Present | Possible | Possible |

IOP, intraocular pressure.

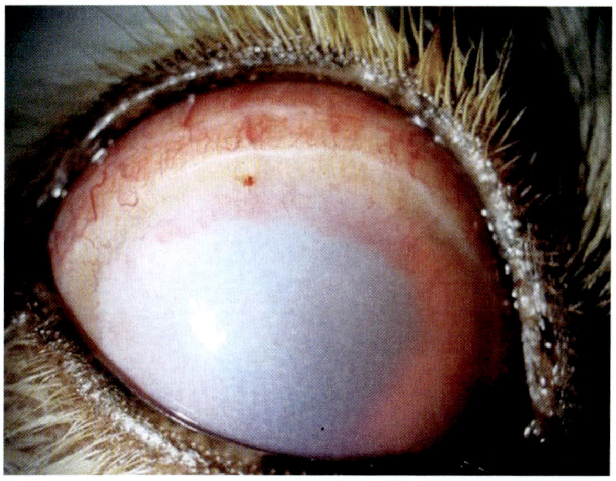

**Figure 8.73.** Uveitis. Note the reddening of the eye, corneal oedema and neovascularization.

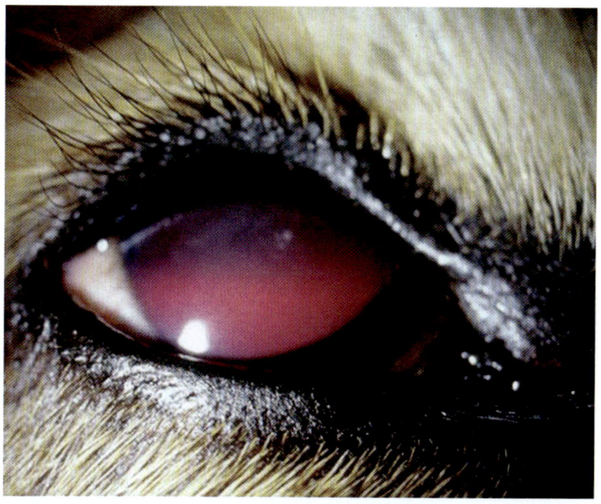

**Figure 8.74.** Hyphaema associated with uveitis.

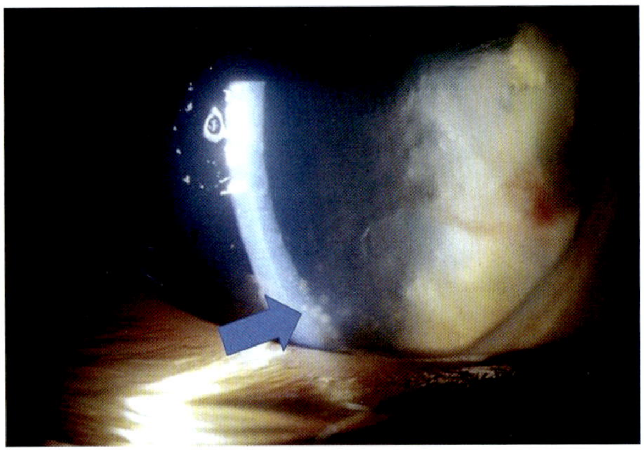

Figure 8.75. Uveitis. Note the presence of corneal precipitates in the endothelium (arrow).

uveitis, this phenomenon also appears in the vitreous, originating from the retinal and the choroid vessels.
- **corneal precipitates**. Inflammatory cells that adhere to the inferior corneal endothelium (Figure 8.75)
- **loss of vision** (in posterior uveitis)
- **retinal oedema** and exudates; chorioretinitis (greyish spots with diffuse edges in the tapetal area)
- **vasculitis and vascular sleeves**, due to accumulation of proteins and cells.

Sequelae of uveitis include:

- **posterior and anterior synechiae**, the union of the iris with the anterior capsule of the lens and with the endothelium of the cornea (Figures 8.76 and 8.77)
- **cataract** due to the action of prostaglandins and abnormalities in the aqueous humour
- atrophy of the pigmentary epithelium and iris stroma
- **atrophy of the ciliary body**, which causes a cease in production of aqueous humour (phthisis bulbi) (Figure 8.78)
- **retinal detachment**

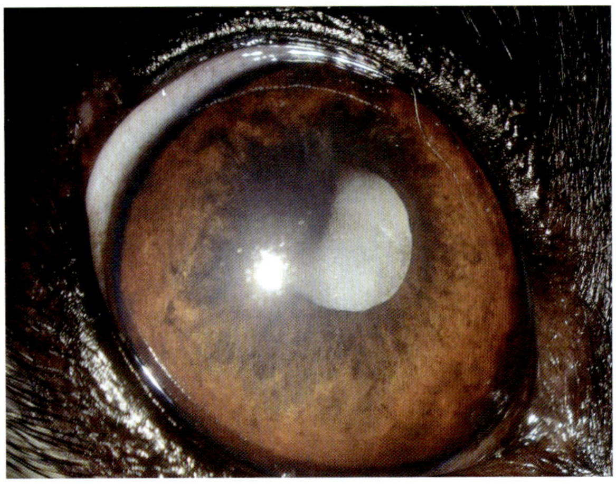

Figure 8.76. Sequelae of uveitis in a dog: posterior synechiae and cataract.

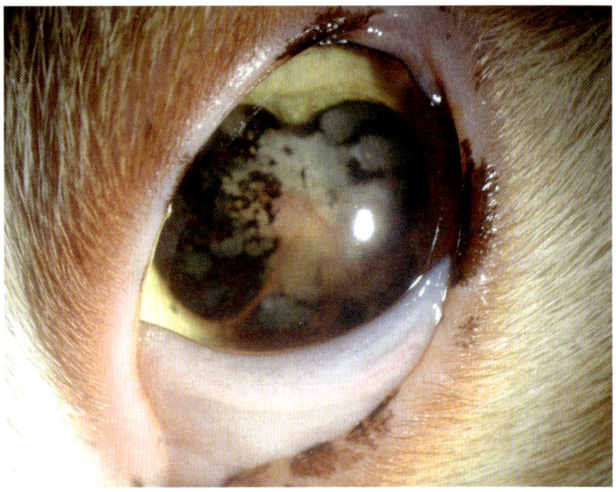

Figure 8.77. Sequelae of uveitis in a cat: posterior synechiae and cataract.

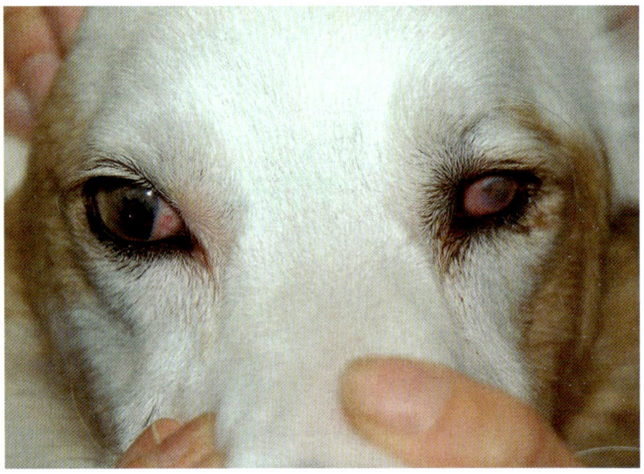

Figure 8.78. Sequelae of uveitis: phthisis bulbi of the left eye.

- **glaucoma** due to synechiae or blockage of the iridocorneal angle by cells (hypertensive uveitis)
- posterior capsular opacities (consequence of the Tyndall effect on the vitreous).

## Diagnosis

A diagnosis of uveitis is made based on:

- clinical history
- clinical signs
- biomicroscopy
- tonometry
- ophthalmoscopy
- investigation into the aetiology.

## Treatment

Treatment consists of:

- **topical** (dexamethasone and prednisolone) and **systemic corticosteroids** (prednisolone 1 mg/kg/d)
- **topical NSAIDs** in combination with corticosteroids (flurbiprofen, ketorolac)

- **mydriatic/cycloplegic agents**. Used to relieve spasm of the ciliary muscle and iris muscle sphincter and help reduce the formation of synechiae. The most commonly used agent is 0.5–1% atropine/12 h for 5 days.
- in cases of **increased IOP**, systemic carbonic anhydrase inhibitors (dorzolamide or methazolamide) and topical beta blockers (timolol) should be used.
- **immunosuppressants**. When there is no response to corticosteroids or the cause is immunopathological, as in phaco-induced uveitis, systemic azathioprine and 2% topical ciclosporine can be used.
- **plasminogen activators** (the aim is to reduce fibrin clots by intracameral (into the eye cavity) injection)
- specific treatment (when possible, identify the cause)
- in some cases, **prophylactic systemic antibiotic therapy** (amoxicillin, trimethoprim, cephalosporins or chloramphenicol).

## Aqueous humour

### *General aspects*

The production and drainage of aqueous humour are influenced by the anatomy of the anterior segment, plus several endogenous components including neurotransmitters, hormones, prostaglandins, proteins, lipids and proteoglycans.

**Aqueous humour is produced in the ciliary body** by:

- **active processes**, that is, selective transport of large or charged molecules against a concentration gradient, thanks to complex enzymatic reactions where carbonic anhydrase plays an important role
- **passive processes**:
  - diffusion (fat-soluble substances)
  - ultrafiltration (water-soluble substances).

Once produced, aqueous humour passes along the following routes:

- **Conventional**. Aqueous humour passes from the posterior chamber, through the pupil, to the anterior chamber. Due to temperature differences between the cornea and the iris, **convection currents** occurring in the anterior chamber cause the aqueous humour to pass through the pectinate ligaments and the ciliary cleft (iridocorneal angle), where the trabecular network is located (mesh of veins that drain into the intrascleral venous plexus and, subsequently, the ciliary, conjunctival and vorticose veins).
- **Non-conventional**. A small percentage of aqueous humour drains by uveoscleral flow, passes through the stroma of the iris and the interstitial spaces of the ciliary muscle to reach the supraciliary space (between the ciliary body and sclera) or the suprachoroidal space (between the choroid and sclera).

For the **IOP to remain stable (15–25 mmHg), the amounts of aqueous humour formed and removed must be equal**.

Any structural, biochemical or cellular alteration that involves an obstruction to the outflow of the aqueous humour leads to an increase in IOP.

**IOP varies**:

- throughout the day:
  - In dogs, it is greater in the morning and decreases until night-time.
  - In cats, it is lower in the morning and increases until night-time.
- with age: IOP decreases as the animal ages.

### *Abnormalities*

#### *Glaucoma*

#### Aetiopathogenesis

Glaucoma is considered as a group of **diverse pathologies** sharing the common presentation of **raised IOP** that is **too high to allow normal functioning** of the optic nerve and retina. Therefore, this causes a progressive deterioration of visual function and even blindness.

Characteristic changes in glaucoma include:

- **optic neuropathy** (damage to the axoplasmic flow in the head of the optic nerve)
- **death of retinal ganglion cells** and their axons
- **excavation of the optic nerve**.

#### Classification

- **Primary glaucoma** is **bilateral**, usually asynchronous, and has a **breed predisposition** and genetic basis. It can be of two types:
  - **Open angle**. Gonioscopy of the angle is normal. Glaucoma is caused by an increase in resistance in drainage channels. Predisposed breed: beagle.
  - **Closed angle**. There is obstruction of the iridocorneal angle due to dysplasia of the pectinate ligament or goniodysgenesis. Predisposed breeds: basset hound, English and American cocker spaniel, husky, chihuahua, miniature poodle.
- **Secondary glaucoma** is associated with other **ocular or systemic pathologies** that alter the dynamics of the aqueous humour. Secondary glaucoma can be unilateral or bilateral, hereditary or non-hereditary.

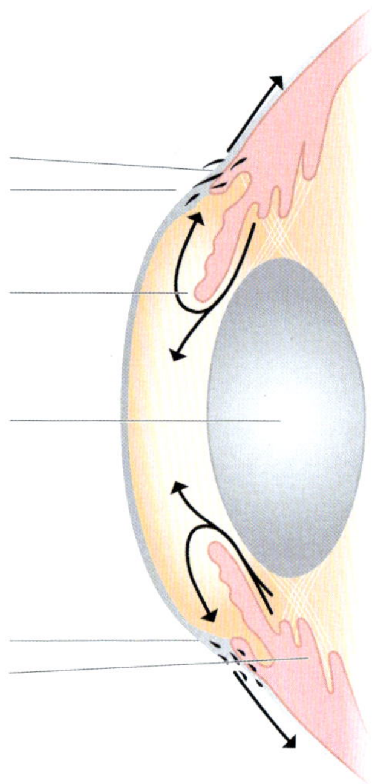


**Figure 8.79.** Causes of secondary glaucoma.

The iridocorneal angle may be open or closed. The most frequent causes are (Figure 8.79):

- **Uveitis**. This is obstruction of the drainage angle due to changes in the aqueous humour (proteins, cells and detritus) due to inflammation, oedema of the trabecular weave, and formation of anterior and posterior synechiae (Figure 8.80).
- Dislocation or **subluxation of the lens**. It causes a pupillary block or displaces the base of the iris, closing the angle. In the case of posterior dislocation, the vitreous is herniated anteriorly blocking the angle.
- **Intumescent cataracts**. The increase in the anteroposterior axis of the lens reduces the space between the lens and pupil.
- **Intraocular neoplasms**. Cause forward shifts in the lens and/or iris that cause closure of the angle. There may also be infiltration of tumour cells into the trabecular space.
- **Intraocular haemorrhages** due to tumours, trauma or uveitis.

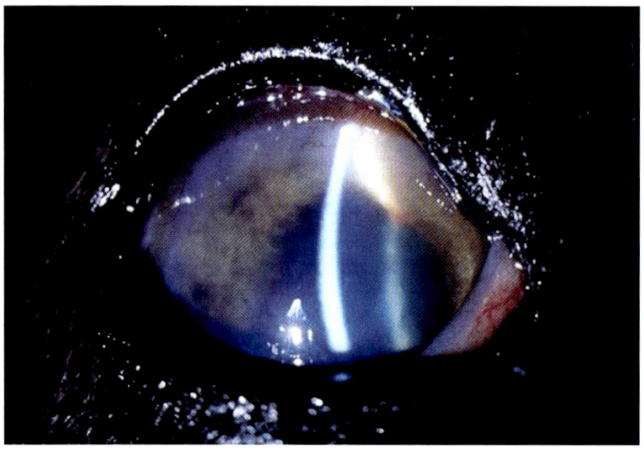

**Figure 8.80.** Blocked iridocorneal angle in hypertensive uveitis.

## Clinical signs

It is essential to consider whether the lesions and clinical signs observed are associated with or are a result of the cause of the pressure increase.

The appearance of one or another clinical sign depends on the duration, intensity and cause of the IOP.

In the early stages of glaucoma (vision sustained), the eye may appear normal and the IOP may or may not be elevated. In some patients there is only a clinical history of intermittent episcleral injection (especially at night) that resolves spontaneously, with normal IOP.

Clinical signs include:

- **pain**. This is characterized by **blepharospasm**, **pain on palpation** and behavioural changes (such as increased sleep and lack of play). If the condition is not treated, it becomes chronic pain, which the owner usually blames on the animal ageing.
- **episcleral congestion**. It consists of increased flow to episcleral veins in the limbus.
- **corneal oedema**. This is significant in acute cases and due to malfunction of the corneal endothelium. Chronic corneal oedema stimulates proliferation of limbal vessels (corneal neovascularization) and the appearance of pigment.
- **buphthalmos** (Figure 8.81) and **Descemet's membrane rupture** (Figure 8.82) occur in chronic cases. These abnormalities are more pronounced in young animals and in the Shar-Pei since the cornea and sclera are more distended than in adults. It is considered irreversible and incompatible with

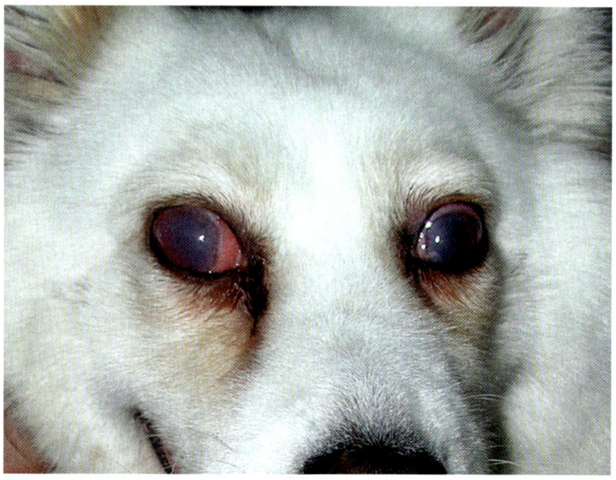

**Figure 8.81.** Glaucoma with bilateral buphthalmos.

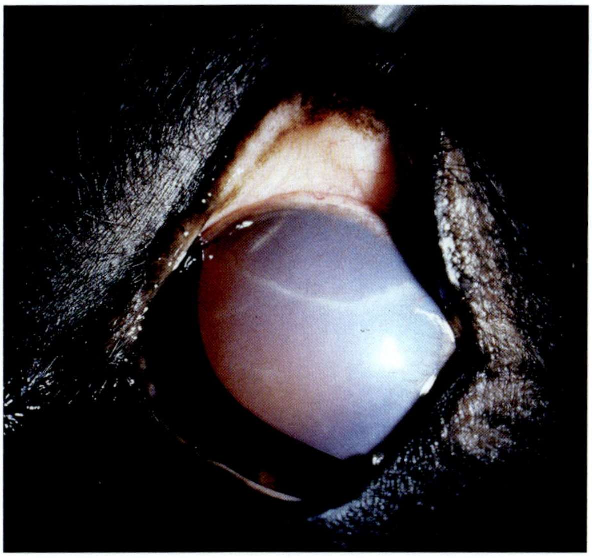

Figure 8.82. Glaucoma. Note corneal oedema and Descemet's membrane rupture (whiter line).

maintaining vision. There may be exposure keratitis due to the inability to close the eyelid and rupture of ciliary zonule fibres (lens dislocation).

- **mydriasis** due to ischaemia of the pupillary constrictor muscle. In chronic cases, **direct and consensual pupillary reflexes disappear**.
- **cataracts** due to metabolic changes caused by aqueous humour accumulation (Figure 8.83).
- excavation and **atrophy of the optic nerve**. It occurs from the early stages of glaucoma.
- **retinal degeneration** occurs in the later stages. It is manifested as **tapetal hyperreflectivity**, attenuation of retinal vessels and peripapillary hyperpigmentation (Figure 8.84).

## Diagnosis

The diagnosis of glaucoma is based on the clinical signs, tonometry, gonioscopy, ophthalmoscopy and OCT (Figure 8.85).

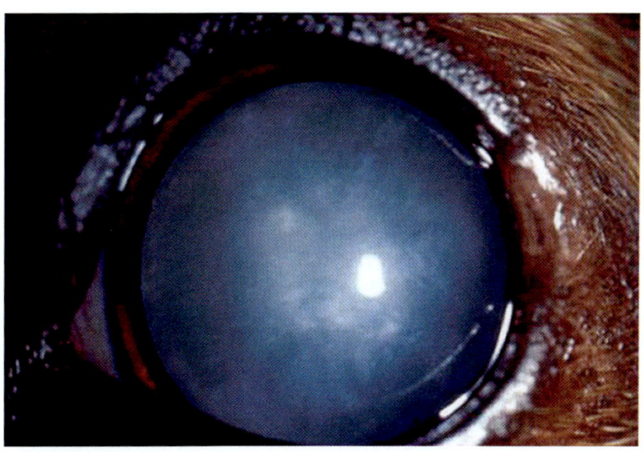

Figure 8.83. Glaucoma with complete mydriasis and cataract formation.

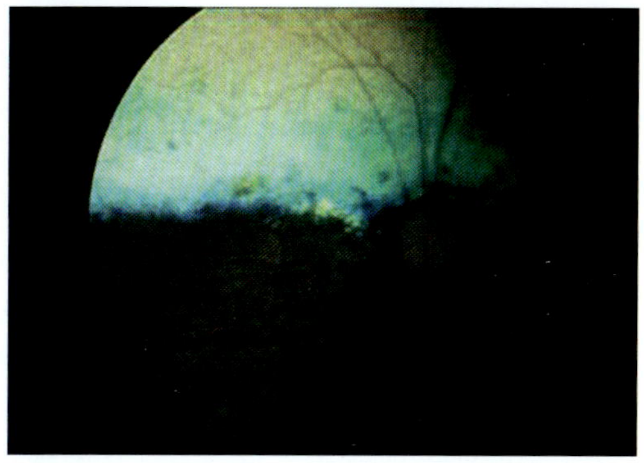

Figure 8.84. Glaucoma with retinal degeneration (tapetal hyperreflectivity and papillary hyperpigmentation).

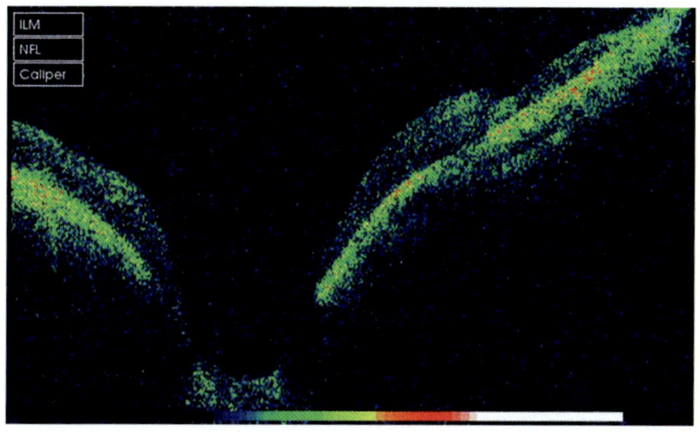


Figure 8.85. Glaucoma. OCT image where excavation of the optic nerve can be appreciated.

### *Tonometry*

To detect early-stage glaucoma, **IOP should be measured when the eye is red**, repeating the measurement 24 hours later.

Care should be taken with animals that are not collaborative since they may have high IOP values without glaucoma simply because they have been held around the neck.

In the presence of clinical signs of glaucoma, a presumptive diagnosis of glaucoma can be made if IOP values are:

- higher than 25 mmHg in dogs
- higher than 27 mmHg in cats.

At pressures greater than 40 mmHg, blindness can occur in 48–72 hours.

## Treatment

There are both medical and surgical treatments in the therapeutic protocol for glaucoma (Figure 8.86).

### *Medical treatment*

Medical treatment involves:

- **osmotic diuresis**. This is achieved with hyperosmolar agents such as **mannitol**, which raise plasma

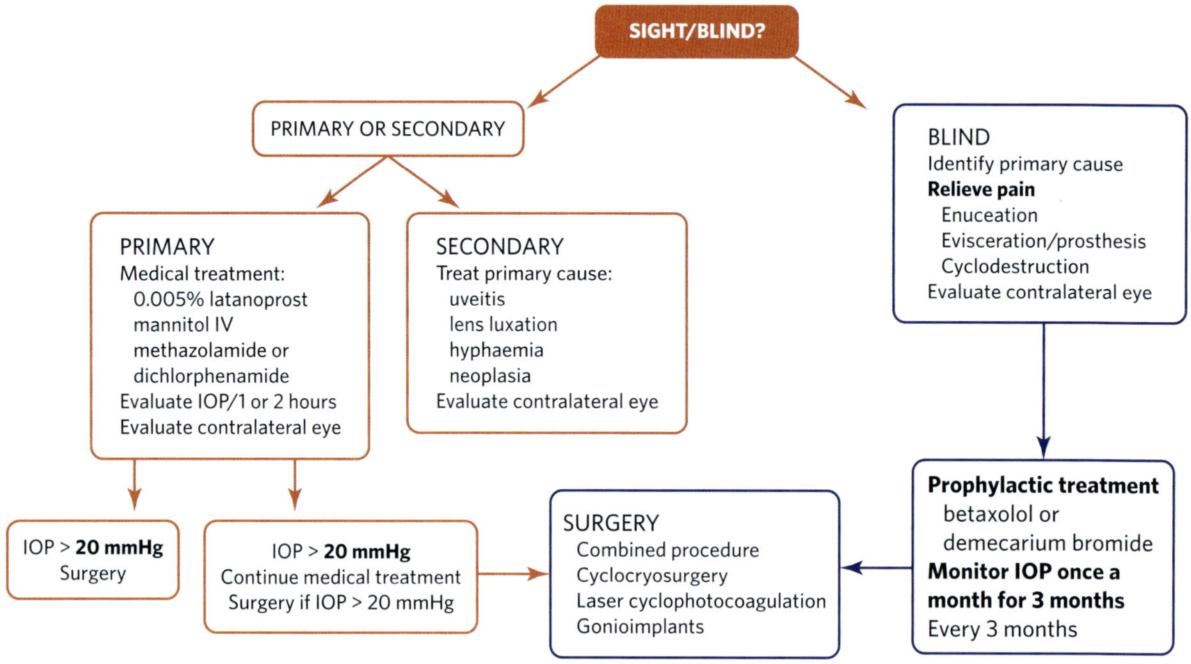


**Figure 8.86.** Glaucoma treatment protocol.

osmolarity, displacing intraocular fluid into the blood vessels. It is used in acute glaucoma. **Dose: 1–2 g/kg intravenously over 20 minutes**, effective 30 minutes after administration. It can be repeated at 4–6 hours, if necessary. Caution should be exercised in patients with congestive heart failure (lung oedema).

- **decreased aqueous humour production**:
  - **carbonic anhydrase inhibitors**. Reduction of aqueous humour production up to 50% within 40 minutes of their administration. Systemic: diclofenamide (2–4 mg/kg/8 h by mouth) and acetazolamide (5–10 mg/kg/8–12 h by mouth). Topical: dorzolamide every 8 hours.
  - **beta adrenergic blocking agents**. They do not affect the pupil. Topical 0.5% timolol maleate/12 h. Its effect is in addition to carbonic anhydrase inhibitors, and cholinergic and adrenergic agonists.
- **increased aqueous humour outflow**:
  - **Cholinergic or miotic agonists**. They contract the ciliary muscle and open the intertrabecular ducts. They are useful in open angle glaucoma; 2% pilocarpine/6 h is used. Contraindicated in uveitis.
  - **Alpha adrenergic agonists**. They act in the trabecular space. Dipivefrin and apraclonidine (additive effect together with beta adrenergic agents).
  - Topical prostaglandins. They increase uveoscleral flow. Topical latanoprost every 24 hours.
  - **Topical corticosteroids**. Pressure-induced ischaemia causes intraocular inflammation. Topical 0.1% dexamethasone/8 h and topical 1% prednisolone/8 h.

### *Surgical treatment*

**This is the treatment of choice in narrow or closed angle glaucoma** when the animal can still see. The following techniques are used:

- gonioimplants
- laser cyclophotocoagulation
- cyclocryotherapy
- combined techniques
- enucleation. When vision loss is irreversible, enucleation or evisceration and placement of an intrascleral prosthesis is recommended.

### Prognosis

**Prognosis is always poor** since lesions affecting the retina and optic nerve are irreversible.

## Lens

### *General aspects*

The intraocular lens is **biconvex, transparent and avascular**. Its anterior surface is less curved than the posterior one. It is formed of:

- **the capsule**. This is **transparent, elastic** and wraps around the lens. It provides the insertion for the zonular fibres, which suspend the lens within the eye. The capsule is impermeable to large molecules (albumin and globulin) but allows the passage of water and electrolytes. The anterior part is thicker than the

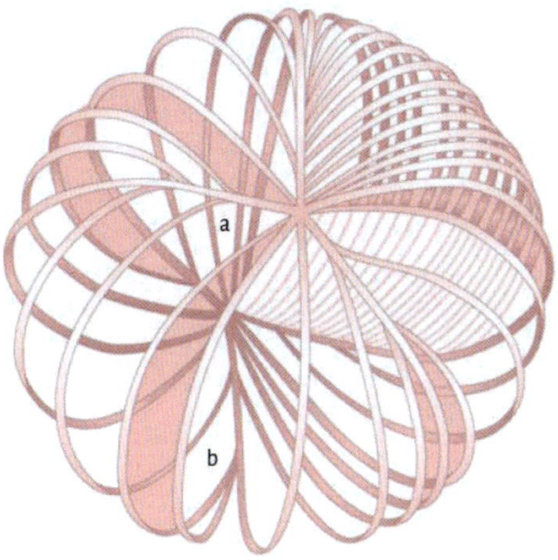


**Figure 8.87.** Concentric layers of the lens converging on the (a) anterior and (b) posterior suture lines.

posterior and has an epithelium on the internal face that reaches the equatorial zone.
- **the lens**. The lens is formed by soluble or crystalline, insoluble proteins (35%) or albuminoids, which form **concentric sheets** that converge in the anterior and posterior parts, constituting **Y-shaped or inverted Y-shaped suture lines**, respectively (Figure 8.87).

## Congenital anomalies

Congenital anomalies are infrequent and include the following:

- **aphakia** (absence of the lens)
- **microphakia** (small crystalline lens that is associated with other ocular malformations)
- **spherophakia** (spherical lens)
- **lenticonus** (anterior or posterior protrusion of the lens capsule, which is usually axial in location). A posterior conus is usually associated with the presence of a persistent hyperplastic hyaloid and primary vitreous artery
- **coloboma** (defects in the lens equator associated with **similar defects in the ciliary body and zonule**)
- **congenital cataract** (lens opacity).

## Cataract

### Aetiopathogenesis

The term cataract includes a group of ocular abnormalities that **manifest with loss of transparency of the lens or its capsule**. These opacities may vary in shape, size, location, aetiology, age of onset and degree of progression.

The biochemistry of the lens is complex; therefore, any abnormality of the following can cause cataract formation:

- nutrition of the lens
- energy and protein metabolism
- osmotic balance.

### Classification

Cataracts are classified according to the **degree of maturation**:

- **incipient**. 10–15% of the lens is opaque (Figure 8.88). Vision is not affected.
- **immature**. Less than 40% of the lens is affected (Figure 8.89). The tapetal reflex is visible but ophthalmoscopically there are partially obscured areas in the fundus. The animal's vision is like looking through dirty glasses.
- **mature**. The lens is completely opaque and the animal is blind (Figure 8.90). There is no tapetal reflex and the fundus cannot be visualized ophthalmoscopically.
- **hypermature**. Some mature cataracts evolve to be hypermature by liquefaction (proteolysis) in the cortex that progresses towards the nucleus (Figure 8.91), causing the appearance of the tapetal reflex. This

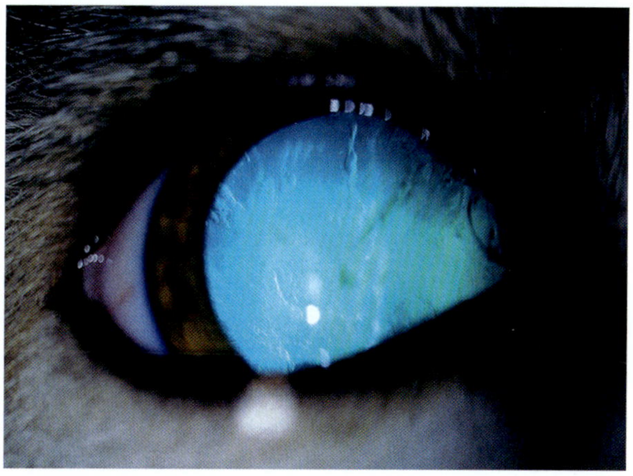

**Figure 8.88.** Incipient cataract.

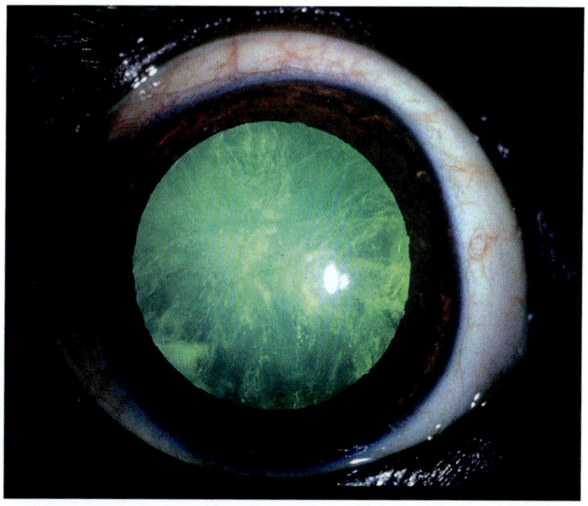

**Figure 8.89.** Immature cataract.

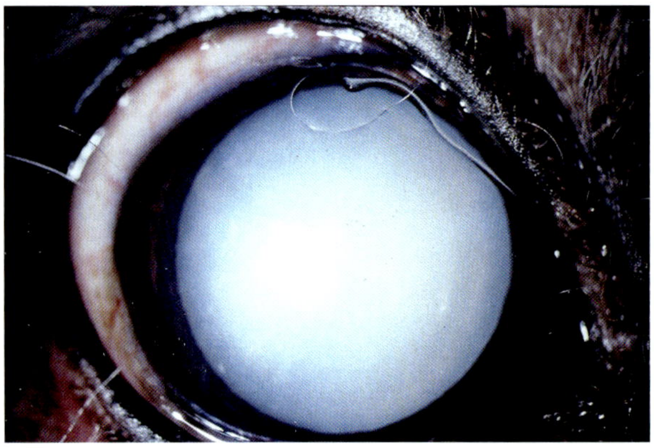

**Figure 8.90.** Mature cataract.

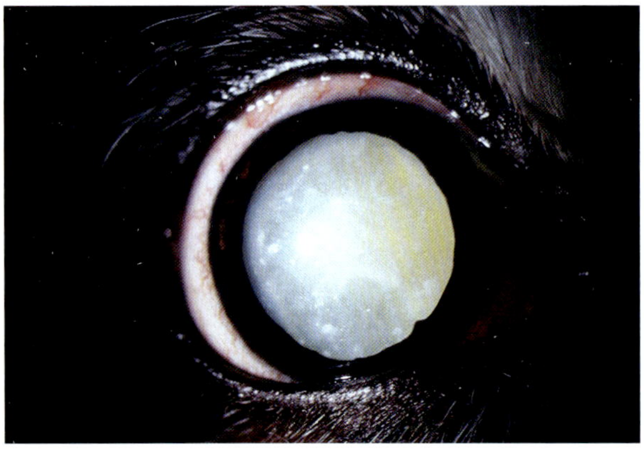

**Figure 8.91.** Hypermature cataract. Note the appearance of a red eye and peripheral liquefaction.

degradation of proteins causes them to leave the anterior chamber, causing inflammation. The **capsule looks wrinkled**.

Depending on the **location of the opacity**:

- anterior or posterior capsular
- anterior or posterior subcapsular
- cortical
- equatorial
- nuclear.

According to **age at the time of appearance**:

- **congenital**. These lens abnormalities occur during foetal development and present at birth. **Not all congenital cataracts are inherited**, they can also be secondary to developmental abnormalities (persistent pupillary membranes, hyperplastic primary vitreous, persistence of the hyaloid artery, microphthalmia) or maternal influence. The breeds of dog with the highest prevalence of hereditary cataracts are the Afghan hound, American cocker spaniel, bichon frise, Boston terrier, German shepherd, golden retriever, Labrador retriever, miniature schnauzer, Old English sheepdog, miniature and toy poodle, and Staffordshire bull terrier. Congenital cataracts are very rare in cats.
- **juvenile**, in animals under 3 years of age
- **adult**, in animals of 3–8 years of age
- **senile**, in animals older than 8 years of age. Progression is extremely slow. There is some controversy over whether they are late-onset hereditary cataracts.

According to the **consistency**:

- fluid
- hard
- soft.

Depending on **aetiology and pathogenesis**:

- **primary (hereditary)**
- **secondary**. **Traumatic**, due to intraocular conditions (uveitis and infections), **nutritional** in origin (hypocalcaemia, hypothyroidism, Cushing's syndrome) or due to progressive retinal atrophy, radiation, diabetes, external toxic agents, congenital or senile anomalies.

### *Clinical signs*

The clinical signs manifest as:

- **visual deficit** that becomes evident when opacity affects more than 50% of the lens (depending on the location of the opacity)
- **white pupil** (leukocoria).

### *Diagnosis*

A diagnosis should be made based on:

- history (white pupils)
- biomicroscopy after pupillary dilation
- tonometry, which is important in lenses with increased anteroposterior diameter
- retroillumination
- ophthalmoscopy, which allows examination of the retina in the presence of incipient and immature cataracts
- ultrasonography
- electroretinography to assess retinal abnormalities that can cause secondary cataracts.

### *Treatment*

#### Medical treatment

The **use of antioxidants** (selenium, vitamin E, orgotein, zinc ascorbate and carnosine) and aldose reductase inhibitors in very early diabetic cataracts is in the experimental stages.

### Surgical treatment

Surgical treatment (Figure 8.92) consists of phacoemulsification and placement of an intraocular lens.

Before proceeding to surgery, the following should be assessed:

- Ensure that the visual deficit is significant.
- Use electroretinography to assess the probability of restoring vision to the patient.
- Treat uveitis if it is present.
- Rule out other eye abnormalities.
- Rule out systemic diseases through preoperative testing and general physical examination.
- Ensure that animals can be managed correctly (collaboration) to administer postsurgical treatments.
- Confirm that the owner can administer postsurgical treatment and cover the cost.
- Explain the surgical and postsurgical risks in geriatric animals to the owner.

## Sclerosis

### Aetiopathogenesis

Throughout life, **new lens cells are produced at the equator**; these new cells move the old cells towards the nucleus, which is compressed, making the nucleus denser and harder.

**Sclerosis is associated with an increase in insoluble proteins and a decrease in soluble (crystalline) proteins in the lens nucleus**.

### Clinical signs

In dogs, after 6 years of age, a kind of **fog or blue-grey reflection** starts to become visible. Advanced sclerosis is often confused, by owners and clinicians, with cataracts. However, in most animals, except in severe cases, visual function is not affected.

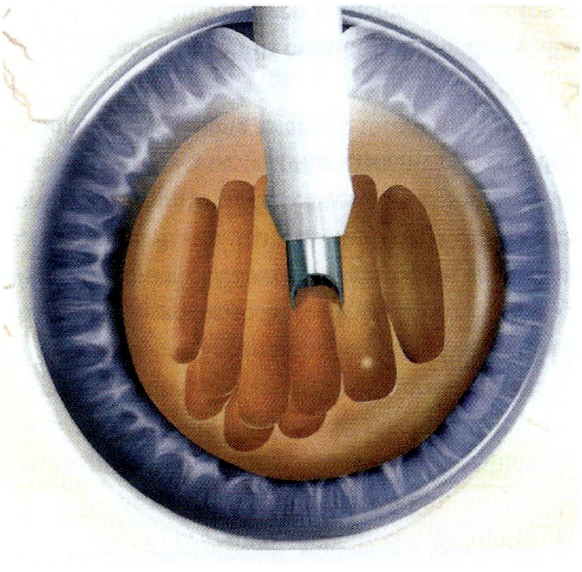

Figure 8.92. Image of phacoemulsification for the surgical treatment of cataracts.

### Diagnosis

Via retroillumination, prior pupillary dilation (there is a reflection of the tapetal area) (Figure 8.93) and **ophthalmoscopic visualization of the fundus**.

## Dislocation/subluxation of the lens

### Aetiopathogenesis

Dislocation of the lens occurs when the **lens becomes detached from the zonule**, which means the hyaloid fossa can be displaced. The lens can **move anteriorly**, **posteriorly and in the vertical** plane.

Dislocation may be **preceded by subluxation** resulting from the breakage of part of the zonule, with partial displacement of the lens.

### Aetiological classification

Dislocation of the lens may be classified as:

- **primary**, due to a weakening of the zonula and its rupture (from 5 years of age onwards). It is more frequent in dogs and hereditary in some terrier breeds, the bull terrier and miniature schnauzer.
- **secondary**:
  - **trauma**
  - **blunt trauma** (violent impacts in the orbital area)
  - **perforation** (e.g. cat scratches)
  - **glaucoma**. In chronic cases, enlargement of the eyeball predisposes to partial (subluxation) or total (dislocation) rupture of the zonule.
  - **uveitis**. Alterations to the aqueous humour and the presence of inflammatory mediators in the posterior chamber can weaken the zonule.

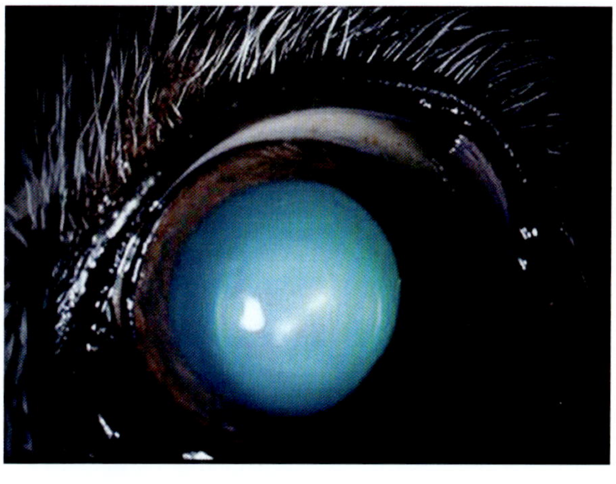

Figure 8.93. Sclerosis of the lens.

- **intraocular neoplasms**. The growth of neoplasms can displace the lens, causing dislocation or subluxation.
- **intumescent cataract**. The increase in lens size can break the zonule.

### *Clinical signs*

Clinical signs include:

- vibration of the iris or **iridodonesis**
- presence of the vitreous in the anterior chamber (Figure 8.94)
- visualization of the **entire lens in the anterior chamber** in the case of anterior dislocation (Figure 8.95)
- visualization of the displaced lens, '**aphakic crescent**' (Figure 8.96)
- observation of the retina and optic nerve without the need for ophthalmoscopy in the case of posterior dislocation (Figure 8.97)
- changes in the of shape of the iris and depth of the anterior chamber (Figure 8.98)

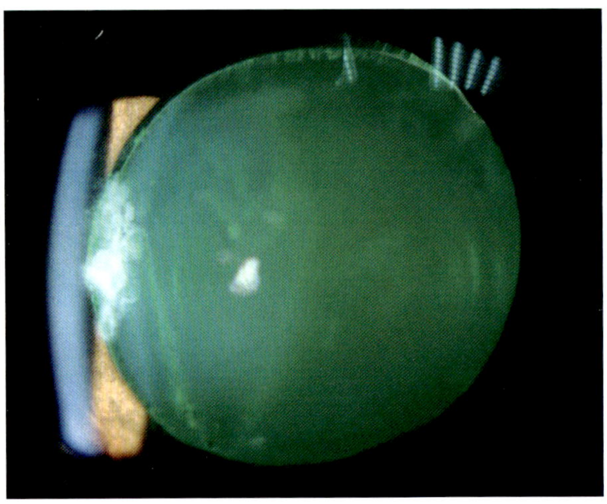

**Figure 8.94.** Presence of the vitreous in the anterior chamber.

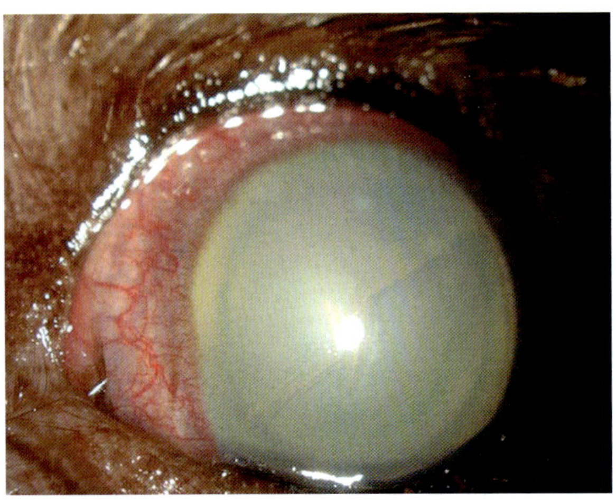

**Figure 8.95.** Anterior luxation of the lens.

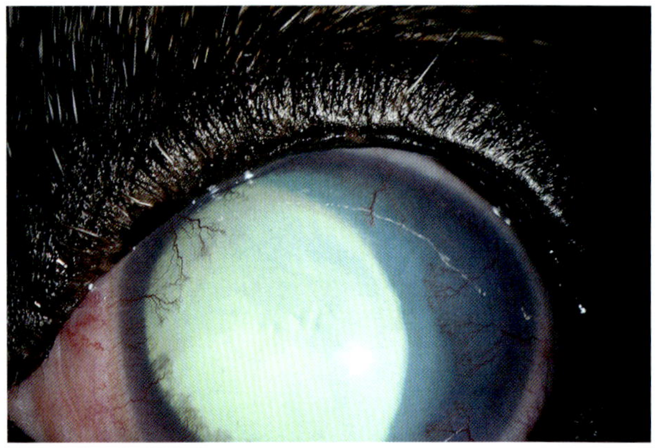

**Figure 8.96.** Subluxation of the lens. Note the aphakic crescent.

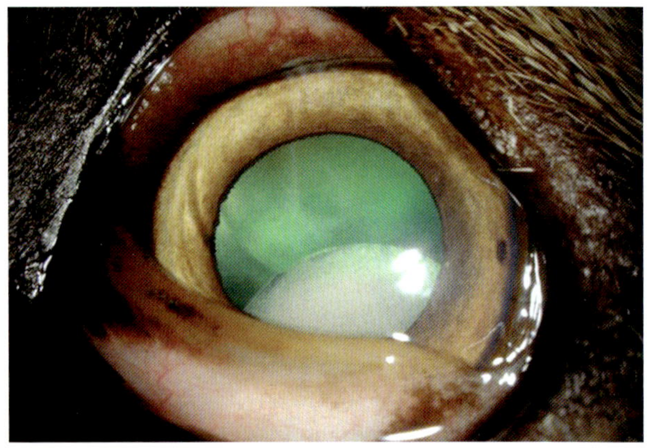

**Figure 8.97.** Luxation of the lens into the vitreous chamber.

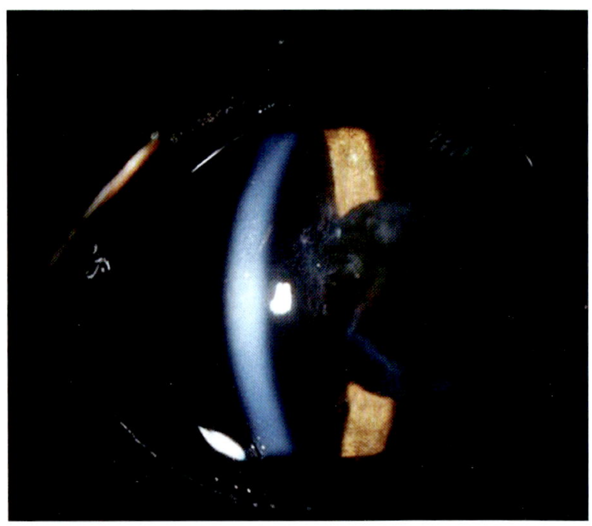

**Figure 8.98.** Posterior luxation of the lens. Appearance of the anterior chamber (very deep), iris displaced posteriorly and presence of the vitreous in the anterior chamber.

- **corneal oedema** (endothelial damage due to the presence of the lens in the anterior chamber)
- **pain** due to impact of the cornea on the lens
- **glaucoma** due to obstruction of the drainage of the aqueous humour.

### Diagnosis
The diagnosis is made based on:

- clinical history (e.g. pain)
- clinical signs
- biomicroscopy (the anterior chamber is reduced in anterior luxation and increased in posterior luxation)
- ultrasound (location of the lens in case of doubt) (Figure 8.99).

### Treatment
There is some debate regarding the most appropriate treatment.

Some clinicians favour performing an intracapsular lens extraction or phacoemulsification in combination with vitrectomy to prevent glaucoma. Other, more conservative clinicians prefer to administer miotics to avoid anterior dislocation in case of subluxation.

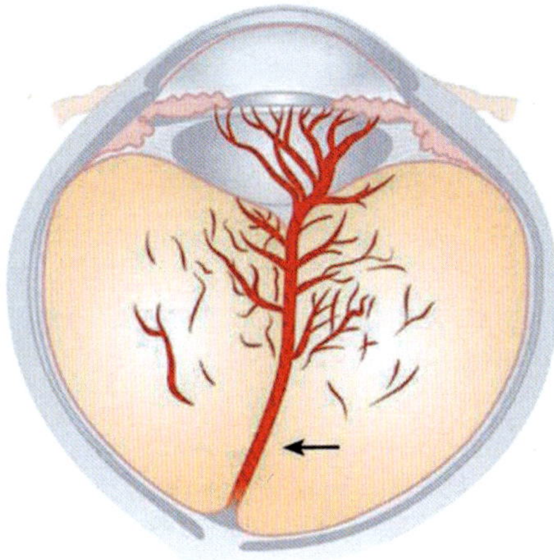

**Figure 8.100.** Drawing showing the primary vitreous. Cloquet's canal (arrow). Inside Cloquet's canal, the hyaloid artery, which generates vessels as it passes through the vitreous body (vasa propia) and on arrival at the lens forms the tunica vasculosa lentis.

## Vitreous humour

### General aspects

The **vitreous is an elastic, transparent hydrogel**. It occupies 80% of the volume of the eye.

During embryonic development it goes through different phases:

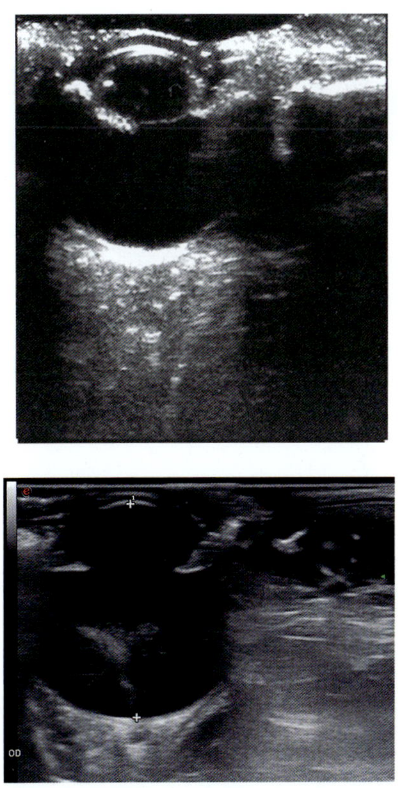

**Figure 8.99.** Ultrasound images of anterior (a) and posterior (b) lens luxation.

- **primary vitreous**, which is associated with the hyaloid vascular system that provides nutrition to the lens during development (Figure 8.100)
- **secondary vitreous** (surrounds the primary vitreous and forms the definitive vitreous)
- **tertiary vitreous**. Contributes to the formation of zonules.

Vitreous and crystalline junctions are formed, through the capsular hyaloid ligament, at the ora serrata and in the peripapillary area.

The vitreous body is divided into the anterior vitreous, posterior vitreous, cortex and central vitreous, which includes Cloquet's canal.

It consists of water (99%), collagen fibres (they serve as skeletons), cells (hyalocytes) and hyaluronic acid.

**Functions of the vitreous**:

- It contributes to the **maintenance of eye volume** and possibly the shape of the eyeball.
- It helps keep the lens and retina in their anatomical positions.
- It is **part of the optical pathways** (passage of light to the retina), although it does not have a significant role in the refraction of light since its refractive index is similar to that of the lens.

### Congenital abnormalities

#### Persistence of the hyaloid artery

##### Aetiopathogenesis

**Remnants of the hyaloid artery** originate from the surface of the optic disc, which is surrounded by glial tissue. This is called Bergmeister's papilla.

It is considered hereditary in the Doberman pinscher.

### Clinical signs

It **does not usually interfere with visual function**, unless it causes subsequent cataracts.

### Diagnosis

The following can be observed with the ophthalmoscope:

- red or white elevations, which originate in the optic disc and extend anteriorly with varying lengths within the vitreous (Figure 8.101)
- in the distal part of the artery, junctions to the posterior capsule of the lens, a Mittendorf dot
- complete persistence of the artery.

## *Persistent tunica vasculosa lentis*

### Aetiopathogenesis

A **failure in the regression** of this network of vessels.

### Diagnosis

It is visible as an **opaque network on the posterior surface of the lens** (Figure 8.102).

The opacification is generally a very fine matrix that does not interfere with vision.

## *Persistent hyperplastic primary vitreous (PHPV)*

### Aetiopathogenesis

This anomaly encompasses foetal and postnatal **hyperplasia of the hyaloid system**, the tunica vasculosa lentis and the primary vitreous. The result is **severe opacification**.

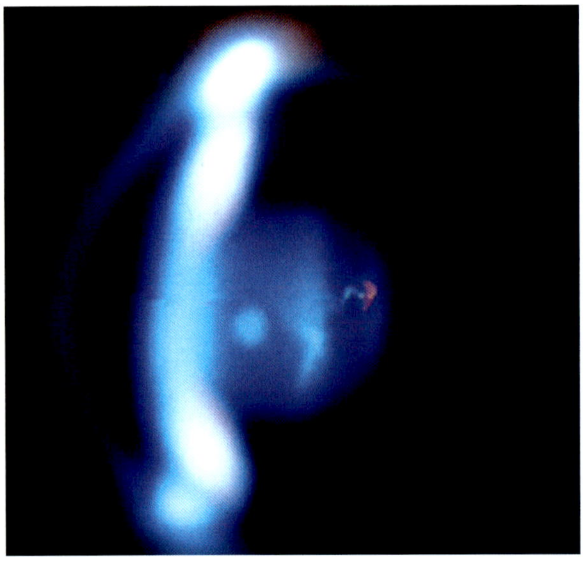

**Figure 8.101.** Route of the hyaloid artery in the vitreous body.

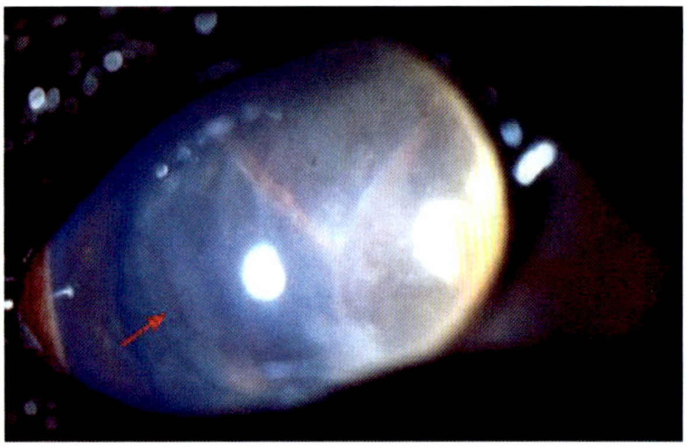

**Figure 8.102.** Primary persistent hyperplastic vitreous. Presence of a cataract and tunica vasculosa lentis (arrow).

### Epidemiology

It can appear in cats and in different breeds of dogs. It is hereditary in the Staffordshire bull terrier, bouvier and Doberman pinscher (Figure 8.103). In this last breed, a 6-stage classification system has been devised (Figure 8.104).

### Diagnosis

Diagnosis is made mainly by biomicroscopy and ultrasonography (Figures 8.105 and 8.106).

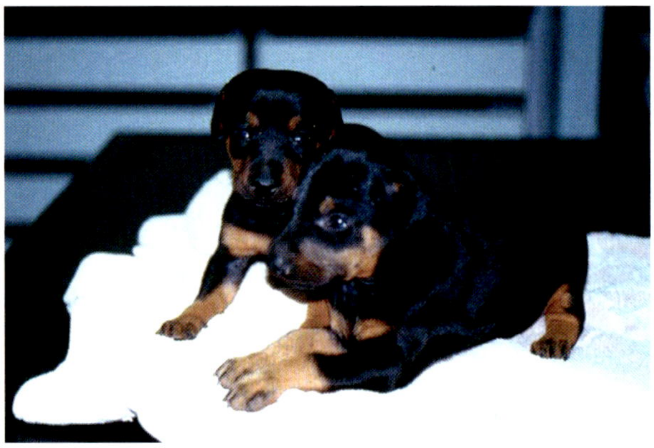

**Figure 8.103.** Doberman puppies with white pupils and a diagnosis of PHPV. PHPV, persistent hyperplastic primary vitreous.

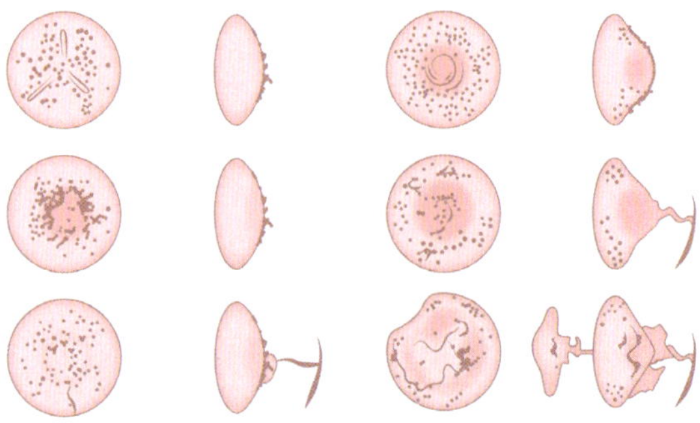

**Figure 8.104.** Drawing showing the classification of the 6 stages of PHPV as devised by Stades.

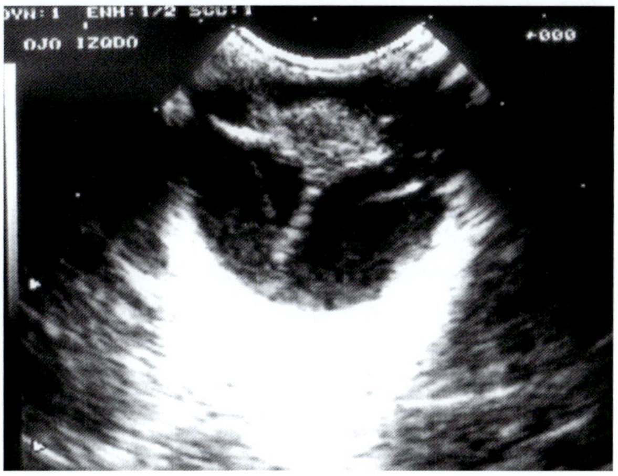

**Figure 8.105.** PHPV. Ultrasound showing cataract with microphakia, lenticonus, hyperechogenic line from the lens capsule to the optic nerve (Cloquet's canal). PHPV, persistent hyperplastic primary vitreous.

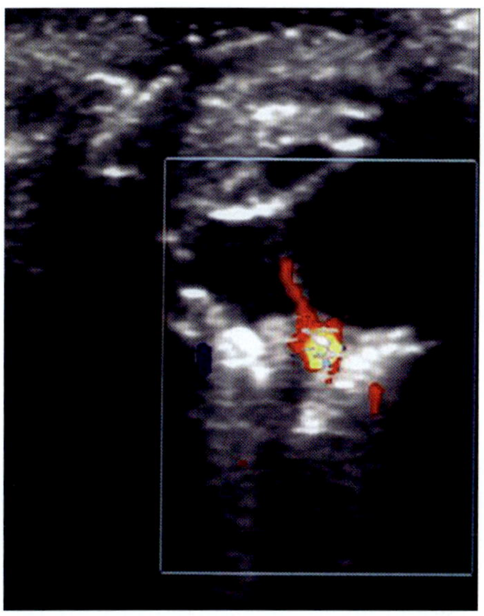

**Figure 8.106.** PHPV. Colour Doppler ultrasound showing persistence of the hyaloid artery. PHPV, persistent hyperplastic primary vitreous.

A white or fibrovascular plaque is seen in the posterior pupil near the posterior capsule of the lens and anterior to the vitreous.

Vascular invasion and haemorrhage in the vitreous and body of the lens, calcium deposits, lenticonus at the back of the lens, microphakia, lens coloboma, intralental pigmentation, progressive cataracts and elongation of the ciliary processes can also be visualized.

### Prognosis

The cataract surgery associated with PHPV has a **reserved prognosis** due to the opacification of the posterior capsule of the lens, the possible existence of blood vessels and the need to combine surgery with vitrectomy.

## *Acquired abnormalities*

### *Vitreous degeneration*

### Aetiopathogenesis

Vitreous degeneration consists of segregation of the fluid and solid components of the vitreous, **causing its liquefaction** (syneresis).

This degeneration, which predisposes the eye to retinal detachment, can occur naturally in geriatric animals or as a result of intraocular inflammation.

### Diagnosis

In dogs with cataracts, vitreous degeneration should be demonstrated on ultrasonography, as a presurgical examination.

The higher incidence of rhegmatogenous retinal detachments in eyes with hypermature cataracts may be related to the higher incidence of these animals suffering from vitreous degeneration.

### *Vitreous inflammation (vitritis or hyalitis)*

### Aetiopathogenesis

Due to the absence of vessels, **primary inflammation per se does not appear in the vitreous**. However, the vitreous may be affected by inflammatory abnormalities in the surrounding tissues (chorioretinitis, optic neuritis and anterior uveitis).

### Clinical signs

Clinical signs include:

- opacifications
- haemorrhage
- syneresis
- cellular exudation.

Vitreous fog is common in inflammatory changes in the posterior chamber; its disappearance is an indicator of the effectiveness of treatment.

### Diagnosis

The primary cause must be identified:

- microorganisms after penetrating trauma
- systemic bacteraemia
- fungal infections.

### Treatment

Treatment is using a combination of treatments:

- aetiological
- symptomatic: anti-inflammatory and cycloplegic
- surgical: vitrectomy.

### *Vitreous opacities*

#### Aetiopathogenesis

Also called **'floaters'**, vitreous opacities are considered **benign findings in geriatric patients**, where they probably represent degenerative changes of the vitreous.

They may be due to the presence of blood or exudates.

#### Diagnosis

Vitreous opacities are shown using ophthalmoscopy.

#### Differential diagnosis

Vitreous opacities must be differentiated from 'flying fly syndrome', where the affected animal sees moving objects in the air. It is currently thought that this syndrome is due to abnormalities in the temporal or occipital lobe of the brain, rather than the eye.

### *Asteroid hyalosis and synchysis scintillans*

#### Aetiopathogenesis

Both conditions are characterized by the appearance of **numerous small refractile bodies through the vitreous** (Figure 8.107).

They may appear:

- spontaneously, in old animals
- with chronic inflammation
- due to degenerative ocular abnormalities.

The composition of the particles is different between the two:

- in asteroid hyalosis: calcium and complex phospholipids
- in synchysis scintillans: cholesterol.

#### Clinical signs

Vision is not affected.

#### Differential diagnosis

The two conditions can be distinguished clinically based on the motility of the particles:

- In **asteroid hyalosis**, the particles are **attached to the vitreous collagen mesh** and move with head and eye movements.
- In **synchysis scintillans**, the particles are free in the liquefied vitreous and **move like snowflakes** with head movements; when these cease, sedimentation occurs.

## Retina

### *General aspects*

The retina is the most complex ocular structure (Figure 8.108) and is responsible for **converting light energy into chemical energy to generate the electrical signal** that is conducted to the brain.

In addition, it is the **most metabolically active tissue in the body**, as proven by oxygen consumption. Loss of retinal blood flow leads rapidly to ischaemia and cell death. This perfusion depends on:

- **choroidal circulation** for the outer layers
- **retinal circulation** for the inner layers.

The processes that result in vision are extremely complex and not fully understood. Electroretinography is used to examine the functionality of cones and rods.

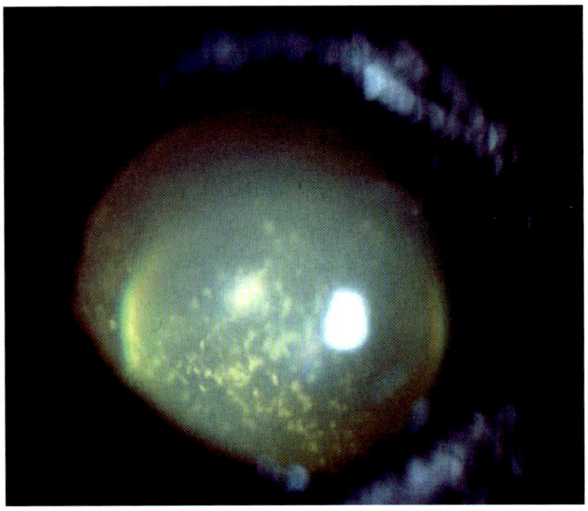

**Figure 8.107.** Asteroid hyalosis. Note the calcium and phospholipid particles in the vitreous.

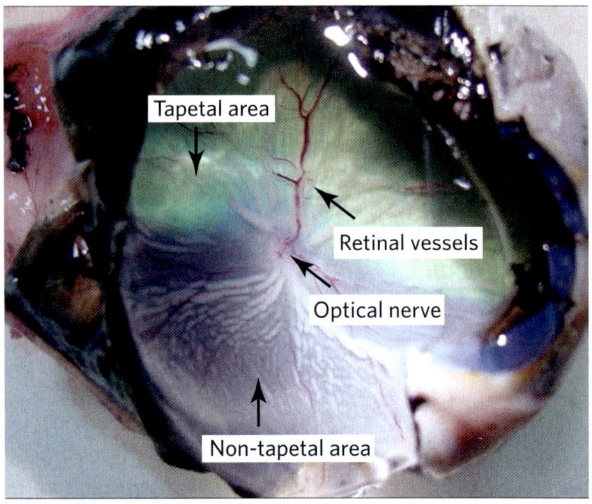


**Figure 8.108.** Anatomical image showing the parts of the retina in the dog.

In brief:

- **Rods are responsible for night** or scotopic vision.
- **Cones** are responsible for **daytime and colour vision**.

Abnormalities that affect the retina are classified as:

- developmental retinopathies
- acquired retinopathies.

The clinical evaluation and diagnosis of these conditions is achieved through a complete history (signalment and clinical history), physical examination and specialized examination methods such as ophthalmoscopy, biomicroscopy, ophthalmometry, ultrasonography, fluorescein angiography, electroretinography and OCT.

## *Developmental retinopathies*

### *Collie eye anomaly (CEA)*

#### Aetiopathogenesis

CEA is a **congenital eye syndrome characterized by defects of the vascular and fibrous tunics in the eye**. The type of transmission was thought to be simple, autosomal recessive but is currently considered polygenic.

It is a consequence of the **abnormal differentiation of the mesoderm**, which causes **abnormalities of varying severities of the choroid, retinal vascularization, optic nerve and sclera**.

The condition is not progressive, except in cases with retinal detachment and intraocular haemorrhage.

#### Epidemiology

There is no sex predisposition.

The dog breeds mainly affected are the rough-haired collie, Border collie and Shetland sheepdog, among others.

#### Clinical signs

Animals have **asymmetric bilateral signs**.

- Many dogs have no visual abnormalities. Those who have **severe colobomas or retinal detachment are blind**.
- **Retinal folds** (retinal dysplasia) and subepithelial corneal opacities (dystrophy) along with **microphthalmia**. These latter lesions may appear in normal dogs; therefore, they are not specific to Collie eye syndrome.
- **Choroidal hypoplasia** (pale area of temporal or supratemporal depigmentation of varying size on the optic disc). In adult dogs, it can be masked by pigment. It occurs bilaterally.
- **Colobomas** of the posterior pole, frequently of the optic nerve (papillary coloboma) or in an adjacent area (peripapillary coloboma). They are almost always located in the medial and lateral limits of the optic disc.
- **Partial or total retinal detachment**. Usually unilateral, although sporadically it can be bilateral.
- **Hyphaemia, retinal or vitreous haemorrhages**. These occur in a very small percentage of cases.

Sometimes, **retinal vascular tortuosity** can be seen, although it is not pathognomonic of the condition, and this may accompany microphthalmia.

#### Diagnosis

A diagnosis of CEA is based on the presence of clinical signs (e.g. coloboma, absence of pigment in a zone temporal to the optic disc). Puppies that are severely affected can be diagnosed by 4–8 weeks of age.

#### Treatment

There is **no effective treatment**.

#### Control of the disease

Control and eradication of CEA are very difficult due to its high prevalence. In addition, it is important to be aware that breeds (within those described) with minimally affected animals can produce severely affected litters.

### *Retinal dysplasia*

#### Aetiopathogenesis

The condition is caused by **abnormal differentiation of the retina**, with proliferation of one or more of its constituent elements.

It affects puppies as an isolated condition or coexists with other ocular abnormalities, such as microphthalmia and coloboma. For example, in the Bedlington terrier, it can be seen in combination with other conditions, resulting in vitreous-retinal dysplasia; in the Labrador retriever, it is possible that it is associated with skeletal dysplasia.

**Retinal dysplasia can be hereditary, with recessive or dominant forms, or acquired**.

The **acquired forms** are secondary to:

In **dogs**:

- intrauterine inflammatory conditions during pregnancy
- canine herpesvirus
- hypovitaminosis A
- X-ray radiation
- certain medications
- intrauterine trauma (Figure 8.109).

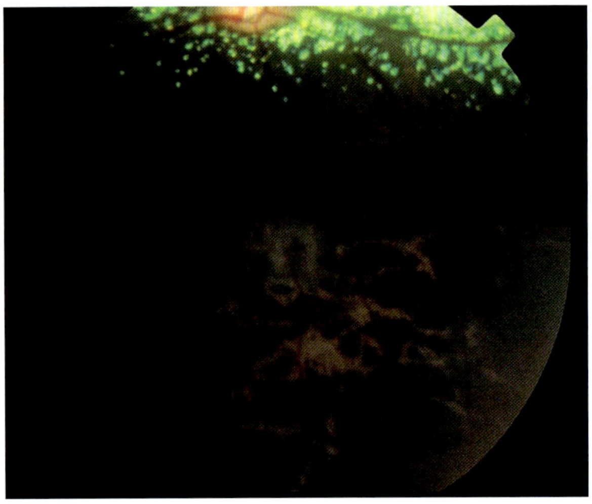

Figure 8.109. Acquired retinal dysplasia.

In **cats**:

- feline panleukopenia
- feline infectious peritonitis
- chronic glomerulonephritis.

### Epidemiology

Retinal dysplasia occurs most frequently in the following dog breeds: the American cocker spaniel, English springer spaniel, beagle, Labrador retriever, Rottweiler, Samoyed and golden retriever.

### Clinical signs

Generally, the condition is not progressive, but **severe dysplasia results in blindness**.

- **retinal folds**. These are observed as V- or Y-shaped lines, points or structures in the tapetal area of the ocular fundus, often around the superior retinal vessels. They are green, grey or dark in colour. They can also be seen in the non-tapetal area (in both grey and black).
- focal degeneration of the retina
- **retinal detachments** with haemorrhage, if dysplasia is extensive
- leukocoria
- microphthalmia
- cataract
- nystagmus.

### Diagnosis

A diagnosis is reached based on the clinical signs and observation of the relevant retinal lesions. Lesions may be seen with an ophthalmoscope from 4 to 8 weeks of age.

### Control of the disease

Disease control implies avoiding the use of affected animals for breeding.

## *Progressive retinal atrophy*

### Aetiopathogenesis

**Retinal photoreceptor dysplasia** can be:

- **hereditary** in young animals (transmission is simple autosomal recessive)
- **degenerative** in mature animals.

In dogs affected at a young age, such as the Irish setter and the collie, the condition is due to the lack of the cGMP-specific phosphodiesterase enzyme and, consequently, to the **accumulation of cGMP, which is toxic to photoreceptors**.

### Clinical signs

It causes a progressive loss of vision, first at night and then during the daytime.

### Epidemiology

The main dog breeds affected are the Irish setter, collie, American and English cocker spaniel, miniature poodle, toy poodle, Norwegian elkhound, Afghan hound, Border collie, Cardigan corgi, beagle, borzoi, dachshund, cairn terrier, English springer spaniel, Gordon setter, greyhound, Labrador retriever, miniature pinscher, pointer, saluki, Siberian husky, Samoyed and Shetland sheepdog, among others.

Among cats, it appears in the Abyssinian breed.

The **age at onset is variable**; in dogs, it depends on the breed:

- In the Irish setter and the collie, it can be diagnosed at 6–8 months of age.
- In the miniature poodle, it can be seen between 3 and 12 years.

In cats:

- The early form is seen in the first few years of life.
- The late form appears between 3 and 6 years.

### Clinical signs

Clinical signs include:

- **night blindness** that progresses to total blindness
- **incomplete pupillary reflexes**
- **tapetal hyperreflectivity** (thinning of the retina) (Figure 8.110)

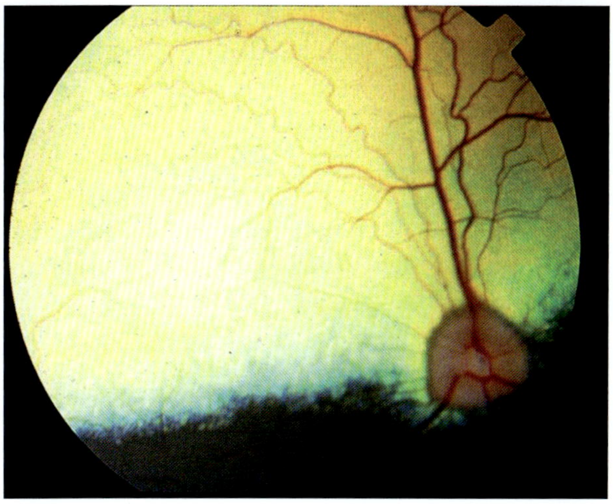

**Figure 8.110.** Progressive retinal atrophy. Early stage. Note the tapetal hyperreflectivity.

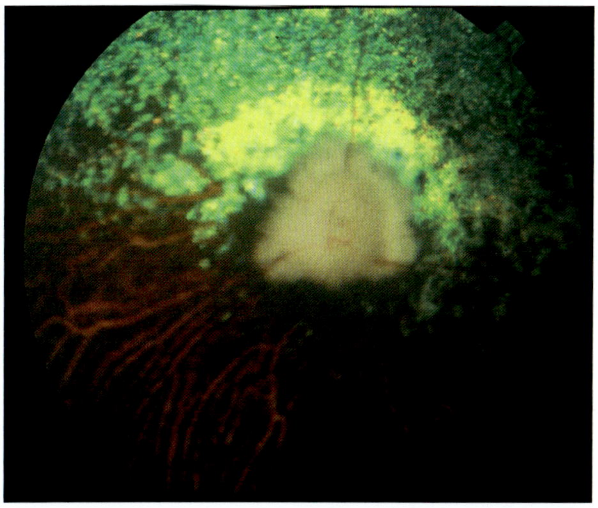

**Figure 8.111.** Progressive retinal atrophy. Note the depigmentation of the non-tapetal area (visualization of the choroid vessels) and the small vessels of the retina.

- depigmentation of the non-tapetal area and clustering of pigment (Figure 8.111)
- thinning of retinal blood vessels, so much that they disappear, especially the arterioles of the peripheral zone (Figure 8.111)
- atrophy of the optic nerve
- **cataracts**, due to toxins released from the damaged retina.

### Diagnosis

A diagnosis of retinal atrophy is based on the history (e.g. animal stumbling), clinical signs, assessing the behaviour of the animal as blindness develops (first nocturnal and then daytime), the labyrinth test, ophthalmoscopy (presence of thinning of retinal vessels and tapetal hyperreflectivity) and electroretinography (assessing cones and rods and observing voltage decreases in the b-wave).

## *Acquired retinopathies of nutritional origin*

### *Retinopathy due to taurine deficiency in the cat*

#### Aetiopathogenesis

**Cats fed on a taurine-deficient diet**, such as foods formulated for dogs, may have retinal degeneration or atrophy as well as dilated cardiomyopathy.

Taurine is stored in the liver, although higher tissue concentrations are found in the heart muscle and retina (photoreceptors). **Taurine is an essential amino acid for cats** since they cannot synthesize it from cysteine. The function of taurine is unclear, but it is thought to act as a neurotransmitter and have protective properties in membranes.

#### Clinical signs

Clinical signs include:

- **blindness**
- observation of localized or diffuse **hyperreflective areas of the retina**.

As for the signs observed in the retina, there are 5 stages:

1. increase in granularity of the area centralis
2. appearance of ellipsoid hyperreflective lesion
3. visualization of a second hyperreflective lesion in the nasal area to the optic papilla
4. the two anterior lesions converge to form a single, band-shaped lesion located dorsally to the optic papilla
5. **generalized degeneration of the retina with attenuation or loss of retinal vessels**.

#### Diagnosis

**Ophthalmoscopic signs begin after 3–7 months of deficiency**, manifesting a complete degeneration of the retina after 9 months.

Evidence such as **low plasma taurine levels**, along with signs of blindness and other symptoms of deficiency. **Falsely elevated readings can occur if blood is not separated immediately** after collection since taurine can be released from platelets.

On **electroretinography**, it manifests initially with **increased latency times in the cones**; in the later stages, it manifests with decreased amplitudes in the cones and rods.

#### Treatment

The **administration of taurine supplements** gives good results for cardiomyopathy but not for advanced retinal degeneration with blindness since **the effects of retinal deficiency are only partially reversible**.

### *Vitamin E deficiency*

#### Clinical signs

**Vitamin E deficiency** in the dog produces **nyctalopia** (impaired ability to see at night).

#### Diagnosis

The ophthalmoscopic appearance is like progressive retinal atrophy; early in the condition, there is a loss of electroretinographic waves.

### *Vitamin A deficiency*

#### Aetiopathogenesis

In dogs, **systemic pathologies that cause problems with fat absorption may cause vitamin A deficiency**. This clinical situation is extremely rare.

#### Clinical signs

It is characterized by **night blindness**.

## *Acquired retinopathies of toxic origin*

### *Drug-induced retinopathy*

#### Aetiopathogenesis

There are drugs that can cause retinal damage:

- **directly** (in the neuroretina or retinal pigment epithelium)
- **indirectly** (through inflammatory reactions with subsequent focal or generalized cell death (degenerative abnormalities)).

These drug-induced retinopathies are usually **symmetrical and bilateral**, depending on the duration of administration of the toxic compound and the dose.

The main drugs that induce retinopathies are:

- **ethambutol**. Drug administered for the treatment of tuberculosis. Causes discoloration of the tapetal area. There are no effects on vision.
- **diphenylthiocarbazone**. Used as a metal chelator. It can cause changes in the ocular fundus, such as a dark red colour and diffuse retinal oedema. High doses cause retinal degeneration.
- **hydroxypyridinone**. Zinc chelator. Causes blindness in dogs as a sequela to tapetal necrosis, oedema and retinal detachment.
- **quinine**. Produces rapid vasoconstriction of retinal arterioles and pale optic disc. Destruction of ganglion cells occurs.
- **enrofloxacin**. Its administration in cats can cause mydriasis and acute blindness due to diffuse retinal degeneration, which is evidenced by increased tapetal reflectivity and vascular attenuation.
- others, such as rafoxanide, chloroquine, azithromycin and closantel.

#### Diagnosis

The **history and clinical signs in animals that have received these drugs** can guide a diagnosis. This information, together with the results of the examination (signs of retinal degeneration), allow confirmation.

#### Treatment

Most of the time, **retinal lesions are severe and irreversible** with no option for treatment.

### *Light- and oxygen-induced retinopathy*

#### Aetiopathogenesis

**Prolonged exposure (>20 minutes) of the retina to intense** light (for example, from an indirect ophthalmoscope) can cause ophthalmoscopic changes to the fundus such as:

- increased granularity of the tapetal area
- increased retinal pigmentation
- tapetal reflectivity
- the non-tapetal area is not affected.

In very advanced cases, degeneration of photoreceptors and atrophy of the retinal pigment epithelium occur.

The administration of high oxygen pressures causes selective damage of the visual cells in the dog. In addition, light and oxygen can interact to produce oxygen free radicals, which cause photosensitization that sometimes leads to retinal dysplasia.

### *Sudden acquired retinal degeneration (SARD) or silent retinal syndrome*

#### Aetiopathogenesis

An **abnormality of the retina of unknown cause** (autoimmune, toxic or endocrine) that results in **sudden and permanent blindness in adult dogs** due to the rapid loss of external segments of photoreceptors (cones and rods), followed by a degeneration of other retinal layers.

#### Epidemiology

It can occur in any breed (predisposition in the dachshund) and even in cross-breeds, around **middle age (8.5–10 years)**.

There is a greater predisposition in **spayed females** and there is a seasonal incidence in the months of December and January.

## Clinical signs

**Sudden loss of vision, within days or 1–2 weeks.**

**Pupillary dilation and absence of photomotor** reflex (Figure 8.112).

In many dogs there are **signs compatible with hyperadrenocorticism**, such as polyuria, polydipsia and polyphagia, as well as weight gain. Likewise, the adrenocorticotrophic hormone (ACTH) stimulation test and the low-dose dexamethasone suppression test show results compatible with hyperadrenocorticism. Complete blood counts and blood biochemistry reveal lymphopenia, neutrophilia and elevated levels of bilirubin, alkaline phosphatase and cholesterol.

## Diagnosis

Ophthalmoscopic examination:

1. Early stages. Absence of abnormalities of the fundus (Figure 8.113).
2. After several weeks or months, alterations in degenerative conditions of the retina (vascular attenuation and tapetal hyperreflectivity) can be observed.
3. The final stage involves generalized atrophy of the retina, which is impossible to distinguish from progressive atrophy of the retina.

Flat electroretinogram.

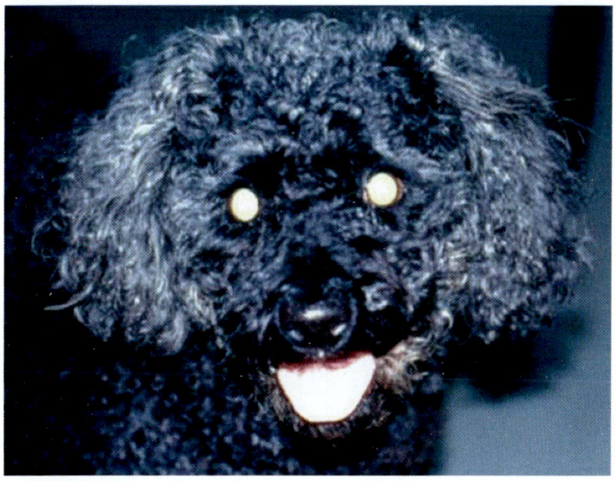

**Figure 8.112.** Bitch with sudden blindness (SARD). Note the presence of bilateral pupillary dilation. (There are no pupillary reflexes.)

## Treatment

There is **no treatment**.

# *Inflammatory conditions of the retina*

## *Retinitis, choroiditis, retinochoroiditis and chorioretinitis*

### Aetiopathogenesis

**Primary inflammatory lesions of the ocular fundus are rare in the dog**; they are usually secondary to conditions that extend from the choroid and, sometimes, from the vitreous humour.

The terms chorioretinitis and retinochoroiditis indicate the primary site and direction of expansion when both choroid and retina are affected.

### Causes

Cause of inflammatory conditions of the retina include:

- **infectious conditions** (canine distemper virus, cryptococcosis, histoplasmosis, blastomycosis, aspergillosis, coccidioidomycosis, protothecosis, geotrichosis, toxoplasmosis, leishmaniasis, dirofilariasis, toxocariasis, ehrlichiosis)
- neoplasms
- foreign bodies
- trauma.

### Clinical signs

They manifest with **different degrees of blindness**.

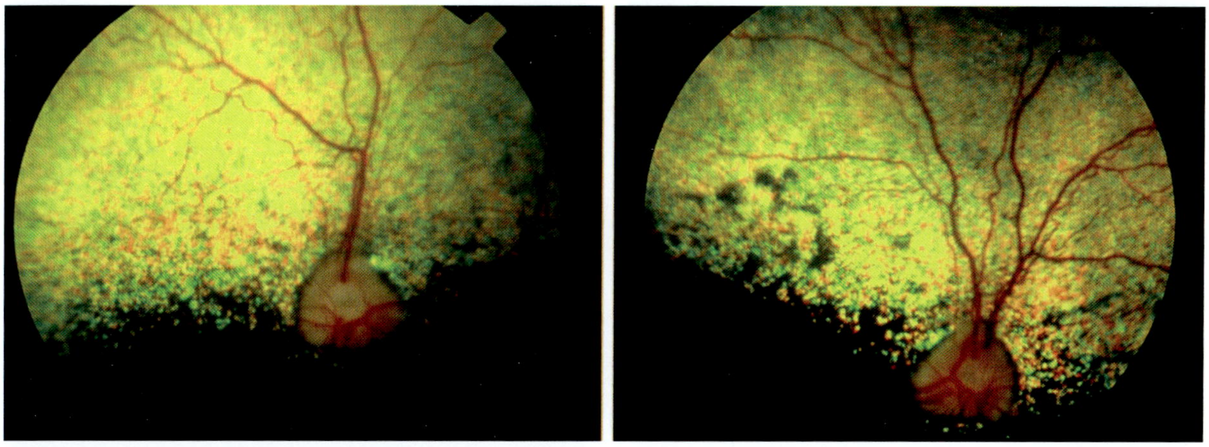

**Figure 8.113.** Ophthalmoscopic images of the retina in a dog with sudden blindness diagnosed as SARD. SARD, sudden acquired retinal degeneration.

## Clinical forms

### *Active form*

Grey exudate in the retina or below it, around the retinal vessels, or also in the vitreous humour, which causes a **blurred appearance and tapetal hyporeflectivity** (Figure 8.114). **Bleeding, retinal detachment and vitreous turbidity** may also be seen. IOP may be lower than normal.

### *Inactive form*

Presence of **focal areas of retinal thinning** (tapetal hyperreflectivity) with dense foci of pigmentation inside as a result of proliferation and migration of the retinal pigment epithelium (Figure 8.115).

## Diagnosis

Clinical signs of the ocular condition, together with the clinical signs of the primary condition, guide the diagnosis. Confirmation requires specific tests to reveal the primary condition.

## Treatment

The cause and uveitis must be treated.

## *Vascular abnormalities of the posterior segment*

The following may be considered.

**Retinal haemorrhage** (Figure 8.116). Most commonly caused by trauma, coagulopathies (warfarin), CEA, retinal detachment, immune-mediated thrombocytopenia, autoimmune haemolytic anaemia, neoplasia (multiple myeloma).

Retinovascular pathologies. These are found in animals since diabetes mellitus rarely causes retinal problems. Vasculitis can be caused by autoimmune problems and drug reactions.

Pathologies in the vessels of the retina:

- **retinal oedema**, flexuous vessels and haemorrhages due to problems with **hypertension** (Figure 8.117)

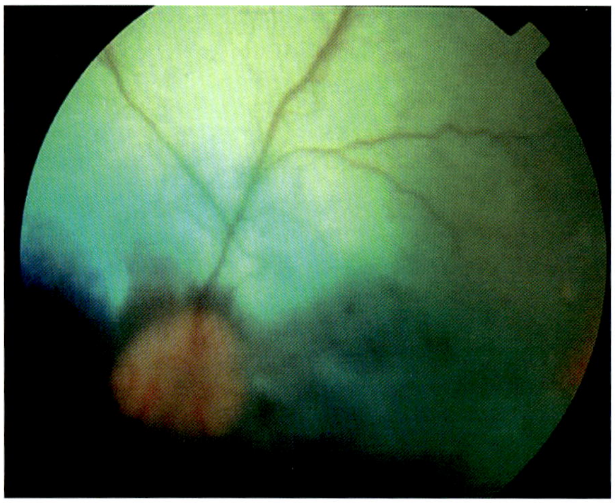

**Figure 8.114.** Chorioretinitis. Active form. Note the blurry image of the retina.

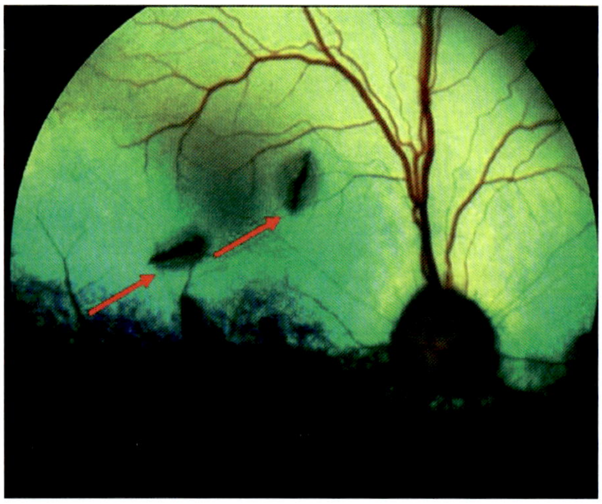

**Figure 8.115.** Chorioretinitis. Inactive form. Note the focal areas with interior pigmentation (arrows).

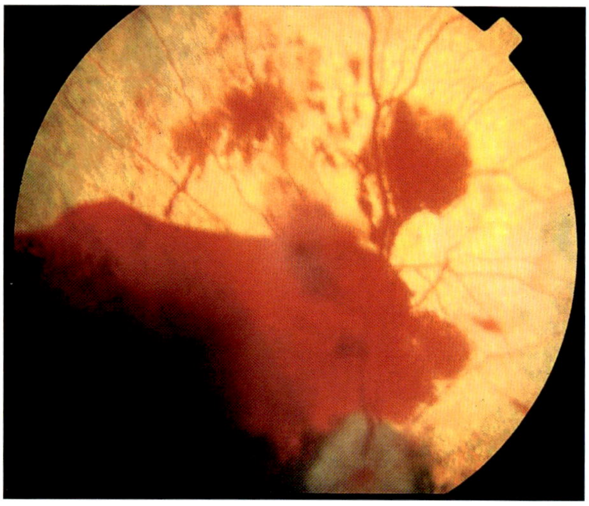

**Figure 8.116.** Retinal haemorrhage.

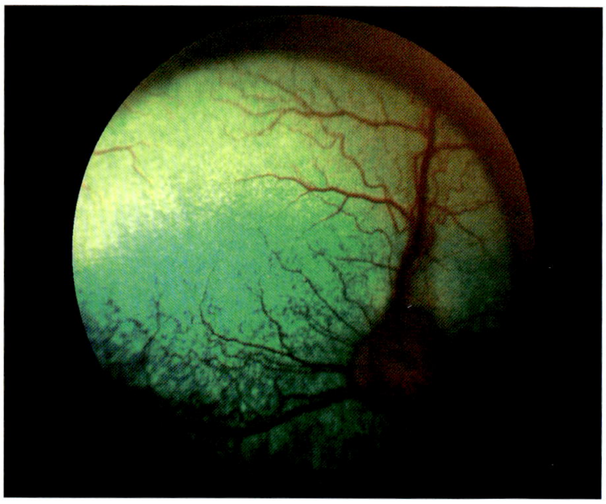

**Figure 8.117.** Systemic hypertension. Flexuous retinal vessels.

- engorged retinal arterioles and venules, and haemorrhages due to hyperviscosity syndrome
- engorgement of the venules due to cardiac abnormalities, such as tetralogy of Fallot and septal defects
- **anaemia** (fine, thin retinal vessels)
- hyperlipidaemia (pink vessels, especially on the periphery of the lower quadrant of the retina)
- polycythaemia (very thickened venules).

## Retinal detachment

### Aetiopathogenesis

Consists of the **separation of the neuroretina from the retinal pigment epithelium**, which implies a discontinuity between the external segments of the photoreceptors and the retinal pigment epithelium. This leads to a loss of function and secondary retinal degeneration in the affected area.

Possible causes may be:

- **traumatic**, even surgical
- **CEA** (congenital)
- vitreous traction bands due to inflammation
- **inflammatory exudates** behind the retina
- neoplasms of the retina or choroid, or orbital tumours that create pressure on the retina
- cyclocryotherapy for glaucoma, which causes exudative choroiditis
- liquefaction of vitreous humour.

### Classification

- Rhegmatogenous detachments. Elevations in the retina are associated with tears or holes through which liquefied vitreous humour has leaked.
- Non-rhegmatogenous detachments. There are no holes in the retina.

### Diagnosis

Made by visualizing the clinical signs using ophthalmoscopy (Figure 8.118) and by ultrasonography.

### Treatment

Serous detachments usually respond to combined therapy with diuretics (furosemide) and systemic corticosteroids.

Other types of therapies used in the treatment of retinal detachment are photocoagulation and laser techniques.

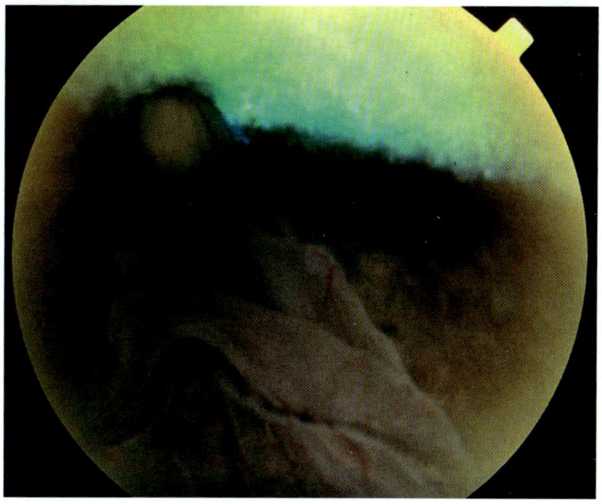

**Figure 8.118.** Retinal detachment. Detachment of the neuroretina and vessels can be observed.

# Optic nerve

## Congenital conditions

### Coloboma and micropapilla

#### Aetiopathogenesis

Coloboma refers to **excavations in the optic papilla** due to a failure in the closure of the optical fissure.

Micropapilla (Figure 8.119) refers to **hypoplasia and aplasia of the optic nerve**. The optic discs and nerve are small but have normal vascularization. There is a lack of ganglion cells in the retina.

#### Clinical signs

The main clinical sign is **blindness to varying degrees**, along with ocular findings by ophthalmoscopy.

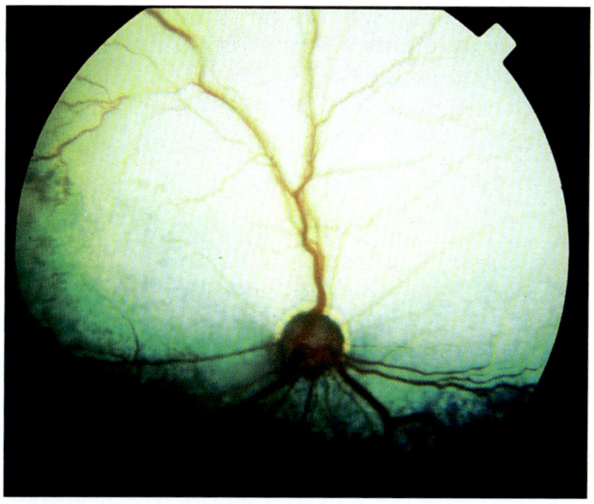

**Figure 8.119.** Micropapilla.

### Diagnosis
It is established through clinical signs, ophthalmoscopic examination and complementary methods, such as OCT.

### Treatment
There is **no treatment**.

## *Acquired conditions*

### *Optic neuritis*
### Aetiopathogenesis
Optic neuritis consists of the **inflammation of the optic nerve either unilaterally or bilaterally**, which can affect both the papilla and the retrobulbar optic nerve.

Causes include:

- viral infections (e.g. canine distemper)
- systemic mycoses (blastomycosis, cryptococcosis)
- neoplasms
- reticulosis
- granulomatous, traumatic and idiopathic meningoencephalitis.

### Clinical signs
Clinical signs include:

- sudden blindness and dilated pupils
- hyperaemia of the disc, oedema and haemorrhages.

When examined with an ophthalmoscope, the optic disc may appear elevated and dark due to **vitreous infiltrates**. However, in cases of retrobulbar optic neuritis, it may be normal.

### Treatment
Aetiological treatment of the infectious cause plus **systemic corticosteroids**.

## Main systemic infections with ocular manifestations in the dog

## *Viral infections*

### *Canine distemper*
### Aetiology
Canine distemper is caused by infection with morbillivirus. Virus is shed in all bodily secretion and infection is spread by aerosols and droplets. The incubation period is 3–5 days, with infection ranging from mild to severe.

### Clinical signs
Ocular signs:

early (Figure 8.120):

- acute serous or **mucopurulent conjunctivitis**
- lacrimal gland adenitis
- decreased tear production (blepharospasm and KCS)
- corneal ulcer.

late:

- anterior and posterior uveitis
- non-granulomatous multifocal chorioretinitis
- retinal detachment
- sudden blindness due to optic neuritis (Figure 8.121).

sequelae:

- hyperreflectivity of the tapetal area and central pigment
- depigmentation of the non-tapetal area.

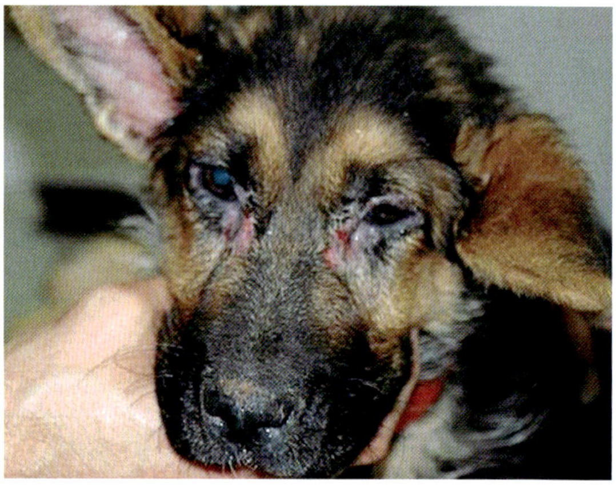

**Figure 8.120.** Canine distemper. Note blepharospasm and acute mucopurulent conjunctivitis.

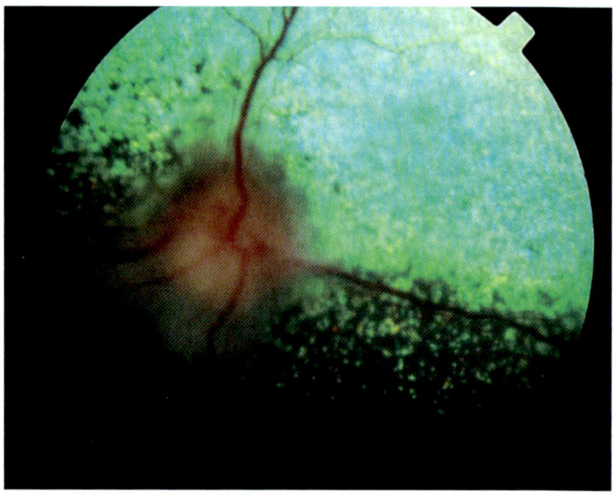

**Figure 8.121.** Canine distemper. Optic neuritis. Blurry image of the optic nerve.

### Diagnosis

Diagnosis is made via:

- conjunctival smears: cytoplasmic inclusion bodies
- immunofluorescence detecting inclusion bodies in cytology
- polymerase chain reaction (PCR) of conjunctival smears.

### Treatment

It depends on the lesions, but administration of the following is usually necessary:

- antibiotics for the control of secondary infections
- artificial tears
- systemic and topical corticosteroids.

## *Canine infectious hepatitis*

### Aetiology

The infection is caused by canine adenovirus type 1. The virus is shed in all bodily fluids and infection is via the oronasal route. Adenovirus may localize in the renal tubules and animals that have recovered may shed virus in the urine for 6–9 months.

### Clinical signs

Ocular signs (days 7–21):

- blepharospasm
- miosis, hypotonia and anterior chamber turbidity
- **bilateral 'blue eye', in 12–28% of cases** (Figure 8.122)
- in severe cases, keratoconus (a thinning of the cornea that leads to a domed appearance).

Systemic signs:

- mild respiratory infection
- hepatomegaly, jaundice and haemorrhages
- disseminated intravascular coagulopathy.

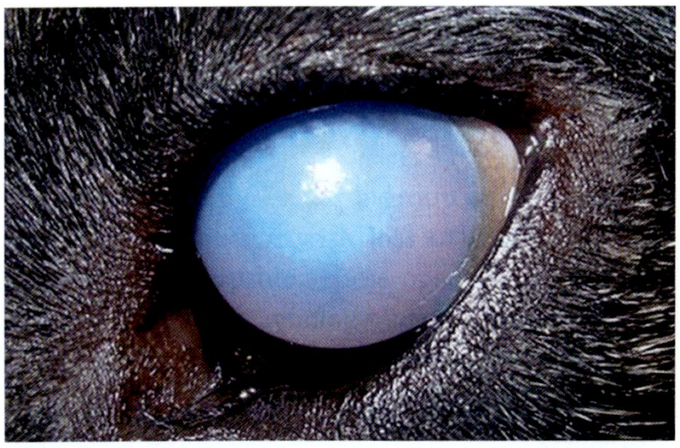

**Figure 8.122.** 'Blue eye' in canine infectious hepatitis.

Vaccination with attenuated canine adenovirus type 1 and 2 strains can cause anterior uveitis and corneal oedema in some dogs.

### Diagnosis

Clinical signs and history.

### Treatment

Topical treatment (corticosteroids, NSAIDs, atropine) and hypertonic solutions.

### Prognosis

In Afghan (Kuchi) shepherd dogs, the condition is chronic and glaucoma develops.

In other breeds, recovery is spontaneous in 2–3 weeks.

Regarding the presence of blue eye caused by canine adenovirus type 1 when animals are vaccinated with attenuated strains of canine adenovirus type 1 and to a lesser extent canine adenovirus type 2, this can cause anterior uveitis and mild corneal oedema in some animals. Recovery is better than in natural infection.

# *Bacterial infections*

## *Brucellosis*

### Aetiology

Venereal disease caused by *Brucella canis*. Infection is spread through body fluids and carries a **zoonotic risk**.

### Clinical signs

Ocular signs (unilateral):

- **anterior uveitis** (bacterial dissemination) (Figure 8.123)
- endophthalmitis (severe inflammation of tissues within the eye).

Systemic signs:

- **apathy**, fatigue, drowsiness and exercise intolerance
- adenopathy

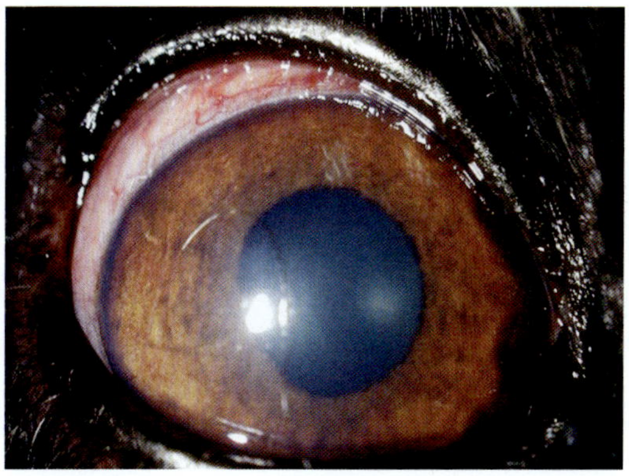

**Figure 8.123.** Uveitis in a dog diagnosed with brucellosis.

- **back pain** (discospondylitis), lameness (arthritis)
- neurological abnormalities (meningoencephalitis)
- **infertility**
- orchitis and testicular atrophy.

### Diagnosis

**Serological tests are sensitive, but false positives are common.** Negative results are generally reliable, but if the suspected infection occurred within two months, then retesting is advised.

### Treatment

Systemic: **tetracyclines** (doxycycline or minocycline).

Topical: **corticosteroids and atropine**.

In cases of endophthalmitis, which does not respond to treatment, enucleation is recommended.

### Prognosis

On discontinuation of treatment, relapses occur with bacteraemia persisting for up to 2 years. Males have chronic problems with fertility.

## *Borreliosis (Lyme disease)*

### Aetiology

Infection caused by the spirochete *Borrelia burgdorferi*. **Borreliosis is spread by the tick vector *Ixodes ricinus***, which needs to attach and feed to spread infection.

### Clinical signs

Ocular signs:

- **conjunctivitis**
- **anterior uveitis**
- chorioretinitis and petechiae (Figure 8.124)
- retinal detachment (see Figure 8.134), haemorrhage and microangiopathies (see Figure 8.135).

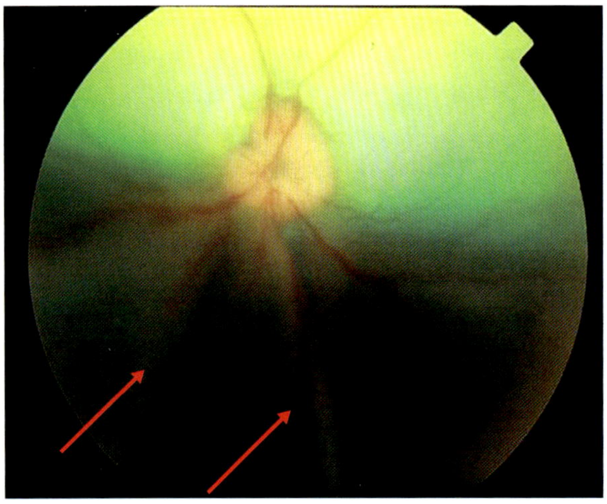

**Figure 8.124.** Chorioretinitis and partial retinal detachment (arrows) in a dog diagnosed with borreliosis.

Systemic signs:

- fever, lack of appetite
- adenopathy
- variable lameness (polyarthritis).

### Diagnosis

Characteristic clinical signs in an endemic area should raise suspicion of borreliosis. Diagnosis is made by:

- PCR on body fluids
- serology is non-specific due to cross-reactions.

### Treatment

**Systemic (14 days minimum)**:

- tetracyclines
- ampicillin
- others.

Topical:

- corticosteroids
- NSAIDs
- atropine.

## *Ehrlichiosis*

### Aetiology

*Ehrlichia canis* infection is spread by tick vectors, in particular *Rhipicephalus sanguineus*.

### Clinical signs

Clinical phases:

acute phase (2–4 weeks):

- thrombocytopenia
- pyrexia
- lymphoid hyperplasia
- vasculitis.

subclinical phase:

- thrombocytopenia
- neutropenia
- anaemia.

chronic phase:

- hyperglobulinaemia
- bone marrow depression (pancytopenia).

**Ocular signs (present in 10–15% of cases)**:

- blindness
- anterior uveitis with hyphaemia (Figure 8.125)

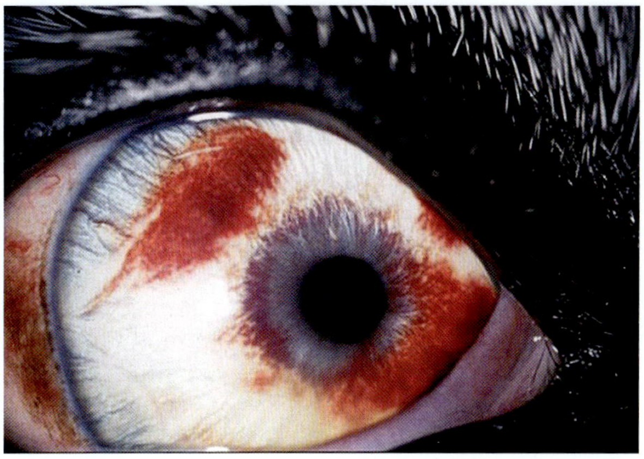

**Figure 8.125.** Uveitis in a dog diagnosed with ehrlichiosis.

- hyphaemia
- retinal haemorrhages
- retinal detachment
- optic neuritis.

### Progression

Glaucoma.

### Diagnosis

A history of tick infestation in an endemic area along with relevant clinical signs should raise suspicion of ehrlichiosis. A complete blood count in the subclinical phase usually shows thrombocytopenia, neutropenia and anaemia; in the chronic phase, it usually shows hyperglobulinaemia and pancytopenia.

PCR and serology can be used to confirm exposure, although serology should be interpreted with caution.

### Treatment

Systemic:

- **tetracycline** of choice:
  - tetracycline 22 mg/kg/8 h for 21 days
  - doxycycline 10 mg/kg/12–24 h for 21 days.
- imidocarb dipropionate.

Topical:

- corticosteroids
- atropine.

## *Parasitic infections*

### *Leishmaniasis*

### Aetiology

Infection caused by the protozoan *Leishmania infantum* and spread by bites from sandflies of the genus *Phlebotomus*.

### Clinical signs

Animals can be asymptomatic or have any of the following systemic signs:

- skin disorders: **exfoliative dermatitis**
- lymphadenopathies
- epistaxis
- splenomegaly
- renal insufficiency
- musculoskeletal abnormalities.

Ocular signs:

- blepharitis (Figure 8.126), conjunctivitis, scleritis and keratitis (Figure 8.127)
- palpebral and conjunctival granulomas (Figure 8.128)
- anterior uveitis, panophthalmitis
- secondary glaucoma.

### Diagnosis

There are several options for diagnosis, including PCR of conjunctival samples or bone marrow aspirates and blood (lower sensitivity than bone marrow). Also, cytology for the visualization of intracellular or free amastigotes has excellent specificity. However, care

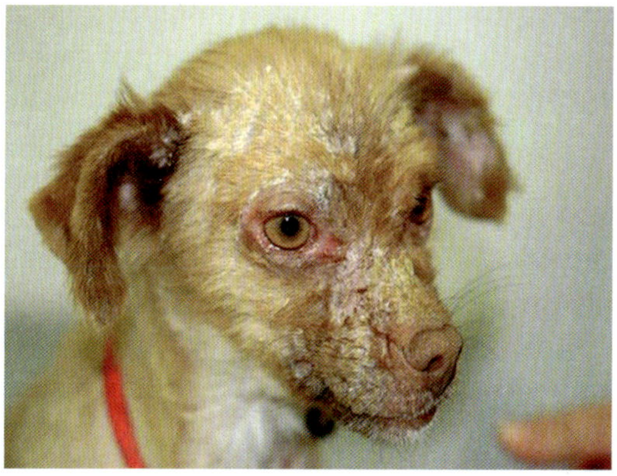

**Figure 8.126.** Blepharitis and skin abnormalities in a dog diagnosed with leishmaniasis.

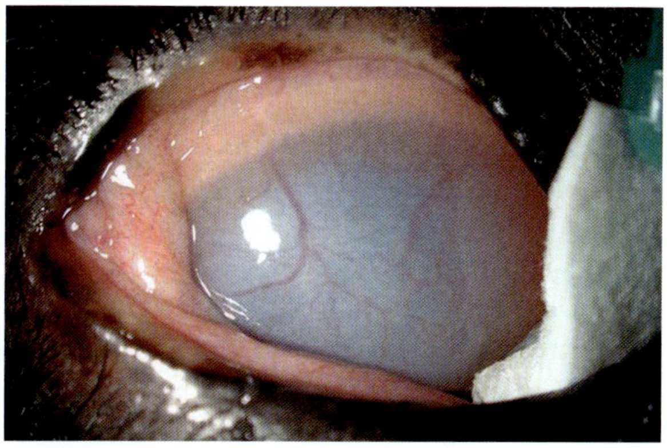

**Figure 8.127.** Conjunctivitis and keratitis in a dog diagnosed with leishmaniasis.

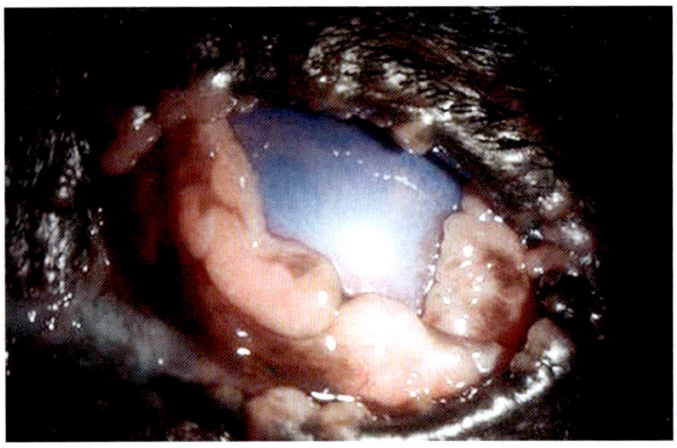

**Figure 8.128.** Palpebral and conjunctival granulomas in a dog diagnosed with leishmaniasis.

should be taken when interpreting serological results since positive results indicate exposure rather than active infection.

### Treatment

Systemic therapy is required:

- meglumine antimonial
- allopurinol.

Topical:

- corticosteroids
- NSAIDs
- atropine.

## *Fungal infections*

### *Cryptococcosis*

### Aetiology

Cryptococcal infections are caused by the **yeast *Cryptococcus neoformans***. Infection is **spread by pigeon faeces**, where the organism can survive for a year or longer.

### Epidemiology

*Cryptococcus* has a worldwide distribution, with infection being more frequent in cats than dogs.

### *Clinical signs*

Ocular signs:

- **anterior uveitis**, granulomatous chorioretinitis (Figure 8.129)
- exophthalmos, retinal detachment, optic neuritis
- **leptomeningitis** of the optic nerve (dog).

Systemic signs:

- granulomas in lung alveoli.

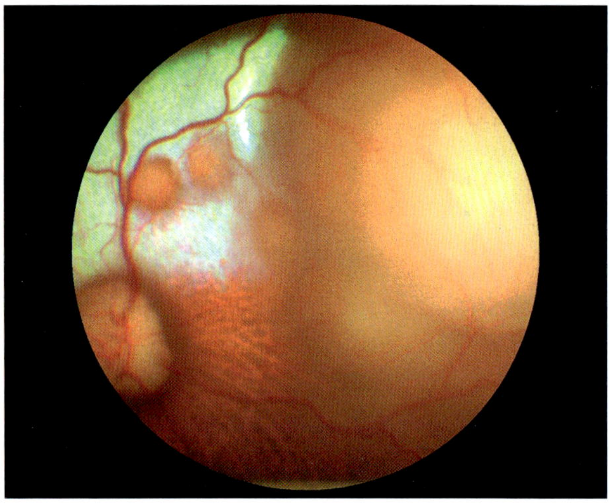

**Figure 8.129.** Granulomatous chorioretinitis in a dog diagnosed with cryptococcosis.

### Treatment

Systemic medication, for example, fluconazole, itraconazole, amphotericin B for 1–10 months.

## Diseases of immune origin

## *Uveodermatological syndrome: Vogt–Koyanagi–Harada disease*

### *Epidemiology*

Uveodermatological syndrome has a breed predisposition affecting principally the Samoyed, bobtail, Siberian husky, St Bernard, Akita, Irish setter, chow chow and golden retriever.

The condition first appears in young adult dogs, with the mean age at presentation being 3 years of age.

### *Clinical signs*

Ocular signs present ahead of dermatological signs; it is thought that ocular symptoms are due to a B cell and macrophage immune response, while cutaneous signs are due to a T cell and macrophage response.

Ocular signs:

- anterior or posterior bilateral uveitis (panuveitis) (Figure 8.130).

**Secondary ocular lesions** and development:

- cataracts
- anterior and posterior synechiae
- glaucoma
- bullous retinal detachment, atrophy of both the retina and optic nerve
- acute blindness

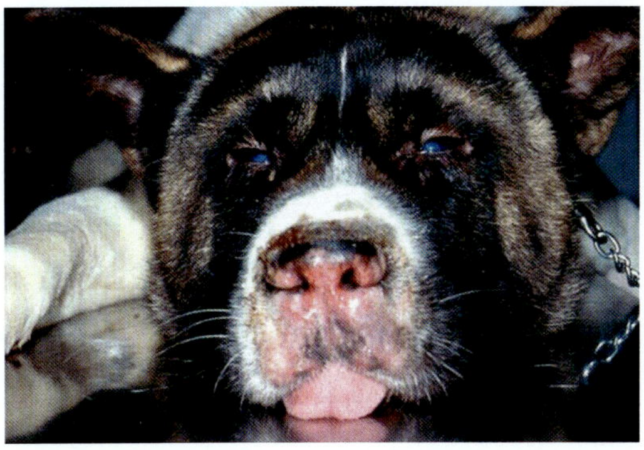

**Figure 8.130.** Uveodermatological syndrome. Bilateral uveitis with blepharospasm and lesions on the nose and lips.

- depigmentation of the non-tapetal retinal pigment epithelium, tapetal hyperreflectivity and vessel attenuation.

The development of secondary glaucoma can cause pain.

**Cutaneous signs**. Skin lesions most commonly affect the head, nose, eyelids, lips, plantar pads and scrotum (Figure 8.130):

- poliosis (the development of white hair)
- vitiligo (loss of skin pigmentation)
- ulceration.

### *Diagnosis*
Diagnosis is based on:

- breed predisposition
- typical clinical presentations such as:
  - **poliosis and vitiligo**
  - lichenoid dermatosis.
- lack of evidence that ocular signs are caused by neoplasia or infection
- histopathological analysis of skin biopsies:
  - infiltration by histiocytes and lymphocytes.

### Treatment
Treatment modalities include:

- systemic: corticosteroids and azathioprine
- topical: corticosteroids, NSAIDs, cyclosporine and atropine
- intravitreal triamcinolone injection
- treat secondary complications:
  - prevent glaucoma (dorzolamide and timolol)
  - 1% indomethacin eye drops.

### Prognosis
The outlook is serious regarding vision, with many **patients becoming blind**. The development of secondary complications such as glaucoma can be painful, making enucleation necessary in some cases.

## Endocrine diseases

### *Diabetes mellitus*

#### *Epidemiology*
Diabetes mellitus is a common condition with an incidence from 1 in 100 to 1 in 500 for both dogs and cats.

Type 1 (insulin-dependent) diabetes mellitus.

#### *Clinical signs*
Ocular signs include:

- **bilateral cataracts**. These develop over days or weeks:
  1. **initial**. Vacuoles in the equatorial cortex (Figure 8.131)
  2. **progression** to anterior and posterior cortex
  3. **mature**. In a short time, fractures appear in suture lines (Figure 8.132). Cataracts prevent light reaching the retina and cause blindness (possibility of secondary glaucoma).

Cataract formation occurs when the activity of aldose reductase is high and the levels of sorbitol, fructose and dulcitol increase. This leads to hyperosmolarity and water enters the lens, forming an intumescent cataract with a reduction of the anterior chamber, blockage of the drainage angle and a risk of glaucoma (Figure 8.133). Cataract progression depends on patient age and blood glucose levels.

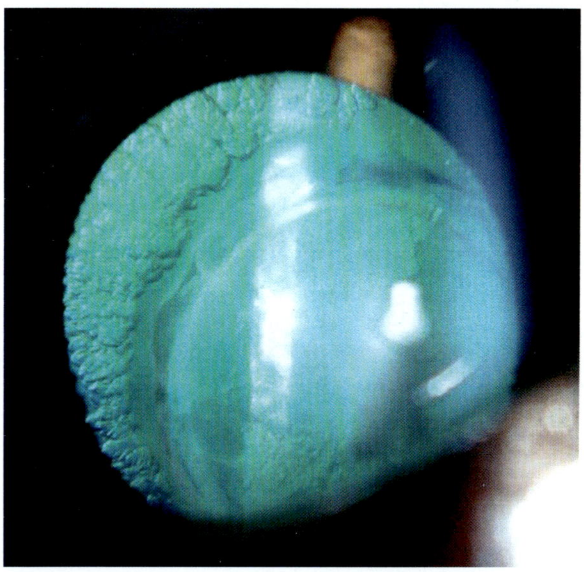

**Figure 8.131.** Diabetic cataract. Initial stage. Note the appearance of vacuoles in the equatorial cortex.

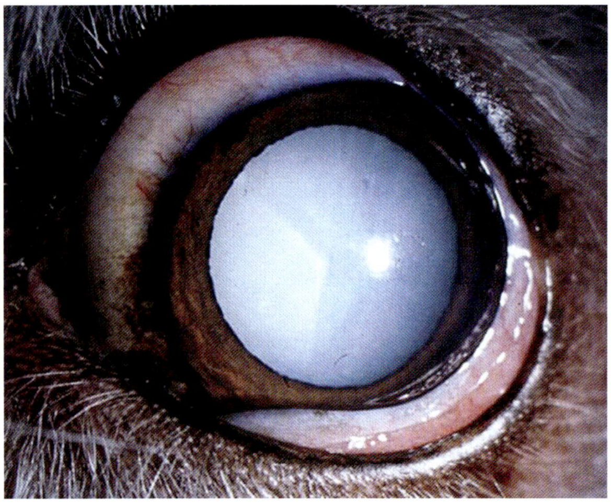

**Figure 8.132.** Mature diabetic cataract with fractures of the suture lines (intumescent).

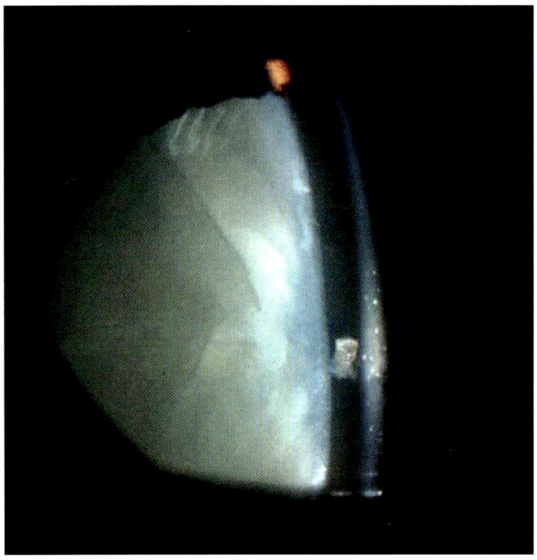

**Figure 8.133.** Biomicroscopic image showing reduction of the anterior chamber in an intumescent diabetic cataract.

- **phaco-induced uveitis**
- **recurrent ulcers**. These are more due to trigeminal dysfunction than corneal sensitivity.
- **diabetic retinopathy** (retinal detachment (Figure 8.134), haemorrhage and microangiopathies (Figure 8.135)).

### *Diagnosis*

In the eye, a diagnosis is established using **biomicroscopy** (reduced anterior chamber, fractures of the lens through the suture lines), **ophthalmoscopy** (inability to visualize the fundus) and **ultrasonography** (lens with anteroposterior enlargement) (Figure 8.136).

A diagnosis of diabetes is reached through measurement of glucose levels in the blood and urine:

- hyperglycaemia, ideally in samples taken at home in a non-stressful environment

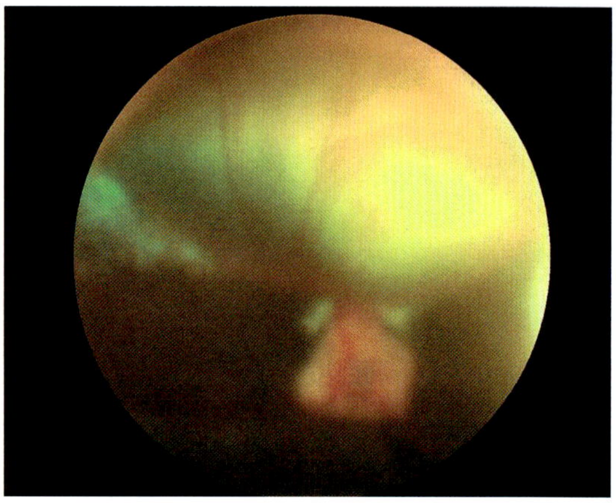

**Figure 8.134.** Retinal detachment in a dog diagnosed with diabetes mellitus.

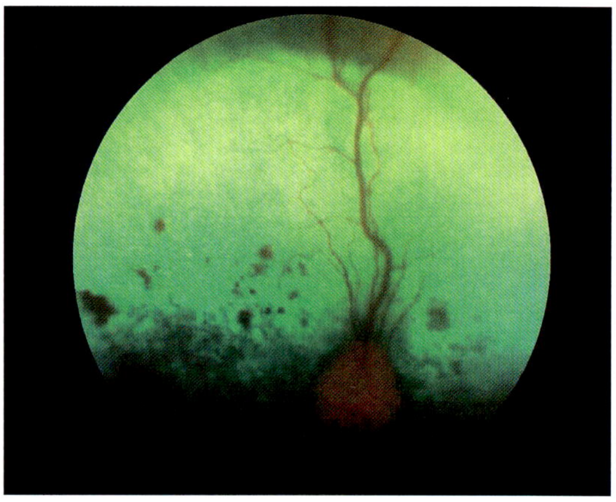

**Figure 8.135.** Diabetic retinopathy. Note the haemorrhages and microangiopathies.

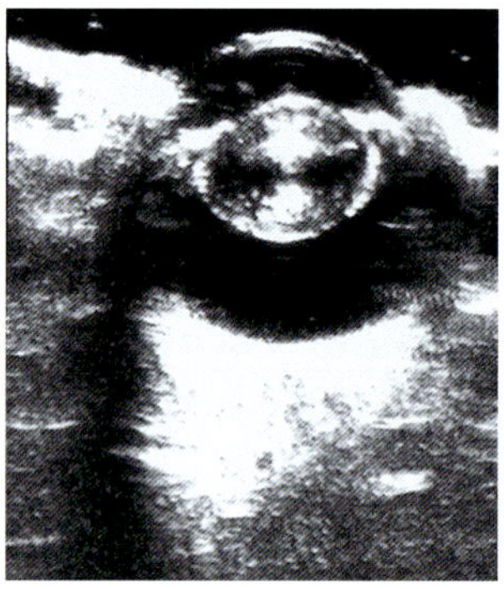

**Figure 8.136.** Ultrasound image of an intumescent diabetic cataract. Note the increase in the diameter of the anteroposterior lens and hourglass shape.

- **persistent fasting glycosuria**
- elevated **serum fructosamine levels**.

There is a complex interaction between the concurrent presence of diabetes mellitus and hyperadrenocorticism, which complicates diabetes control. Therefore, patients with diabetes should be tested for the presence of hyperadrenocorticism.

### Treatment

Both the underlying cause (diabetes) and ocular presentation (cataract) should be treated. This includes stabilization with insulin therapy and dietary adjustment, and careful assessment of retinal function, followed in appropriate cases by phacoemulsification of the cataract.

After surgery, replace corticosteroids with NSAIDs.

## Hyperadrenocorticism or Cushing's syndrome

### Aetiopathogenesis

Hyperadrenocorticism is due to an **excess of natural glucocorticoid production or exogenous administration**.

### Causes

There are three causes:

- hyperplasia or neoplasia of the pituitary gland (ACTH)
- tumour in the adrenal cortex (cortisol)
- iatrogenic.

### Clinical signs

Ocular signs:

- progressive and indolent ulcers
- corneal calcification (Figure 8.137)
- KCS
- accumulation of lipids in the aqueous humour
- lipaemia retinalis
- hypertensive retinopathy
- silent retinal syndrome (SARD).

### Diagnosis

Diagnosis is reached by:

- detecting cortisol/creatinine in urine. A negative result rules out hyperadrenocorticism. A positive result cannot be used as the sole means of diagnosis; it suggests that further investigation is warranted.
- using an ACTH stimulation test
- using a dexamethasone suppression test
- measuring endogenous ACTH to identify the origin.

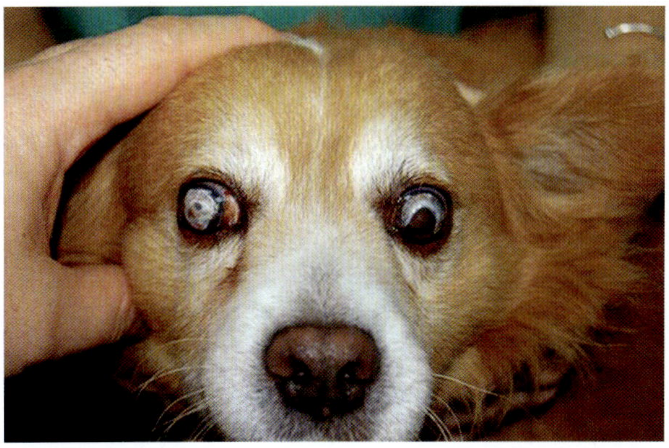

Figure 8.137. Corneal calcifications in a dog diagnosed with Cushing's syndrome.

### Treatment

The mainstay of treatment is the **oral administration of trilostane**. However, in cases resulting from an adrenal gland tumour, surgical adrenalectomy may be appropriate.

For the ocular complications associated with hyperadrenocorticism, symptomatic treatment is warranted, along with stabilization of the underlying condition.

## Hypothyroidism

### Aetiopathogenesis

Hypothyroidism results from a **decrease in $T_3$ and $T_4$ production**. The most common form is primary hypothyroidism due to lymphocytic thyroiditis or idiopathic thyroid atrophy.

### Clinical signs

Ocular signs (due to hyperlipidaemia):

- lipid dystrophy (Figure 8.138)
- corneal ulcers
- secondary uveitis
- accumulation of lipids in the aqueous humour (Figure 8.139)
- lipaemia retinalis
- haemorrhage
- retinal detachment
- KCS (in 20% of cases) (Figure 8.138).

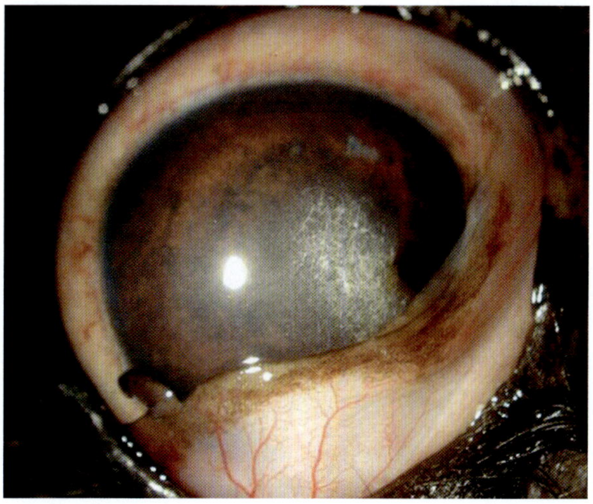

Figure 8.138. Corneal dystrophy and KCS in a dog diagnosed with hypothyroidism. KCS, keratoconjunctivitis sicca.

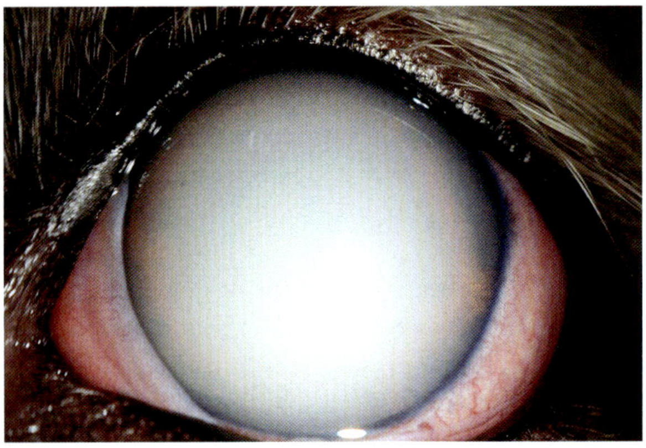

**Figure 8.139.** Lipids in the anterior chamber of a dog diagnosed with hypothyroidism.

### Diagnosis

Serum total $T_4$ and thyroid-stimulating hormone levels are used to diagnose hypothyroidism. Care should be taken to differentiate sick thyroid syndrome from true hypothyroidism. To this end, a thyroid-stimulating hormone stimulation test can help differentiate primary hypothyroidism from euthyroid disease. With the latter, if the hypothalamic–pituitary–thyroid axis is intact, the thyroid responds with an increase in total $T_4$ production.

CT and MRI are required, if there are pituitary and hypothalamic lesions.

### Treatment

Hypothyroidism is a readily treatable condition that responds well to daily oral administration of levothyroxine. In some cases, it is beneficial to restrict lipids and cholesterol in the diet.

In ocular cases, where lipid plaques are present, surgical keratectomy is contraindicated since it predisposes to the formation of larger plaques. Those patients with KCS should be managed appropriately with topical therapies.

## Cardiovascular diseases with ocular involvement

## Systemic hypertension

### Aetiology

Conditions linked to the development of hypertension include:

- chronic nephropathies
- hyperadrenocorticism, pheochromocytoma
- primary aldosteronism
- hyperkinetic cardiac syndrome
- hypercalcaemia, hypo-oestrogenism.

Predispositions to hypertension include obesity and sex (77% are male).

### Clinical signs

Ocular signs:

- oedema in the retina and papilla
- retinal vessel tortuosity and retinal haemorrhages (also in the anterior chamber) (Figure 8.140)
- secondary retinal degeneration
- bullous retinal detachment (blindness) (Figure 8.141).

### Diagnosis

Measurement of **systolic and diastolic pressure**, with diagnostic figures being >180/100 mmHg.

**Stress** causes artificial elevation of blood pressure, so care should be taken to ensure the patient is as relaxed and comfortable as possible when measurements are taken. Several readings should be taken and an average value used.

### Treatment

It is important to **address underlying conditions**, such as renal disease. If this fails to normalize blood pressure, then start systemic therapy. In cases with significant

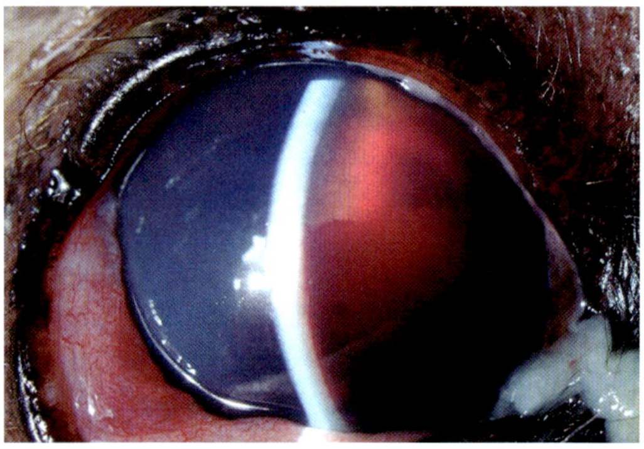

**Figure 8.140.** Hyphaemia in a dog with systemic hypertension.

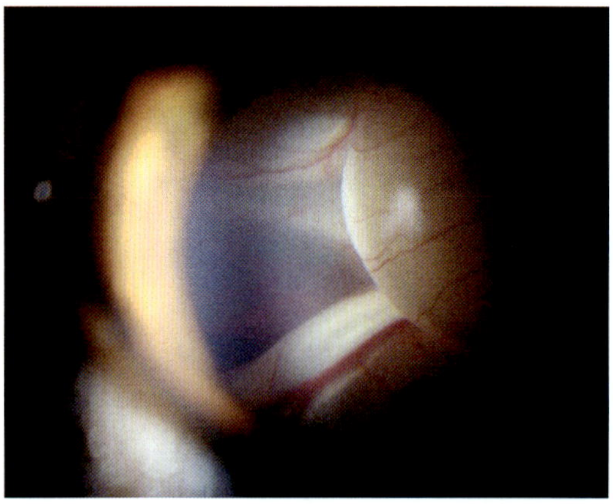

**Figure 8.141.** Biomicroscopic image of bullous retinal detachment in a dog with systemic hypertension.

hypertension, systemic hypertensive medication should be started immediately, but organ function should be monitored.

Systemic treatments:

- angiotensin-converting enzyme inhibitors (enalapril, benazepril)
- calcium antagonists (amlodipine)
- beta blockers (atenolol)
- vasodilators (hydralazine)
- diuretics (furosemide).

Topical treatment:

- manage secondary uveitis with topical steroid application and atropine
- prevent or manage glaucoma with the use of topical prostaglandin analogues, beta blockers or carbonic anhydrase inhibitors, plus pain relief where appropriate.

## Systemic infections with ocular complications in the cat

### *Viral infections*

#### *Feline herpesvirus (feline viral rhinotracheitis)*

#### Aetiopathogenesis

**Feline herpesvirus is a common viral infection in cats.** It can be a contributing agent to 'cat flu'. The virus is shed in oronasal secretions with **cross-infection by sneezing and short-distance aerosol contact.** Infection predisposes the cat to secondary infection with *C. felis*.

Recovered cats become long-term carriers and some kittens may enter a carrier status without ever showing symptoms.

#### Epidemiology

Feline herpesvirus infections are seen in domestic cats, with **colonies and catteries** especially at risk due to the method of transmission.

#### Clinical signs

Ocular signs include:

- conjunctivitis with hyperaemia (Figure 8.142)
- ocular discharge
- **chemosis** (Figure 8.142)
- blepharospasm in adult cats without respiratory symptoms
- dendritic and geographic corneal ulcers
- **KCS**
- stromal keratitis
- symblepharon
- **corneal sequestration** (Figure 8.143)
- eosinophilic keratitis
- corneal vascularization (Figure 8.144)
- pain.

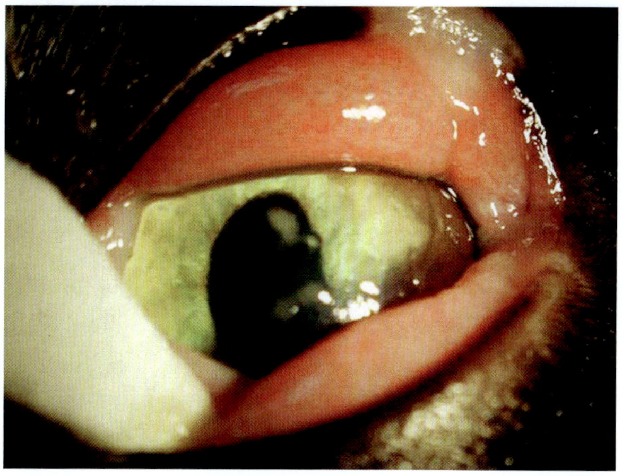

**Figure 8.142.** Feline herpesvirus. Note the presence of conjunctivitis and chemosis.

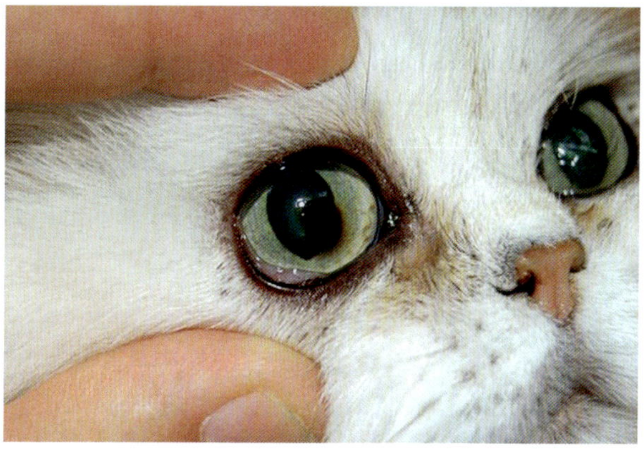

**Figure 8.143.** Feline herpesvirus. Note the presence of chemosis and corneal sequestration.

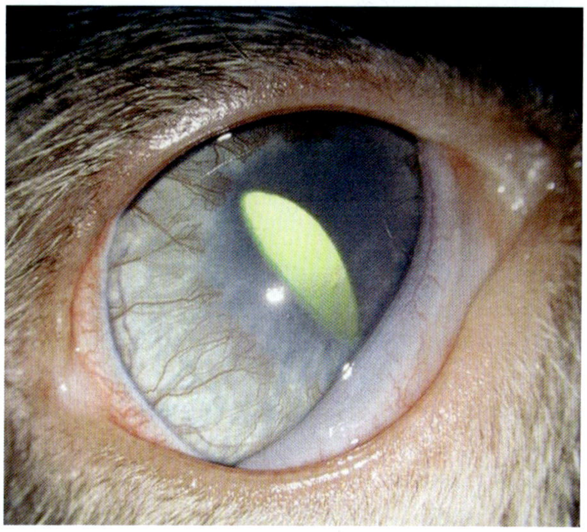

**Figure 8.144.** Corneal vascularization in a cat diagnosed with herpesvirus.

## Diagnosis

The most reliable means of diagnosis include **virus isolation from oropharyngeal swabs** sent in viral transport medium to specialist laboratories. However, be aware that feline herpesvirus is shed intermittently; negative samples in cats with suggestive symptoms should be interpreted with caution. An alternative method of detection is submission of cytological preparations for immunofluorescence analysis.

PCR tests are of limited value due to the high prevalence of herpesvirus in the feline population.

## Treatment

Stress can induce carrier cats to actively shed feline herpesvirus; thus, **stress should be avoided**.

Systemic treatment:

- effective **antiviral drugs**: trifluridine, 5-iododeoxyuridine, vidarabine, ganciclovir
- L-lysine
- interferon alpha and omega
- topical treatment over several weeks to prevent recurrences
- **topical tetracycline** in coinfections with *Mycoplasma* and *C. felis*
- **surgical treatment in corneal necrosis** (corneal sequestration)
- **corticosteroids are contraindicated**.

## *Feline calicivirus*

## Aetiopathogenesis

**Feline calicivirus is one of several infectious agents (including feline herpesvirus) that cause upper respiratory tract disease**. Cats become infected through the oronasal route and pathogenicity varies widely across a range of strains. A high percentage of recovered cats go on to become **persistent carriers** and concurrent infection with FIV enhances secretion of calicivirus by carriers.

## Epidemiology

Domestic cats are infected, especially when **living in groups**.

## Clinical signs

Ocular signs:

- **mild conjunctivitis**.

Systemic signs vary according to the virulence and tropism of the virus:

- fever
- anorexia
- lameness
- oral and lingual ulceration (chronic gingivitis)
- mild respiratory signs (sneezing, runny nose).

## Diagnosis

Clinical signs:

- **virus isolation** from oropharyngeal smears
- PCR performed on oropharyngeal samples.

## Treatment

Treatment is **largely supportive** with the use of broad-spectrum antibiotics for those cases with secondary bacterial infections. Any conjunctivitis should be treated symptomatically with topical antibiotics and regular eye cleaning.

## *Feline leukaemia*

## Aetiopathogenesis

**Feline leukaemia virus is a retrovirus** infection with worldwide distribution. This infectious agent causes anaemia and immunosuppression and is responsible for feline cancer due to cellular transformation.

Infection is spread via **saliva or other bodily secretions** but **close contact** is required to acquire infection. Infected cats can overcome the disease or remain as persistent carriers.

Ocular signs are due to lymphoma and transformed lymphocytes invading the eyeball.

## Clinical signs

Ocular signs:

- **mild uveitis** (corneal precipitates)
- **masses in the iris** (thickening and distortion (Figure 8.145))
- **glaucoma** secondary to obstruction of the iridocorneal angle.

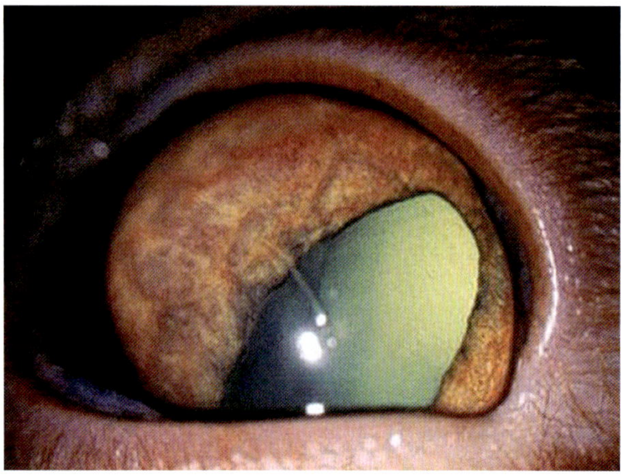

**Figure 8.145.** Mass in the iris and pupillary distortion in a cat with feline leukaemia virus.

Systemic signs vary depending on the viral subtype responsible for the infection and the affected organ system.

### Diagnosis

Diagnosis is made using:

- serological tests: enzyme-linked immunosorbent assay, immunofluorescence
- PCR on tissue samples, including from the cornea.

### Treatment

Treatment consists of:

- **chemotherapeutic protocols** (vincristine, cyclophosphamide, prednisolone) for lymphomas
- **interferon omega** has been shown to increase longevity in some cases
- symptomatic treatment of ocular manifestations
- enucleation in cases of:
  - uveitis that is refractory to treatment
  - secondary glaucoma.

### Prophylaxis

The vaccine is protective.

## *Feline immunodeficiency virus*

### Aetiopathogenesis

**The infection is caused by lentiviruses**, A–D subtypes, with worldwide distribution. Infection occurs **most commonly through bites** and less commonly via placental transfer. The virus cannot survive in the environment and **direct transfer is required** for infection.

### Clinical signs

FIV infection has a **long incubation period**, with infected cats often remaining healthy for long periods of time. Signs of primary disease include:

- fever
- leukopenia
- lymphadenopathy
- weight loss
- neurological disorders
- susceptibility to secondary infections.

Ocular signs include:

- conjunctivitis
- **anterior uveitis** (Figure 8.146)
- pars planitis (inflammation between the iris and choroid)
- glaucoma with or without uveitis
- **focal retinal degeneration**

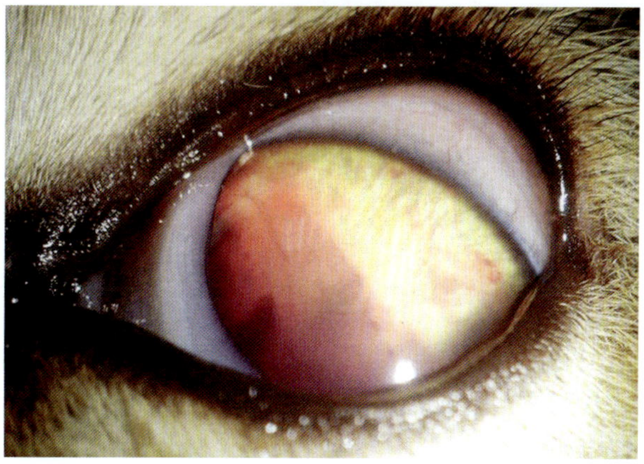

**Figure 8.146.** Anterior uveitis with hyphaemia in a cat diagnosed with FIV. FIV, feline immunodeficiency virus.

- retinal haemorrhage
- concurrent *Toxoplasma* and FIV infection resulting in **anterior uveitis** and chorioretinitis.

### Diagnosis

Serological tests: enzyme-linked immunosorbent assay, immunofluorescence, western blotting and virus isolation.

For seronegative cats in the acute phase of infection, **tests should be repeated at the 6–8-week** point to confirm they are truly negative.

### Treatment

Systemic treatment:

- clindamycin, with the addition of steroids in cases with posterior uveitis.

Topical treatment:

- atropine or tropicamide
- corticosteroids if there is anterior uveitis.

## *Feline infectious peritonitis*

### Aetiopathogenesis

Feline infectious peritonitis (FIP) is an infection caused by **feline coronaviruses** with a worldwide distribution. There are **two serotypes**, which are associated with a range of symptoms from diarrhoea to fulminant FIP:

- **enteric feline coronavirus**, which affects enterocytes
- **FIP virus**, a mutated form of enteric feline coronavirus that affects macrophages.

Stress can predispose to disease, with infection spread via **infected faeces** or less commonly by saliva during mutual grooming. The virus can remain viable in cat faeces for several weeks.

FIP is due to the formation of **immune complexes** when the virus interacts with specific antibodies and inflammatory cells. Ultimately, this results in **granulomatous vasculitis** that affects organs irrigated by these vessels, as occurs in the retina.

## Epidemiology

Most cats affected are **under 2 years of age**, with a higher incidence among multi-cat households, catteries and shelters.

## Clinical signs

There are two types of FIP:

- **effusive (wet)**
- **non-effusive (dry)**.

Ocular signs in dry FIP include:

- iritis with **iris colour change** (Figure 8.147)
- bilateral **anterior uveitis** (Figure 8.148)

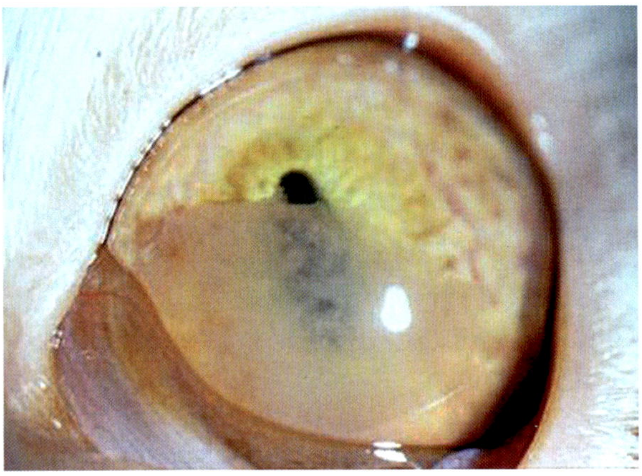

Figure 8.147. Iritis with colour change of the iris and presence of fibrin in the anterior chamber in a cat diagnosed with FIP. FIP, feline infectious peritonitis.

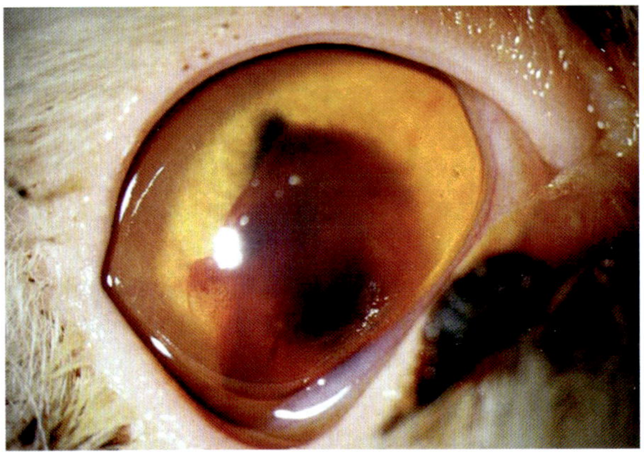

Figure 8.148. Anterior uveitis with hyphaema in a cat diagnosed with FIP. FIP, feline infectious peritonitis.

- corneal precipitates
- **fibrin** in the anterior chamber (Figure 8.147)
- haemorrhage in the anterior chamber (Figure 8.148)
- chorioretinitis
- haemorrhages and retinal detachment
- optic neuritis.

## Diagnosis

Diagnosis is complicated and requires careful consideration of multiple factors, such as clinical history, clinical signs, laboratory test abnormalities, ultrasound and serological results, as well as cytological, biochemical, histopathological and immunohistochemical findings of biopsies and bodily fluids, and PCR results.

## Treatment

Symptomatic, systemic supportive treatment, the nature of which varies depending on the stage of the disease:

- immunosuppressive drugs (glucocorticoids, melphalan)
- human interferon alpha
- vitamins (A, $B_1$, C)
- acetylsalicylic acid
- anabolic steroids
- antibiotics.

Topical treatment:

- corticosteroids (topical or subconjunctival)
- atropine.

## Prognosis

Poor, despite treatment.

# *Bacterial infections*

## *Bartonellosis*

## Aetiopathogenesis

Bartonellosis is caused by *Bartonella henselae* and *Bartonella clarridgeiae*. The route of infection is unclear but is linked to the **cat ingesting infected fleas or flea excreta**.

**Bartonellosis is a zoonosis**. People acquire infection via transfer of *Bartonella* spp. through **broken skin**, often as a result of a cat scratch, hence the popular name **'cat scratch fever'**.

## Epidemiology

Cats that live outside or have **contact with fleas and flea faeces** are at the greatest risk of infection.

## Clinical signs

Most cats are **asymptomatic**. Those experiencing **waxing and waning bacteraemia** may exhibit systemic signs such as:

- **mild febrile state**
- transient neurological disorders.

### *Ocular signs*

Ocular signs include:

- anterior blepharitis
- conjunctivitis
- keratitis
- corneal ulcers
- **uveitis**
- **chorioretinitis**.

## Diagnosis

- **Growth of *Bartonella* from blood or tissue culture** is considered the criterion standard. However, false negative results occur due to the transient nature of bacteraemia, and many laboratories do not perform these tests.
- specific serological tests
- PCR.

## Treatment

To eliminate the infection: rifampicin plus doxycycline for 14–21 days.

To confirm successful elimination of infection, cultures should be repeated three weeks after treatment cessation.

Ocular manifestations of bartonellosis are managed with symptomatic treatment.

## *Chlamydia*

## Aetiopathogenesis

**Cats can become infected with *C. felis*** (up to 45% of healthy cats are seropositive).

*C. felis* is an obligate intracellular bacterium that may be present in the ocular, gastrointestinal, respiratory and urogenital mucous membranes. Cats can enter a **carrier state**, with clinical disease reactivated by stress.

## Clinical signs

It rarely causes systemic symptoms, which when present are mild respiratory signs. Clinical cases usually present with **ocular symptoms** including:

- **conjunctivitis** with conjunctival **hyperaemia and chemosis**
- serous or mucopurulent ocular discharge (Figure 8.149)
- blepharospasm (Figure 8.149).

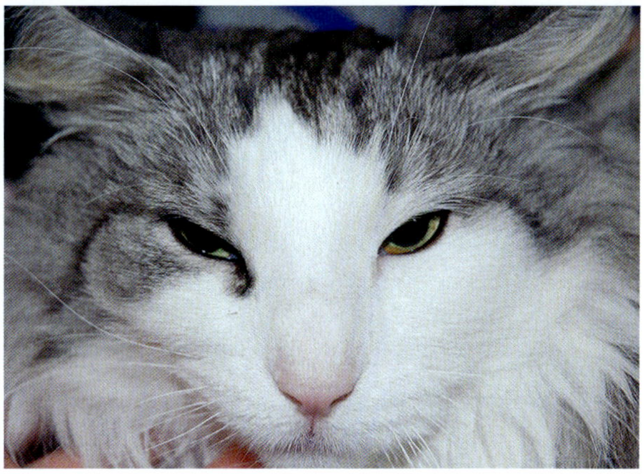

**Figure 8.149.** Presence of serous ocular secretion and severe blepharospasm in a cat diagnosed with chlamydia.

## Diagnosis

A diagnosis is made via:

- **chlamydial culture**. A moistened swab is rolled over the inner aspect of the nictitating membrane (third eyelid) and transported to the laboratory in chlamydial transport media.
- **conjunctival cytological** analysis looking for intra-epithelial cell inclusions
- serological tests (only demonstrate exposure rather than proving active disease)
- PCR on a sample collected similarly as for chlamydial culture.

## Treatment

Systemic treatment:

- oral tetracyclines for 6 weeks (doxycycline).

Topical treatment:

- **tetracycline in ophthalmic ointment**.

## Prophylaxis

The best protection is achieved with **modified live vaccines**. However, vaccination does not prevent colonization or spread of the microorganism but attenuates the clinical signs in infected animals.

## *Mycoplasmosis*

## Aetiopathogenesis

Infection is caused by *Mycoplasma felis*, *Mycoplasma gateae* and *Mycoplasma arginini*. These have been isolated from the **upper respiratory tract of both healthy and diseased cats**, and the organs of diseased and weakened cats. These may act as **secondary opportunistic pathogens** in pneumonia and viral infections.

## Clinical signs

There are many species of *Mycoplasma* that vary in clinical significance. Those referenced here are the most likely to cause ocular signs, including:

- **conjunctivitis in young cats**
- **complicated conjunctivitis** caused by other infections (feline herpesvirus or chlamydiosis).

## Diagnosis

Diagnosis is made by:

- observation of cytoplasmic inclusion bodies
- PCR on nasal smears placed in transport media.

## Treatment

Topical tetracycline.

## *Toxoplasmosis*

## Aetiopathogenesis

Infection by the protozoal parasite *Toxoplasma gondii*.

The cat is the definitive host; part of this parasite's life cycle involves the host shedding oocysts in their faeces.

Cats acquire infection via:

- ingestion of meat contaminated with oocysts (the most common method of transmission among hunting cats)
- transplacental transmission
- lactogenic transmission

*Toxoplasma* has a cellular tropism for:

- brain
- liver
- lungs
- skeletal muscle
- eyes.

## Epidemiology

Toxoplasmosis affects all mammals, although it is more frequent in the cat which is the definitive host. Humans can acquire accidental infection from cats via contact with sporulated oocysts. Should this occur during pregnancy, infection can result in foetal malformations.

## Clinical signs

Systemic signs are vague and include:

- pyrexia
- diarrhoea
- weight loss
- jaundice
- dyspnoea
- peritoneal effusion.

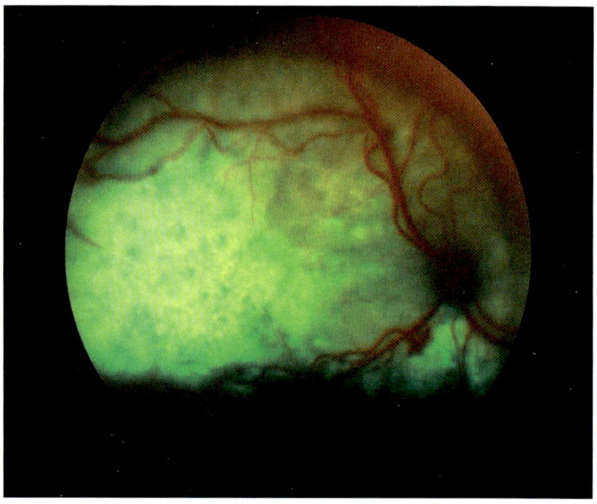

**Figure 8.150.** Posterior uveitis in a cat diagnosed with toxoplasmosis.

Ocular signs (present in 82% of cases) include:

- anterior or posterior bilateral uveitis (Figure 8.150)
- secondary dislocation of the lens
- glaucoma
- retinal detachment.

## Diagnosis

Diagnosis is made by:

- cytology of body fluids (tachyzoites)
- positive serological tests (these do not confirm active disease but indicate exposure)
- PCR on tissue samples and body fluids.

## Treatment

### *Systemic treatment*

Antimicrobials that inhibit the microorganism rather than eliminate it; this means that infected animals do not eliminate it:

- drug of choice: clindamycin 25 mg/kg/12 h VO for 21–30 days
- combination: sulphonamides plus pyrimethamine plus trimethoprim
- folic acid supplements.

Treatment of eye involvement:

- topical corticosteroids and atropine
- if there is posterior uveitis: clindamycin and systemic corticosteroids.

## Cardiovascular disease

### Systemic hypertension

#### Aetiopathogenesis

Systemic hypertension may be secondary to:

- renal disease. In cats, systemic hypertension is more frequent in those suffering from chronic kidney disease.
- hyper- and hypothyroidism
- hyperoestrogenism
- hyperkinetic cardiac syndrome (anaemia, polycythaemia)
- cardiomyopathies.

#### Clinical signs

Ocular signs:

- oedema of the retina and papilla
- retinal vessel tortuosity
- preretinal, intraretinal and subretinal haemorrhages (Figure 8.151)
- secondary retinal degeneration due to ischaemia or inflammation
- sudden blindness. Fixed, dilated pupils are observed.

#### Diagnosis

Blood pressure measurement (repeat several times).

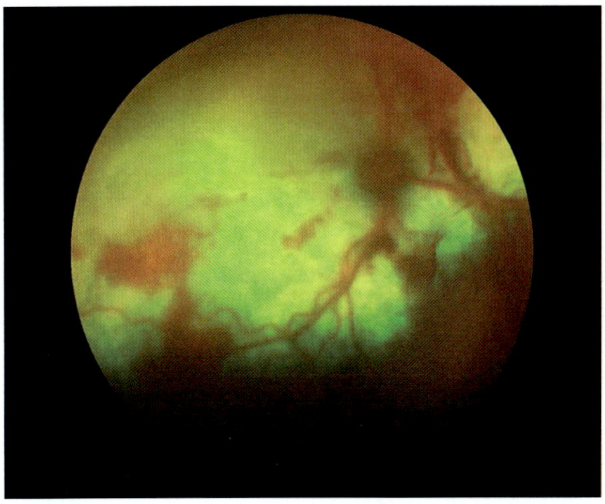

**Figure 8.151.** Retinal haemorrhages in a cat diagnosed with systemic hypertension.

Interpretation of results:

- 180/100 mmHg (high)
- 200/110 mmHg (clinical importance).

#### Treatment

Aetiological treatment of the underlying cause.

Systemic treatment includes:

- carbonic anhydrase inhibitors, such as amlodipine
- angiotensin-converting enzyme inhibitors.

Treatment of eye conditions includes:

- prevention of glaucoma and secondary uveitis
- application of topical and/or systemic corticosteroids.

## Bibliography

### Books


Barnett, K.C. (1992). *Atlas de Oftalmologia Veterinaria*. Grass, Barcelona.

Barnett, K.C. and Crispin, S.M. (1998). *Feline Ophthalmology: an Atlas & Text*. W.B. Saunders Company, London.

Featherstone, H. and Holt, E. (2011). *Small Animal Ophthalmology. What's your diagnosis?* Wiley-Blackwell, Chichester, UK.

Gelatt, K.N., Gilger, B.C. and Kern, T.J. (2013). *Veterinary Ophthalmology*, 5th edn. Wiley-Blackwell, Ames, IA.

Gelatt, K.N. (2014). *Essentials of Veterinary Ophthalmology*, 3rd edn. John Wiley & Sons, Ames, IA.

Gelatt, K.N. and Plummer, C.E. (2017). *Color Atlas of Veterinary Ophthalmology*, 2nd edn. Wiley, Chichester.

Maggs, D.J., Miller, P.E. and Ofri, R. (2018). *Slatter's Fundamentals of Veterinary Ophthalmology*, 6th edn. Elsevier, St Louis, MO.

Martin, C.L. (2009). *Ophthalmic Disease in Veterinary Medicine*. CRC Press, Boca Raton, FL.

Peiffer, R.L. and Petersen-Jones, S.M. (2002). *Oftalmología de Pequeños Animales*, 3rd edn. Harcourt, Madrid.

Stades, C., Wyman, M. and Boevé, M.H. (2007). *Ophthalmology for the Veterinary Practitioner*. Schlütersche, Hannover.


### Journals


*Veterinary Ophthalmology*. Blackwell Publishing.

*Veterinary Clinics of North America: Small Animal Practice*. Elsevier.

## Test

1. **The secondary causes of conjunctivitis in dogs and cats are:**
   A) presence of a foreign body
   B) bacterial problems
   C) mechanical irritation, tear film abnormalities, systemic conditions
   D) viral conditions.
2. **Clinical signs of keratoconjunctivitis sicca:**
   A) mucopurulent ocular discharge, very sticky and greenish-yellowish, blepharospasm and red eye
   B) deep ulcers with negative fluorescein test
   C) dermatitis of the lower eyelid
   D) positive fluorescein test in all cases.
3. **In relation to corneal healing, indicate which statement is correct:**
   A) Stromal repair mechanisms can be due to vascular or avascular scarring or combinations of both.
   B) Descemet's membrane and endothelium undergo regeneration after damage, at any age.
   C) Stromal repair is rapid, as is that of the epithelium.
   D) Corneal repair is faster when topical NSAIDs are applied, regardless of the cause of the corneal condition.
4. **Treatment guidelines for deep collagenase ulcers:**
   A) topical antibiotic application every hour and topical 1% atropine
   B) topical use of NSAIDs
   C) collagenase-inhibiting agents and application of specific topical antibiotic every 1 or 2 hours
   D) use of healing ointments.
5. **Indicate the incorrect answer regarding the clinical picture of anterior uveitis:**
   A) photophobia, tearing, exophthalmia
   B) blindness and corneal precipitates
   C) miosis, ciliary injection, corneal precipitates
   D) Tyndall effect, neovascularization of the iris.
6. **Immature cataracts consist of:**
   A) full lens opacity with blindness
   B) lens opacity greater than 40%
   C) lens opacity less than 40%
   D) liquefaction of the lens.
7. **Vision loss syndrome where no abnormalities are present in the fundus is:**
   A) progressive retinal atrophy
   B) daytime blindness
   C) silent retinal syndrome
   D) retinal degeneration.
8. **The most representative ocular signs of feline leukaemia virus are (indicate which answer is false):**
   A) mild uveitis with presence of keratic precipitates
   B) presence of hyphaemia and fibrin in the anterior chamber
   C) presence of masses in the iris
   D) secondary glaucoma due to obstruction of the iridocorneal angle.
9. **Systemic causes of symblepharon in the cat are (indicate the incorrect answer):**
   A) feline herpesvirus type 1
   B) chlamydia
   C) feline immunodeficiency virus
   D) all of these.
10. **Regarding the ocular signs and evolution of canine infectious hepatitis, indicate the answer that is incorrect:**
    A) Appearance of blepharospasm and miosis.
    B) Bilateral blue eye in 12–28% of cases, which evolves into keratoconus in complicated cases.
    C) In the Afghan shepherd dog, it becomes chronic and frequently causes glaucoma.
    D) Recovery is never spontaneous.

**11. Ocular signs in the retina in uveodermatological syndrome include (indicate which answer is incorrect):**
   A) bullous retinal detachment
   B) tapetal hyperreflectivity with normal vessel gauges
   C) depigmentation of the retinal pigment epithelium in the non-tapetal area
   D) atrophy of the retina and optic nerve.

**12. Regarding diabetes mellitus, point out which statement is incorrect:**
   A) There is appearance of recurrent ulcers due to trigeminal nerve dysfunction.
   B) Rapidly forming bilateral cataracts are present due to high aldose reductase activity.
   C) Appearance of secondary glaucoma is due to the increase in the anteroposterior diameter of the lens.
   D) Phacoclastic type uveitis is present.

## Clinical case 1

**Signalment:** 9-year-old mixed breed, spayed female dog weighing 10 kg. Housing: a flat.

**Reason for consultation:** sudden loss of vision in January (4 days ago). The owners comment that lately the animal drinks and urinates more. They also comment that it seems to have white pupils.

**Physical examination:** body condition 7/9. The rest of the physical examination is normal.

**Eye examination:** absence of bilateral threat response. Direct and consensual photomotor reflexes very diminished, maintaining semi-mydriasis in both eyes. Schirmer's test 16 mm/min in the right eye and 18 mm/min in the left eye. Tonometry 15 mmHg in the right eye and 13 mmHg in the left.

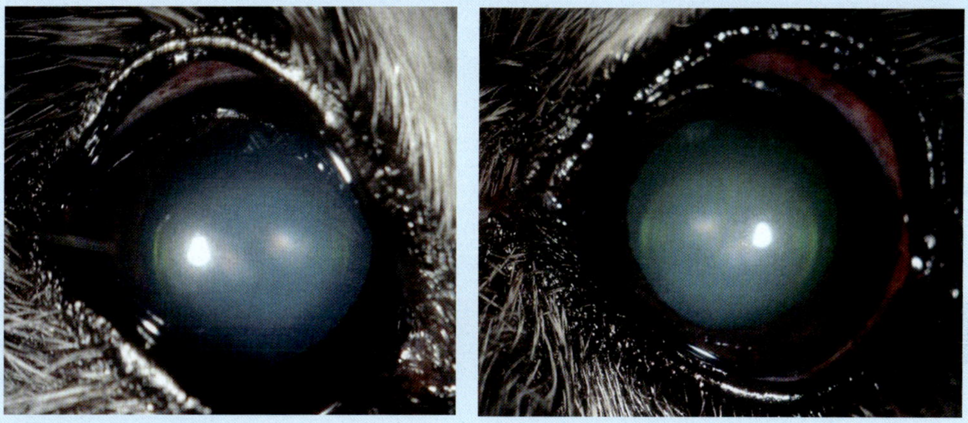

**Figure case 1.1a,b**

**1. What ocular signs can be seen in Figure case 1.1?**
   A) bilateral cataracts
   B) conjunctival hyperaemia and lens sclerosis
   C) conjunctival hyperaemia and buphthalmia
   D) subluxation of the lens and corneal oedema.

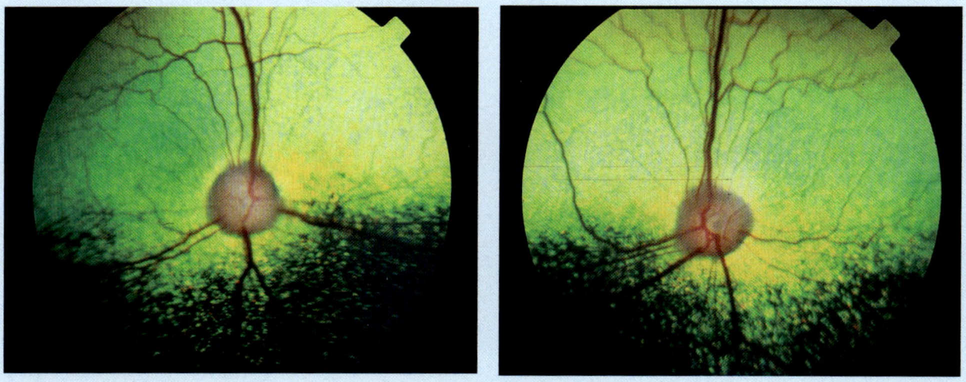

**Figure case 1.2a,b**

2. **Which clinical signs can you point out in the ophthalmoscopic images in Figure case 1.2?**
   A) retinal detachment
   B) presence of an optic disc with signs of inflammation
   C) depigmentation of the retinal pigment epithelium with visualization of the choroid
   D) slight thinning of retinal vessels but without any other remarkable sign.
3. **Which complementary test in addition to ocular examination would be necessary to reach a diagnosis?**
   A) ocular ultrasound
   B) electroretinography
   C) CT of the head
   D) MRI of the head.
4. **Based on what was observed in Images 1 and 2, what is the most likely diagnosis?**
   A) systemic hypertension with secondary retinal detachment
   B) progressive retinal atrophy
   C) chorioretinitis and/or optic neuritis
   D) sudden acquired retinal degeneration.
5. **Would you recommend any further tests to the owner based on the aetiology of the condition that has been diagnosed?**
   A) blood tests aimed at diagnosing hyperadrenocorticism and adrenal ultrasound
   B) blood tests aimed at diagnosing diabetes mellitus
   C) blood tests to detect toxins
   D) abdominal radiology.
6. **The prognosis of visual function is:**
   A) favourable after topical and systemic treatment (immunosuppressive doses) with anti-inflammatory therapy
   B) unfavourable because there is no treatment for the condition
   C) reserved with specific treatment
   D) only favourable by administering topical anti-inflammatory treatment.

## Clinical case 2

**Signalment:** 3-year-old, unspayed retriever from Burgos. Housing: farm.
**Reason for consultation:** eye problems for the last two years. According to the owner, the condition began with a red eye. He comments that the dog is used for hunting and observes a certain clumsiness. The problem has continued progressing to the present day, at which point she has become blind. She is being treated with topical tobramycin and dexamethasone.
**Physical examination:** body condition 5/9 (24 kg). There is nothing remarkable on physical examination.
**Eye examination:** threat response in both eyes. The photomotor reflexes could not be assessed. Schirmer's test 18 mm/min in the right eye and 19 mm/min in the left eye. Tonometry of 46 mmHg in the right eye and 12 mmHg in the left eye. Both eyes were fluorescein-negative. Both had conjunctival hyperaemia, although it was more obvious in the right eye.

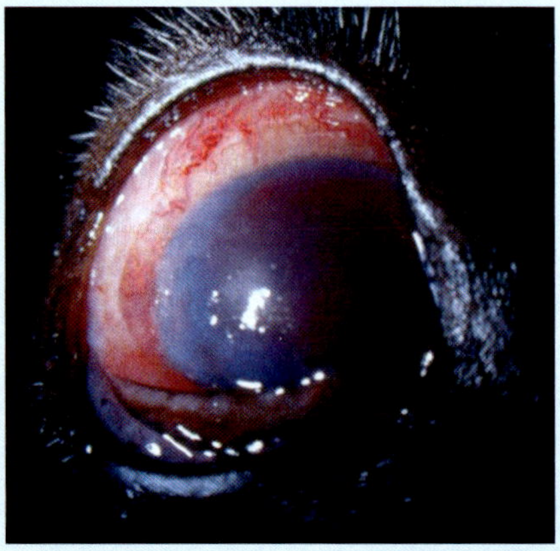

Figure case 2.1

**1. Description of the ocular signs seen in Figure case 2.1:**

A) buphthalmos
B) corneal oedema
C) hyphaemia
D) all of these.

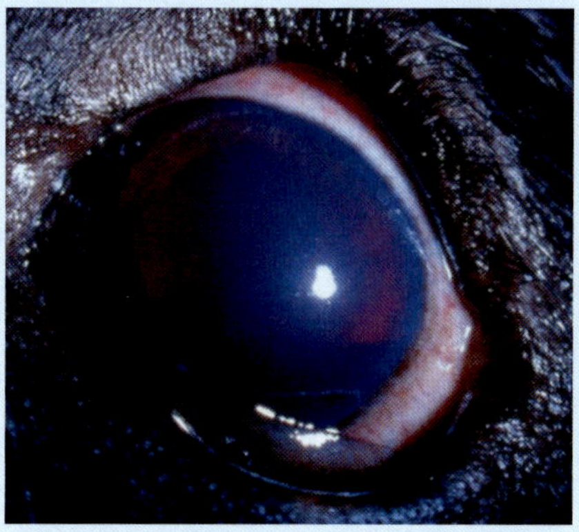

Figure case 2.2

**2. Description of the ocular signs seen in Figure case 2.2:**

A) hyphaemia
B) buphthalmos
C) corneal oedema
D) hypopyon.

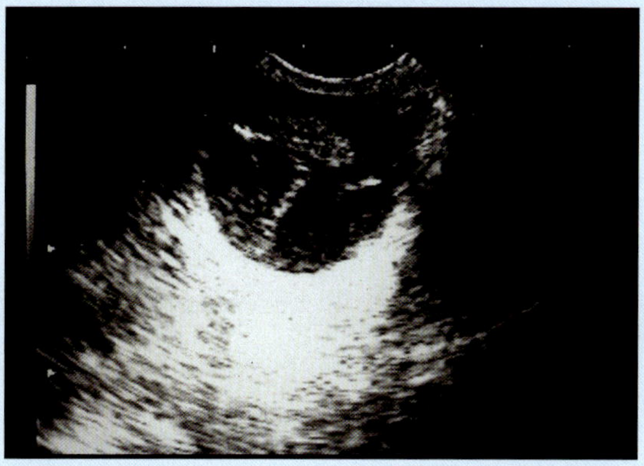

Figure case 2.3

**3. Ultrasound signs seen in Figure case 2.3:**

A) microphakia, presence of retrolental tissue and hyperechogenicity of the lens
B) vitreous hyperechogenic lines, compatible with retinal detachment
C) hyperechogenic line that connects the lens with the optic nerve
D) all of these.

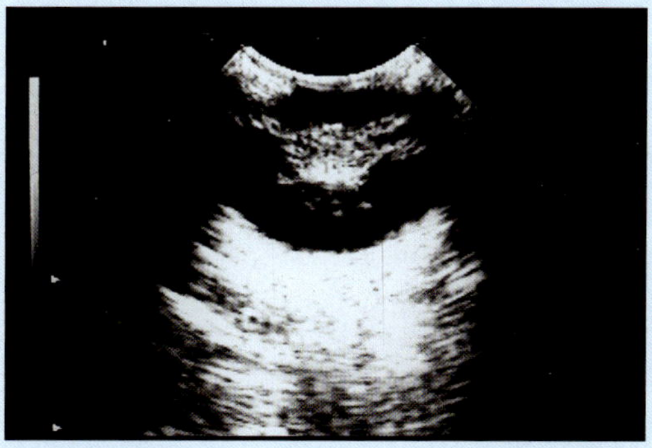

Figure case 2.4

4. **Ultrasound signs seen in Figure case 2.4:**
   A) microphakia, microphthalmia, hyperechogenic lens and retrolental tissue
   B) microphthalmia
   C) presence of hyperechogenic mass in vitreous chamber compatible with haemorrhage
   D) only hyperechogenicity of the lens.
5. **Based on what was observed in Images 1 and 2, what would be the most likely diagnosis?**
   A) persistence of grade 4 hyperplastic primary vitreous in the left eye and grade 6 in the right eye
   B) bilateral cataracts
   C) bilateral uveitis
   D) bilateral glaucoma.
6. **What is the most appropriate approach in this patient?**
   A) surgical treatment of cataracts
   B) medical treatment with topical and systemic anti-inflammatories
   C) evisceration and intraocular prosthesis in both eyes
   D) treatment for glaucoma in the right eye and anti-inflammatory treatment in the left eye.

## Answers

### Test

| | |
|---|---|
| 1. C | 7. C |
| 2. A | 8. B |
| 3. A | 9. C |
| 4. C | 10. D |
| 5. B | 11. A |
| 6. C | 12. D |

### Clinical case 1

1. B
2. D
3. B
4. D
5. A
6. B

### Clinical case 2

1. D
2. A
3. D
4. A
5. A
6. C

# 9

# Cytology

Nick Marsh

## Chapter summary



## Introduction

Although to the uninitiated, cytology often appears to be a mass of blue and purplish-red blobs, to the skilled cytologist it is an extremely useful tool for evaluating swellings, growths, inflammation and other cellular changes within the skin, subcutis, viscera and fluids. It is relatively simple to perform, cheap and cost effective. It also has the added bonuses of being fascinating, very rewarding and, occasionally, extremely beautiful.

Although it should be realistically regarded as a screening test (to evaluate the presence of neoplasia, inflammation, infectious agents or other non-neoplastic lesions) it can, with proper techniques, often provide a specific diagnosis with the advantages of being quick, comparatively safe and minimally invasive.

As with any tests, there are limitations: cytological specimens do not preserve tissue architecture, which makes evaluation of complex or heterogeneous lesions (such as mammary neoplasms) challenging. Cells degenerate rapidly within fluid, making their identity challenging or impossible to assess if examination is delayed. Some lesions exfoliate cells very poorly, whereas some contain very friable cells that may rupture on aspiration.

Some lesions (particularly neuroendocrine neoplasms) have a benign cytological appearance that belies their aggressive clinical behaviour. Inflammation, necrosis or cell degeneration within fluid can all cause cytological changes that mimic malignant change. Additionally, the presence of multiple pathological processes (such as inflammation within a tumour, or multiple neoplastic processes) can be confusing cytologically.

However, many of these pitfalls can be avoided, or at least alleviated, with good planning, good technique, careful sample preparation as well as consideration of the broader clinical picture. The aim of this chapter is to help the reader to make sense of those bluish-purple blobs and, perhaps, start to share the fascination that many cytologists develop for the unique insight that their microscopes provide.

### Key learning points

- Understand the principles and practical aspects of cytological sample collection, storage and preparation.
- Learn how to approach cytological specimens in a stepwise fashion.
- Understand the principles of routine cytological examination.
- Recognise the different cytological characteristics of effusions, aspirates and lavage samples.
- Recognise conditions most commonly diagnosed by cytology.

## Sampling techniques

The most commonly harvested specimens are lesions within the skin, subcutaneous tissues and lymph nodes, and the liver and spleen are the most commonly harvested internal viscera, but decent and often diagnostic samples can usually be safely taken from many others including lung, thyroid, kidney, intestine, bladder and the reproductive organs – if a lesion is visible on imaging, it can usually be successful aspirated with at least some chance of a quick, definitive diagnosis.

The most frequently examined fluids are blood and pleural or abdominal effusions, but other fluid specimens that can be usefully assessed include urine, joint fluid, cerebrospinal fluid and washes from a variety of locations (nasal, BAL, prostatic).

Impression smears from ulcerated or inflamed cutaneous lesions often harvest predominantly surface inflammation only, but they can occasionally provide helpful clues to underlying disease processes (such as acantholytic cells and non-degenerate neutrophils, raising suspicion for immune-mediated disease). Additionally, impression smears of swabs taken from the external ear canals, conjunctiva/cornea and sinus tracts, as well as smears of surgical biopsies, can provide limited information on infections and neoplastic processes more quickly than microbiological or histopathological examinations.

The diagnostic reward from these samples depends on the quality and preservation of the preparations – selecting the most appropriate sampling method greatly improves the chance of taking a diagnostic sample. **Table 9.1** summarises the most appropriate sampling and preparation methods for a variety of different tissues, based upon the author's and others' experience – although note that, in most cases, using a variety of sampling methods where possible (e.g. **both suction and non-suction preparations for most solid lesions, direct, concentrated (or squash) and cytocentrifuged preparations for fluid**) will improve diagnostic chances.

Table 9.1. Recommended sampling and preparation techniques for different lesions.

| Lesion or specimen | Sampling method | Preparation technique |
|---|---|---|
| Hard masses, bone lesions | FNAB – suction | 'Squash', 'blood smear'* |
| Soft masses, lymph nodes, vascular lesions/organs | FNAB – non-suction | 'Squash', 'blood smear'* |
| Effusions (bloody) | Fluid collection | Direct or buffy coat |
| Effusions (turbid), abscesses | Fluid collection | Direct or concentrated** |
| Effusions (clear), CSF, urine, other poorly cellular fluids | Fluid collection | Cytocentrifuge preparation |
| Viscous fluid (e.g. synovial) | Fluid collection | Direct or squash |
| Surgical biopsy, ulcerated lesions | Impression smear | Imprint |
| Conjunctiva/cornea, very firm cutaneous lesions, plaque-like lesions | Scraping | Imprint or roll |
| Mucosae, ear canals, sinus tracts | Rolled swab | Roll |
| Respiratory tract, prostate*** | Wash | Direct, concentrated or cytocentrifuged** |

*Where sufficient fluid/blood is present

**Depending on cellularity

***Although prostatic washes eliminate the risk of needle-tract metastasis from prostatic neoplasia, in the author's experience the diagnostic quality is generally inferior to direct prostatic aspirates.

## Safety of cytological techniques and recommended precautions

Cytology is minimally invasive and, in the majority of cases, can be carried out without sedation. The risk associated with aspiration of lesions is negligible in the majority of cases. Situations with slight risk of complications include:

- Aspiration of haemorrhagic lesions (e.g. thyroid masses, vascular neoplasms such as haemangiosarcomas).
- Aspiration of vascular organs (e.g. liver or spleen) in patients with impaired coagulation ability.
- Aspiration of mast cell tumours leading to histamine release.
- Aspiration of lesions in highly excitable patients.
- Failure of sterility (risk of implantation of infection).
- Aspiration of intra-thoracic lesions (slight risk of pneumothorax).
- Aspiration of adrenal masses with suspected phaeochromocytoma (hypertension followed by paradoxical hypotension has been reported).
- Aspiration of neoplastic lesions that may seed along the needle tract.

Recommended precautions in these cases are as follows:

- When aspirating lesions suspected to be haemorrhagic, or from patients with impaired coagulation ability, close monitoring of the patient for half an hour to an hour following sampling to assess for bleeding is recommended.
- Pre-sampling treatment of patients with suspected mast cell disease with antihistamines may be prudent, and having equipment and medication for anaphylaxis treatment close to hand is recommended.
- Highly excitable, stressed or aggressive patients may be sedated prior to sampling.
- High standards of sterility should be maintained as much as possible during sampling.
- Pneumothorax is extremely rare following sampling of intrathoracic masses, but appropriate equipment should be nearby to deal with the complication if it arises.
- Similarly, the risk of hypotension following aspiration of suspected phaeochromocytoma appears to be very rare, but caution, as above, is advised when attempting aspiration of these lesions*.

*Needle-tract metastasis has been reported in transitional cell carcinomas, renal carcinomas and pulmonary adenocarcinomas, but it is extremely rare. The risks of needle-tract implantation neoplasia must be weighed against the value of rapid diagnosis and the limited treatment options available for these neoplasms.

## Fine needle aspirate biopsy (FNAB)

Clipping of the area may be warranted where it will aid visualisation of the lesion, or where internal organs or body cavities are to be entered and where sterility or contamination is more of a concern. An alcohol swab is recommended for most lesions to clean the area, and to reduce the risk of contamination with surface commensal organisms where infection is suspected. If ultrasound contact gel or anaesthetic cream is used, then excess gel/cream should be wiped away as this can have a significant effect on the diagnostic quality of samples.

### Suction versus non-suction

The simple answer to whether lesions should be biopsied with suction applied or without is usually 'both', as each technique has advantages and disadvantages. Unfortunately, limitations of time and patient patience often mean that one or the other must be chosen.

The non-suction technique (also known as **fenestration**) is slightly easier to perform, and tends to reduce blood contamination and improve the preservation of fragile cells (such as lymphocytes). Cellular yield may be increased or decreased compared to suction techniques, depending on the type of lesion sampled.

The suction technique is most useful for lesions that do not exfoliate well, and may be easier (or at least kinder) to perform in more sensitive areas, as adequate samples can often be obtained with a single needle penetration of the skin.

The choice of technique depends to some extent on experience and personal preference – as a general rule, the firmer the lesion is on palpation the more likely it is to exfoliate poorly. Vascular lesions will usually produce haemodiluted samples when aspirated. **Overall, soft lesions and vascular lesions will generally produce better samples without aspiration, whereas firmer lesions may require suction to be applied**, although it should be noted that many firm lesions will exfoliate well enough with the non-aspiration technique to produce diagnostic samples.

### FNAB without suction (fenestration technique)

- Set aside a 5 or 10 ml syringe containing 4–6 ml of air.
- Select a needle – 23–25 gauge is recommended (the softer or more vascular the lesion, the smaller the needle required).

- Introduce the tip of the needle into the lesion, holding the lesion firmly with the non-dominant hand.
- Gently rotate and redirect the needle within the lesion to collect a core of cells within the needle hub.
- Remove the syringe from the needle, withdraw 4–6 ml of air then reattach the needle and express the sample onto a slide (see below).

### *FNAB with suction (aspiration technique)*

- Select a 5 or 10 ml syringe.
- Select a needle – 21–23 gauge is recommended (the softer or more vascular the lesion, the smaller the needle required) and attach to the syringe.
- Introduce the tip of the needle into the lesion, holding the lesion firmly with the non-dominant hand.
- Apply a small amount of negative pressure and release 1–3 times (redirecting the needle slightly each time may increase cellular yield) – the appearance of material within the hub of the needle is a good indicator of successful sampling, but is not necessary.
- Release pressure on the syringe and withdraw the needle from the lesion.
- Withdraw the needle, attached the preprepared syringe and express the sample onto a slide (see below).

### *General tips for FNAB*

- If blood is noted in the syringe hub at any point, stop the current sample and prepare the slide – further sampling is only likely to increase the degree of blood contamination.
- If fluid is aspirated, place in an EDTA tube (for better preservation) and a plain tube (if culture may be required – EDTA has mild antibacterial properties) then repeat aspiration to attempt to retrieve soft tissue.
- The core of larger lesions may be necrotic – sampling the periphery of these lesions is more likely to be useful; bony lesions, however, are often surrounded by peripheral osteomyelitis – sampling the centre of these lesions is more likely to be rewarding; sampling from multiple sites of larger lesions (centre, periphery, different anatomic locations) may be useful.
- Mammary lesions in particular often have complex and mixed pathology, and are often challenging to interpret cytologically; histopathological examination is usually more useful for mammary masses (especially in dogs).
- The use of smaller-gauge needles, where possible, will reduce blood contamination and minimise pain/discomfort associated with the procedure.

### *Slide preparation*

Expel a small drop of sample, roughly the same amount as that required for the production of a blood smear, onto a clean slide. Again, similar to a blood smear, the sample should be placed approximately one-third of the way along the slide rather than directly in the centre.

The sample now needs to be spread so that the cells within it can be examined. Ideal spreading creates many areas of monolayer – that is, areas on the slide where cells are in a single layer, so that they can be easily assessed – **without rupturing them**.

There are several techniques described to obtain this ideal outcome; the author's preferred methods are summarised below, along with several techniques that generally produce poor samples.

### *'Squash' preparation (slide over slide)*

- Place sample on a clean slide, as above.
- Take a second clean slide (the 'spreader').
- With the spreader at right angles to the sample slide, lay the spreader on top of the sample material on the sample slide. **Do not press the slides together as this may lead to cell rupture***.
- Lightly move the spreader slide across the length of the sample slide – **again with no downward pressure***.
- Both sample slide and spreader slide can now be stained for examination.

*Very thick or viscous samples may require slight downward pressure to help spread them, however, this must be kept to a minimum to reduce cell rupture.

### *'Blood smear' preparation*

This technique is suitable for more fluid samples and is often very useful for lymph node aspirates.

- Place sample on a clean slide, as above.
- Take a second clean slide (the 'spreader').
- Incline the spreader to 45° and place on the sample slide in front of the specimen.
- 'Reverse' the spreader gently onto the specimen so the material spreads along the edge of the spreader slide.
- In a single smooth motion, slide the spreader forward across the sample slide.
- The sample slide is now ready to be stained.

Note: for fluid samples with low cellularity, the 'line smear' variant is useful; rather than spreading the fluid all the way across the slide, the movement is stopped abruptly to concentrate the cells in a thin line.

### General tips for slide preparation

- Avoid placing or spreading the specimen to the very end of the slide – the edges of samples are often the best areas of monolayer and may be lost if they 'fall off the cliff'; also, many automated stainers (used in most commercial labs) do not stain 1–2 cm at either end of the slide.

### Not recommended: 'shotgun' and 'starfish' preparation

Despite their more exciting names, these techniques are not recommended unless other techniques are not possible as they usually produce thick, dense areas of material with only small areas of monolayer at the periphery of the specimen.

The 'shotgun' technique involves blasting the specimen in multiple small droplets across the preparation without further spreading. Although it is sometimes necessary due to limitations of time or the specimen sampled, it is to be avoided where possible.

The 'starfish' technique is a method of spreading material across the slide using the tip of a needle. Although cell preservation is often better than might be expected, the technique does a poor job of spreading the material. Figure 9.1 illustrates the results of some of the above techniques.

## Fluid and wash preparations

Fluid collection is straightforward for most samples, although specialist techniques (beyond the scope of this chapter) and great attention to sterility are required for synovial fluid, cerebrospinal fluid (CSF) and some other fluid samples.

Preparation of fluid samples is dependent on the amount of material aspirated. With an ample harvest, the fluid should be divided between EDTA and plain tubes. EDTA is most suitable for cytology and cell counts as it preserves cells, but it has a mild antibacterial effect (due to prevention of biofilm formation) – sterile plain tubes are more useful if culture is to be performed, and if biochemistry is required on the submitted fluid. **Do not routinely add formalin, as it has significant effects on cell staining for most techniques**.

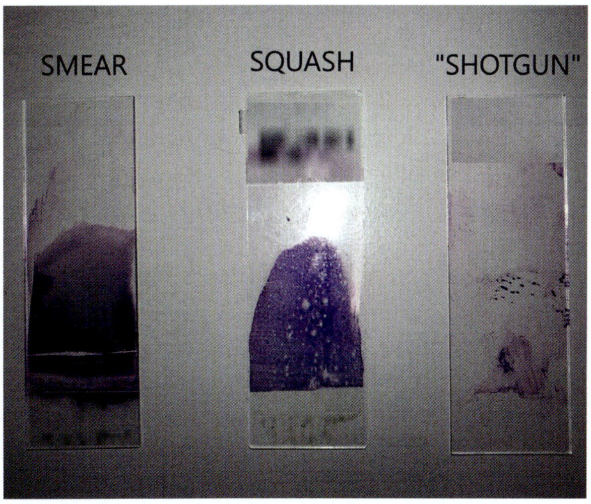


**Figure 9.1.** Well-prepared stained smear and squash techniques, and an example of 'shotgun' preparation.

Even if the sample is not going to be processed immediately, **fresh fluid preparations should always be made where possible**. Direct smears of fluid (prepared in an identical fashion to the 'blood film' technique above) are most useful for cellular smears and fluids where cellularity is unknown, although these should be performed on all fluids to give a broad assessment of appearance and overall cellularity. Concentrated preparations are useful for less cellular fluids – the 'line smear' variant of the blood smear technique is useful for this. Alternatively, a clean wooden, plastic or glass stick can be drawn through the droplets of fluid to spread them across the slide.

Cytocentrifuges are used in commercial labs to concentrate fluid with very low cellularity (such as CSF, urine or BAL samples). Although these are expensive and impractical in general practice, several papers have described the use of kitchen salad spinners instead to similarly concentrate samples, with encouraging results (see Bibliography). As an alternative, using centrifuges at low levels (roughly 1500 rpm) for ten minutes should help to concentrate samples without excessive cell lysis.

For highly blood-contaminated samples, a buffy coat preparation can be made: the sample is placed in a microhaematocrit tube and centrifuged at high speed. The tube is then cut at the thick buffy coat, containing the concentrated cells, and this material is placed upon a slide and prepared as with other specimens.

### Impression smears

Impression smears of ulcerated lesions are frequently unrewarding, as they often only exfoliate surface inflammation and infection rather than material from deeper lesions, but they can occasionally be helpful in identification of infectious agents (Figure 9.2).

Impression smears from surgical biopsies, in contrast, can provide rapid, valuable and often diagnostic information while awaiting histopathology results. The recommended procedure is as follows:

- Cut the surface of the excised tissue and blot with paper towel or filter paper to clear excess blood and fluid.

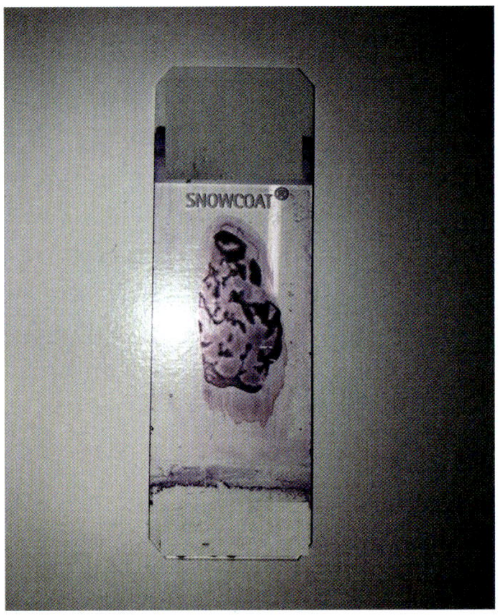


**Figure 9.2.** Surgical impression smear from testicular neoplasm.

- Press the cut surface of the tissue firmly onto a clean slide in several places (the yield increases with each press – the final preparation is often the best).
- For very fibrous tissues, scarifying the surface of the sample with a scalpel blade will help to improve yield.
- No further spreading is required.

### *Scrapings*

Used for very firm lesions, as well as surfaces that cannot readily be aspirated (such as the cornea).

- Clean the surface of the lesion with a cotton swab or by flushing with saline to remove surface inflammation (which is often secondary).
- Using a sterile spatula (such as a Kimura spatula) or the blunt edge of a sterile scalpel blade, gently scrape the surface of the lesion, ideally along the margin, in one direction, until a small drop of the specimen appears.
- Transfer to a slide and smear as above.

### *Rolled swabs*

Used for difficult-to-reach areas and lesions where the superficial inflammatory pattern or micro-organism is of prime interest (e.g. ears, mucosae).

- A plain cotton swab is suitable for most lesions.
- For dry areas, moisten the swab prior to sampling (to improve adhesion to the swab).
- Gently swab the lesion and roll over the centre of a slide (rolling, rather than dragging, will reduce cell rupture) in one direction (do not roll back and forth over the same area).

### *Drying*

Samples must be completely dry prior to staining or placing in slide containers (to avoid drying artefact and poor preservation) – air drying is suitable for preserving most cytological specimens and, once dried, the slides will remain usable for many months. The majority of specimens will dry very quickly in air but, for some samples (such as synovial fluid), a hair dryer set to cold or a fan can speed up the process. **Avoid blowing on the slides** as this can lead to droplets of saliva contaminating the sample, as well as allowing the cytologist to judge the sampler's oral hygiene regimen.

### *Tips to improve preservation*

- Use the non-aspirate (fenestration) technique wherever possible, especially lymph nodes, as this will reduce cell rupture.
- Always be gentle when smearing samples; in particular, avoid downward pressure when using the 'squash' technique except in firm or gritty samples.
- Clear excess ultrasound/anaesthetic gel prior to sampling.
- Sample the margins of larger lesions that may be necrotic, rather than the centre (exception: bone lesions).
- Avoid talking over or blowing on specimens, to reduce saliva contamination.
- Ensure that specimens are completely dry prior to staining/placing in slide boxes.
- **Never place histopathological and cytological specimens in the same package** – formalin fumes ruin cytological samples!

Figure 9.3 shows a slide with damaged, unidentifiable cells.

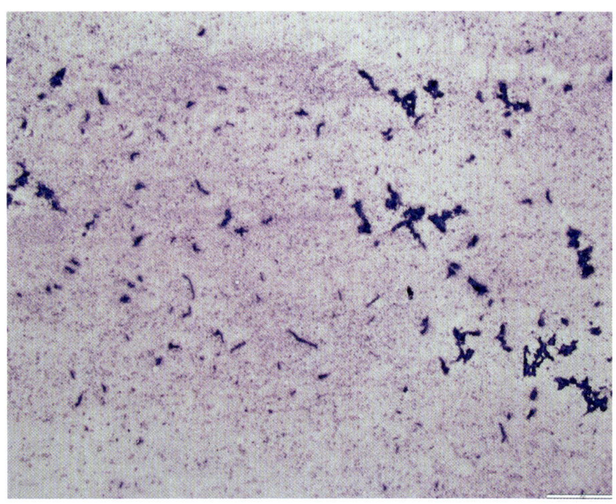

**Figure 9.3.** Rolled, unidentifiable cells damaged during spreading.

## Staining

Most standard cytological examinations use Romanowsky (MR) stains – material on the slide takes up different material depending largely on the pH; acids take up red (eosinophilic) stain, whereas bases take up blue–purple (basophilic) stain.

Most commercial labs use methanol MR stains such as Wright or Wright–Giemsa, but in practice the use of aqueous Romanowsky (AR) stains such as Diff-Quik is more common. Both stains involve methanol fixation, although in MR stains the dyes are dissolved in methanol whereas in AR stains they are dissolved in water and the methanol fixation is a separate step (the first 'dip').

There are some differences between MR and AR: principally, **AR stains do not reliably stain cytoplasmic granules such as mast cell granules, basophil granules and lymphocyte granules, and this should be borne in mind when examining specimens**.

Details of Romanowsky staining techniques, as well as other more specialist staining techniques, are given in the Appendix.

## Submissions to external laboratories

Although much can be learned by examining cytological specimens in-house, cytology is a broad, complex and occasionally confusing subject. In difficult cases, submitting samples to a pathologist can greatly aid the interpretation. Here are some tips to improve diagnostic yield from external laboratory submissions:

- Include concise history, including the *precise* location of lesions (rather than 'neck' or 'back end'), as well as whether a mass in internal or external, cutaneous or subcutaneous.
- Label *all* slides, rather than using labelled slide boxes, with the name of the patient and location of the lesion (for easy correlation with the location described on the submission form); pencil written on ground glass edges is preferable.
- Avoid pre-staining all of the most cellular submitted preparations as this will affect in-house staining.

## Stepwise approach to evaluation of cytology smears

Cytological specimens can have an infinite variety of appearances, and examining them can feel overwhelming at first, particularly in samples with highly mixed cellularity. A stepwise and logical approach to each slide helps to apply some order to the chaos and, with practice, allow a cytologist to rapidly and efficiently assess specimens.

### *Objectives*

Objectives work with the magnification of the microscope eyepieces (typically 10×) to magnify the image – so a 4× objective with a 10× eyepiece will produce a final image magnified forty times, and a 100× objective will magnify the image 1000-fold.

Common objectives used are 4×, 10×, 20× (dry – oil immersion is not required), 40× (wet or dry) and 50× and 100× (wet – these objectives require oil immersion). Most microscopes have space for four or five objectives to be rotated through. The author finds that a combination of 4×, 10×, 50× and 100× is suitable for most purposes, although the choice of objectives is largely down to personal preference as there is no 'correct' set-up.

### *Initial examination and assessment of cellularity/preservation*

On low power (4× or 10× objective), scan the specimen whilst asking yourself the following questions:

- Does the sample have sufficient cells or other material (such as keratin) to draw a meaningful conclusion on its contents?
- Is the material in the sample likely to be representative of the lesion given the collection technique? For example, adipocytes present on a sample taken from a cutaneous mass are more likely to reflect inadvertent aspiration of subcutaneous fat than be a true representation of the lesion.
- Is the cellular material adequately preserved? Are the cells present ruptured, rolled or otherwise unidentifiable?
- Has the material on the preparations taken up adequate amounts of stain?
- Is the material evenly spread throughout the preparations? Are there suitable areas of monolayer for examination?
- Is there abundant ultrasound gel, drying artefact, damage from formalin fumes or other contaminants (such as fingerprints/saliva) that is obscuring the detail of the preparations?

If the material is of sub-optimal quality or preservation, then it may be more useful to take another sample, if feasible.

Once cellularity and preservation are assessed, a stepwise approach to assessing the material can begin. Again, scan the slide from low power to high power whilst asking yourself a series of logical questions – the author finds the following simple approach to be useful:

- Is this lesion predominantly inflammatory or neoplastic (or is it mixed)?
- If inflammatory, what are the predominant leukocytes (neutrophils, macrophages, eosinophils, lymphocytes) or is this a mixed inflammatory pattern?
- If neoplastic, what is the predominant cell type present (epithelial, mesenchymal or round cells)?
- Is there any relevant acellular material present (keratin, extracellular matrix, crystals, fat droplets)?
- Are there any visible infectious agents?

The following flowchart summarises this process in more detail.

**Stepwise approach to cytological specimens**

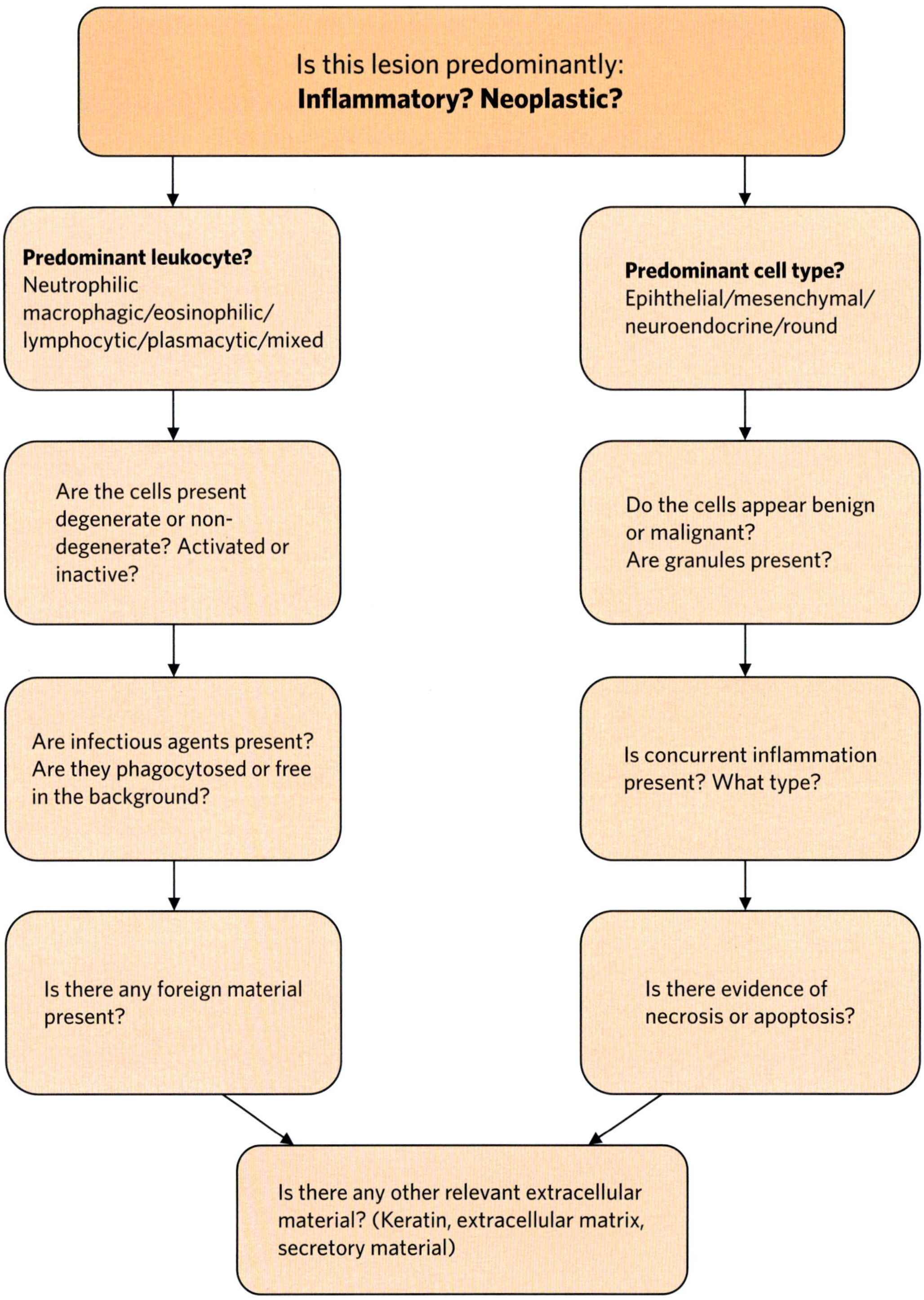

## *Backgrounds*

Some information about a specimen can be gleaned from the background to the material. Assessments should be made of the colour (eosinophilic (red), basophilic (blue-purple), amphophilic (a mixture of both colours)), intensity (faint, mid, deep/intense) and texture (smooth, lightly stippled, heavily stippled).

**Proteinaceous fluids, such as from a seroma, tend to have highly stippled eosinophilic to amphophilic backgrounds, often with small clefts (see Figure 9.49)**. Aspirates from fatty areas are usually clear and smooth, with numerous fat spaces (fat is dissolved by methanol, and therefore is clear with Romanowsky stains). Haemodiluted samples often have a smooth eosinophilic background.

# Cytology of inflammation

Almost all inflammatory patterns are mixed to some extent, but in most cases there is a predominant cell type present, or increased numbers of cells less commonly seen (such as eosinophils).

Although leukocytes have varied and distinctive morphologies, they often condense in high-protein environments (such as joint fluid and exudates), appearing as small, round, dense nuclei with small amounts of pale eosinophilic cytoplasm; distinguishing between leukocytes in such fluids can be difficult.

## *Neutrophilic inflammation*

Also known as 'suppurative' or 'purulent' inflammation, inflammation is defined as neutrophilic when 85% or more of the observed leukocytes are neutrophils. They are often accompanied by low numbers of macrophages (Figure 9.4).

In samples taken from tissues with a relatively benign environment (most tissues except for bile, urine and some other fluids), neutrophils are usually *non-degenerate* – **non-degenerate neutrophils have sharply defined nuclear borders with dark, dense nuclear chromatin and well-segmented nuclei**. Their overall appearance is similar to mature neutrophils in peripheral blood.

In more toxic environments, particularly those created by bacterial toxins, neutrophils undergo hydropic change as the cells begin to lose their membrane integrity and swell up. These ***degenerate* neutrophils contain paler, swollen nuclei with fewer distinct segments (*karyolysis*)** (Figure 9.5). In contrast, neutrophils with shrunken, rounded, very dense nuclei (*pyknosis*) or with nuclei fragmented into multiple small, dense dots (*karyohexis*) with intact membranes are more likely to be ageing *in situ* rather than degenerating due to toxins. However, pyknotic neutrophils and those displaying karyohexis are often seen in low numbers amongst degenerate neutrophils.

When neutrophils are poorly preserved, especially when this is due to delayed processing of fluid samples, they can closely resemble degenerate neutrophils; for this reason, **great care should be taken in interpreting degenerate neutrophils in poorly preserved samples**.

Although bacteria should be considered in all predominantly neutrophilic inflammatory lesions, **the presence of degenerate neutrophils should raise the cytologist's suspicions and prompt a search for bacterial organisms** (see below); note that some septic diseases (especially septic arthritis) exhibit almost no degenerate change.

There are many other causes of neutrophilic inflammation, including necrosis, foreign body reaction (although this is more commonly associated with a mixed inflammatory pattern including numerous

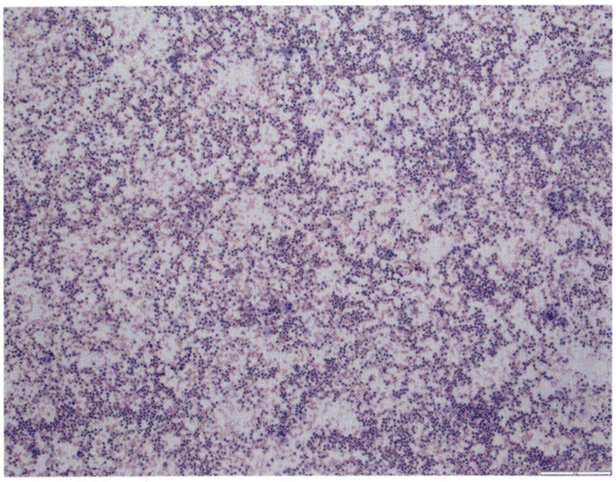

**Figure 9.4.** Neutrophilic inflammation (abscess) (100×).

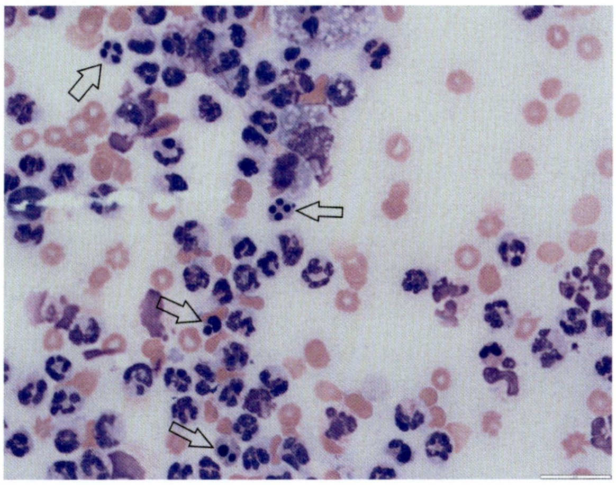

**Figure 9.5.** Degenerate neutrophils; note also karyohexis (open arrows) (400×).

macrophages), immune-mediated diseases, neoplasia (such as squamous cell carcinomas), trauma and ischaemia.

## Bacteria

It is important to try to get samples prior to starting antibiotics – the chance of finding bacteria rapidly reduces afterwards. Failing to find bacteria on cytology does not exclude bacterial infection, and culture should be carried out on all suspect samples.

Searching for bacteria is possible only on higher magnifications (using at least 50×5 and usually 100× objectives). Stain precipitate (small, dense blobs of dye) often strongly resembles bacterial cocci, although there are several differences that can help distinguish between the two:

- Stain precipitate is often refractile (it will change in colour and intensity as the focus is slightly altered) – true bacterial organisms usually aren't.
- Stain precipitate is often slightly variable in size – true bacteria are usually nearly identical size, staining intensity and shape.
- Bacteria are often found in chains, pairs or small colonies whereas stain precipitate is usually distributed randomly across the slide.

In genuine infection, bacteria are often found in the areas of the preparation where the neutrophils appear most degenerate. The presence of bacteria phagocytosed within neutrophils (or occasionally eosinophils or macrophages) is diagnostic of bacterial infection, although care must be taken not to confuse karyohexis with bacterial organisms (Figure 9.6). Additionally, cases where all bacteria are observed within neutrophils and with no free organisms present are often associated with a negative bacterial culture despite the cytological appearance. Finally, remember that in fluid samples, limited bacterial phagocytosis can occur within the sample if there is a delay in processing.

### Contamination

When bacteria are not seen within leukocytes, it can be challenging to distinguish between true infection and contamination from the skin surface or oral cavity. As a general rule, pure growths of a single organism are likely to be infection whereas the presence of multiple different organisms is more likely to reflect contamination (although anaerobic infections such as pyothorax often contain a mixed population of bacilli and cocci). Additionally, where there are frequent bacteria present but no significant inflammation, contamination is more likely.

## Eosinophilic inflammation

Eosinophils are a less common, albeit more eye-catching, leukocyte, and so their presence in smaller proportions is considered significant; **when >10% of inflammatory cells are eosinophils, inflammation is described as eosinophilic**. Recruitment of eosinophils is one of the chief functions of mast cells, and so they are commonly found together (Figure 9.7).

They are often seen in more unusual conditions, occasionally collectively called 'worms, wheezes and weird diseases' (Raskin). Eosinophils respond to parasitic infestations and are one of the key cells involved in type 1 hypersensitivity ('immediate hypersensitivity', including allergies). They can be found in eosinophilic plaques, and are also one of the more common leukocytes found in neoplasia-related inflammation (usually mast cell tumours, although several other neoplasms, notably some lymphomas, also attract eosinophils).

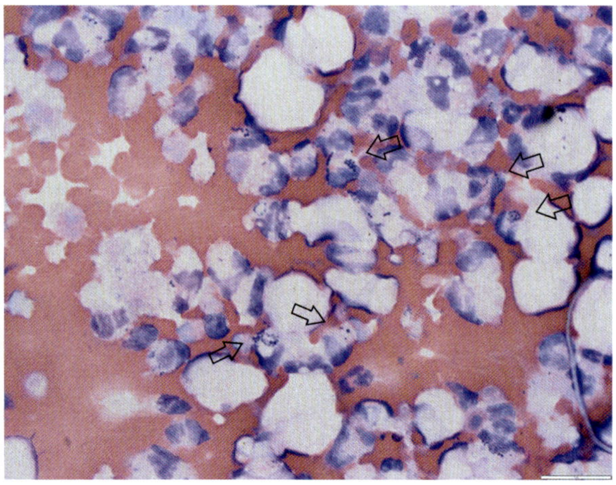

**Figure 9.6.** Bacterial phagocytosis (open arrows) within highly degenerate neutrophils, confirming infection (septic exudate) (1000×).

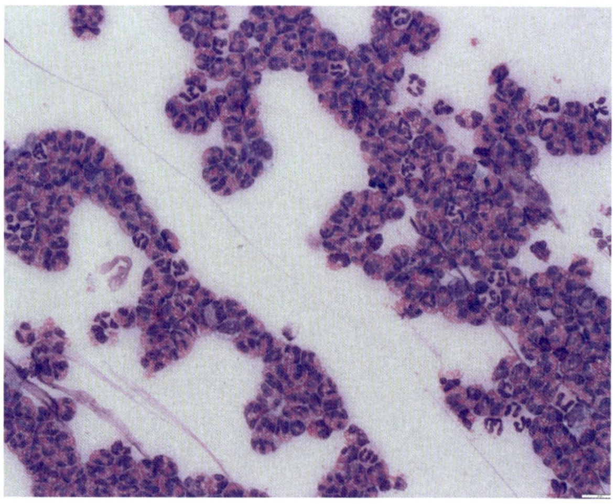

**Figure 9.7.** Eosinophilic inflammation (canine BAL with *Angiostrongylus* infection) (400×).

More rarely, eosinophils can be found in foreign body reactions and fungal infections.

## *Macrophagic inflammation*

Macrophages are the 'big guns' of the inflammatory world. They have great versatility, can phagocytose infectious organisms and debris or secrete cytokines to aid in fighting infection or healing. **Inflammation containing >50% macrophages is described as macrophagic or 'granulomatous', whereas mixtures of neutrophils (60–70%) and macrophages (20–30%) are described as 'pyogranulomatous'** (Figure 9.8).

The versatility of macrophages can make them harder to identify as it gives them a varied appearance – they can occasionally be mistaken for neoplastic cells. Most macrophages have pale grey cytoplasm, with variably sized nuclei. 'Inactivated' macrophages and histiocytes are the smallest. 'Activated' macrophages have more abundant cytoplasm, frequently containing vacuolation, and are found in chronic inflammatory lesions. Given their major role in phagocytosis, it can be rewarding to check the cytoplasm of activated macrophages to see whether they contain leukocytes or infectious organisms. The presence of **phagocytosed leukocytes (leukophagia) confirms that inflammation is present, and this can be useful in preparations heavily contaminated with blood, where it is not clear whether the leukocytes present are from the tissue sampled or the blood** (Figure 9.9).

In more intense or long-standing inflammatory lesions, the cytoplasm can darken to a deep blue and 'epithelioid' macrophages, clustered together in a manner similar to epithelial cells, may be present (Figure 9.10). These cells are more associated with cytokine secretion than phagocytosis. Multi-nucleated 'giant' macrophages are similar, and are more commonly associated with foreign body reactions (such as stick injuries, ruptured keratin-containing lesions or suture reactions).

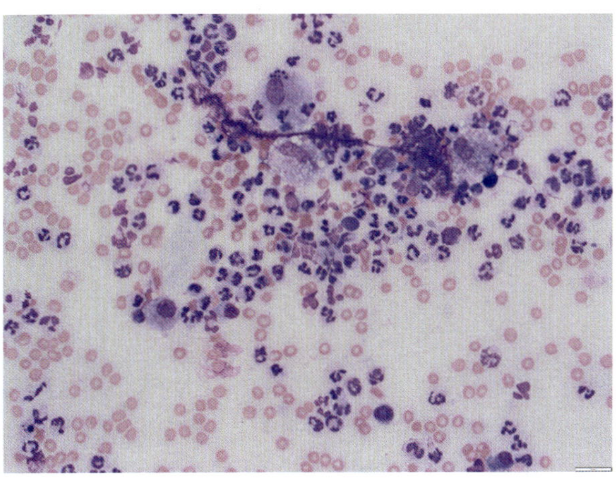

**Figure 9.8.** Pyogranulomatous inflammation; note frequent non-degenerate neutrophils and leukophagia (400×).

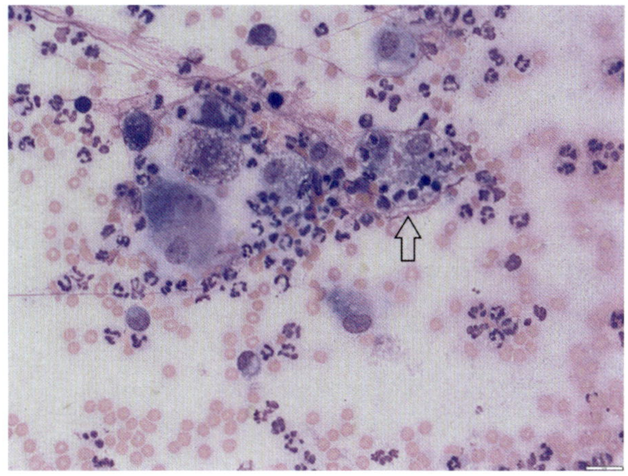

**Figure 9.9.** Marked leukophagia (open arrow), as well as activated basophilic macrophages with vacuolated cytoplasm (400×).

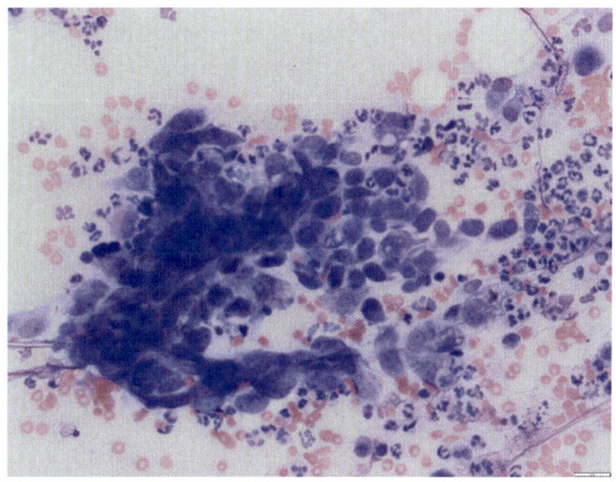

**Figure 9.10.** Epithelioid macrophages in a foreign body reaction (400×).

## *Lymphocytic and lymphoplasmacytic inflammation*

Primarily lymphocytic inflammation is relatively uncommon in small animals – lymphocytes are found much more commonly in mixed inflammatory responses. **Purely lymphocytic inflammation should be interpreted with caution, as lymphoma is also a consideration for the presence of high numbers of lymphocytes.**

Lymphocytes are classified according to their size – small lymphocytes are smaller than a neutrophil (and roughly 1–1.5 erythrocytes in diameter) with dark, dense chromatin and no nucleoli, intermediate lymphocytes are about the same size as neutrophils (about 1.5–2 erythrocytes) with more 'open' (paler) nuclear chromatin, and large lymphocytes are larger than neutrophils (usually 2.5–3.5 erythrocytes) with even more open chromatin and frequently containing nucleoli (Figure 9.11).

A genuine reactive population of lymphocytes should contain predominantly small cells (>60% of observed cells), with progressively fewer intermediate and large lymphocytes. In contrast, a monomorphic population of similarly sized cells (especially intermediate to large cells) raises concern for a clonal, and often neoplastic, population – lymphoma.

Reactive populations often contain scattered plasma cells – these are mature B lymphocytes that produce antibodies and are one of the natural end points of a population of reactive lymphocytes – the complete absence of plasma cells amidst high numbers of lymphocytes again raises concern for lymphoma (Figure 9.12).

Common causes for true lymphocytic inflammation include antigenic stimulation – such antigens could originate from vaccines, foreign bodies, insect bites and viral infections, amongst many other sources. Lymphocytes are often also found in regressing histiocytomas and type IV sensitivity reactions (delayed-type hypersensitivity).

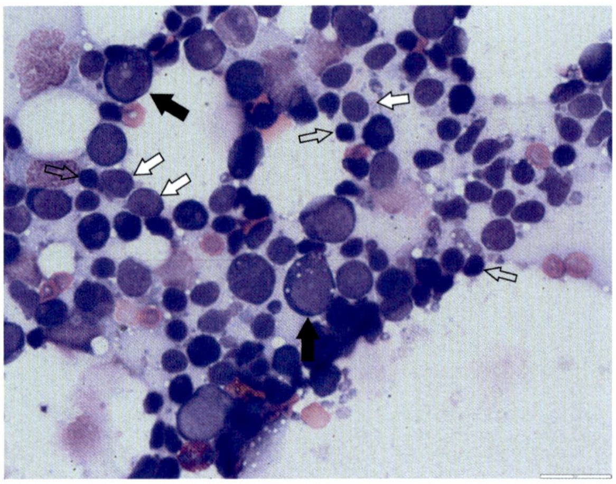

**Figure 9.11.** Examples of small (clear arrows), intermediate (white arrows) and large (black arrows) lymphocytes – note that the nuclear chromatin becomes progressively paler as the cells mature and become more active (1000×).

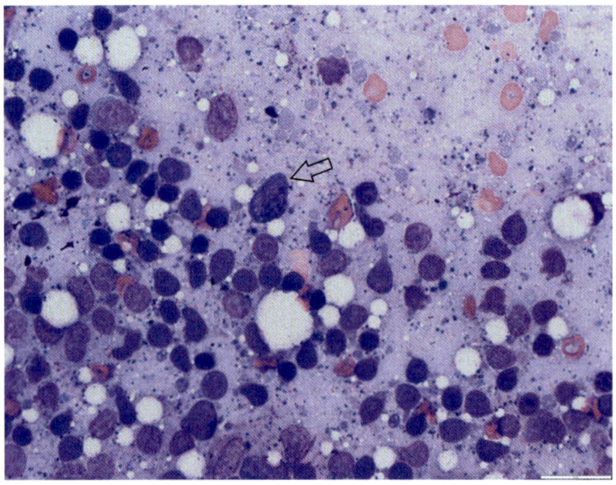

**Figure 9.12.** Reactive lymphoid population (mostly small and intermediate) with well-preserved plasma cell (open arrow); note also melanin pigment granules in the background ('melanin incontinence', common in nodes draining skin disease) (400×).

## Plasma cells

Plasma cells are mature and fully differentiated B lymphocytes specialised in the formation of antibodies specific to a single antigen (Figure 9.13). They are easily recognisable (and, in the author's opinion, extremely beautiful) – they have densely 'clumped' chromatin (often described as appearing like a dried-out river bed) with expanded, deeply basophilic cytoplasm, often containing a clearer area adjacent to the nucleus; this perinuclear clear zone represents the well-developed Golgi apparatus possessed by plasma cells in order to produce antibodies.

Mott cells are variants of plasma cells packed with pale basophilic or eosinophilic structures, usually circular (although many different shapes can be observed), representing packets of immunoglobulins (Figure 9.14).

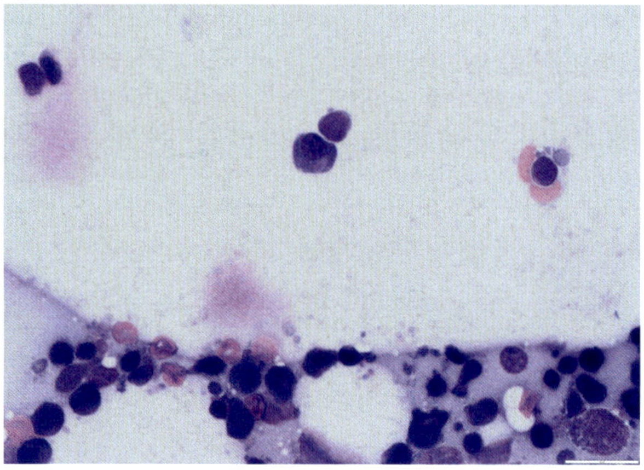

**Figure 9.13.** Plasma cell (left) adjacent to an intermediate lymphocyte (1000×).

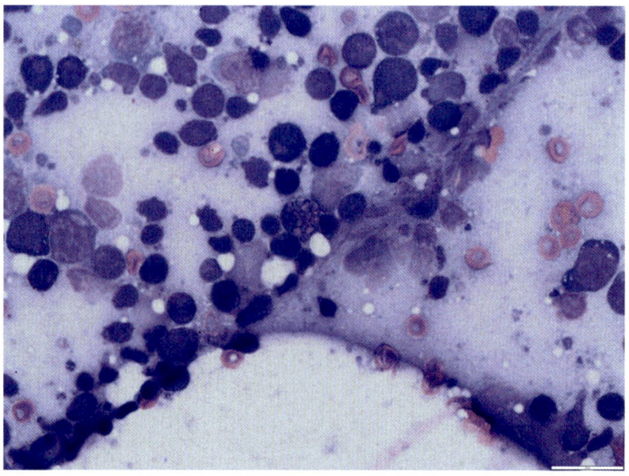

**Figure 9.14.** Mott cell (centre) with eosinophilic immunoglobulin packets; note also plasma cell (top centre) (1000×).

'Flame cells' are plasma cells with a reddish-pink border and a somewhat 'spiky' outline. This border is again thought to represent precipitated immunoglobulins.

### *Mixed inflammation*

Mixed inflammatory patterns are amongst the most commonly encountered in cytology – many different leukocytes are present with no clear predominance. In these cases, differentials include all of the possibilities for the various leukocytes present. Consideration of the history, location and the proportion of different inflammatory cells present will help to narrow the differential list in these cases.

### *Other cells present in inflammation*

Aside from plasma cells, Mott cells and flame cells (see above), fibroblasts are commonly seen, particularly in marked or long-standing inflammatory lesions. These cells are fusiform (spindle-shaped) mesenchymal cells and can be numerous (depending upon the degree of fibroplasia present). **As fibroblasts are highly active cells, they can display several criteria of malignancy (in particular, pleomorphism and variable nuclear features) that can lead to misdiagnosis of a neoplastic population (e.g. sarcoma).**

Additionally, in the presence of significant inflammation, other cells (such as epithelial cells) can undergo dysplastic (reversible atypia) change that can mimic malignancy.

## Cytology of neoplasia

When a lesion comprises predominantly tissue cells, rather than leukocytes, ask yourself these questions:

- Are the tissue cells present appropriate for the tissue sampled?
- Is the number of cells appropriate for the tissue sampled?
- Is the morphology of the cells normal for the tissue sampled?

If the answer to any or all of these questions is 'no', then neoplasia is likely. At this stage, you have two more important questions to attempt to answer: what is the origin of the cells present, and is this lesion likely to behave in a benign or malignant fashion?

### *Tissue types*

Neoplasms are grouped into four main types according to their cytological appearance (Table 9.2). The groups are broad and varied (especially 'round' cell tumours), but help to predict the clinical behaviour.

#### *Epithelial neoplasms*

Epithelial tumours arise from the cells lining organs, glands and most other tissues. These cells are involved in protection, secretion and absorption, and generally have very tight cell–cell junctions – these junctions are often preserved during aspiration and, for this reason, the cells are often found adherent to each other in dense **clusters** and flattened sheets in cytological specimens (Figure 9.15). Epithelial clusters usually have rounded, well-defined edges and contain tightly packed cells. When found in fluids, they have a tendency to curl up into 'balls' of cells.

Epithelial tumours are described as 'adenomas' when benign or 'carcinomas' when malignant; 'adenocarcinoma' refers to a malignant neoplasm of glandular origin. Due to the preservation of cell junctions, architectural patterns reflecting the origin of the cells are most readily recognised in epithelial tumours. Common patterns include:

- Palisading – cells arranged in regular rows (like a picket fence); usually seen in basilar cell tumours (basal cell tumours) such as trichoblastomas or apocrine ductular adenomas (Figure 9.16).

Table 9.2. Characteristics of the four tumour groups.

| Epithelial | Mesenchymal | Neuro-endocrine | 'Round' cell |
|---|---|---|---|
| Tightly cohesive 'clusters' and sheets of cells | Loosely cohesive 'aggregates' | Cohesive clusters with poorly defined borders and many bare nuclei | Individual cells with little cohesion, occasional groups |
| Cuboidal, columnar and squamous cells with distinct borders | Spindle, caudate or stellate cells with 'wispy', indistinct borders | Round but indistinct cells, often appearing as bare nuclei within a sea of cytoplasm | Round or polygonal cells with distinct borders |
| Round nuclei | Slender to plump oval nuclei | Round, often bare, nuclei | Round to polygonal nuclei |
| Adenoma, carcinoma | Sarcoma | Adenoma, carcinoma | Variety (see below) |

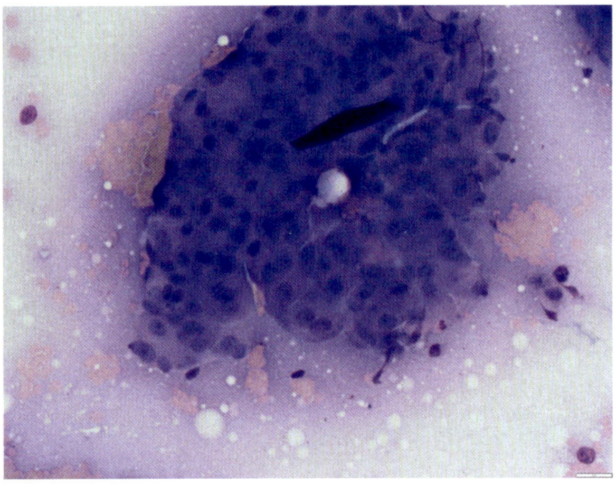

**Figure 9.15.** Cluster of 'hepatoid' epithelial cells from a perianal adenoma; the term 'hepatoid' refers to the finely granular eosinophilic cytoplasm, reminiscent of hepatic epithelium. Note the close cohesion of the cells and the smooth, rounded cluster edges (400×).

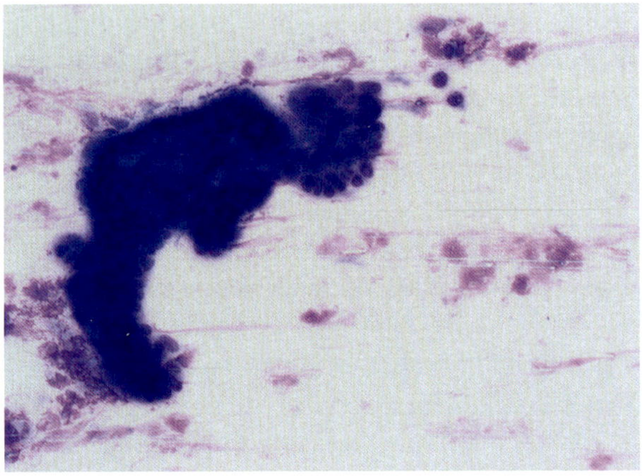

**Figure 9.16.** Palisading epithelium in a trichoblastoma (benign tumour of basal epithelium); cells are tightly packed and arranged with nuclei closely adjacent and often in rows, sometimes reminiscent of a picket fence (400×).

- Honeycomb – polygonal cells in a regular, tessellated pattern (like a mosaic); seen most commonly in aspirates from the prostate or intestinal tract (particularly the stomach wall) (Figure 9.17).
- Papillary – cells arranged in rows around a central vascular or stromal core (this core is not always apparent cytologically), usually with finger-like rounded projections; often seen in pulmonary and mammary epithelium (Figure 9.18).
- Pavement – thin layers of polygonal and often angular cells; usually seen with squamous epithelium lining mucosae and skin.
- Trabecular – branching and often wide, cohesive clusters of cells; reminiscent of trabecular bone, and often seen in liver and perianal aspirates (Figure 9.19).

Glandular tumours (adenocarcinomas) often contain **acinar structures** – rings of cells around a central area

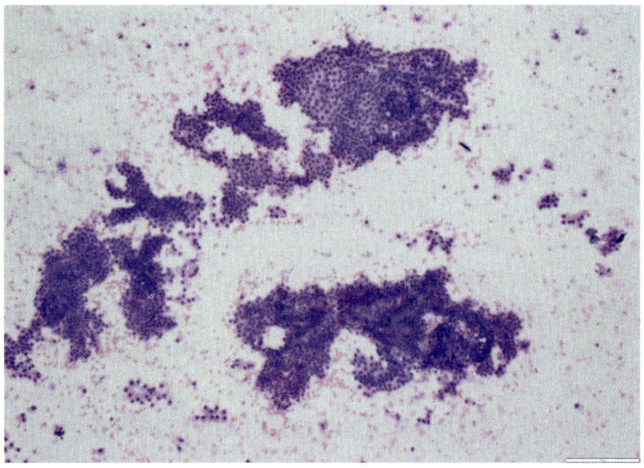

**Figure 9.17.** Distinctive honeycomb pattern of prostatic epithelium (cuboidal to columnar cells) (100×).

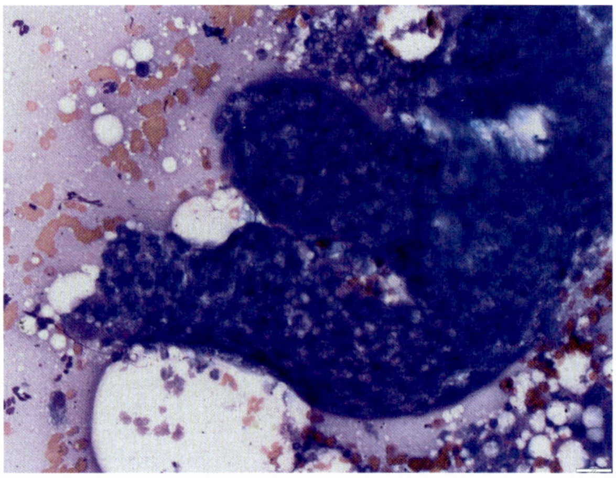

**Figure 9.18.** Papillary epithelial cluster in a pulmonary adenocarcinoma (400×).

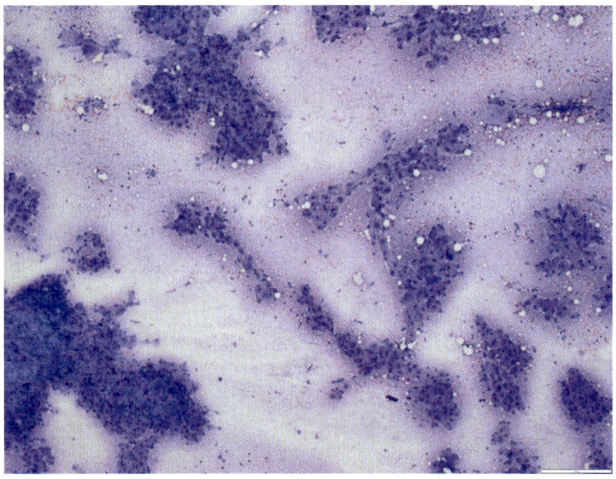

**Figure 9.19.** Trabecular pattern of hepatic epithelium (100×).

that may contain secretory product (Figure 9.20). Secretory products are variable but are often small patches, or lakes, of pale eosinophilic (occasionally basophilic) amorphous, rounded material.

Epithelial cells usually have a round central nucleus (basal in columnar epilthelium) with abundant cytoplasm

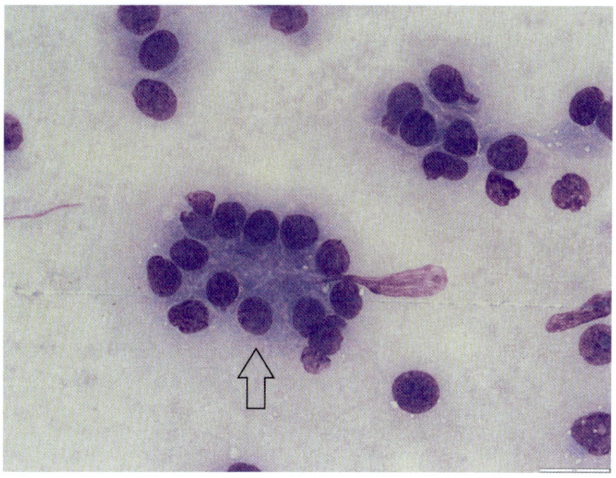

**Figure 9.20.** Acinar structure in anal sac adenocarcinoma (open arrow) (a neuroendocrine neoplasm, but epithelial acini appear similar; no central secretory product visible in this example) (1000×).

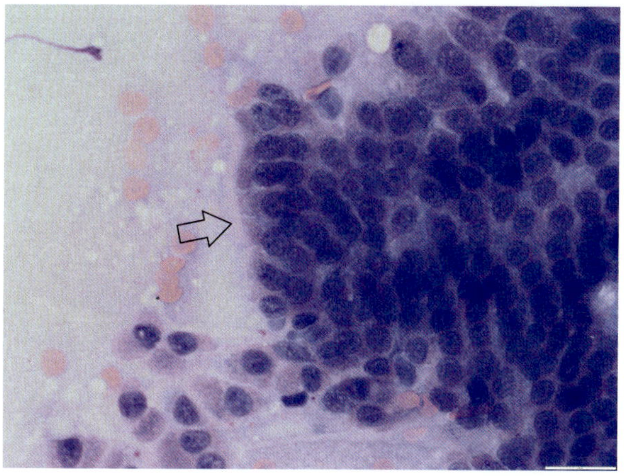

**Figure 9.22.** Columnar epithelial cells from small intestine; note the basal nuclei, most obvious at the edge of the cluster (open arrow) (1000×).

(although see 'Features of malignant tumours', below). Where observable, the cell shape can also provide a clue to the origin of the cells:

- Cuboidal – small squarish, rounded or polygonal cells; found most often in renal aspirates, basilar epithelium or intact neuroendocrine neoplasms (see below).
- Squamous – larger irregular polygonal cells, angular when keratinised; seen usually in cutaneous or mucosal aspirates (Figure 9.21).
- Columnar – rounded rectangular cells with a 'basal' or paracentric nucleus (at one end of the cell); seen in respiratory epithelium (with cilia), intestine, prostate (cuboidal to columnar) and secondary to self-trauma in cutaneous lesions (a metaplastic change) (Figure 9.22).
- Transitional – cell shape varies between cuboidal (usually at the centre of clusters) to columnar or squamous (at the periphery); found lining the urethra, bladder and ureters.

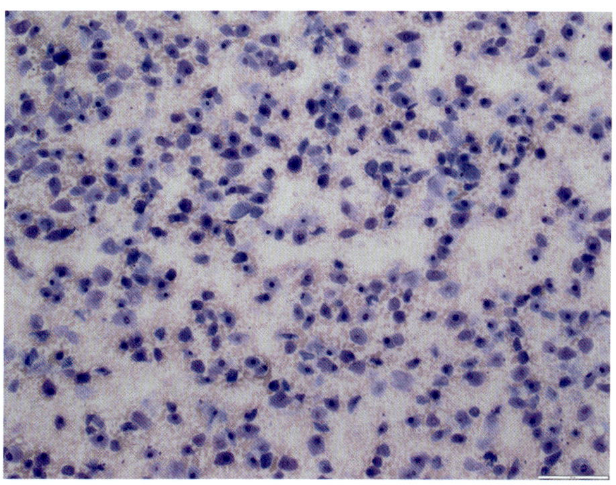

**Figure 9.21.** Individual keratinised squamous epithelial cells in a papilloma (100×).

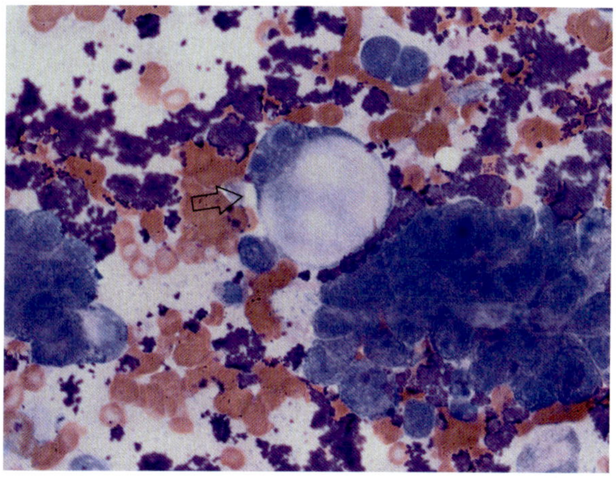

**Figure 9.23.** Large binucleate signet ring cell (open arrow) in a pulmonary adenocarcinoma (100×).

Individual cells from glandular neoplasms often contain vacuoles within the cytoplasm, usually clear; these can vary from multiple small 'punctate' vacuoles with clear borders to a large single vacuole, displacing the nucleus to the periphery of the cell ('signet ring' cells, a feature of malignancy (see below; Figure 9.23)).

The most commonly aspirated cutaneous epithelial neoplasms include basilar epithelial neoplasms (previously called 'basal cell tumours'), perianal ('hepatoid') neoplasms (see above for examples) and squamous cell carcinomas (Figure 9.24).

Malignant epithelial neoplasms (carcinomas) often have high potential to metastasise – initially to local lymph nodes, and from there through the lymphatics to many other body tissues.

### *Neuroendocrine neoplasms*

These neoplasms derive from neuroendocrine tissue and appear cytologically somewhat similar to epithelial tumours, in that they are often cohesive and contain round, dense nuclei. Unlike many epithelial tumours,

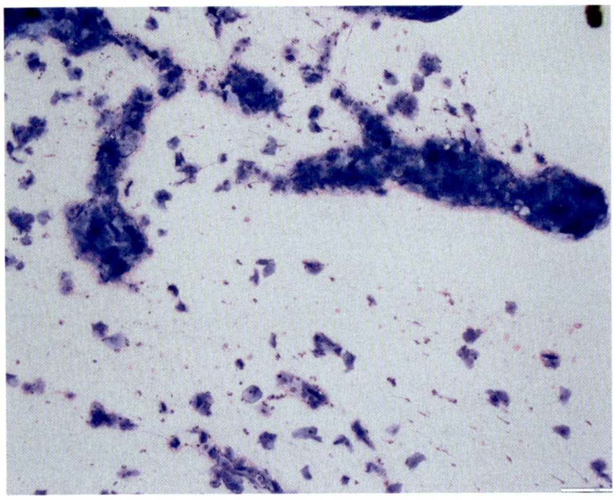

**Figure 9.24.** Squamous cell carcinoma: note the irregular clusters and the atypical keratinised epithelial cells (nuclei large and prominent when they should be regressing) (100×).

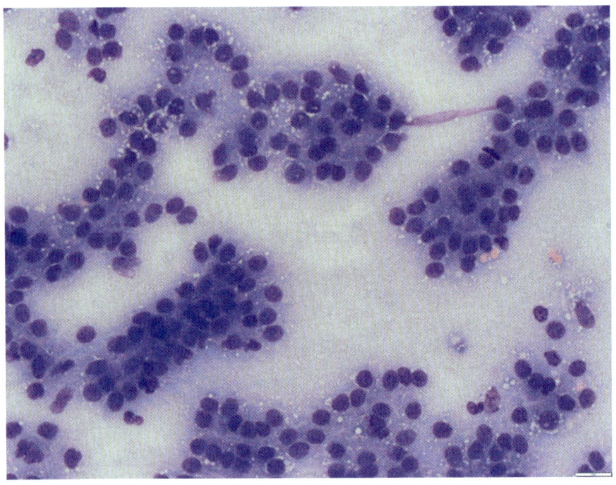

**Figure 9.25.** Neuroendocrine tumour (anal sac apocrine gland adenocarcinoma; epithelial-like clusters containing cells with indistinct borders and minimal malignant features) (400×).

they are extremely fragile and frequently rupture during aspiration, so that they often contain high numbers of bare nuclei. Again, unlike carcinomas, the cytoplasmic borders of these cells are indistinct; when intact, the clusters of cells look like free nuclei within a pool of pale cytoplasm (Figure 9.25).

Despite their frequently innocuous cytological appearance, neuroendocrine tumours often follow an aggressive clinical course and often metastasise. The most commonly encountered neuroendocrine tumours are anal sac adenocarcinomas (see above) and thyroid tumours (Figure 9.26).

### *Mesenchymal neoplasms*

Mesenchymal cells form the connective tissues of the body – bone, cartilage, fibrous tissue, muscles, fat and vascular tissue. Although they are somewhat cohesive, the cell-to-cell junctions are not as strong as in epithelial cells. Consequently, although their architecture is

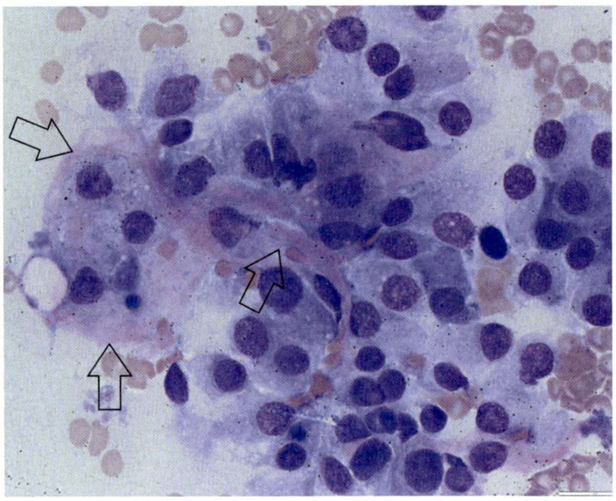

**Figure 9.26.** Thyroid carcinoma containing colloid (pale pink material interspersed with cells, open arrows); again, malignant features are largely absent (400×).

occasionally preserved on cytological samples, these looser **aggregates** are less distinctive than the patterns seen in epithelial tumours and many individual cells are often concurrently present (Figures 9.27 and 9.28).

Benign mesenchymal neoplasms carry the suffix '-oma', similar to some other benign tumours (and, confusingly, some more aggressive tumours such as lymphoma); examples include lipomas, fibromas, myxomas, chondromas and haemangiomas. Malignant versions are described as sarcomas.

As with the architecture, the individual cell shape is less specific in mesenchymal neoplasia, but some information can still be gained from a close inspection:

- Fusiform – 'spindle'-shaped cells, tapering at both ends with central nuclei; these are the most commonly observed mesenchymal cell, found in many sarcomas, but most often seen in soft tissue sarcomas.

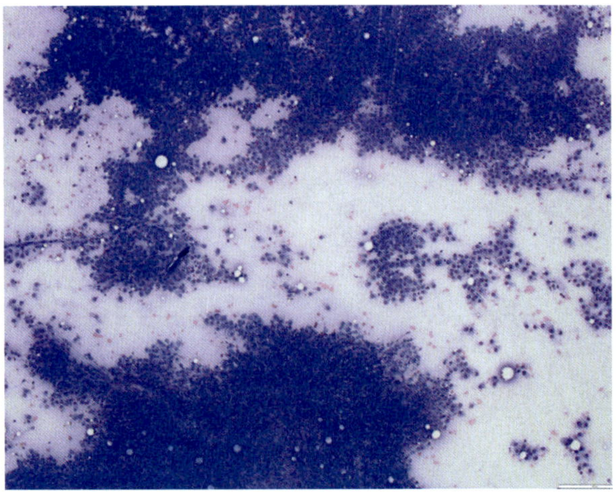

**Figure 9.27.** Mesenchymal aggregates in a soft tissue sarcoma; note the looser 'frayed' appearance and scattered individual cells.

- Stellate – like a star, with three or more tapering projections with central nuclei; again, not specific but often seen in soft tissue sarcomas.
- Caudate – eccentric nuclei, similar to columnar epithelial cells, although tapering to a rounded end or point opposite the nucleus; seen most commonly in osteoblasts and chondroblasts (the neoplastic cells in osteosarcomas and chrondrosarcomas respectively (Figure 9.28).

Lipomas are a common neoplasm (Figure 9.29).

The cytology of mesenchymal neoplasms is complicated by the fact that fibroblasts and other mesenchymal cells proliferate as a response to inflammation or injury, and it can be challenging to distinguish between a reactive and neoplastic population of cells. **In general, high numbers of mesenchymal cells with no evidence of inflammation and no previous history of trauma should raise the cytologist's suspicions for neoplasia**.

Despite the looser cell–cell junctions, mesenchymal cells are usually well embedded within their surrounding matrix, which can be abundant (Figure 9.30). Due to this, mesenchymal tumours are often grossly firmer than epithelial tumours and generally do not exfoliate as well. Individual cells are elongated, with oval nuclei, and the cytoplasmic borders are indistinct (often described as 'wispy') and blend into the background.

Although there are exceptions, the majority of sarcomas behave in a similar clinical fashion – they are locally invasive but slow to metastasise. When metastasis occurs it is usually via invasion of blood vessels, in contrast to the lymphatic spread most commonly seen in carcinomas and round cell tumours. **Metastasis to lymph nodes is very rare for sarcomas**.

It is often difficult to distinguish between different types of sarcoma cytologically but, given their similarities, the clinical behaviour can often be predicted.

The most commonly encountered mesenchymal neoplasms presenting as skin and subcutaneous masses are lipomas (Figure 9.31) and soft tissue sarcomas

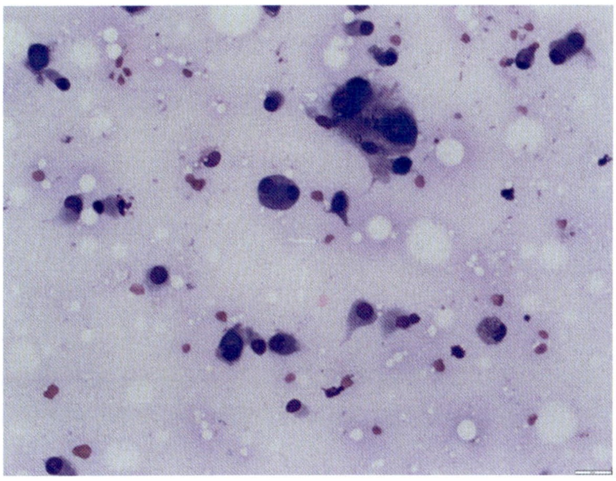

**Figure 9.28.** Individual mesenchymal cells (fusiform and caudate) with indistinct borders from a soft tissue sarcoma (STS); note the indistinct borders and the binucleate 'alien head' cell, commonly seem in STS (500×).

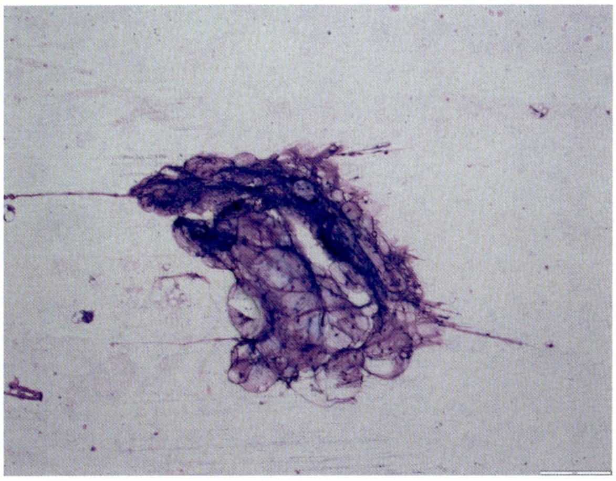

**Figure 9.29.** Aggregate of adipocytes in a lipoma (500×).

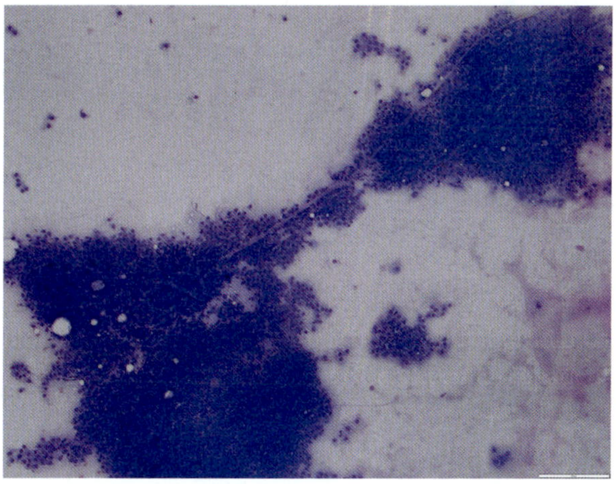

**Figure 9.30.** Perivascular arrangement of mesenchymal cells in a soft tissue sarcoma (100×).

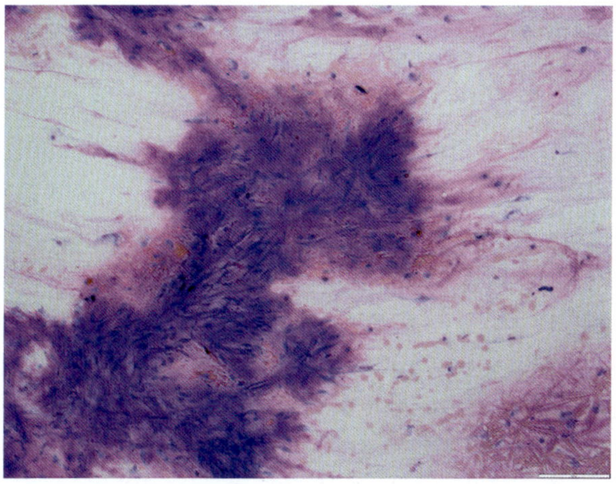

**Figure 9.31.** Marked matrix production in a mesenchymal neoplasm (100×).

(including perivascular wall tumour and peripheral nerve sheath tumours); distinguishing between them has no prognostic value.

### Extracellular matrix

Aspirates from mesenchymal cells often include the extracellular matrix they produce; this is due to the presence of lakes and clumps of granular or fibrillar (containing thin strands of fibrils) material, and mesenchymal cells are often closely associated or embedded within it. The colour and appearance of the matrix varies with its nature; it is most commonly pink to eosinophilic, although can vary from a reddish appearance (in fibromas/fibrosarcomas), pink fluid material resembling joint fluid (in myxomas/myxosarcomas; Figure 9.32), intense purple (chondroid from chondromas/chondrosarcomas) or intense pink (osteoid from osteomas/osteosarcomas), although sarcomas can produce matrix atypical for their original cell line.

The presence of material resembling matrix lends support for mesenchymal neoplasia, but is not absolutely specific – secretory material from glandular epithelial tumours, basement membrane associated with basilar epithelial cells and amyloid from plasma cell tumours can all closely resemble matrix on Romanowsky stains.

## *Round cell neoplasms*

Tumours in this broad, and slightly unsatisfactory, category vary greatly in clinical behaviour and prognosis; rather, they are linked by their cytological appearance. Round cell tumours are a collection of tumours containing, unsurprisingly, round cells with round nuclei. They are not usually cohesive (although they may appear in groups due to high numbers), and mostly exfoliate well – specimens often contain high numbers of individual cells with distinct cell borders.

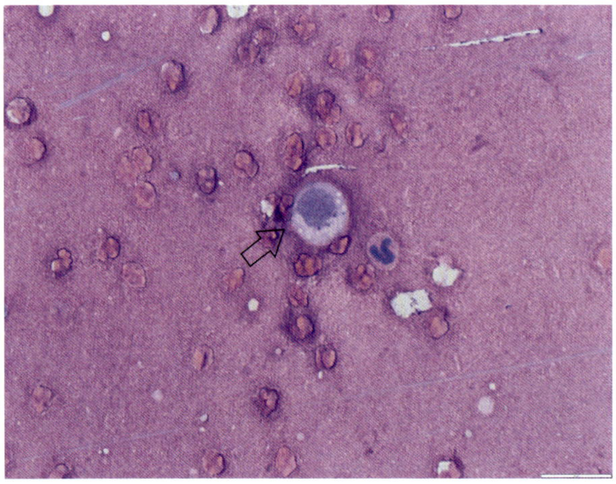

Figure 9.32. Granular pink matrix with embedded mesenchymal cell ('lacuna', open arrow) from a chondrosarcoma (1000×).

Due to the varied appearance and behaviour of the neoplasms in this section, it is easier to discuss them separately rather than as a whole group.

### Mast cell tumour

Mast cells (Figure 9.33) are readily recognisable on cytological specimens, as they usually appear as rounded cells packed with purple granules (**although note that cytoplasmic granules, including mast cell granules, stain unreliably using aqueous Romanowsky stains (such as Diff-Quik)**).

Mast cells appear in low numbers as part of normal inflammatory processes and trafficking, but their presence in high numbers is strongly suggestive of aspiration of a mast cell tumour (MCT); these tumours are a common cytological diagnosis in aspirates from skin and subcutaneous tissues (more commonly in dogs), but are also encountered in the viscera (especially the spleen, liver and GI tract; the spleen is a relatively common site of primary mast cell tumours in cats, whereas visceral mast cell tumours in dogs are usually secondary). Boxers, Staffordshire bull terriers, Golden Retrievers and Labrador Retrievers are reported to have an increased incidence of MCT. Siamese cats are reported to have increased occurrences of cutaneous MCT, whereas other cat breeds more commonly suffer from visceral disease.

Due to the cytokines produced by mast cells, MCT aspirates also frequently contain significant numbers of eosinophils. Many MCTs also contain mesenchymal cells, representing the supporting stroma of the tumour – these mesenchymal cells can be markedly pleomorphic (variably shaped) and of atypical appearance, due to their high activity. Aspirates from MCTs can also contain ribbons of collagen due to the collagenolytic activity of mast cells.

The grade of MCT is of great clinical importance but, unfortunately, grading has historically been unreliable

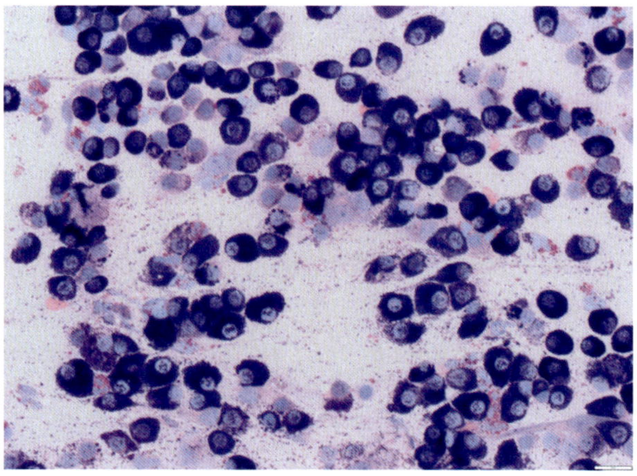

Figure 9.33. Mast cell tumour, canine, probably low-grade (400×).

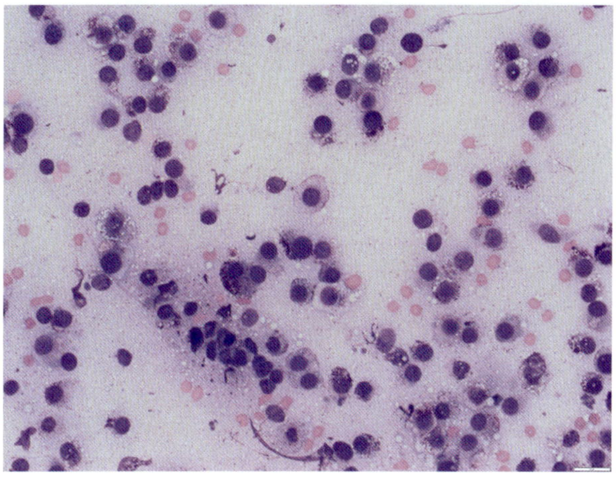

**Figure 9.34.** High-grade canine MCT; note poor granulation, frequent binucleation and anisokaryosis (500×).

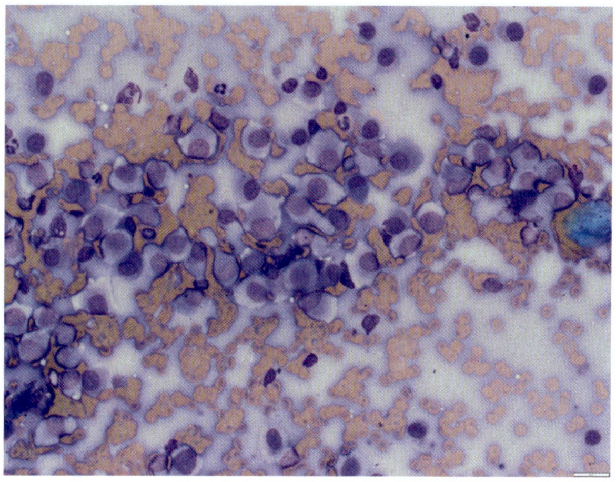

**Figure 9.35.** Canine histiocytoma with frequent 'fried eggs'; note the basophilic background and occasional small lymphocytes present (500×).

based on cytological appearance alone. Recent work, however, has identified several key features that correlate well with high-grade canine neoplasms on histopathology (these are neither consistent nor confirmed in feline mast cell neoplasia; Figure 9.34). These features are:

- granulation
- mitotic index
- bi-/multinucleation
- anisokaryosis (>50%, i.e. some cells with nuclei 50% larger than others)
- nuclear pleomorphism (variably-shaped nuclei).

Of these features, poor granulation is the most likely to be correlated with higher-grade tumours. For well-granulated tumours, if two of the remaining four features are present, a higher-grade tumour should also be suspected.

## Histiocytoma

This is a common benign lesion in the dog, frequently occurring in young patients, arising from dendritic cells in the epidermis (large mononuclear cells related to macrophages but involved more with antigen recognition and presentation than phagocytosis). They are usually solitary, raised, rounded and frequently reddened lesions (sometimes called 'button tumours'), often found around the head and pinnae. They generally regress spontaneously within three months.

Aspirates are often highly cellular, and frequently have a deeply basophilic background. Individual cells usually have large (1.5–3 erythrocyte diameters) central nuclei with round, indented or kidney-shaped nuclei, occasional nucleoli and abundant pale cytoplasm; often they have a characteristic 'fried egg' appearance (Figure 9.35). Although most cells are individual, the cells can occasionally be found in groups that appear quite cohesive (presumably via mechanisms similar to those involved in the formation of epithelioid macrophages). There is often some mitotic activity present. When well preserved with their classical appearance, they are a relatively simple cytological diagnosis but, in some cases, they can appear surprisingly similar to plasmacytomas. Additionally, epitheliotropic lymphoma can on first examination appear very similar although the differences are apparent on close inspection (lymphoma usually has a higher nuclear/cytoplasmic ratio, with denser chromatin).

Histiocytomas are often inflamed, which can complicate the cytological pattern – frequently they contain lymphocytes (probably cytotoxic lymphocytes involved in regression of the lesion), which can occasionally outnumber histiocytes.

## Plasma cell tumour (plasmacytoma)

This neoplasm is more common in the older dog and generally appears as a single, raised cutaneous lesion, again frequently on the pinnae or the lips. Single cutaneous plasmacytomas are usually benign, although local recurrence has been reported following surgical excision.

Cytologically they usually contain high numbers of plasma cells, although they often contain high numbers of binucleate cells and can display quite marked variation in cell size (anisocytosis). Nuclei are usually eccentric, and the presence of eccentric nuclei and moderate numbers of binucleate cells can help to distinguish them from histiocytomas in less clear-cut cases (also, in the author's experience, plasmacytomas more commonly have eosinophilic or clear backgrounds, rather than basophilic, which is more common in histiocytomas; Figure 9.36).

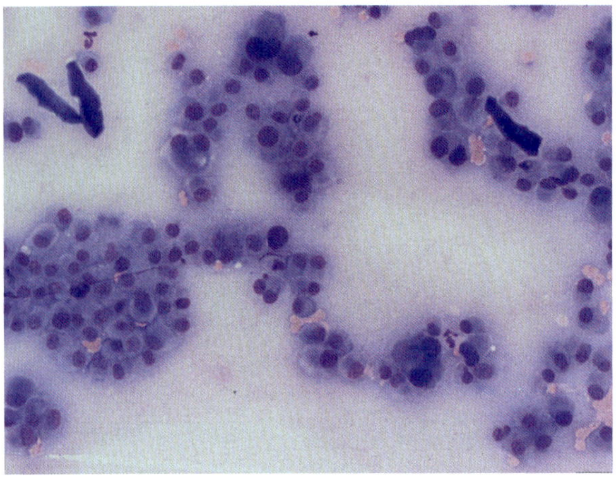

**Figure 9.36.** Canine plasmacytoma; differences from histiocytoma include eccentric nuclei, clumped chromatin and occasional binucleation (400×).

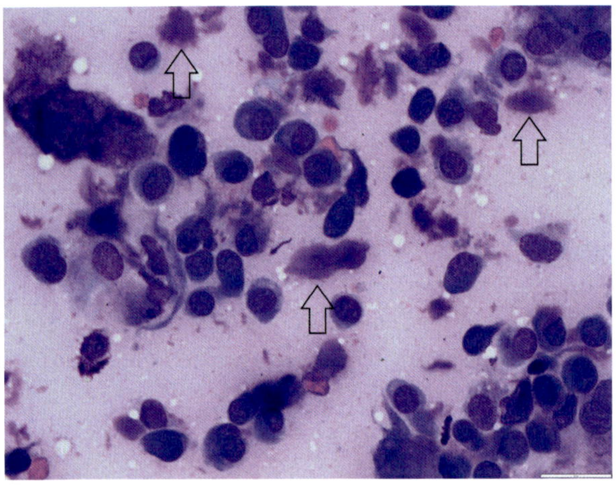

**Figure 9.37.** Plasmacytoma containing amyloid (purple, amorphous and slightly wispy material, open arrows) (1000×).

Some plasmacytomas (approximately 10%) also contain small patches of amyloid protein, due to immunoglobulin production; these usually appear as a small, smooth, purple, wispy clump of material (Figure 9.37).

## Lymphoma

Lymphoma will be covered in more detail later but, when present as a cutaneous mass, it can have a very variable appearance. Cutaneous lymphoma is not automatically epitheliotropic lymphoma – this is a specific subtype of lymphoma (also called mycosis fungoides) with a characteristic appearance somewhat similar to histiocytoma (see histiocytoma, above, for a summary of the differences).

When large cell lymphoma is present the diagnosis is relatively simple – the appearance is similar to the disease observed within lymph nodes (see later). When small cells predominate, the diagnosis is challenging and hard to distinguish from lymphocytic inflammation. Further investigation (such as histopathology or PCR for antigen receptor gene rearrangements (PARR) analysis) is often required in these cases (Figure 9.38).

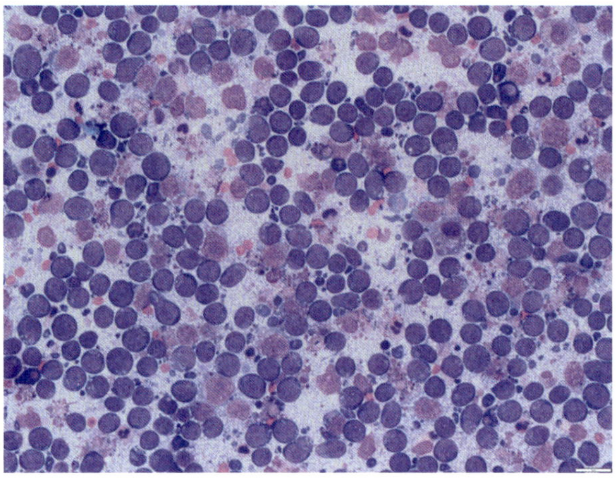

**Figure 9.38.** Large cell lymphoma in canine lymph node (400×).

## Melanocytic tumours (melanocytoma/melanoma)

Although melanocytes are technically mesenchymal cells, they are often included in the round cell category due to their cytological appearance. Melanocytes are the great imitators of cytology – when the lesions are benign (melanocytomas) the diagnosis is more straightforward, as the cells appear as heavily pigmented individual cells within which cytological details cannot be observed. These 'black holes' are quite easy to identify, although it can be challenging to distinguish them from melanophages – macrophages packed with melanin granules – which are often also present.

However, malignant melanocytic tumours ('melanomas', confusingly – they are often called 'malignant melanomas' for clarity) can be very challenging to identify (Figure 9.39). Their appearance can vary greatly, from individual round cells to aggregates of cells and even occasionally cohesive clusters. When melanin is observed within the cytoplasm, the diagnosis can be made more confidently but in poorly pigmented tumours the melanin is often present only as a light dusting in a few cells, and is sometimes not present at all. They often have a quite open ('stippled') chromatin pattern, and many cells have a single large nucleolus, often larger than an erythrocyte (macronucleolus – a feature strongly correlated with malignancy (see below)). Given that malignant melanomas are one of the most aggressive neoplasms encountered in veterinary medicine, with frequent metastasis to lymph nodes and distant sites, it is frustrating that they can be difficult to identify. Poorly pigmented melanoma should be on the differential list for any cutaneous or mucocutaneous lesion that is otherwise challenging to classify.

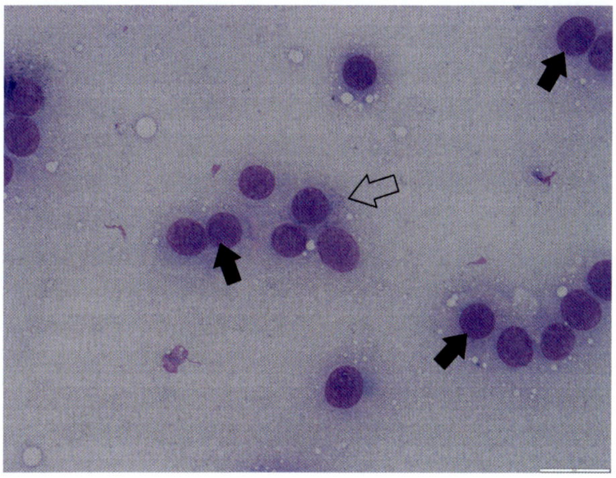

**Figure 9.39.** Malignant melanoma; note the open chromatin and large, usually single, nucleoli (filled arrows) and the scattered melanin pigment in the central cell (open arrow) (1000×).

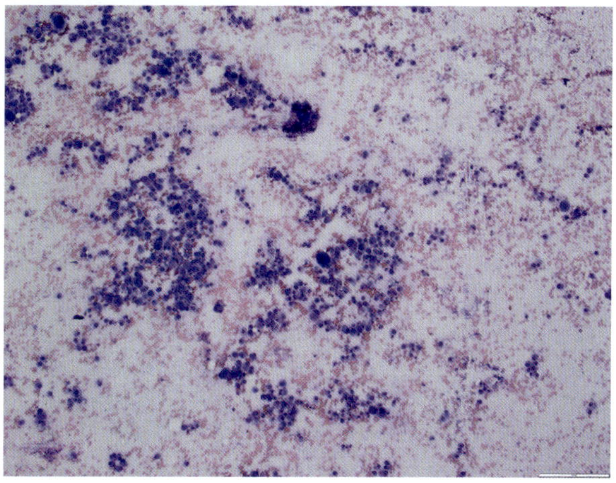

**Figure 9.41.** Canine histiocytic sarcoma; note the marked pleomorphism apparent even at low magnification (100×).

## Transmissible venereal tumour

This is a canine tumour rarely diagnosed in the UK, usually found in imported patients. It is a rare and fascinating example of infectious neoplasia in which tumour cells are transplanted into a new host via direct contact with the previous patient. Due to the nature of these tumours they are usually found in the genital region, but they are occasionally found on the nose or other areas of skin.

They generally exfoliate well on both aspirates and impression smears, and have a characteristic cytological pattern – they contain high numbers of round cells with a central nucleus and abundant pale cytoplasm, somewhat similar to histiocytomas, but the cells contain high numbers of round, clear and distinct vacuoles (Figure 9.40).

## Histiocytic sarcoma

This aggressive histiocytic neoplasm can present as either localised or generalised disease – local lesions appear as firm cutaneous or subcutaneous masses, frequently on the limbs. Despite the name, they are round cell tumours although occasional aggregates of cells can be found. Cytologically the cells frequently display extreme pleomorphism and often contain very large multinucleate cells. Chromatin is open and frequently 'ropey' (see below), and mitotic figures are frequent (Figure 9.41).

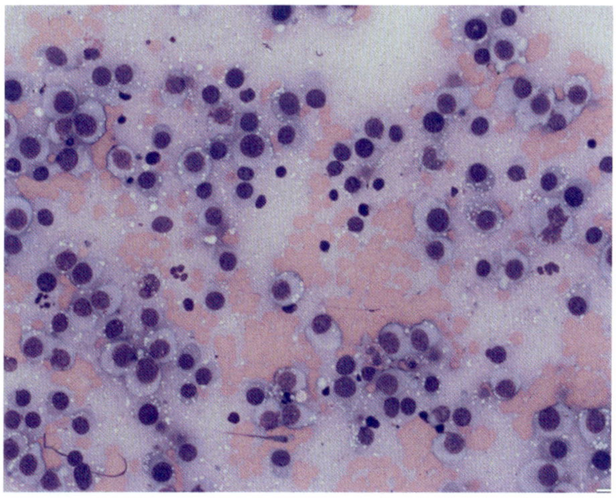

**Figure 9.40.** Transmissible venereal tumour; cytoplasmic vacuolation is characteristic of this neoplasm.

It can sometimes be challenging to distinguish between histiocytic sarcoma and intense granulomatous inflammation, although in the former there are usually occasional cells displaying features too atypical for even markedly reactive macrophages. Malignant features are common (see below, and images in 'Features of malignant tumours'). These neoplasms frequently metastasise to local nodes. Localised disease is more common in the dog, and generalised in the cat. **Bernese Mountain Dogs and Flat-coated Retrievers are strongly predisposed to these lesions, and histiocytic sarcoma should be considered as a differential in any granulomatous-appearing lesion from these patients.**

## *Features of benign and malignant tumours*

Probably the most important question to answer during the examination of neoplastic tissues is whether the neoplasm is likely to follow a benign or malignant clinical course. There follow some broad general features of benign and malignant neoplasms, although there any many exceptions to these general rules – most notably, neuroendocrine tumours (such as thyroid carcinomas and anal sac adenocarcinomas) can have a relatively benign appearance but are often extremely aggressive biologically. Similarly, lymphoma usually appears as a uniform collection of cells rather than the markedly pleomorphic population that characterises many other malignant neoplasms.

### *General features of benign tumours*

Benign tumours display only limited changes from their tissue of origin, and typically closely resemble the original tissue. The cells present are usually homogenous and of a size similar to that of normal cells from the original tissue.

Benign cells often have a low nuclear to cytoplasmic ratio (N/C ratio) – that is, they usually have small nuclei with moderate to abundant amounts of cytoplasm, although there are exceptions in tumours derived from cells with a naturally high N/C ratio (such as basal epithelium). Their nuclei are usually small and uniform, with dense chromatin. If nucleoli are present, these also tend to be small, uniform, well defined and with similar numbers and shapes in each nucleus. Binucleate and multinucleate cells are usually uncommon (exception: plasmacytomas and benign tumours of liver tissue – normal hepatocytes commonly display binucleation).

### *Features of malignant tumours*

As cells accrue mutations moving them genetically, behaviourally (and crucially, from a cytological perspective, morphologically) further away from their original tissue, they tend to behave more aggressively. **Cells become more individualised and less uniform; variations in shape (pleomorphism) and the size of both cells (anisocytosis) and their nuclei (anisokaryosis) become more common**. Increase in cell size is termed cytomegaly (Figure 9.42).

Malignant features can be broadly divided into changes noted within three categories: cellular, nuclear and cytoplasmic.

#### Cellular criteria for malignancy

- **Abnormal location**: Cells found in a location distant to their original tissue, such as cutaneous lymphoma (high numbers of dermal lymphocytes) or epithelial/neuroendocrine cells found within a lymph node).
- **Variations in cell size and shape**: Anisocytosis and pleomorphism. Benign lesions often display mild anisocytosis, but twofold or higher variation is more suggestive of malignancy.
- **Loss of cohesion**: One feature of more aggressive neoplastic behaviour is decreased cell–cell adhesion, which increases the likelihood of metastasis, leading to increased sample cellularity. Epithelial and mesenchymal tumours often exfoliate in smaller clusters or aggregates, with more individual cells (Figure 9.43).
- **Disorderly arrangement**: As cells change in size and shape and lose cohesiveness, the overall appearance of groups becomes more disordered. Epithelial clusters become crowded and disorganised, with nuclear moulding occasionally visible (nuclei become 'moulded' around the shape of larger, adjacent nuclei; this can occur between adjacent cells or within multinucleate cells; Figure 9.44).

#### Nuclear criteria for malignancy

- **Variations in nuclear size and shape**: Anisokaryosis, nuclear pleomorphism and macronucleosis (nuclei larger than RBCs) are all features of malignancy, and lead to variations (usually increases) in the N/C ratio.
- **Nucleolar changes**: Nucleoli are the site of ribosome construction within the nucleus, and are therefore more prominent and more numerous in active cells; as neoplastic cells are usually highly active, they frequently display increased numbers of them. Variations in the size, shape and number of nucleoli is also criteria for malignancy (Figure 9.45). **The**

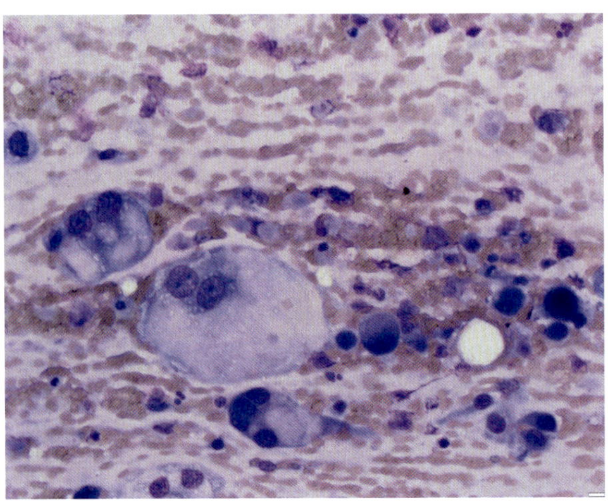

Figure 9.42. Marked cytomegaly in an anaplastic cutaneous canine neoplasm (400×).

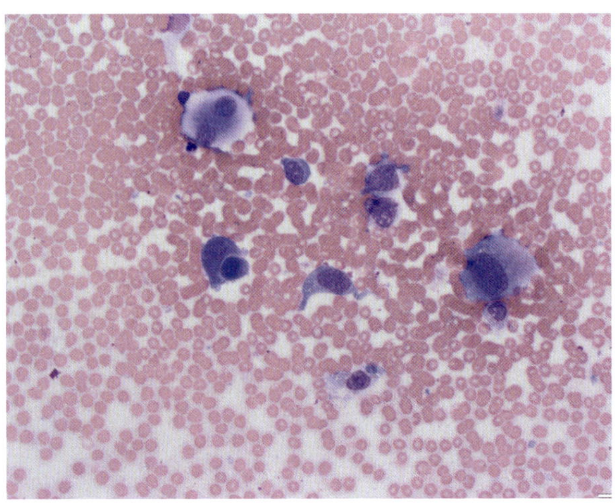

Figure 9.43. Pleomorphic cells from a canine transitional cell carcinoma; note also the poor cohesion of these cells (400×).

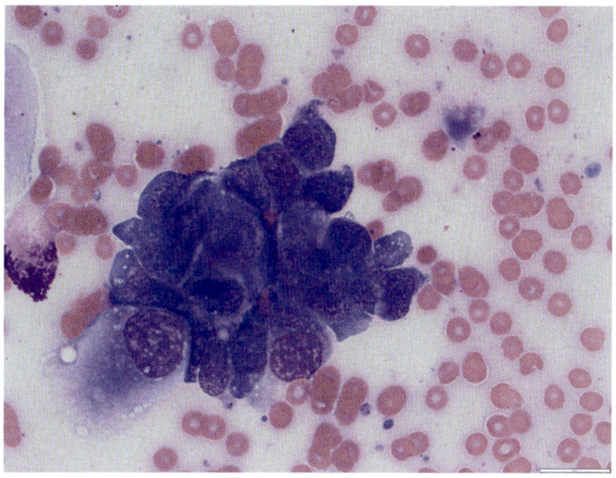

**Figure 9.44.** A disorganised and crowded cluster from a pulmonary adenocarcinoma; many nuclei appear 'squeezed' by adjacent cells (nuclear moulding) (1000×).

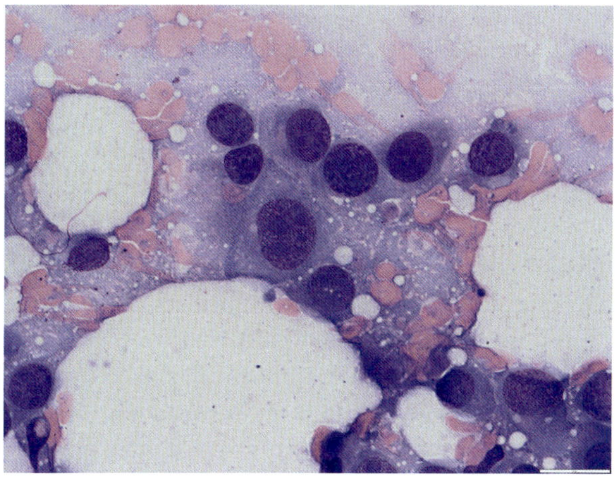

**Figure 9.45.** Multiple, variably-sized nucleoli in cells from a histiocytic sarcoma; note also the irregular 'ropey' chromatin (1000×).

**presence of macronucleoli is a feature strongly associated with malignancy**.

- **Mitotic figures**: Mitotic figures are visible as cells replicate DNA ready for division – a population of cells containing mitotic figures indicates actively replicating tissue; small numbers may be seen in reactive or hyperplastic tissues such as lymph nodes or mesothelial cells, but high numbers are more commonly associated with malignancy (Figure 9.46). In addition, the presence of atypical mitotic figures (tripolar or multipolar division, 'scattered' chromatin due to fragments lagging behind the axis of division, asymmetry) raises significant concern for a malignant tumour.
- **Chromatin changes**: Dense chromatin with no discernible pattern (commonly seen in small lymphocytes or basal epithelium) indicates tightly packed chromosomes and, usually, inactivity; **the more 'open' the chromatin (i.e. paler with discernible patterns), the more active the cell**; malignancy is

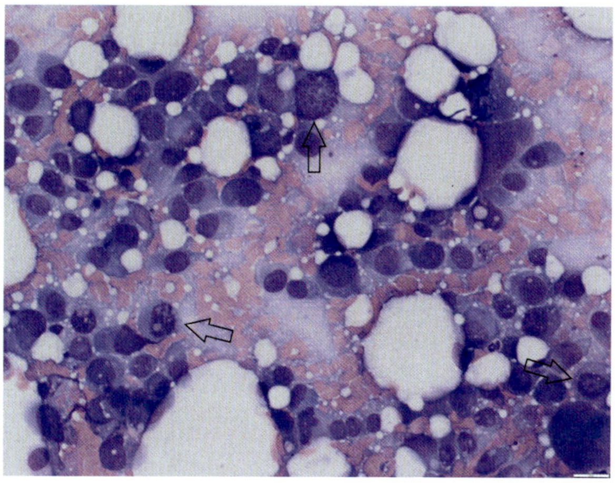

**Figure 9.46.** Multiple mitotic figures (arrows) in cells from a histiocytic sarcoma (400×).

associated with 'coarse' or 'ropey' chromatin, with irregular patches and clumps visible within the nuclei.

## Cytoplasmic criteria for malignancy

Of the three criteria, these changes are the least specific; the changes below indicate increased cellular activity, including hyperplasia, reactivity and benign neoplasia, not necessarily malignancy.

- **Cytoplasmic basophilia**: As cells accrue organelles and synthesise protein and secretory products, their cytoplasm becomes more basophilic (blue); in contrast, cells with shrunken eosinophilic cytoplasm are likely to be inactive, or potentially apoptotic or necrotic.
- **Cytoplasmic vacuolation**: Proteins and other products can accumulate in vacuoles within the cytoplasm, especially when production is excessive or aberrant; vacuoles are most commonly found in the perinuclear area (as this is the location of the Golgi apparatus); 'signet ring' cells, found within adenocarcinomas, are cells with a large single vacuole containing secretory product, displacing nucleus to the side of the cell (see Figure 9.23).

## *Common pitfalls and useful points to remember in neoplasia cytology*

- Inflammation causes hyperplasia and dysplasia in tissues, which can mimic neoplasia – be cautious when diagnosing tumours in the presence of inflammation.
- The prognosis of many tumours is dependent on their grade; because grading of tumours often involves examining their invasiveness to adjacent tissues, cytological schemes for grading have not been established; histopathology is required for the grading of many neoplasms.

- Despite the general guidelines for the appearance of malignant tumours, several tumours (particularly neuroendocrine tumours such as thyroid carcinomas and anal sac apocrine gland adenocarcinomas) behave much more aggressively than their cytological appearance suggests.
- Similarly, the behaviour of complex tumours – particularly mammary tumours – is often poorly correlated with their appearance on cytology preparations, and mammary neoplasia may be better examined histopathologically than cytologically.
- Fibroblasts present due to reactivity can display many features consistent with malignancy, and are often extremely challenging to distinguish from poorly cellular aspirates from sarcomas, particularly when inflammation is also present.
- Similarly, due to their highly plastic nature, macrophages can appear very variable in cytological specimens, displaying anisocytosis, anisokaryosis, multi-nucleation and pleomorphism; examining the N/C ratio can be helpful in these cases, as the larger active cells will usually also have expanded cytoplasm, keeping the N/C ratio low, but macrophages provide a constant challenge even for the experienced cytologist.
- Reactive mesothelial cells, which can be found in areas lined with mesothelium (i.e. the pleural, pericardial and peritoneal cavities) can also take on multiple features of malignancy, particularly if an effusion is long-standing or markedly inflammatory. Mesothelial cells can be challenging to distinguish from exfoliating carcinomas in effusions; mesothelial cell harvests can be particularly high in pericardial effusions, or in pleural effusions from patients with history of pericardial disease or pericardectomy (see later).

## Cytology of non-inflammatory and non-neoplastic lesions

Not every pathological process is inflammatory or neoplastic: there are a variety of other causes for fluid-filled or solid masses, many of which can still be recognised or at least suspected on cytological examination. Below are some of the most commonly encountered lesions.

### *Epidermal inclusion cyst/follicular cyst*

Although there are histological differences between these lesions, they are cytologically identical and have a good prognosis – excision is expected to be curative, when required. Aspiration of these lesions usually produces variable amounts of thick, off-white material which, when examined cytologically, is usually a mixture of keratin, keratin bars and scrolls, and cholesterol crystals (Figure 9.47).

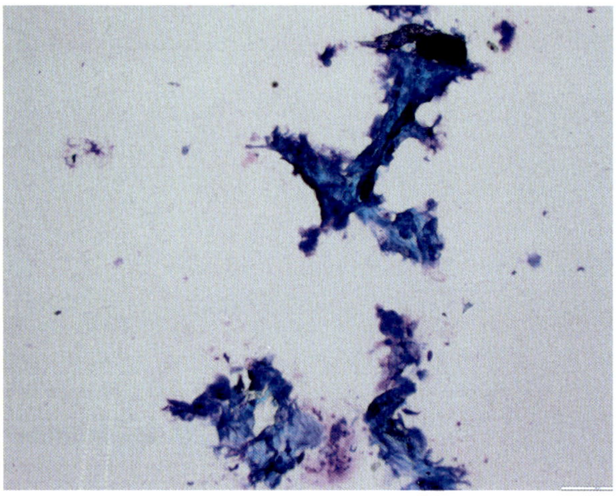

**Figure 9.47.** Clumps of keratin (100×).

Keratin is angular, anucleate and palely to deeply basophilic, or (less commonly) slightly purple. Keratin bars and scrolls are small, linear, angular structures with pale (scrolls) or deep (bars) basophilic staining. Cholesterol crystals are formed from the breakdown of cell membranes and are clear, square or rectangular. 'Ghost cells' are also commonly encountered – these are anucleate cellular-shaped structures with a pale central area, and have been associated with pilomatricomas (benign hair follicle tumours; Figure 9.48).

**Keratin is highly irritant to surrounding tissue** – when these lesions rupture, they commonly produce a marked neutrophilic, macrophagic or mixed inflammatory pattern, often with multinucleate macrophages (consistent with a foreign body reaction – see above). Ruptured keratin-containing lesions can be challenging to resolve medically, and surgical excision often proves the fastest route to resolution in these cases. However, care should be taken when interpreting inflamed lesions containing keratin, as the cytological

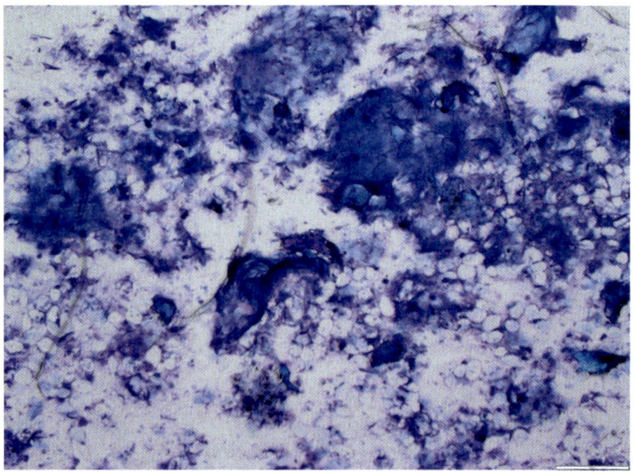

**Figure 9.48.** Keratin and embedded 'ghost cells', associated with pilomatricomas (100×).

appearance of squamous cell carcinomas can be similar to that of ruptured keratinising cysts, particularly where high numbers of neutrophils are present.

## Apocrine cyst

This common lesion forms due to occlusion of apocrine (sweat) glands. It is a firm dermal mass filled with pale yellow–brown fluid. Cytologically, this fluid is usually acellular with a clear background.

## Seroma/haematoma

The cytological appearance of these lesions is somewhat similar – both contain low to moderate numbers of macrophages, usually activated, within a fluid background. Seromas contain proteinaceous fluid that appears cytologically as a markedly stippled pale-to-mid-eosinophilic or amphophilic background, often with protein clefts – crescent-shaped folds within the fluid (Figure 9.49). Haematomas usually have a far less stippled, often eosinophilic, background and contain moderate to high numbers of erythrocytes with evidence of previous haemorrhage (see below).

## Blood contamination versus previous haemorrhage

When cytological samples yield large amounts of blood, it is valuable to distinguish between fresh blood contamination during sampling and bleeding prior to sampling. Platelets are present for only a few minutes following haemorrhage, and their presence on cytology almost always indicates accidental contamination.

In lesions with pre-existing haemorrhage, macrophages are often seen containing phagocytosed red blood cells or (after several days) red cell breakdown products – haemosiderin (dark granular pigment; Figure 9.50) or haemotoidin (golden-brown rhomboid crystals). Note that red cell phagocytosis (erythrophagia) can occur while fluids are in sample tubes, which is why it is important to make fresh fluid preparations as soon as possible after sampling.

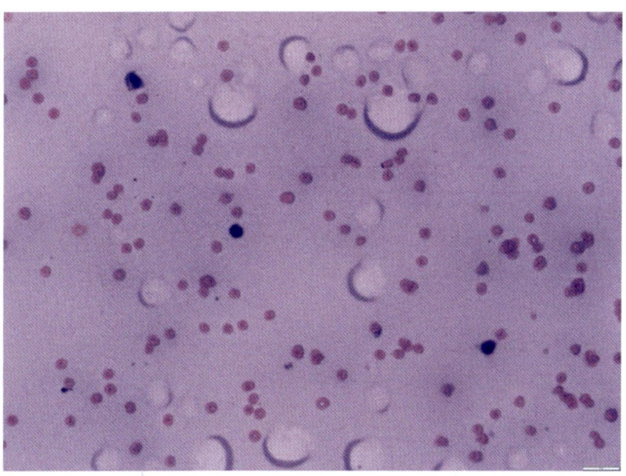

**Figure 9.49.** Stippled purple fluid with protein clefts (crescent-shaped objects), indicative of high-protein fluid (400×).

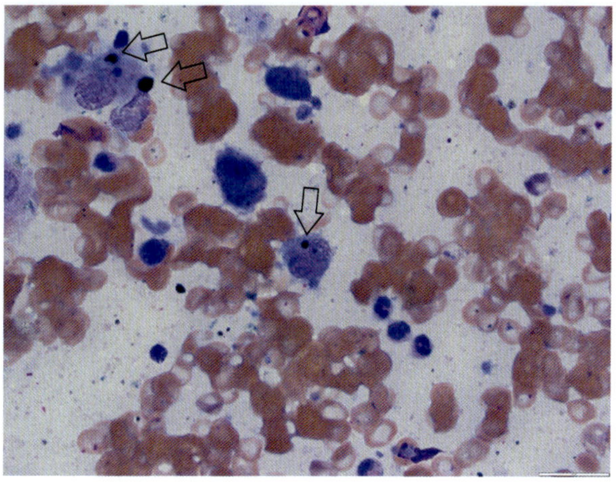

**Figure 9.50.** Macrophages containing haemosiderin (arrows), indicating haemorrhage prior to sampling (1000×).

## Calcinosis

Dystrophic mineralisation is often readily recognisable grossly on cytological specimens. Calcinosis circumscripta is seen at pressure points and in areas of repeated trauma, uncommonly in dogs and rarely in cats. Calcinosis cutis is more usually seen in dorsal regions, especially over the neck, and is associated with glucocorticoid administration (and therefore is occasionally seen in Cushing's disease).

The conditions appear cytologically identical – on the slide, the stained material often has a chalky pale blue to lilac appearance. Under the microscope the material has a darker and often brownish appearance, with a granular irregular background, sometimes containing rounded calcium carbonate crystals; this background (and the crystals) dissolves when immersion oil is applied to the slide. Due to the irritation associated with mineralisation, macrophages, sometimes multinucleate, are often seen, as well as other leukocytes and fibroblasts.

When unexpected mineralisation is found in a cytological preparation, evaluation of the patient's serum calcium may be prudent (Figure 9.51).

## Hyperplasia

Hyperplasia is a reversible, non-neoplastic proliferation of tissue (usually epithelial) in response to stimuli. The cells have normal morphology and hyperplasia cannot be definitively confirmed cytologically, but the

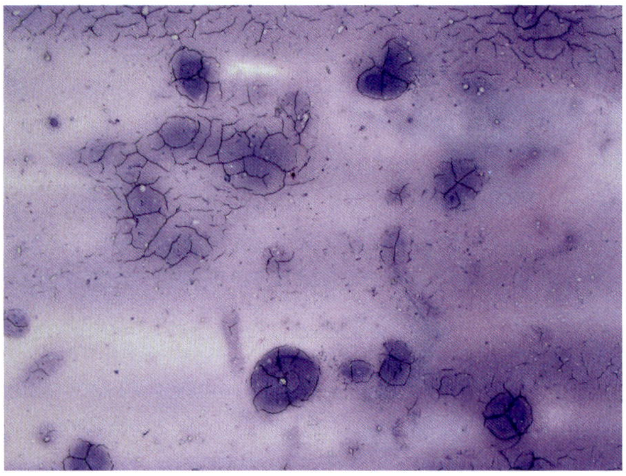

**Figure 9.51.** Dystrophic mineralisation: granular and brownish-purple background (100×).

presence of high numbers of morphologically unremarkable cells in an enlarged organ or tissue is strongly suggestive; hyperplastic prostate gland and lymph nodes are the most commonly seen tissues. In cutaneous lesions, sebaceous epithelial hyperplasia and mammary hyperplasia can be challenging to distinguish from well-differentiated neoplastic lesions such as sebaceous and mammary adenomas.

### *Necrosis*

Necrosis appears as greyish-blue amorphous material, found in wide swathes and often containing indistinct and blurred necrotic cell ghosts, or degenerating clusters or aggregates of cells. Neutrophils and macrophages are often embedded, as necrosis stimulates an inflammatory response.

Necrosis is not a specific finding, as it can be caused by intense inflammation or infarction, but the otherwise unexplained presence of necrosis in a lesion often raises concern for underlying neoplasia (Figure 9.52).

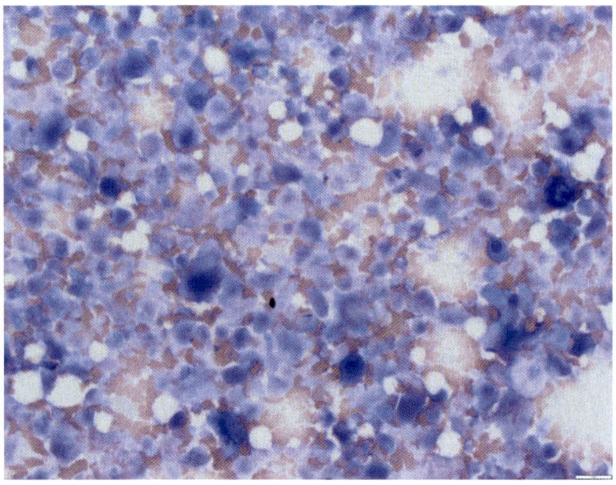

**Figure 9.52.** Marked necrosis within a prostatic carcinoma; note the blurred/smudged indistinct shapes that once were living cells (400×).

## Cytology of lymph nodes

Lymph nodes are aspirated for a number of different reasons:

- Assessment of whether enlarged lymph nodes are neoplastic or hyperplastic / reactive.
- Assessment of the type and (ideally) cause of inflammation.
- Staging of nearby neoplasms by checking for metastatic disease.
- Monitoring of ongoing lymphoma.

Aspiration of lymph nodes is challenging when they are not enlarged; frequently, attempted aspiration of normal-sized lymph nodes harvests only peri-nodal adipose tissue. Lymphocytes are fragile cells, and a slide containing only ruptured cells cannot be usefully assessed; for this reason, the non-suction (fenestration) technique, or at least a combination of techniques including non-suction samples, is recommended.

When multiple lymph nodes are enlarged, sampling of multiple nodes spanning the diaphragm is recommended to assess whether all nodes are enlarged for the same reason, and to help stage lymphoma, where present. In these cases, the submandibular nodes should be avoided as these are often enlarged due to persistent antigenic stimulation (from the oral cavity), and due to the close proximity of the submandibular salivary glands (which are very difficult to distinguish from lymph nodes with palpation or ultrasound). **The prescapular and popliteal nodes are preferred sampling sites for generalised lymphadenopathy**.

As with other large lesions, the very centre of greatly enlarged nodes should be avoided when sampling to avoid necrosis or poorly preserved material.

### *Assessment of lymph nodes*

As with other areas of cytology, a stepwise and logical approach greatly aids evaluation of lymph node aspirates: first assess the lymphoid population and then concentrate on non-lymphoid cells.

#### *Lymphoid component*

Although lymphocytes can be classified into multiple different categories and subdivisions (i.e. centrocytes, immunoblasts, etc.), **from a practical perspective the most useful task is to assess the proportions of small, intermediate and large lymphocytes** (see earlier section on lymphocytic inflammation for more details on this).

It is also important to assess whether the lymphocytes are atypical or morphologically unremarkable (see later section on lymphoma for examples). In some cases, a differential count of these cells may be helpful for assessment of the total population, although uneven spread of cells and difficulty achieving absolute accuracy in assessment of cell size in densely packed preparations render its usefulness very limited.

In a quiescent, normal (and therefore rarely aspirated) node, unremarkable small lymphocytes should be the dominant cell found (>90% of lymphocytes), alongside occasional intermediate cells and occasional large lymphocytes.

### *Non-lymphoid component*

Other 'normal' resident nucleated cells of lymph nodes include low numbers of plasma cells and 'tingible-body' macrophages (activated macrophages containing phagocytosed cellular debris). Lymph node aspirates also frequently contain high numbers of 'lymphoglandular bodies' – small, irregular, pale grey fragments of cytoplasm stripped from fragile lymphocytes (Figure 9.53). When observed in the presence of high numbers of unidentifiable cells, lymphoglandular bodies strongly suggest (but don't absolutely confirm) that the ruptured cells were once lymphocytes.

Other cells, including other leukocytes, epithelial and mesenchymal cells, are not expected to be found in significant numbers within 'normal' lymph nodes.

### *Reactive/hyperplastic lymph nodes*

Small lymphocytes remain the predominant cell in reactivity, but proportions are decreased as the cells mature. Intermediate–large lymphocytes can reach 30% of the total lymphocyte total or, rarely, even higher proportions in markedly reactive nodes – these nodes can be extremely difficult to distinguish from early lymphoma. Plasma cells also increase, as well as (in some cases) melanin pigment (particularly in nodes draining areas of skin disease); the pigment can be found both free in the background and phagocytosed within macrophages – **'melanin incontinence'** (Figure 9.54).

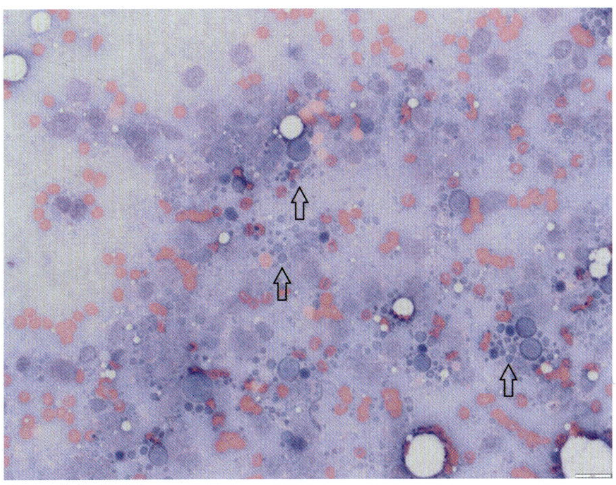

**Figure 9.53.** Pale grey, rounded lymphoglandular bodies in canine lymphoma (arrows indicate several few groups; many more are present in the image) (400×).

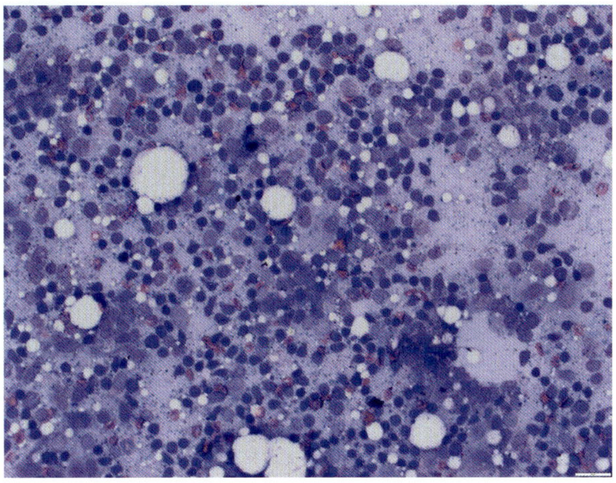

**Figure 9.54.** Reactive lymph node with expanded intermediate and large lymphocytes; note the mixed nature of the lymphoid harvest. Melanin pigment is also present scattered throughout the background (400×).

There are many causes for reactivity or hyperplasia of nodes, the most common including draining sites of inflammation or neoplasia. **Generalised lymphadenopathy is not exclusive to lymphoma** – it is also seen with generalised or systemic inflammation (such as FIV or leishmania) and immune-mediated disease. **In feline patients (unlike dogs), generalised lymphadenopathy is more commonly associated with inflammation than with lymphoma.**

### *Lymphoma*

Lymphoma (interchangeably termed lymphosarcoma) is caused by uncontrolled clonal expansion of lymphocytes; because the neoplastic cells are clones, they are morphologically similar. **For many neoplasms, a population of cells displaying marked differences to each other raises significant concerns for malignancy, whereas with lymphoma, a population of lymphocytes appearing nearly identical, rather than the mixed pattern found in reactive nodes, raises the cytologist's suspicion of cancer** (Figure 9.55).

The many subclassifications of lymphoma that have been described are beyond the scope of this chapter; the majority do not have specific treatment protocols currently developed for them, and are mainly useful for prognostic purposes (those interested are directed to Valli et al. (2010)). Again, for practical purposes, the important thing is to recognise that a homogenous population of lymphocytes, particularly when plasma cells and other indications of reactivity are absent or greatly reduced, is consistent with lymphoma. This is relatively straightforward when the neoplastic cells are

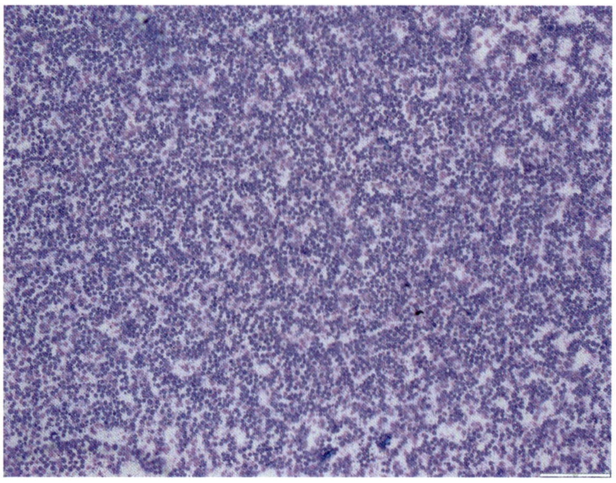

**Figure 9.55.** Large cell lymphoma; even at low power, the homogenous nature of the lymphocytes can be appreciated (100×).

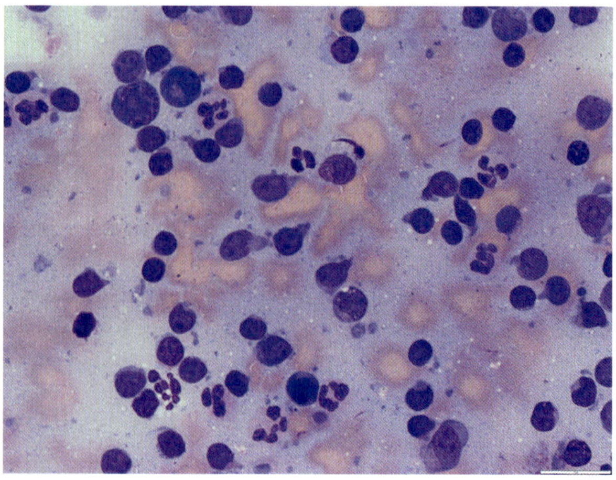

**Figure 9.57.** Small–intermediate cell lymphoma: cells have slightly atypically clumped chromatin and frequent hand-mirror forms; note there are also occasional plasma cells (upper left) and, although these suggest reactivity, they do not exclude lymphoma (1000×).

large and present in high numbers, but can be more challenging in early disease or when the cells are small.

Diffuse large cell lymphoma is the most common lymphoma observed in dogs; clinically the disease generally presents as generalised lymphadenopathy, and cytologically the specimens contain >30% (and often >50%) monomorphic large lymphocytes, usually with open or 'dispersed' chromatin, and frequently with prominent nucleoli. Mitotic figures may be increased (Figure 9.56).

Identification of clonal expansions of small lymphocytes is much more challenging cytologically – the cells often appear as unremarkable small lymphocytes although they are often slightly larger than typical small cells, and occasionally have slightly more open or clumped chromatin patterns. High numbers of 'hand-mirror' lymphocytes, with a tapering cytoplasmic projection, are concerning but not absolutely exclusive for lymphoma (because certain types of hyperplasia also produce this pattern). As above, high numbers of small lymphocytes with limited evidence of reactivity (i.e. very few intermediate to large cells, reduced or no plasma cells) raise suspicion for lymphoma (Figure 9.57).

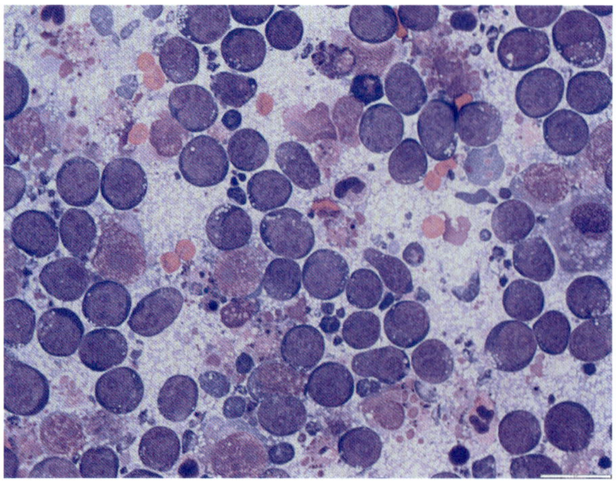

**Figure 9.56.** Large cell lymphoma (same case as Fig. 9.54); the lymphocytes are dominated by a population of large cells (>2.5% erythrocytes) with dispersed chromatin and multiple prominent nucleoli, as well as multiple small, clear cytoplasmic vacuoles. There are also bare nuclei and a single macrophage (centre right) (1000×).

Atypical lymphocyte features are less common in lymphoma than in other neoplasms, but when present – and particularly when replicated many times across the observed cell population – raise concerns for neoplasia. Such features include:

- Atypical mitotic figures.
- Irregular, convoluted or 'cleaved' nuclei.
- Binucleate or multinucleate cells.
- Prominent cytoplasmic vacuolation.
- Prominent cytoplasmic granulation (particularly when granules are large and irregular).

## Further testing

Several further tests are available for lymphoma, to confirm the diagnosis in more challenging cases or to further characterise the neoplasm. PARR can be performed on pre-stained slides and can confirm the presence of a clonal (as opposed to mixed) population of cells. Immunophenotyping (e.g. immunocytochemistry, which again can be performed in some laboratories on pre-stained preparations) can confirm the neoplasm's lineage (i.e. B or T cell). Histopathological examination, as with many other neoplasms, provides further information but is a more invasive test.

### *Lymphadenitis*

The assessment of inflammation in lymph node aspirates can be challenging, as these often also contain moderate to marked blood contamination. When significant numbers of other leukocytes are found interspersed with the lymphocytes, especially with minimal blood contamination, inflammation can be confirmed – inflamed lymph nodes are divided into three broad categories with causes similar to those in other areas of the body.

#### Neutrophilic lymphadenitis

Neutrophils are usually the most numerous leukocyte found in dogs and cats, which makes this pattern of inflammation especially difficult to interpret when there is a large amount of peripheral blood present. As with other tissues, neutrophilic inflammation within the node is often caused by bacterial infection, either within the node itself or in an area drained by the node. Neutrophils may be degenerate or non-degenerate (see earlier section on neutrophilic inflammation), and bacteria may or may not be present. Other causes include immune-mediated disease or underlying neoplasia (again, either in a region drained by the node or metastatic within the node itself).

#### Eosinophilic lymphadentis

The most common reason for eosinophilic inflammation within a node is either hypersensitivity or external parasites; more specifically, it is seen in nodes draining areas of skin disease (such as atopy or flea-allergy dermatitis), and often accompanied by melanin incontinence. Other causes include eosinophilic granuloma, hyper-eosinophilic syndrome (accompanied by a significant circulating eosinophilia) and paraneoplastic syndrome (most commonly due to mast cell tumours or lymphoma).

#### Granulomatous lymphadenitis

Low numbers of tingle-body macrophages are normal residents within lymph nodes, but increased numbers, or the presence of multinucleate or epithelioid macrophages, indicate granulomatous or 'histiocytic' inflammation. Causes in dogs include fungal infections, leishmaniasis and immune-mediated disease (particularly in the Springer Spaniels), whereas in cats infections by mycobacteria, viruses (such as feline infectious peritonitis (FIP), particularly abdominal nodes) or fungi are more commonly encountered.

Well-differentiated histiocytic sarcoma can sometimes be challenging to distinguish from granulomatous inflammation; histopathological examination of nodes containing an otherwise unexplained large population of macrophages is worthwhile in susceptible dog breeds (e.g. Flat-coated Retrievers and Bernese Mountain Dogs, and also Rottweilers and Schnauzers).

## Metastatic disease

Tumour metastasis is suspected when cells are present that are not normally observed within lymph nodes (such as epithelial cells) or when cells normally present only occasionally are found in high numbers (such as mast cells). The cytological appearance of metastatic disease can vary, from finding occasional small clusters of atypical cells to complete effacement of the node with atypical cells and no obvious lymphoid component. In the latter case, it is important to know exactly from where (anatomically) the aspirate was taken because it is no longer possible to confirm lymph node aspiration on cytological appearance.

**Common metastatic tumours within lymph nodes include carcinomas, mast cell tumours and melanomas – sarcomas rarely invade lymph nodes (except via local invasion)**. The presence of the invading neoplasm often produces a reactive population of lymphocytes and, occasionally, inflammation. Necrosis can also be found, although this is not specific for neoplasia as it can also be found in very inflamed nodes (Figure 9.58).

Mast cell tumour metastasis in particular can be difficult to identify in the early stages, as low numbers of mast cells can be found in reactive nodes, particularly those draining areas of skin disease or mast cell tumours. Atypical features (such as reduced granulation, binucleation and pleomorphism) and/or the presence of mast cells in aggregates, rather than individually, should raise the cytologist's suspicion of metastatic disease.

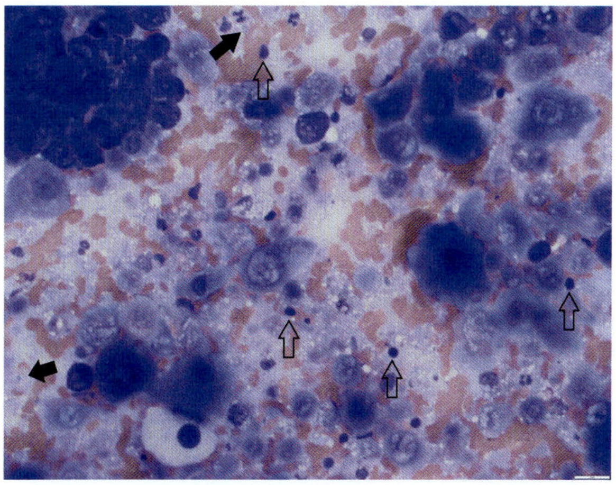

**Figure 9.58.** Metastatic squamous cell carcinoma in a lymph node; there are scattered small lymphocytes (open arrows) and lymphoglandular bodies (black arrows), but the node is dominated by large, atypical epithelial cells (400×).

## Body cavity fluid analysis

Fluid accumulates in body cavities (principally the peritoneum, pleural and pericardial cavities) for a number of reasons; the main purpose of fluid analysis is to distinguish between transudates (formed due to alterations in hydrostatic forces) and exudates (formed by changes in vascular permeability due to inflammation). In certain cases, more specific causes (e.g. chylothorax) or definitive diagnoses (e.g. neoplastic effusions) can be made.

### *Fluid analysis*

This technique assesses the following:

- **Macroscopic appearance**: Including colour, turbidity and viscosity; pH assessment can also be useful.
- **Cell count**: This can be broadly assessed from the cytological preparations, but some haematology machines can give cell counts; the manufacturer's advice should be sought, but **do not attempt on very thick or flocculent fluids**.
- **Protein**: Refractometry gives a broad indication of protein content, although it can underestimate at lower values; more accurate values can be achieved using well-spun supernatant using an in-practice automated chemistry analyser.
- **Other biochemistry**: As above, other biochemical values can be calculated by many in-practice analysers: evaluation of triglycerides, bilirubin, glucose and others can aid interpretation, especially when compared with serum values.

### *Mesothelium*

The body cavities are lined with mesothelium – cells derived from embryonic mesoderm that are arranged as a thin sheet attached to a basement membrane, and they express both epithelial and mesenchymal markers (Figure 9.59).

Cytologically, this is a diagnostic challenge because cells become markedly reactive in the presence of inflammation or in long-standing fluids, and the reactive changes strongly mimic features of malignancy. These are large mononuclear cells, usually found individually or in small sheets. Their nuclei are usually central and they have a clear to reddish-magenta fringe with 'wrinkled' borders. When reactive, their mitotic rate increases dramatically, the cells enlarge and bi- and multinucleate cells become common. Reactive mesothelial cells are frequent and markedly reactive in pericardial effusions and, in the author's experience, in pleural effusions from patients that have had pericardial disease or undergone pericardectomy.

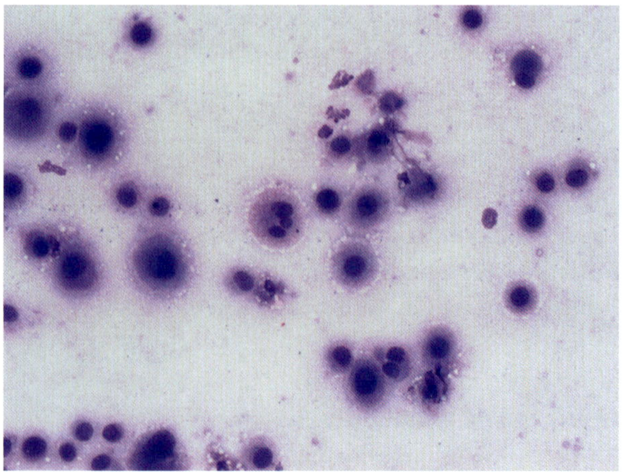

**Figure 9.59.** Reactive mesothelial cells in canine pericardial effusion; note the pleomorphism and multinucleation (400×).

**For this reason, neoplasia should be diagnosed with caution in body cavity fluids, especially in pericardial fluid.**

### *Fluid classification*

'Normal' fluid is rarely assessed, as there is too little to collect in the absence of pathology. When assessed experimentally it has a clear/pale straw colour, with low cellularity and low to moderate protein.

Pathological fluids are classified according to their protein and cellularity and, as with many biological processes, because there is considerable overlap between classifications the interpretation needs to take the history and clinical picture into consideration.

#### *Transudates*

- macroscopic appearance, clear
- S.G. <1.015
- total protein, <25 g/l
- nucleated cell count, very low ($<1 \times 10^9$/l) – mesothelial cells, macrophages, neutrophils.

'Pure' transudates have very low protein and cellularity. Thsey are usually caused by reduced oncotic pressure due to low serum albumin (<14 g/l, more often <10 g/l), often in combination with increased hydrostatic pressure. Severe liver disease, such as cirrhosis, combines reduced albumin production with increased portal venous pressure and so this is a common cause of peritoneal transudate. Other causes include renal disease (nephrotic syndrome due to renal protein loss), protein-losing enteropathy and underlying neoplasia (although this is a relatively uncommon cause).

**Finding a transudate should prompt assessment of a patient's serum protein levels.**

### 'Modified' or 'high-protein' transudates

- macroscopic appearance, yellow to clear, occasionally slightly turbid
- S.G. 1.015–1.025
- total protein, >25 g/l
- nucleated cell count, moderate (1–5 × $10^9$/l) – mesothelial cells, macrophages, neutrophils, occasionally lymphocytes and other leukocytes.

Although still formed by transudation (alterations in hydrostatic forces), these effusions are 'modified' by increased protein and, usually, increased cellularity. Many of these effusions represent transudates that have been present long enough to elicit mild irritation/inflammation (hence the increased cellularity). The most common causes include heart disease, increased venous pressure (often due to liver disease) and underlying neoplasia or inflammation (such as pancreatitis, hepatitis or lung lobe torsion).

## *Exudates*

- macroscopic appearance, turbid and usually opaque, red–pink–yellow
- S.G. >1.025
- total protein, >25 g/l (often much higher)
- nucleated cell count, usually high (>5 × $10^9$/l, often significantly higher).

Exudates are formed from increased vascular and mesothelial permeability due to inflammation, allowing large proteins and cells to enter the cavity. Sepsis (septic peritonitis, pyothorax) is the most common cause, and in these cases the majority of cells present will be degenerate neutrophils, alongside activated macrophages and reactive mesothelial cells. Free bacteria may be present, and the presence of phagocytosed bacterial organisms confirms bacterial infection. **For suspected exudates, always take a sample in a sterile plain tube for culture**. The bacterial morphology may guide empirical therapy – mixed-morphology bacteria, including cocci and long rods, suggests anaerobic infection and GI rupture.

Sterile exudates contain non-degenerate neutrophils or, occasionally, other leukocytes; causes include underlying neoplasia, inflammation and foreign body. **The presence of an otherwise unexplained sterile exudate raises significant concern for underlying neoplasia**, and a careful search of the fluid for neoplastic cells is recommended (although note the above section on mesothelial cells).

Note: as the protein in exudates reflects the patient's serum protein, significantly hypoproteinaemic patients can have low-protein exudates.

### Poorly cellular exudates and FIP

In some situations, an effusion can have significantly high protein but a relatively low cell count (<1 × $10^9$/l). Although this could equally be classified as a 'high-protein, poorly cellular transudate', the underlying cause is often an increase in vascular permeability. The cytological appearance is a fluid with a highly stippled background containing scattered and usually poorly preserved cells.

FIP is the most common cause of this effusion, and is described in some sources as unique for this disease, although the author has also occasionally encountered it in cases of poorly exfoliative underlying inflammatory disease, particularly pancreatitis, or in other causes of vasculitis.

These effusions will often have a low albumin/globulin ratio, consistent with inflammation. **An albumin/globulin ratio <0.4 is strongly suggestive of (but not pathognomic for) FIP**. Identifying coronavirus within the fluid (either via PCR or immunohistochemistry) lends further strong support for FIP.

## *Specific effusions*

### Haemorrhagic effusions

- macroscopic appearance, turbid red
- protein and cell count, varied but usually high (compare with peripheral blood)
- PCV usually >5% (often much higher – again, varies and depends upon peripheral blood value)
- cellularity, mostly RBCs with neutrophils, macrophages and mesothelial cells.

It is crucial to distinguish between true haemorrhagic effusions (with erythrophagia and possibly haemosiderin/haematodin) and blood contamination caused during sampling (containing platelets – see earlier). Note that, due to the fibrinolytic activity of mesothelium, haemorrhagic effusions will not form clots after sampling (unlike in accidental sampling of peripheral blood).

Causes of haemorrhagic effusions include bleeding disorders (e.g. infectious causes such as *Angiostrongylus vasorum* or *Dirofilaria immitis*, trauma, torsion (e.g. liver or spleen, followed by rupture) or underlying haemorrhagic neoplasia (most commonly haemangiosarcomas)). Aspirates of pericardial effusions are most commonly haemorrhagic, and these effusions frequently contain high numbers of reactive mesothelial cells, often displaying multiple features resembling malignant neoplasia.

### Chylous effusions

- macroscopic appearance, milky/opaque
- total protein, variable but usually high (>25 g/l)

- triglyceride > serum level (and usually >1.1 mmol/l (100 mg/dl))
- cholesterol < serum level
- nucleated cell count – moderate to high ($>1.5 \times 10^9$/l) – mostly small lymphocytes (early) with neutrophils and macrophages (later), variable mesothelial cells.

Chylous effusions form due to either reduced lymphoid drainage or rupture of lymphatic ducts, and in small animals are most commonly found within the thoracic cavity. The elevated triglyceride arises from chylomicrons, formed from intestinal lipids and absorbed into the lymphatics, and which also give chyle its characteristic milky opacity (Figure 9.60).

Cytologically, chyle often has a background containing high numbers of small, indistinct vacuoles (only usually appreciated on higher-power magnification) and contains high numbers of lymphocytes, most of which should be unremarkable small lymphocytes (Figure 9.61). In more established chylous effusions, the irritant effects of chyle result in a mixed inflammatory influx (mostly macrophages and neutrophils) along with reactive mesothelial cells.

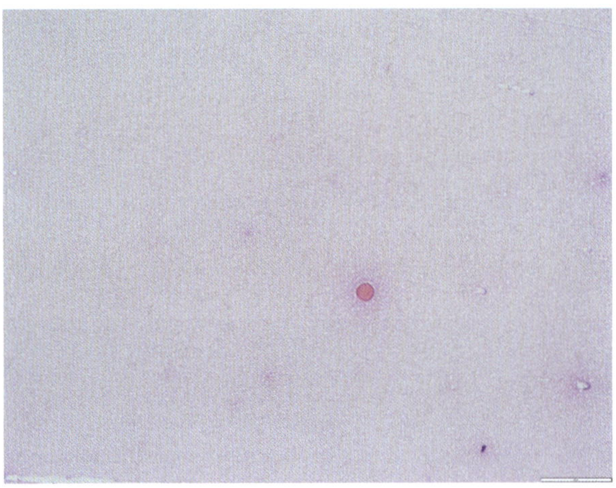

**Figure 9.60.** Background of chylous effusion; note the high numbers of faint, clear vacuoles (1000×).

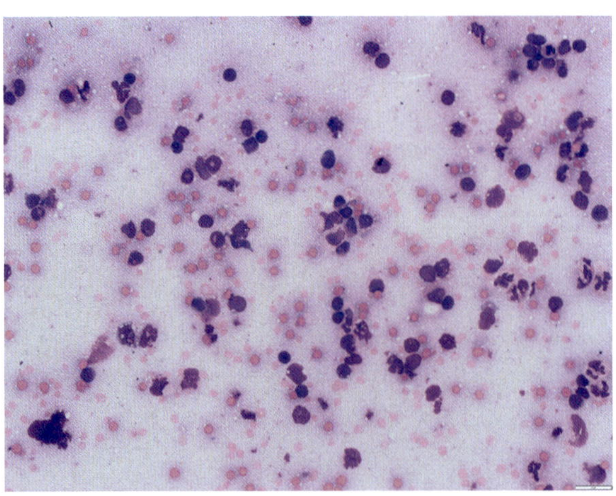

**Figure 9.61.** Mixed lymphocytes and bare nuclei in chylous effusion (concentrated preparation) (400×).

Heart disease, underlying neoplasia and trauma are the most common causes of chylous effusions.

### *Lymphorrhagic (lymphocyte-rich) effusions*

These uncommon effusions are formed via reduced drainage following rupture of lymphatics not containing chylomicrons (i.e. that do not drain the intestine), or in patients with markedly reduced food intake. They have characteristics similar to modified transudates but contain high numbers of small lymphocytes.

Both lymphocyte-rich types of effusion can sometimes be challenging to distinguish from lymphoma, especially small cell lymphoma. Further testing (especially PARR or flow cytometry) is sometimes required for definitive information.

### *Pseudo-chylous effusions*

These effusions are rare in veterinary practice. Although they appear grossly similar to chyle, they are rich in cholesterol rather than triglycerides (the cholesterol is formed from the breakdown of cell membranes), often due to chronic inflammation of the serosa.

## Bile peritonitis

- macroscopic appearance, yellow–orange, occasionally greenish, variably turbid
- protein and cellularity high (as with exudate)
- bilirubin high (>serum level, often much higher).

Bile is strongly irritant and quickly elicits an inflammatory response – the influx of fluid often masks the initial greenish colour of the fluid. Bile peritonitis can be suspected from the history, or if bile is observed on cytological examination. It may be seen as a greyish-blue to black material, free in the background or phagocytosed within macrophages, although in fluids of longer duration much of the bile will have been converted to rhomboidal golden pigment crystals. In some cases, the bile effusion also contains amorphous, cloudy, bluish-grey mucinous material (sometimes termed 'white bile') – if this is the only material present, bilirubin in the fluid may not be increased (Figures 9.62 and 9.63).

The inflammatory response typically comprises high numbers of neutrophils and macrophages, as well as reactive mesothelial cells.

## Uro-abdomen

- macroscopic appearance, clear to pale yellow
- protein and cellularity low (as transudate or modified transudate)
- urea and creatinine high (>serum level, usually much higher).

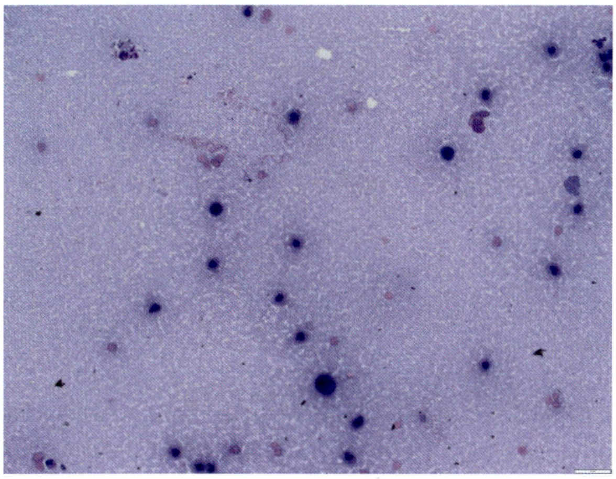

**Figure 9.62.** Greyish-blue background in bile peritonitis: the actual amount of bile can be considerably less than this as it is diluted by influxes of fluid from the exudate that it stimulates; note the poorly preserved and largely unidentifiable leukocytes (direct preparation, 100×).

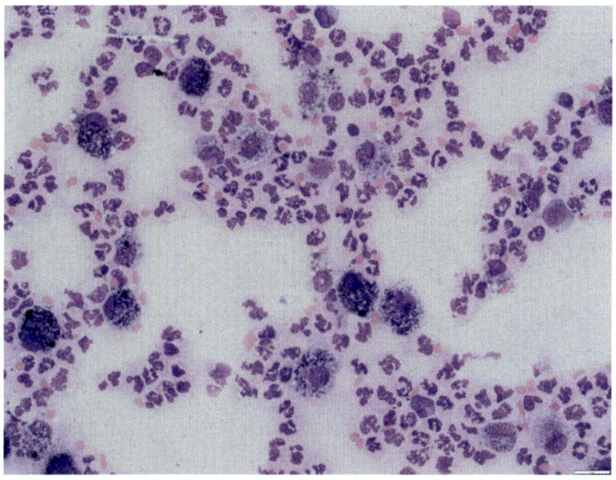

**Figure 9.63.** Bile peritonitis, concentrated preparation; bile pigment is phagocytosed within macrophages, which appear similar to haemosiderophages because bile pigments and haemosiderin are analogous substances (400×).

Urine is also irritant to the abdomen but there is a continued influx of urine, diluting cellularity and protein; an exudate will eventually form in long-standing uroabdomen. Occasionally, urine crystals may be present.

Creatinine equilibrates more slowly than urea and so is more likely to be elevated, although usually both urea and creatinine are significantly increased from serum values.

### Neoplastic effusions

Most neoplasms exfoliate poorly into fluid, so the majority of effusions secondary to neoplasia do not contain neoplastic cells. The most common exceptions are lymphoma (in cats) and carcinomas (in dogs), although care must always be taken to avoid misdiagnosing reactive mesothelial cells as neoplastic (see earlier text; Figure 9.64).

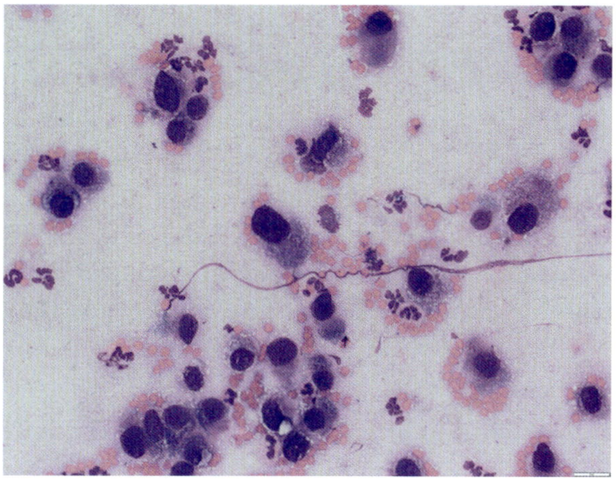

**Figure 9.64.** Carcinoma in canine peritoneal fluid; compare with mesothelial cells (Figure 9.48) – cells of the former have eccentric nuclei, smooth rounded borders and displaying some cohesion (although mesothelium can also be somewhat cohesive) (500×).

## Airway samples

### *Anatomy*

The external nares are covered in keratinised squamous epithelium, which rapidly transitions through non-keratinised squamous epithelium to columnar epithelium, with characteristic cilia, persisting down to the terminal alveoli. For the majority of samples from the airway, ciliated columnar epithelial cells are expected.

### *Sampling techniques*

It is beyond the scope of this chapter to give comprehensive descriptions of airway sampling techniques, but brief descriptions follow.

#### *Nasal flush*

Samples can be taken using a catheter inserted into the external nares, and flushing and aspirating small volumes (5–10 ml) of warmed saline whilst advancing and retracting the catheter. Sample yield is often improved by making a small nick in the side of the catheter, providing a rough surface that can help dislodge tissue.

#### *Trans-tracheal wash (TTW)*

Tracheal washes are achieved by inserting a catheter into the trachea through the cricothyroid ligament or between tracheal rings. The samples produced have slightly different constituents to broncho-alveolar lavage (BAL) samples as they often represent higher airway, although they are often broadly comparable.

The main advantage of TTW is that it can be performed in a conscious patient under local anaesthetic, although it is most commonly used in larger animals (particularly horses).

### BAL

BAL samples are achieved via insertion of a catheter into an endotracheal tube. Concurrent use of bronchoscopy greatly augments sampling technique and aids visualisation of focal lesions; 5 ml/kg of warmed sterile saline can be safely instilled, and the re-aspirated fluid can then be examined.

## Oropharyngeal contamination

Even in normal situations, the oropharnyx contains high numbers of both mixed bacteria and neutrophils. Contamination of airway samples with material from the oropharnyx therefore makes assessment very challenging, and can lead to misinterpretation of inflammation or bacterial infection (Figure 9.65).

The presence of keratinised squamous epithelial cells or mixed-morphology bacterial organisms should raise the cytologist's suspicion of oropharyngeal contamination. *Simonsiella* organisms are oropharyngeal commensals with almost no pathogenic potential; they have a distinctive large, tablet-like shape (which actually comprises high numbers of closely associated rod-shaped bacteria), and their presence confirms an oropharyngeal origin. Note that samples from cases of aspiration pneumonia can resemble oropharyngeal contamination, although there is usually an intense inflammatory response in these cases.

## Cytological findings

Cytological examination of airway samples is useful in identifying patterns of inflammation and, less commonly, aetiological agents (including bacteria, fungi and parasites). Additionally, neoplastic lesions (most commonly squamous cell carcinoma, lymphoma and malignant melanoma in the upper respiratory tract, and primary bronchial carcinoma and lymphoma in the lower) occasional exfoliate into the respiratory tract.

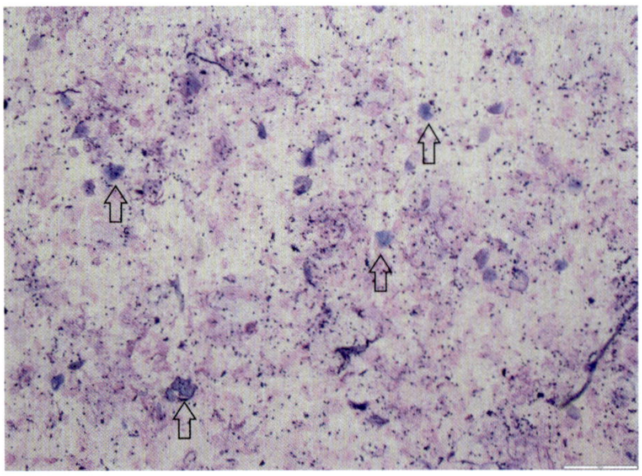

Figure 9.65. Squamous epithelial cells in BAL (open arrows are examples), indicating probable oropharyngeal contamination; mixed-morphology bacteria were also present (100×).

Table 9.3. 'Normal' BAL leukocyte proportions.

| Leokocytes | Dog | Cat |
|---|---|---|
| Macrophages (%) | 70–80 | 70–80 |
| Lymphocytes (%) | 6–14 | <5 |
| Neutrophils (%) | <5 | <5 |
| Eosinophils* (%) | <5 | <25 |

Note: *See text on eosinophilic inflammation.

Cytology is less useful for non-inflammatory conditions. In addition, exfoliation is somewhat variable and slightly unpredictable; leukocytes embedded in mucus may not be truly representative of the inflammatory population. For this reason, differential counts and 'normal' cell numbers and proportions (such as those listed in Table 9.3) should be interpreted with caution.

### 'Normal' BAL values

Cell counts of 250–500/ml have been reported in clinically normal patients (although see above regarding exfoliation of samples).

Other normal cytological findings include variable numbers of ciliated columnar epithelial cells, found individually or in small clusters and often interspersed with low numbers of goblet cells (columnar to slightly cuboidal epithelial cells containing large blue–purple rounded droplets of mucus; Figure 9.66). In some samples the cilia detach from the surface of the cell and can be mistaken for rod-shaped bacteria, but they are paler and more irregular than true bacterial organisms, however.

Mucus may also be seen as patches of amorphous, bluish-purple material, often containing embedded leukocytes.

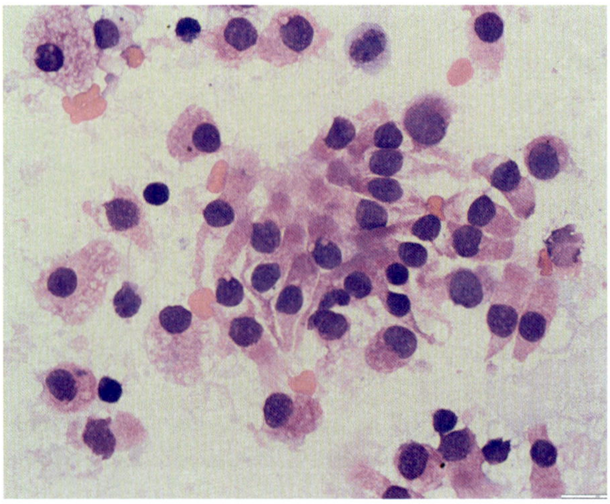

Figure 9.66. Typical ciliated columnar respiratory epithelial cells.

## Inflammation

Inflammatory patterns are similar to those in other areas of the body, with similar causes. Other findings consistent with chronic inflammatory irritation include increased amounts of mucus and/or goblet cell hyperplasia (denoted by increased numbers of goblet cells) and Curschmann's spirals (inspissated mucus appearing as dense basophilic spirals on cytology).

### Neutrophilic inflammation

As with other cytological specimens, the presence of degenerate neutrophils raises suspicion for infection although this can be harder to assess due to the frequently poor preservation of airway samples. Phagocytosed bacteria confirm the suspicion (although remember that a delay in sample preparation can lead to this occurring *in vitro*).

The normally pale granulation of neutrophils can become darker and more prominent in airway samples; added to the fact that eosinophil granules occasionally become paler brown and slightly harder to visualise, it can sometimes be surprisingly difficult to distinguish between neutrophils and eosinophils on airway preparations. Spending time finding both types of leukocyte in the same visual field greatly helps in identification.

### Eosinophilic inflammation

See above for some of the difficulties encountered in identification of eosinophils on airway samples. Eosinophils are found in higher proportions in feline airway samples – up to 25% are reported to be normal (although many clinical pathologists consider this figure to be higher than their experience with BAL preparations suggests). In dogs, >5% is considered abnormal.

As elsewhere in the body, eosinophils are associated with parasitism and hypersensitivity. The presence of lungworm larvae confirms infestation; even in the absence of larvae, high numbers of eosinophils, as well as evidence of prior haemorrhage in canine BAL samples, should raise suspicion for *A. vasorum* (Figure 9.67).

Eosinophilic inflammation is commonly associated with feline asthma and canine eosinophilic bronchopneumopathy, although it is worth remembering that the use of corticosteroids prior to sampling will drastically reduce eosinophil numbers. Mixed inflammatory patterns comprising neutrophils and eosinophils are sometimes associated with bacterial infection secondary to hypersensitivity (particularly *Mycoplasma*, which is extremely challenging to identify on cytology samples due to its small size).

### Granulomatous, pyogranulomatous and mixed inflammation

Macrophages are normal residents of the lower airway but their presence in increased numbers – particularly

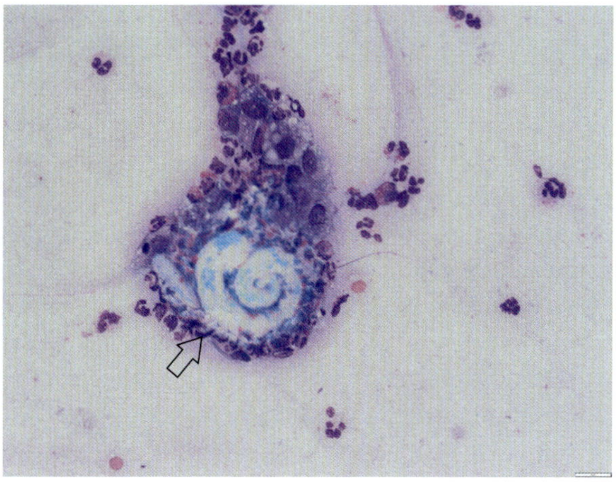

**Figure 9.67.** Lungworm larval stage (open arrow) in BAL, surrounded by eosinophils and macrophages; as is common, the larva is curled, making challenging identification via tail morphology (400×).

when highly activated (with expanded and often vacuolated cytoplasm, rare multinucleation) and when alongside other leukocytes – suggests macrophagic (granulomatous) inflammation. This is associated with chronic inflammation and raises concerns for more challenging infectious organisms. Mycobacterial infection is a significant concern in feline patients, especially due to its zoonotic potential, and suspected cases should have air-dried samples submitted for closer examination and Ziehl–Neelsen staining. Fungal organisms can also cause this inflammatory pattern in both dogs and cats, and there are other causes of prolonged inflammation.

## Haemorrhage

Evidence of prior haemorrhage includes the presence of red blood cells, especially when phagocytosed within macrophages, as well as haemotoidin crystals and haemosiderin granules. Macrophages containing haemosiderin granules are consistent with haemorrhage prior to sampling, and have occasionally been described as 'heart failure' cells due to their perceived association with cardiac disease, although recent studies have shown that the finding is not very specific, especially in cats – nearly 65% of feline BAL samples were reported to contain haemosiderophages. These are present in high numbers, and heavily laden, in equine patients with exercise-induced pulmonary haemorrhage.

Possibilities for haemorrhage into the airway include lungworm, heart disease (presumably due to lung congestion), bleeding disorders and other inflammatory causes.

## Neoplasia

Neoplasia is occasionally observed in upper airway samples but it a relatively uncommon finding in the lower airway (direct aspiration of pulmonary masses is often more rewarding). Criteria for malignancy are similar to elsewhere in the body, although airway samples are often complicated by concurrent inflammation, mucus and poor preservation. Additionally, inflammation within the confined space of the nasal cavities often produces markedly dysplastic change in the respiratory epithelium, meaning that carcinomas should be diagnosed with caution in these cases.

### Infectious agents

Bacteria (and oropharyngeal contamination) are discussed elsewhere. Fungal infections are very rare in the UK, but the presence of organisms phagocytosed within macrophages is diagnostic. Helminth parasites (most commonly *Angiostrongylus* and *Crenosoma* in dogs, *Aleurostrongylus* in cats) have large larvae that are easier to identify on lower power, and often elicit significant eosinophilic inflammation (Figure 9.67).

Protozoal infections are occasionally seen, although they can be hard to identify cytologically. *Toxoplasma gondii* tachyzooites are small, banana-shaped organisms found free in the background and phagocytosed within macrophages. *Pneumocystis carinii* has small, elongated tachyzoites and bradyzoites, which are round structures with central and radial dots – these are relatively easily mistaken for large platelets. This organism is usually found in the Cavalier King Charles Spaniels and Dachshund, and is usually associated with an inherited immune disorder.

## Appendix: aqueous Romanowsky staining (e.g. Diff-Quik, Rapi-Diff)

These are convenient and highly useful stains that are readily utilised in-house. Nuclear detail is not generally as good as with methanol-based stains, and cytoplasmic granulation (e.g. mast cell granules) can be harder to appreciate. They are also relatively expensive, so the use of small dipping jars is recommended.

### Technique

- Create smear and air-dry.
- Dip 5× (1 s each) in fixative (pale blue), allowing excess to drain after each dip.
- Dip 5× (1 s each) in stain solution 1 (pink), wiping excess off before proceeding.
- Dip 5× (1 s each) in stain solution 2 (dark blue).
- Rinse with distilled water.

### Tips

- As stains age, slides require longer immersion; keep an eye on the colour of the slide throughout the process.
- The methanol fixative will rapidly evaporate if left open.
- The pink dye must be wiped off or it will form a precipitate with the next solution.
- If surface precipitate forms on the deep blue dye, it can be safely removed with filter paper.
- In general, samples are easier to examine if slightly more basophilic dye is applied than eosinophilic (i.e. dip in the deep blue dye a few more times than the pink).
- Keep a 'clean' set for general use and a 'dirty' set for samples likely to contain bacterial organisms (i.e. ears, skin).

## Bibliography

### Textbooks

Barger, A. and MacNeill, A. (2016). *Small Animal Cytologic Diagnosis*, 1st edn. CRC, Boca Raton, FL.

Cowell, R., Tyler, R., Meinkoth, J. and DeNicola, D. (2008). *Diagnostic Cytology and Hematology of the Dog and Cat*, 3rd edn. Mosby Elsevier, St. Louis, MO.

Dunn, J. (2014). *Manual of Diagnostic Cytology of the Dog and Cat*. John Wiley & Sons, Inc., Chichester, UK.

Raskin, R. and Meyer, D. (2016). *Canine and Feline Cytology*, 3rd edn. Elsevier, St. Louis, MO.

### Journals

Arai, S., Rist, P., Clancey, N., Gilroy, C., Stryhn, H. and Amsellem, P. (2019). Fine-needle aspiration of cutaneous, subcutaneous, and intracavitary masses in dogs and cats using 22- vs 25-gauge needles. *Veterinary Clinical Pathology* 48(2), 287–292.

Camus, M., Priest, H., Koehler, J., Driskell, E., Rakich, P., Ilha, M. and Krimer, P. (2016). Cytologic criteria for mast cell tumor grading in dogs with evaluation of clinical outcome. *Veterinary Pathology* 53(6), 1117–1123.

Han, K., Ha, H., Kong, J., Myung, J., Park, S., Kim, J., Shin, M., Seol, H., Koh, J. and Lee, S. (2018). Importance of individual ghost cells in fine-needle aspiration cytology diagnosis of pilomatricoma. *Journal of Pathology and Translational Medicine* 52(1), 45–50.

Marcos, R., Santos, M., Marrinhas, C., Correia-Gomes, C. and Caniatti, M. (2016). Cytocentrifuge preparation in veterinary cytology: a quick, simple, and affordable manual method to concentrate low cellularity fluids. *Veterinary Clinical Pathology* 45(4), 725–731.

Masserdotti, C. and Ubbiali, F. (2002). Fine needle aspiration cytology of pilomatricoma in three dogs. *Veterinary Clinical Pathology* 31(1), 22–25.

Sapierzyński, R., Czopowicz, M. and Ostrzeszewicz, M. (2016). Factors affecting the diagnostic utility of canine and feline cytological samples. *Journal of Small Animal Practice* 58(2), 73–78.

Sumner, J., Lacorcia, L., Rose, A., Woodward, A. and Carter, J. (2018). Clinical safety of percutaneous ultrasound-guided fine-needle aspiration of adrenal gland lesions in 19 dogs. *Journal of Small Animal Practice* 59(6), 357–363.

Valli, V., Myint, M., Barthel, A., Bienzle, D., Caswell, J., Colbatzky, F., Durham, A., Ehrhart, E., Johnson, Y., Jones, C., Kiupel, M., Labelle, P., Lester, S., Miller, M., Moore, P., Moroff, S., Roccabianca, P., Ramos-Vara, J., Ross, A., Scase, T., Tvedten, H. and Vernau, W. (2010). Classification of canine malignant lymphomas according to the World Health Organization criteria. *Veterinary Pathology* 48(1), 198–211.

Vignoli, M., Rossi, F., Chierici, C., Terragni, R., De Lorenzi, D., Stanga, M. and Olivero, D. (2007). Needle tract implantation after fine needle aspiration biopsy (FNAB) of transitional cell carcinoma of the urinary bladder and adenocarcinoma of the lung. *Schweizer Archiv für Tierheilkunde* 149(7), 314–318.

Warland, J. and Dobson, J. (2013). Breed predispositions in canine mast cell tumour: A single-centre experience in the United Kingdom. *The Veterinary Journal* 197(2), 496–498.

## Website

eClinpath. (2020). *eClinPath|A Resource for Veterinary Clinical Pathology*. Available at: http://eclinpath.com/ (accessed 27 January 2020).

## Test

1. **A stippled, amphophilic fluid background to a specimen, containing frequent crescent-like structures indicates what?**
   A) calcification
   B) chylous effusion
   C) high-protein fluid
   D) necrosis.
2. **Degenerate neutrophils (with paler, swollen nuclei and fewer distinct segments) are commonly associated with what?**
   A) bacterial infection
   B) foreign body reactions
   C) neoplasia
   D) trauma.
3. **Which of the following statements is not true regarding activated macrophages?**
   A) Activated macrophages contain increased amounts cytoplasm, frequently with vacuolation.
   B) Activated macrophages usually have high nuclear/cytoplasmic ratios.
   C) Chronic inflammatory patterns usually include activated macrophages.
   D) Macrophages can form epithelioid clusters with prolonged inflammation.
4. **Which of the following statements is true regarding plasma cells?**
   A) Derive from mature T lymphocytes.
   B) Are usually absent in reactive lymph nodes.
   C) Occasionally produce amyloid when neoplastic.
   D) Have intensely eosinophilic cytoplasm with Romanowsky staining.
5. **Which of the following statements is true regarding mesenchymal cells?**
   A) Have rounded nuclei.
   B) Form loosely cohesive 'aggregates'.
   C) Are termed 'carcinomas' when neoplastic.
   D) Frequently metastasise to lymph nodes when neoplastic.
6. **Which of these neoplasms is not derived from mesenchymal cells?**
   A) fibroma
   B) histiocytic sarcoma
   C) lipoma
   D) osteosarcoma.
7. **Which of the following statements is true regarding prostatic epithelium?**
   A) cuboidal to columnar
   B) squamous
   C) transitional
   D) anaplastic.

**8. Primary thyroid tumours (carcinomas and adenomas) are classified as what?**

A) epithelial
B) mesenchymal
C) neuroendocrine
D) round cell.

**9. Which feature of mast cell tumours is not associated with higher-grade tumours?**

A) heavy granulation
B) binucleation
C) nuclear pleomorphism
D) high mitotic index.

**10. Which of these features is most strongly associated with malignancy?**

A) cytoplasmic basophilia
B) cytoplasmic vacuolation
C) macronucleoli (nucleoli larger than an erythrocyte)
D) mitotic figures.

**11. Accidental blood contamination during sampling can be distinguished from previous haemorrhage by what?**

A) the number of erythrocytes present
B) erythrocytes phagocytosed within macrophages
C) platelets and platelet clumps
D) macrophages containing haemosiderin pigment.

**12. Reactive lymph nodes contain what?**

A) mostly intermediate lymphocytes
B) mixed but predominantly small lymphocytes
C) scattered clusters of epithelial cells
D) high numbers of neutrophils.

**13. Increased hydrostatic pressure (such as increased portal venous pressure), coupled with decreased oncotic pressure (such as reduced serum albumin), is likely to produce which of the following abdominal effusions?**

A) chylous
B) exudate
C) modified transudate
D) transudate.

**14. Chylous effusions can be confirmed by which of these findings?**

A) increased cholesterol within fluid compared with serum value
B) increased triglyceride within fluid compared with serum value
C) decreased glucose within fluid compared with serum value
D) increased total protein within fluid compared with serum value.

**15. Which classification of lymphoma is most commonly found in canine patients?**

A) diffuse large cell lymphoma
B) intestinal small cell lymphoma
C) Hodgkins-like lymphoma
D) epitheliotropic lymphoma.

**16. Ziehl–Neelsen staining is used to identify what?**

A) acid-fast organisms such as *Mycobacterium*
B) amyloid
C) iron
D) mucus and fungal organisms.

## Clinical case 1

A 12-year-old entire male Jack Russell Terrier presents with a history of lethargy, polyuria and polydipsia, and a firm subcutaneous mass to the right of its anus. Below is a low-power (100× magnification) image of material aspirated from this mass.

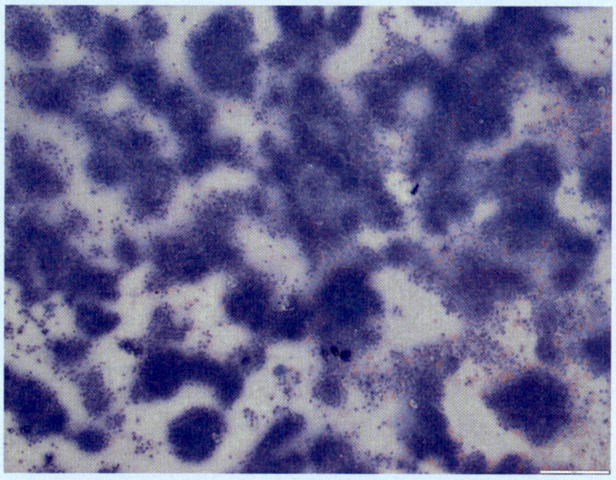

**1. Does this lesion appear to be inflammatory or neoplastic? If inflammatory, what is the pattern? If neoplastic, what broad type of neoplasm is present?**

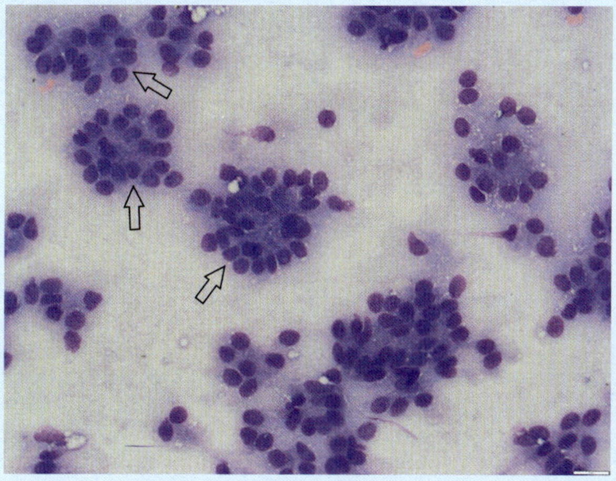

Higher-power evaluation (400×) of the preparations reveals numerous structures similar to those indicated by the arrows.

**2. What are the structures, and what does their presence indicate?**

**3. What is the likely diagnosis?**

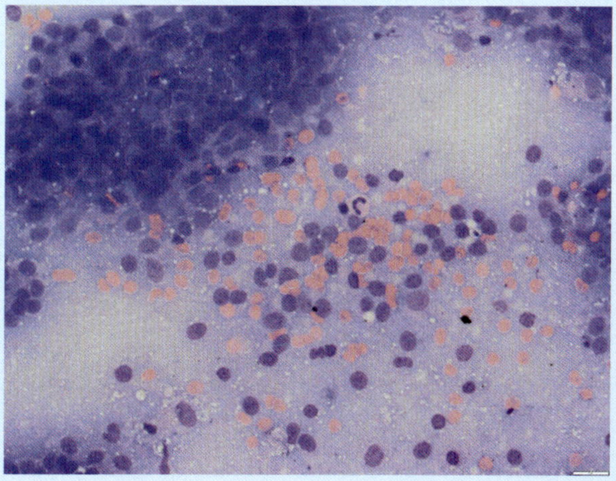

Imaging of the abdomen revealed an enlarged, rounded structure in the mid-caudal dorsal abdomen. A fine-needle aspirate biopsy from this lesion had the above appearance (400×).

4. **Given the interpretation of the previous mass, what is the most likely explanation for this cytological appearance?**
5. **What further tests would you recommend?**

## Clinical case 2

A 2-year-old mixed-breed dog presents with a firm cutaneous mass over the left shoulder. The owner reports that it has been present for several months but has recently doubled in size. Below is a low-power (100×) image of an aspirate from this lesion.

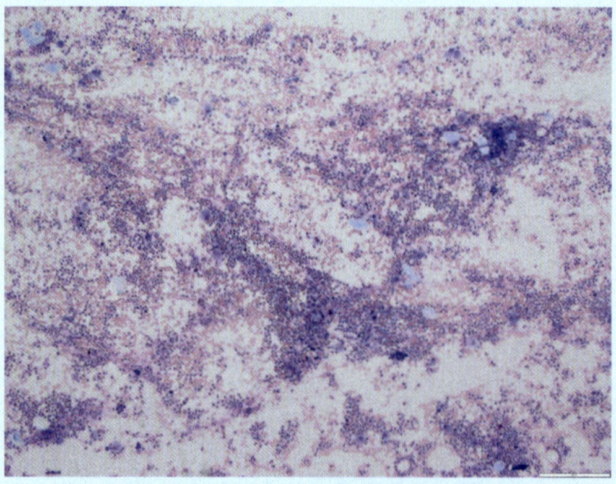

1. **Is the low-power appearance more consistent with inflammation or neoplasia?**

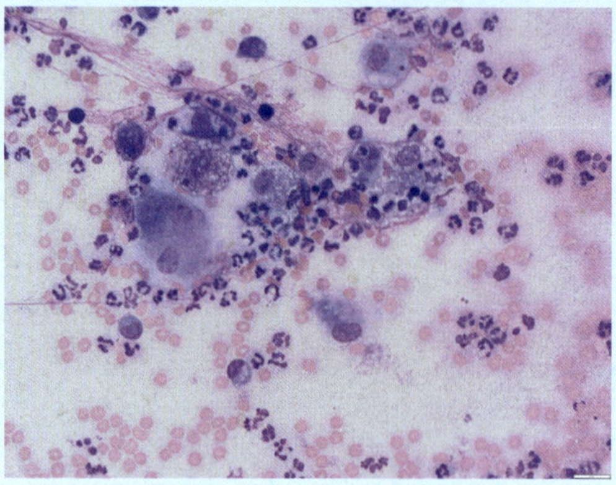

2. **What is the probable identity of the large and occasionally binucleate cells?**
3. **What does the presence of neutrophils within these cells indicate?**

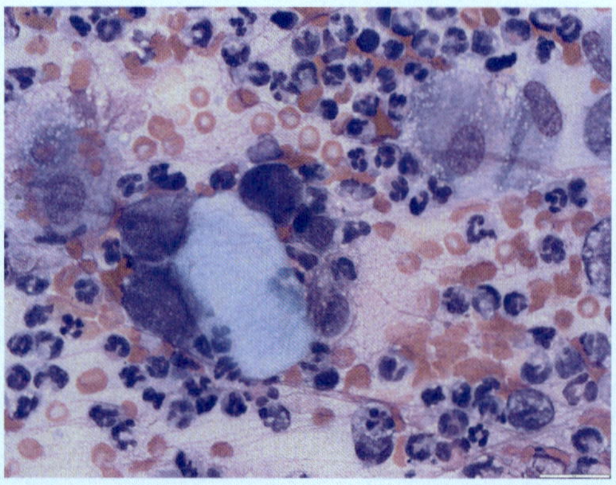

4. **What is the likely identity of the pale blue material?**
5. **Characterise the cytological pattern (type of inflammation or type of neoplasia) further and suggest possible causes.**

## Answers

### Test

1. C
2. A
3. B (although they can resemble malignant cells, activated macrophages rarely have high N/C ratios)
4. C (plasmacytomas are occasionally associated with amyloid due to aberrant immunoglobulin production)
5. B
6. B (despite their name, histiocytic sarcomas derive from macrophages or dendritic cells)
7. A
8. C
9. A (reduced granulation is associated with higher-grade mast cell tumours)
10. C (although the other findings are observed in malignant tumours, they are also commonly found in dysplastic or active tissue; macronucleoli are rarely seen, except in malignancy)
11. C
12. B
13. D
14. B
15. A
16. A

### Clinical case 1

1. **Neoplasia** (high numbers of cohesive clusters of cells and scattered, bare nuclei with little evidence of inflammation). **Neuroendocrine origin is most likely** (although there is a slight mesenchymal appearance at low power, because the clusters do not have well defined borders the nuclei are rounded rather than oval, and the edges of the clusters are indistinct rather than frayed – overall the clusters resemble bare nuclei in seas of cytoplasm, a pattern usually associated with neuroendocrine tumours).
2. **Acinar structures; these indicate a glandular origin (i.e. adenoma or adenocarcinoma)**.
3. **Anal sac apocrine gland carcinoma (ASAC)** (based upon the location, the neuroendocrine appearance and the presence of acini).
4. **Metastasis to lymph node** (there are scattered, small lymphocytes but the preparation is otherwise similar to the aspirate of the original mass; ASACs behave aggressively and frequently metastasise, often to the **medial iliac lymph node** initially).
5. **Evaluation of serum calcium** (hypercalcaemia is a common paraneoplastic effect); **further imaging of the chest and abdomen to further stage the tumour**.

### Clinical case 2

1. **Inflammation** (high numbers of neutrophils are visible at low power, as well as larger cells which may be macrophages).
2. **Activated macrophages with abundant vacuolated cytoplasm; binucleate cells are present**.
3. **Phagocytosis of neutrophils by macrophages confirms active inflammation**.
4. **The appearance in consistent with keratin**.
5. The inflammatory pattern is **pyogranulomatous (neutrophilic/macrophagic)**, and the presence of keratin and multinucleate macrophages is suggestive of a **foreign body reaction in response to keratin**. A ruptured **keratin-containing lesion (such as a cyst or benign hair follicle tumour)** is the most likely explanation.

# Index

**D**



**E**